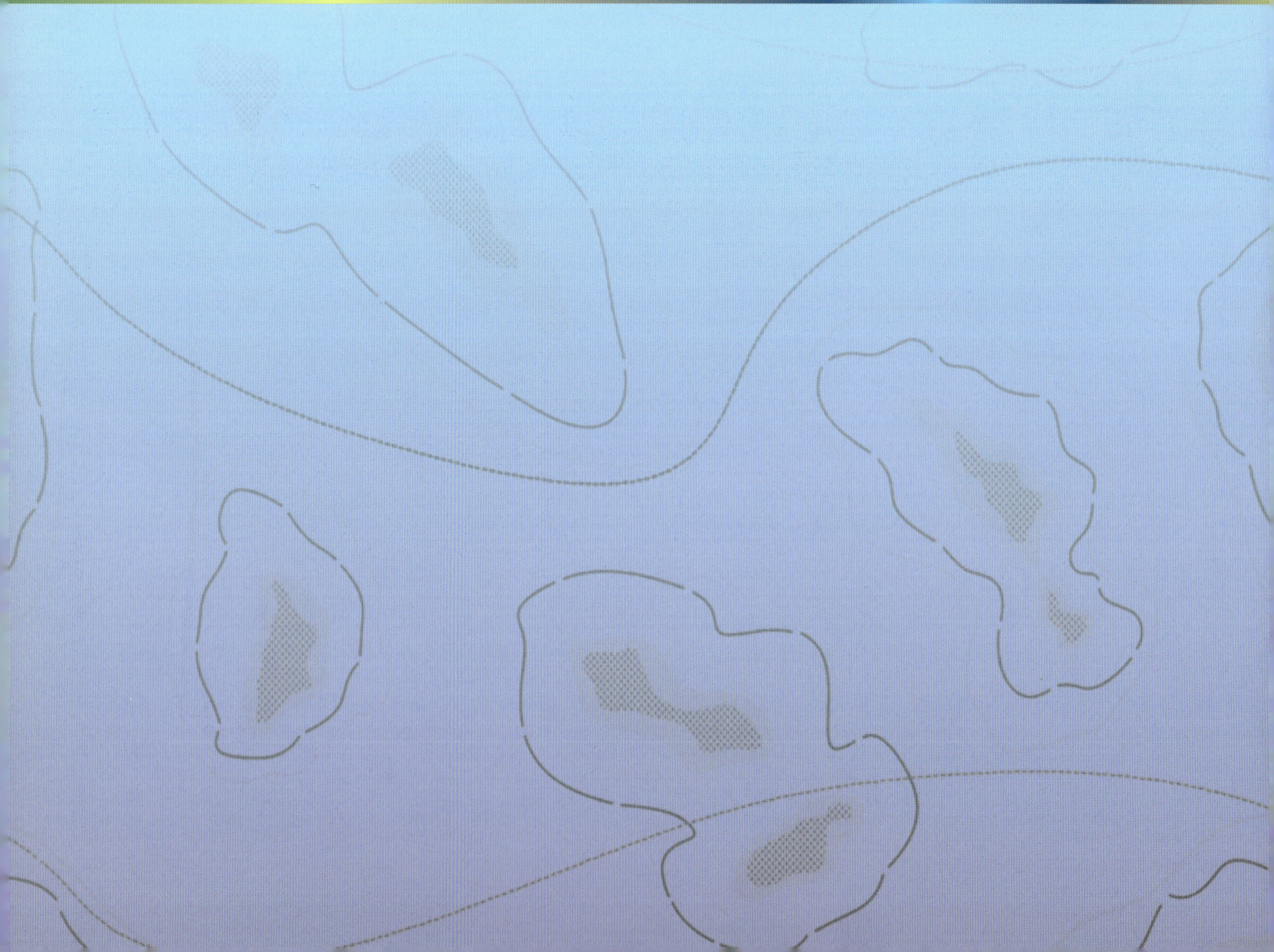

全国高等医药院校精品图书

供临床、基础、预防、口腔、护理、麻醉、影像、药学、检验等专业使用

英汉皮肤性病学

（第2版）

English-Chinese Dermatovenereology (Second Edition)

主　编◎黄长征
副主编◎郑　敏　陈思远　程　波

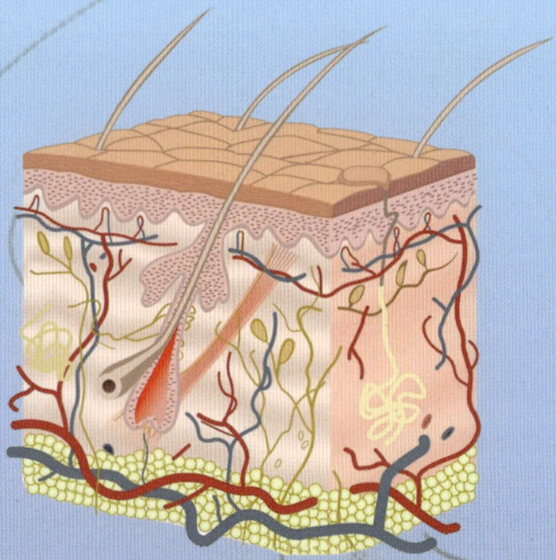

華中科技大學出版社
http://www.hustp.com
中国·武汉

内 容 简 介

本书为高等医药院校精品教材《英汉皮肤性病学》第 2 版。全书分为两部分：第一部分共 4 章，为皮肤性病学的基础知识、基本理论、技术和方法，包括皮肤的基本结构和功能，皮肤病的症状、体征和基本诊断方法，皮肤组织病理及皮肤性病治疗学的基本知识；第二部分共 23 章，介绍皮肤科常见病和多发病、部分少见疑难性皮肤病、性传播疾病，包括病因、发病机制、临床表现、诊断与鉴别诊断、预防和治疗。全书共有图片 405 幅，其中彩色照片 396 幅，彩色示意图 6 幅，黑白照片 3 幅。

本书为华中科技大学立项精品课程教材，适合五年制、六年制和八年制医学生以及来华留学生英文教学使用，也适合中文教学和皮肤科专科医师及规培生使用。

图书在版编目(CIP)数据

英汉皮肤性病学/黄长征主编. —2 版. —武汉：华中科技大学出版社，2017.11
ISBN 978-7-5680-2572-0

Ⅰ.①英… Ⅱ.①黄… Ⅲ.①皮肤病学-医学院校-教材-英、汉 ②性病学-医学院校-教材-英、汉
Ⅳ.①R75

中国版本图书馆 CIP 数据核字(2017)第 034034 号

英汉皮肤性病学(第 2 版)
English-Chinese Dermatovenereology(Second Edition)　　黄长征　主编

策划编辑：荣　静
责任编辑：荣　静　秦　曌
封面设计：原色设计
责任校对：张　琳
责任监印：周治超
出版发行：华中科技大学出版社(中国·武汉)　　电话：(027)81321913
　　　　　武汉市东湖新技术开发区华工科技园　　邮编：430223
录　　排：华中科技大学惠友文印中心
印　　刷：湖北新华印务有限公司
开　　本：889mm×1194mm　1/16
印　　张：29
字　　数：996 千字
版　　次：2017 年 11 月第 2 版第 1 次印刷
定　　价：198.00 元

Editorial Board Members and Contributors
(编委及编写者)

Editor-in-Chief(主编)

Chang-zheng HUANG(黄长征)

Associate Editors-in-Chief(副主编)

Min ZHENG(郑敏)　Si-yuan CHEN(陈思远)　Bo CHENG(程波)

English Editors(英文主审)

Dong-mei LI, M. D., Ph. D., Assistant Professor, Department of Microbiology and Immunology, Georgetown University Medical Center, USA(美国华盛顿特区乔治城大学微生物和免疫系)

You-wen ZHOU, M. D., Ph. D., Professor, Department of Dermatology and Skin Science, University of British Columbia, Canada(加拿大不列颠哥伦比亚大学皮肤科)

Associate English Editor(英文副主审)

Jia-ying ZHOU, BSc, Doctor of Pharmacy Program, Faculty of Pharmaceutical Sciences, University of British Columbia, Canada(加拿大不列颠哥伦比亚大学药学院)

Chinese Editor(中文主审)

Chun-sen WANG(王椿森), M. D., Professor, Department of Dermatology, Union Hospital, Tongji Medical College, Huazhong University of Science and Technology(华中科技大学同济医学院附属协和医院皮肤科)

Editorial Board members(listed in the order of the editor's first name in Pinyin):编委(按名字拼音的首字母排列)

Bo CHENG(程波)　The First Affiliated Hospital, Fujian Medical University(福建医科大学附属第一医院)

Chang-zheng HUANG(黄长征)　Union Hospital, Tongji Medical College, Huazhong University of Science and Technology(华中科技大学同济医学院附属协和医院)

Chao JI(纪超)　The First Affiliated Hospital, Fujian Medical University(福建医科大学附属第一医院)

Dan LUO(骆丹)　The First Affiliated Hospital, Nanjing Medical University(南京医科大学第一附属医院)

Guan-qing WANG(王官清)　Shanghai General Hospital, Shanghai Jiaotong University(上海交通大学附属第一人民医院)

Hong-xiang CHEN(陈宏翔)　Union Hospital, Tongji Medical College, Huazhong University of Science and Technology(华中科技大学同济医学院附属协和医院)

Hua ZHAO(赵华)　Chinese PLA General Hospital(中国人民解放军总医院)

Lie-hua DENG(邓列华)　The First Affiliated Hospital, Jinan University(暨南大学附属第一医院)

Lin WANG(王琳)　West China Hospital, Sichuan University(四川大学华西医院)

Min ZHENG(郑敏)　The Second Affiliated Hospital, Zhejiang University, School of Medicine(浙江大学医学院附属第二医院)

Si-yuan CHEN(陈思远)　Union Hospital, Tongji Medical College, Huazhong University of Science and

Technology(华中科技大学同济医学院附属协和医院)

Song-mei GENG(耿松梅) The Second Affiliated Hospital, Xi'an Jiaotong University(西安交通大学第二附属医院)

Sui-qing CAI(蔡绥勍) The Second Affiliated Hospital, Zhejiang University, School of Medicine(浙江大学医学院附属第二医院)

Wei HE(何威) Xinqiao Hospital, Third Military Medical University(第三军医大学新桥医院)

Wei SHI(施为) Xiangya Hospital, Central South University(中南大学湘雅医院)

Xing-hua GAO(高兴华) The First Hospital of China Medical University(中国医科大学附属第一医院)

Xing-ping CHEN(陈兴平) Tongji Hospital, Tongji Medical College, Huazhong University of Science and Technology(华中科技大学同济医学院附属同济医院)

Ya-ting TU(涂亚庭) Union Hospital, Tongji Medical College, Huazhong University of Science and Technology(华中科技大学同济医学院附属协和医院)

Yang WANG(汪旸) Peking University First Hospital(北京大学第一医院)

Ye-qiang LIU(刘业强) Shanghai Skin Disease Hospital Affiliated to Tongji University(同济大学上海市皮肤病医院)

Yu-xue GAO(高玉雪) The Second Affiliated Hospital, Dalian Medical University(大连医科大学附属第二医院)

Contributors(listed in the order of the first name of the contributors' institutes in Pinyin):编写者(按编写者单位名称首字拼音排序)

北京大学第一医院(Peking University First Hospital):Yang WANG(汪旸)

大连医科大学附属第二医院(The Second Affiliated Hospital, Dalian Medical University):Yu-xue GAO(高玉雪)

第三军医大学新桥医院(Xinqiao Hospital, Third Military Medical University):Wei HE(何威)

福建医科大学附属第一医院(The First Affiliated Hospital, Fujian Medical University):Bo CHENG(程波), Chao JI(纪超), Guan-nan ZHU(朱冠男)

广东医科大学附属深圳南山医院(Affiliated Shenzhen Nanshan Hospital, Guangdong Medical University):Bao CHAI(柴宝), Ming WANG(王明)

华中科技大学同济医学院附属同济医院(Tongji Hospital, Tongji Medical College, Huazhong University of Science and Technology):Hui CHEN(陈辉), Xing-ping CHEN(陈兴平), Yong-chu HUANG(黄永初)

华中科技大学同济医学院附属协和医院(Union Hospital, Tongji Medical College, Huazhong University of Science and Technology):Chang-zheng HUANG(黄长征), Hong-xiang CHEN(陈宏翔), Juan TAO(陶娟), Meng-wen HE(何蒙文), Ming-jing LI(李明静), Si-yuan CHEN(陈思远), Song ZHANG(张颂), Ya-ting TU(涂亚庭), Yan LI(李延)

暨南大学附属第一医院(The First Affiliated Hospital, Jinan University):Lie-hua DENG(邓列华)

南京医科大学第一附属医院(The First Affiliated Hospital, Nanjing Medical University):Bing-rong ZHOU(周炳荣), Dan LUO(骆丹), Yang XU(许阳)

上海交通大学附属第一人民医院(Shanghai General Hospital, Shanghai Jiaotong University):Guan-qing WANG(王官清)

四川大学华西医院(West China Hospital, Sichuan University):Lin WANG(王琳)

同济大学上海市皮肤病医院(Shanghai Skin Disease Hospital Affiliated to Tongji University):Ye-qiang LIU(刘业强)

西安交通大学第二附属医院(The Second Affiliated Hospital, Xi'an Jiaotong University):Jin-gang AN(安金刚), Song-mei GENG(耿松梅)

厦门大学附属中山医院(Zhongshan Hospital, Xiamen University): Zhen-ling LU(卢珍玲)

浙江大学医学院附属第二医院(The Second Affiliated Hospital, Zhejiang University, School of Medicine): Hua-li CAO(曹华莉), Jiong ZHOU(周炯), Min ZHENG(郑敏), Sui-qing CAI(蔡绥勍)

中国人民解放军总医院(Chinese PLA General Hospital): Hua ZHAO(赵华)

中国医科大学附属第一医院(The First Hospital of China Medical University): Lan ZHANG(张岚), Xing-hua GAO(高兴华)

中南大学湘雅医院(Xiangya Hospital, Central South University): Jiang-lin ZHANG(张江林), Wei SHI(施为), Xiang CHEN(陈翔)

Editorial Secretaries(编写秘书)

Li ZHU(朱里), Xiang-jie AN(安湘杰): Union Hospital, Tongji Medical College, Huazhong University of Science and Technology(华中科技大学同济医学院附属协和医院)

Color Illustration(彩色示意图制作)

Yong-kang LU(鲁永康): Union Hospital, Tongji Medical College, Huazhong University of Science and Technology(华中科技大学同济医学院附属协和医院)

Acknowledgements(特别致谢)

Throughout the preparation of this book, Mr. Ernest Allen has kindly provided invaluable comments and suggestions regarding English grammar and conventions of word usage.

非常感谢 Ernest Allen 对本教材中的英文用词、拼写和语法提出的宝贵意见!

序　　言

近几年来，专业英文教学在我国高等医学院校中普遍开展，很多院校有全英文班或开展了全英文教学以及来华留学生专业英文教学，专业英文教学日益受到重视。2008年我们组织了国内13个单位的专家编写了《英汉皮肤性病学》教材第1版，于2009年正式出版，第1版出版后得到了广大读者的肯定和好评，同时也指出了其中的不足并提出了宝贵的意见，在此，向各位读者表示衷心的感谢！第1版全体编委及编写人员为本教材的出版付出了艰辛的劳动，特别是美国华盛顿特区乔治城大学微生物和免疫系的李冬梅教授作为本教材的英文主审所做出的巨大努力是难以想象的，在此向她深表谢意！

7年过去了，皮肤性病学领域在学科理论、疾病分类、实验技术、临床诊治方面都有了新的进展，为适应学科的发展和新世纪医学人才培养的需要，特对本教材进行修订。本次修订保持了本教材第1版的总体特色，即全书分为两部分，第一部分为皮肤性病学的基本知识，第二部分为各论，介绍皮肤科常见多发病，并根据学科的发展需要和疾病病种发病率的改变对部分章节及内容进行了增补和删减，对部分疾病进行了更合理和科学的章节归类及采用了更科学的命名：第一章更名为“皮肤的基本结构和功能”；第三章增加了“皮肤镜检查”等新的诊断方法；增加了第四章“皮肤病的外用药治疗和物理治疗”；第五章中将“鲍温样丘疹病”删除，其内容移入尖锐湿疣鉴别诊断中；第六章细菌感染性皮肤病增加了“非典型分枝杆菌所致的皮肤病”；第九章中将“化妆品皮炎”并入“接触性皮炎”一节中；第十五章新增了“原发性免疫缺陷病”；第十六章增加了“青斑样血管病”；第十八章中的“类脂质渐进性坏死”移至“非感染性肉芽肿”章节；新增第二十五章“非感染性肉芽肿”等。新概念、新理论、新技术、新的疾病分类、诊断标准及鉴别诊断和治疗的进展将体现在各章节中。同时对第1版中的绝大部分照片进行了更换或调整，多数为近几年来新拍摄的质量较好和典型的照片，如此种种读者从中可以了解。

参加第2版编写的编委及编写人员基本上都参加了第1版的编写，他们具有第1版的写作经验，并曾在国外学习或工作1年以上，具有较好的英文基础及丰富的临床经验；为加强写作力量，我们新增了7位编委：南京医科大学第一附属医院骆丹教授，浙江大学医学院附属第二医院蔡绥勍教授，西安交通大学第二附属医院耿松梅教授，华中科技大学同济医学院附属协和医院陈宏翔教授，中南大学湘雅医院施为教授，北京大学第一医院汪旸教授，福建医科大学附属第一医院纪超教授。

同时，我们再次邀请了美国华盛顿特区乔治城大学微生物和免疫系的李冬梅教授及加拿大不列颠哥伦比亚大学皮肤科的 You-wen Zhou 教授作为本教材的英文主审、加拿大不列颠哥伦比亚大学药学院的 Jia-ying Zhou 作为英文副主审，并请 Ernest Allen 先生对英文用词进行把关，以保证本教材的质量，我们希望第2版能比第1版编写得更出色。

教材中的图号两位数字分别表示章、图序号。示意图图1-1、图1-2、图1-7、图1-10、图1-11和图1-24由我院影像科的鲁永康女士制作；图17-1、图24-2由第四军医大学皮肤科提供；图2-24、图21-3、图21-5、图21-11和图21-12由北京大学第一医院皮肤科陈喜雪教授提供，其他照片由本人及各参编单位提供。在本教材的编写过程中，两位英文主审特别是李冬梅教授、英文副主审、各位副主编、编委以及编写者付出了大量的心血和辛勤劳动；同时得到华中科技大学及华中科技大学出版社有限责任公司各级领导的关心和支持，华中科技大学同济医学院附属协和医院皮肤科陶娟主任、前任主任涂亚庭教授及全体同仁给予了热情鼓励和帮助，本科室的博士和硕士研究生赵梦洁、冉艺、赖艇、孙艳虹、谢蒙、安湘杰、吴士迪以及 Abdul-fattah Bilal, Al-Muriesh Maher, Nabatanzi Amelia, Hageb Omar 等在教材的资料整理及校对工作中也付出了艰辛的劳动，在此一并表示感谢！

虽然我们尽力而为之，但是，毕竟对所有作者而言，英文都不是我们的母语，疏漏谬误之处难以避免，敬请各位同道和读者指正和谅解！

黄长征

2016年8月12日

目　　录

Contents

Part One　第一部分

Part Two　第二部分

Part One 第一部分

Chapter One Basic Structure and Function of the Skin

第一章 皮肤的基本结构和功能

Section One Basic Structure of the Skin

第一节 皮肤的基本结构

The skin is the largest human organ and completely covers the body. It accounts for about 15 percent of a human's weight, and has an area about 0.2 m^2 for a newborn and approximately 1.6 m^2 for an adult. It performs many vital functions and is an important component of the immune system.

The entire surface of the skin is covered by alternating sets of fine grooves and ridges which are known as the *sulci cutis* and the *cristae cutis* respectively. The orientation and density of these dermal ridges and valleys varies according to the specific area of the body. The openings for the sweat pores are located exclusively in the ridges. Although it is unknown precisely how the conditions of human development determine the orientation of these ridges, it is well known that the swirled pattern on the palms and soles, also known as the "fingerprints" when it comes to modern crime analysis dramas, is not only unique to the person but also unchanging over a person's life. The terminal hairs or tiny vellus hairs also cover most parts of the body. In addition, some characteristic lines known as "Blaschko lines" can manifest themselves in cutaneous mosaicism as a symptom of certain skin diseases.

The color of the skin depends upon race, age, gender, nutrition and environment, and even varies with specific location on the body.

The skin is composed of three anatomically distinct layers. From the surface inward, these are the epidermis, dermis, and subcutaneous tissue (fat-storing cells) (Fig. 1-1).

皮肤覆盖于人体表面，是人体最大的器官，约占总体重的15%，成人和新生儿的皮肤总面积约分别为1.6 m^2和0.2 m^2。皮肤具有许多重要功能，是人体的重要免疫器官之一。

皮肤表面有呈网状深浅不一和方向不同的沟和嵴，分别称为皮沟和皮嵴。身体上不同部位的皮嵴和皮沟的起始方向不同，汗孔开口于皮嵴。虽然还不清楚人类在发育时是如何决定这些不同皮嵴的起始的，但众所周知的是，掌跖部位的皮沟和皮嵴的漩涡状形态，即现代犯罪案例分析中的指纹，不仅对每个人而言是独特的，并且终生不变。皮肤表面大多被覆有毛发和毳毛。此外，皮肤表面可有许多呈特殊分布和走向的不规则分界线，称为Blaschko线。某些具有镶嵌特征的皮肤病可以呈现Blaschko线分布。

皮肤的颜色因种族、年龄、性别、营养以及外在环境而异，甚至同一个人不同部位的颜色也有深浅的差别。

在解剖学上，皮肤都是由表皮(epidermis)、真皮(dermis)、皮下组织(subcutaneous tissue)或皮下脂肪(subcutaneous fat)三层所组成(图1-1)。

Epidermis

The epidermis is the outmost layer of the skin, which interacts directly with the external environment. The thickness of the epidermis varies significantly from site to site on the body, from less than 0.1 mm on the eyelids to 1.5 mm on the palms of the hands and soles of the feet. The epidermis is composed of keratinocytes, Langerhans cells, α-dendritic cells (also known as indeterminate cells), melanocytes, Merkel cells and unmyelinated neurons. It also contains the cuboidal epithelial cells that form the

表皮

表皮(epidermis)位于最外层，直接与外界接触。不同部位的皮肤其相对厚度有显著差异，掌跖部位的表皮最厚，约为1.5 mm，眼睑部位则不到0.1 mm。表皮由角质形成细胞、朗格汉斯细胞、α-树枝状细胞(未定类细胞)、黑素细胞、Merkel细胞及无髓鞘神经元构成。表皮中还含有形成小汗腺导管的末端螺旋汗

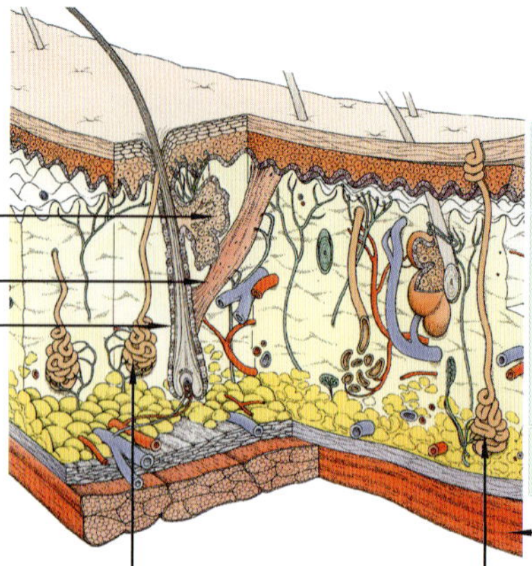

Fig. 1-1　Illustration of the skin structure(图 1-1　皮肤的组织结构示意图)

spiral acrosyringia of the eccrine sweat ducts. In about 10% of the population, the so-called Toker cells can be found in the epidermis of the nipple. Toker cells are clear cells with light staining cytoplasm, vesicular nuclei and prominent small nucleoli. These cells can express molecular markers for CK7, AE1, CAM5.2, cerB2, EMA, ER, PR, but not for P53 and CD138 in contrast to Paget's cells which do not express ER or PR but are positive for P53 and CD138 staining.

管的立方形上皮细胞;在约 10%的个体的乳头表皮中可发现有 Toker 细胞。Toker 细胞也是一种透明细胞,呈多角形或卵圆形,胞质淡染,核呈空泡状,有显著小核仁。该细胞阳性表达 CK7、AE1、CAM5.2、cerB2、EMA、ER、PR,而不表达 P53 和 CD138,与之相反的是,Paget's 细胞则不表达 ER 和 PR,而表达 P53 和 CD138。

1. Keratinocytes

The epidermis is composed primarily of well-ordered cells called keratinocytes (or squamous cells). The name is derived from the fact that the basic function of such cells is to synthesize keratin. Keratinocytes account for 95% of the epidermal cell mass.

At the microscopic level, if we were to slice into the epidermis, we would see it divided into four layers. From the innermost layer to the outermost, these are known as the basal cell layer (*stratum basalis*), the prickle cell layer, or suprabasal cell layer (*stratum spinosum*), the granular cell layer (*stratum granulosum*), and the horny cell layer (*stratum corneum*)(Fig. 1-2, Fig. 1-3). Sometimes a pink layer can be found between the granular cell layer and the horny cell layer in the skin of the palms and soles. This layer is called the *stratum lucidum*.

The plane of contact between the epidermis and dermis is not smooth and flat, but is an undulant interface. The rete ridges of the epidermis grow down into the dermis and alternate with interdigitated projections of the dermal connective tissue (the latter are the so-called dermal papilla). The basement membrane zone (BMZ) is situated just between the epidermis and the dermis.

一、角质形成细胞

表皮主要由有规则排列的细胞即角质形成细胞(keratinocyte)(又称鳞状细胞)构成,其基本功能是合成角蛋白。表皮的细胞 95%是角质形成细胞。

显微镜下,在二维切片中,表皮由内到外可以分为四层:基底细胞层(或基底层)、棘细胞层(或基底上细胞层,或棘层)、颗粒细胞层(或颗粒层)和角质细胞层(或角质层)(图 1-2,图 1-3)。在掌跖部位,颗粒层与角质层之间尚有一粉红色的透明层。

表皮和真皮之间的接触面不是平整的,而是高低不平呈起伏状,表皮嵴伸入真皮内,并与真皮内的结缔组织呈指状突起(后者称为真皮乳头)相互交织,基膜带位于表皮与真皮之间。

1) Basal cell layer(*stratum basalis*)

(1) Basal cells: the basal cells are also called epidermal matrix

(一) 基底细胞层(基底层)

(1) 基底细胞　基底细胞又称为表

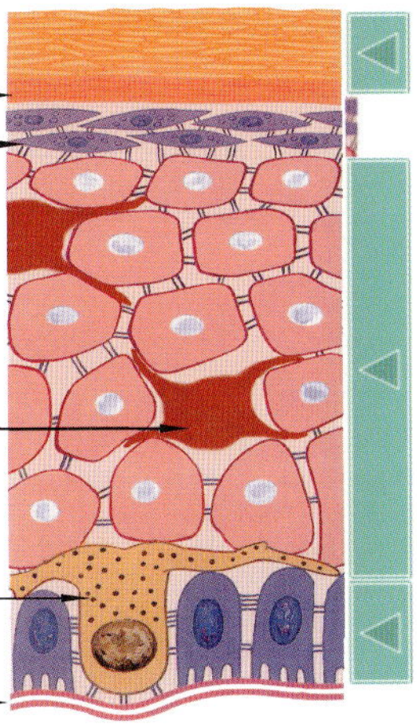

Fig. 1-2　Illustration of the epidermal layers(图 1-2　表皮的层次示意图)

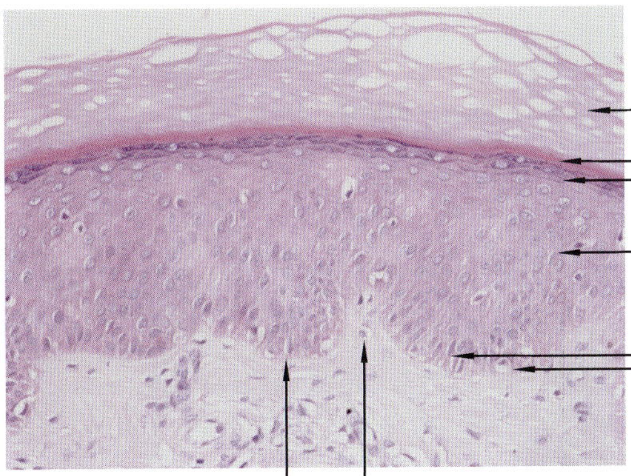

Fig. 1-3　The epidermal layers, HE staining(图 1-3　表皮的层次, HE 染色)

cells or epidermal germinative cells. They proliferate, differentiate, and then move upward through the full thickness of the epidermis, layer by layer. The mitotic activity in the epidermis is mainly confined to the basal cell layer. The time spanning from differentiation of keratinocytes in the basal cell layer to the exfoliation process in the horny cell layer is known as the epidermal transit time or epidermal turnover time. In normal skin, this takes about 28 days.

The epidermal stem cells are predominately located at the tips of the epidermal rete ridges, but also in the bulge regions of the hair follicles, and at the base of the sebaceous glands. Epidermal stem cells are characterized by their high expression levels of β1-integrin, α6-integrin, Lrig1, Rac1 and P63, their low expression of desmoglein 3 and by the lack of markers for terminal differentiation of epidermal cells. Hair follicle stem cells in the bulge areas can generate cells of the outer root sheath, differentiate into sebocytes and interfollicular epidermal cells and express the cell surface

皮母质细胞(epidermal matrix cells)或表皮生发细胞(epidermal germinative cells)。基底层细胞发生增殖、分化，并逐步向表皮上部移行于表皮全层。表皮的分裂活性主要发生于基底层。基底细胞从基底层发生增殖到表皮角质层脱落的时间称为表皮通过时间(epidermal transit time)或表皮更替时间(epidermal turnover time)，正常人约为 28 天。

表皮干细胞(epidermal stem cells)主要位于表皮嵴的顶端，在毛囊的隆突处、皮脂腺的底部也有类似的细胞。表皮干细胞的特征是高表达 β1 整合素、α6-整合素、Lrig1、Rac1 和 P63，而桥粒芯糖蛋白 3 的表达水平低，并缺乏终末分化标记。毛囊隆突处的干细胞能产生外毛根鞘细胞，分化为皮脂腺细胞、毛囊间表皮细胞，并表达细胞表面分子 CD34、

molecules such as CD34, VdR and transcription factors TCF3, Sox9, Lhx2 and NFATc1. Therefore, these stem cells play an important role in maintaining the homeostasis of the pilosebaceous unit. When sebocyte stem cells differentiate into sebocytes, the cells become full of lipid and express Blimp1.

VdR 及转录因子 TCF3、Sox9、Lhx2 和 NFATc1。这些干细胞在维持毛囊皮脂腺单位的自稳中发挥重要的作用。皮脂腺干细胞能分化为充满脂质的皮脂腺细胞并表达 Blimp1。

The basal cell layer is grouped into a series of rectangular or columnar shaped keratinocytes, which contain relatively large round-oval nuclei dominated by chromatin, and which contain slightly more basophilic cytoplasm than the keratinocytes above it. By aligning in the manner of a series of palisades, the basal cells keep their long axes perpendicular to the plane of the basal membrane. The melanin in basal cells is obtained from adjacent melanocytes that govern the color and shades of the skin.

基底细胞呈长立方形或圆柱形，胞质嗜碱性，核呈椭圆形，深染色质。基底层由单排呈栅栏状排列的基底细胞构成，其长轴与表皮和真皮间的分界线垂直。基底细胞胞质内含有从临近的黑素细胞输送而来的黑素颗粒，其含量的多少与肤色相匹配。

The cytoplasm of the basal cells and the keratinocytes above it are packed with intermediate keratin filaments arranged as bundles of threads (tonofilaments). This structure runs from the peripheral area of the nuclei to the specialized attachment plaques, desmosomes or hemidesmosomes, which are described below.

基底细胞及其上面的角质形成细胞的胞质内含有角蛋白中间丝，即张力细丝，张力细丝呈束状聚集在核周，并终止于胞质膜的特异化结构附着板，即桥粒或半桥粒。

(2) Desmosome, hemidesmosome, and gap junction: epidermal cells are joined to one another by desmosomes (specialized intercellular bridges as shown in Fig. 1-4). They are joined horizontally between adjacent basal cells, vertically between basal cells and prickle cells above and also transversely between prickle cells themselves. The detailed view of desmosome structure reveals an electron-lucent space in the central part of the desmosomes, and an electron-dense central lamina (Fig. 1-4 inset) just in the middle of this intercellular matrix. The hemidesmosomes attach the basal-cell membrane to the basal membrane. The gap junctions also allow communication between adjacent basal cells.

(2) 桥粒、半桥粒、间隙连接　相邻的基底细胞之间以及基底细胞与其上面相邻的棘细胞之间、相邻的棘细胞之间通过细胞间桥(intercellular bridges)即桥粒(desmosome)(图 1-4)联系，桥粒中央为电子透明间隙，间隙内细胞间黏合物质的中央为电子密度致密的中央层(图 1-4 插入图)。基底层与其下的基膜则通过半桥粒(hemidesmosome)相互联系。基底细胞之间尚有用于细胞通讯的间隙连接(gap junction)。

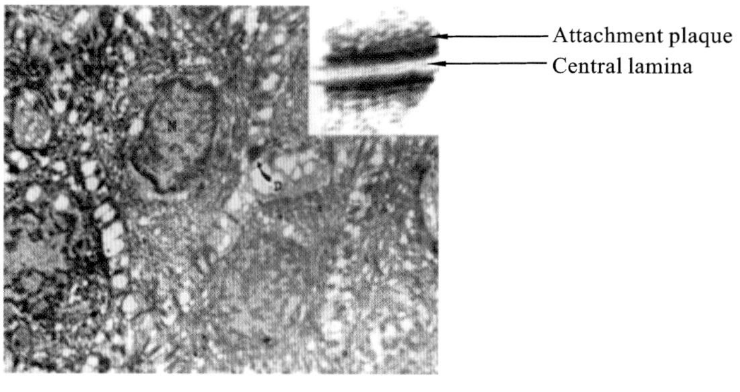

Fig. 1-4　Electron microcopy of desmosome. D: desmosome. Inset is the magnification of desmosome

(图 1-4　桥粒电镜照片。D:桥粒，插入图为桥粒放大)

① Desmosomes: desmosomes are composed of attachment plaque and transmembrane proteins that set up a bridge between cell surface and intracellular filaments. The attachment plaque is

①桥粒由附着板和跨膜蛋白构成，在细胞表面与细胞内的细丝之间起桥梁作用。前者的主要成分是桥粒斑蛋白

where desmoplakin attaches to the keratin fibers, and is also the place for transmembrane proteins, desmogleins and desmocollins to attach to desmoplakin via plakoglobin and plakophilin. Then the extracellular domains of desmogleins and desmocollins bind to each other in order to bridge the space between adjacent epidermal cells. In general, desmoglein 3 is common (and easily detected) in suprabasal keratinocytes and desmoglein 1 is in the group of keratinocytes just beneath the horny cell layer.

(desmoplakin),并与角蛋白纤维相连。后者主要是桥粒芯糖蛋白(desmoglein)和桥粒黏蛋白(desmocollin)。桥粒芯糖蛋白和桥粒黏蛋白通过桥粒斑珠蛋白(plakoglobin)和桥粒斑菲素蛋白(plakophilin)连接到桥粒斑蛋白。桥粒芯糖蛋白和桥粒黏蛋白的细胞外域彼此以相邻的表皮细胞间隙相连接。正常情况下,桥粒芯糖蛋白3比较常见且易于检测,位于基底层上的角质形成细胞间,而桥粒芯糖蛋白1主要位于角质细胞层下的角质形成细胞间。

With the use of electron microscopy, each desmosome is seen to be made of three parts: the trilaminar plasma membrane structure of the adjacent keratinocytes, the electron-dense attachment plaque in each adjacent keratinocyte's cytoplasm, and an intercellular matrix betneen the two.

This trilaminar plasma, 8 nm in width, presents as three layers of differing density under electron microscopy. The inner layer (inner leaflet) is a fine electron-dense line along the cytoplasmic side of the plasma membrane adjacent to the attachment plaque; an electron-lucent central lamina stands in the middle, and finally the electron-dense outer layer (outer leaflet) interfaces to the intercellular matrix between the epidermal cells. The densest material of such intercellular matrix tends to be deposited on the surface of outer leaflet, and is known as cell surface coat. However, it is not easy to clarify the boundary between the cell surface coat and outer leaflet of the plasma membrane because of their similar density.

电镜下,每一个桥粒包括两个相邻的角质形成细胞的三层胞质膜(trilaminar plasma membrane)及各自胞质内的1个电子致密的附着板以及细胞间黏合物质。

胞质膜:胞质膜厚约8 nm,显示有三层结构,内层或内小叶(inner leaflet)表现为一道纤细的电子致密线,与附着板紧密相邻,中层为一电子透明线,外层或外小叶(outer leaflet)也为一电子致密线,表面直接与细胞间黏合物接触,这一覆盖于外小叶表面的黏合物质最致密的部分称为细胞表衣(cell surface coat),因细胞表衣和外小叶的致密度相差不多,所以通常不易在二者之间分出界限。

②Hemidesmosomes: as the name implies, hemidesmosomes are half desmosomes. This structure is important for connecting the basal cells to the lamina densa of the basal membrane. It is known that those intermediate filaments of the cytoskeleton at the hemidesmosomes that protrude from the basal keratinocytes are keratin 14 and keratin 5. A number of important molecules or antigens have been linked to hemidesmosomes including bullous pemphigoid antigen 1 (BPAG1, 230 kD), bullous pemphigoid antigen 2 (BPAG2, 180 kD), $\alpha6\beta4$integrin, and other molecules such as $\alpha3\beta1$ integrin, $\alpha2\beta1$ integrin, IFAP300, P200, etc(Fig. 1-7).

②半桥粒,顾名思义,是桥粒的一半,是连接基底细胞与基膜的致密板的重要结构。基底层角质形成细胞内插入到半桥粒内的细胞骨架中间丝主要是角蛋白14和角蛋白5。半桥粒含有大疱性类天疱疮抗原1(BPAG1,230 kD)、大疱性类天疱疮抗原2(BPAG2,180 kD)、$\alpha6\beta4$整合素及其他分子如$\alpha3\beta1$整合素、$\alpha2\beta1$整合素、IFAP300、P200等(图1-7)。

③Gap junctions: these are 2-4 nm wide intercellular spaces between adjacent cells composed mainly of connexin units on the cell membrane. A total of 13 connexins have been described so far that can be classified into three groups: α、β and γ. The key function of these proteins is to connect adjacent cells by transporting small

③间隙连接:在间隙连接处相邻细胞间有2～4 nm的缝隙,间隙连接的主要成分是间隙连接蛋白,迄今已发现有13种连接蛋白,并分为3组即α、β和γ,其主要功能是连接细胞和转运小分子和

molecules and ions. The size limit for passing molecules is less than 1.5 kD(1 D=1 u).

(3) Basement membrane zone (BMZ): the BMZ is usually not visible with hematoxylin-eosin (HE) stain. However, it can be exhibited as a violaceous homogenous band of 0.5-1 μm thickness when stained with PAS (Periodic acid-Schiff)(Fig. 1-5). The main components of the BMZ are neutral mucopolysaccharides.

离子。间隙连接的通道可以允许分子量小于 1.5 kD(1 D=1 u)的分子通过。

(3) 基膜带(basement membrane zone,BMZ) 基膜带在 HE 染色切片中通常看不见,但用 PAS(过碘酸-雪夫)染色在表皮与真皮连接处则可以见到厚 0.5～1 μm、呈紫红色均质性的条带(图 1-5),其主要成分是中性黏多糖。

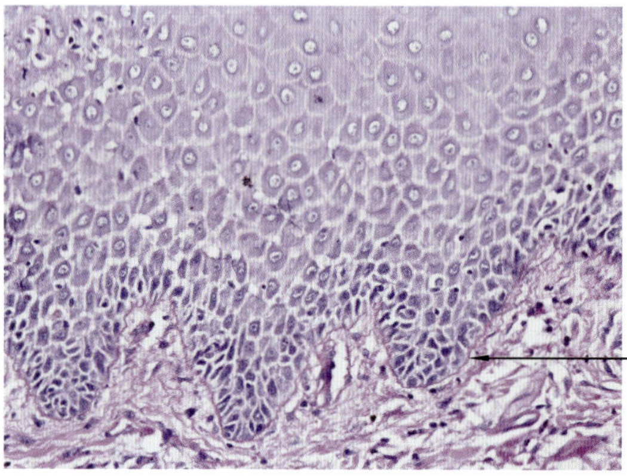

Fig. 1-5 Basement membrane zone, PAS staining(图 1-5 基膜带:PAS 染色)

With the electronic microscope, the BMZ is divided into four layers (Fig. 1-6).

在电镜下基膜带分为四层(图 1-6)。

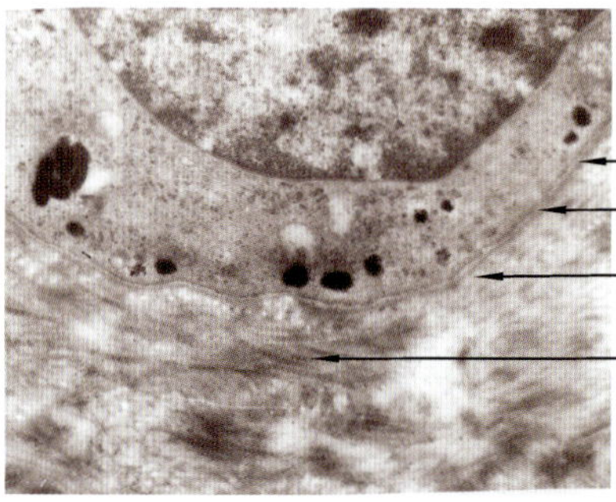

Fig. 1-6 Electron microscopy of the basement membrane zone(图 1-6 基膜带电镜照片)

① The lower border of the basal-cell plasma membrane: the attachment plaque on the plasma membrane, and the cytoplasmic tonofilaments that attach to the attachment plaque are well illustrated in a hemidesmosome.

②Lamina lucida: this is a 20-40 nm thick electron-lucent zone beneath the plasma membrane of the basal cells. The additional electron-dense band, 7-9 nm in width, paralleling the attachment plaque of hemidesmosomes, is seen within the lamina lucida area running underneath the attachment plaque of hemidesmosomes. The main components of the lamina lucida are laminin 332 (known in earlier texts as laminin 5).

③Lamina densa: also known as basal lamina, it is a 60-80 nm wide band-like structure. It is synthesized by the basal cells of the

①基底细胞真皮侧的胞质膜:胞质膜上有一个附着板,附着板上附着有张力细丝(tonofilaments),构成半桥粒(hemidesmosome)。

②透明板(lamina lucida):是一厚 20～40 nm、位于基底细胞的胞质膜层下方的电子密度比较透明的区域。在每一个半桥粒附着板下方的透明板内可见与附着板平行的厚 7～9 nm 的基底细胞下致密板。透明板的主要成分是层粘连蛋白 332(以往称为层粘连蛋白 5)。

③致密板(lamina densa):又称为基底板(basal lamina),厚 60～80 nm 的带

epidermis. The main components of the lamina densa are type Ⅳ collagens. Other ingredients include fibronectins, heparan sulfate proteoglycans, nidogen (also called entactin), and laminin 332. It has been observed that Type ⅩⅦ collagen (or BP180), a 180 kD bullous pemphigoid antigen, spans the lumina lucida and then connects to the lamina densa and the hemidesmosomes.

状结构。致密板由表皮的基底细胞合成。其主要成分为Ⅳ型胶原及其他成分如纤维连接素、硫酸肝素蛋白聚糖、巢蛋白(以往称为内功素)和层粘连蛋白332。ⅩⅦ型胶原，即BP180，是一种180 kD的大疱性类天疱疮抗原，横跨透明板，并连接致密板和半桥粒。

④Reticular lamina: fibers beneath the basal lamina are derived from the papillary dermis layer and include anchoring filaments, dermal microfibrils, and collagen fibers. These fibrous components constitute the so-called PAS-positive BMZ under microscopy, in which the anchoring filaments are 5-7 nm thick fibrils that are believed, at least in part, to originate from the dermis, and their main components are type Ⅶ collagen. The anchoring fibrils form the semi-circular loop structure that surrounds type Ⅰ and type Ⅲ collagens and also produce a tight connection with the latter collagen; meanwhile both ends of anchoring fibril are inserted into the lamina densa. Therefore, the main function of anchoring filaments, as the name suggests, is to create firm attachments between the epidermis and the dermis.

④网板(reticular lamina)：由位于基底板下方、来自乳头真皮的纤维成分组成，包括锚丝、真皮微纤维和胶原纤维。特别需要注意的是光学显微镜下PAS染色阳性的基膜带是由纤维成分组成的。锚丝是5～7 nm厚的纤维，锚纤维至少一部分来源于真皮，其主要成分是Ⅶ型胶原。锚纤维呈半环形，其两端插入致密板，而其弧形端围绕Ⅰ型和Ⅲ型胶原并与后者紧密连接。锚纤维的主要功能是有效地锚定表皮和真皮。

The BMZ permits the exchanges of cells and fluids between the epidermis and dermis.

基膜带能允许表皮和真皮间进行细胞和液体的交换。

Structural molecules are abundant in the desmosomes, hemidesmosomes, gap junctions and BMZ. Recent findings have associated some diseases with these molecules either through encoding gene mutations or autoantibody mechanisms (Fig. 1-7, Tab. 1-1).

桥粒、半桥粒、间隙连接及基膜带有许多结构分子，当编码这些结构分子的基因发生突变或存在针对这些结构分子的自身抗体时会导致相应的疾病(图1-7，表1-1)。

2) Prickle cell layer (suprabasal cell layer, or *stratum spinosum*)

(二) 棘细胞层(或基底上细胞层，或棘层)

The prickle cell layer, also known as the squamous cell layer, is composed of 5-10 layers of cells which are larger than the basal cells, characterized by vacuolar nuclei, one or several nucleoli and eosinophilic cytoplasm. The prickle cells are named due to the delicate "spine" that may be seen, with light microscopy, to cross the narrow intercellular spaces. Toward the surface, polyhedral cells of the suprabasal spinous layer assume a gradually more flattened aspect and the cells' long axes are correspondingly transformed from a vertical to a horizontal orientation as they get closer to the surface of the skin.

棘细胞层又称为鳞状细胞层，由5～10层细胞构成，细胞较基底细胞大，胞质嗜酸性，具有泡状核和一至数个核仁。棘细胞有此称谓是因为在光学显微镜下，通过狭窄的细胞间隙可以看到很细的"棘"。下面的细胞呈多角形，上部的细胞相对扁平，其长轴与表皮平行。

The tonofilaments in the cytoplasm of the prickle cells are 7-8 nm in diameter and shown as loose bundles of thread which are highly electron-dense under electron microscopy. One end of the tonofilaments in prickle cells is inserted into the cytoplasm nearby the nucleus while the other converges upon the attachment plaque of the desmosomes. The tonofilaments are one important ingredient of the cytoskeleton.

电镜下，棘细胞的胞质内含有张力细丝(tonofilaments)，7～8 nm直径大小，为疏松束状的电子致密细丝，这些张力细丝的一端游离于细胞核附近的胞质内，另一端附着在桥粒的附着板上。张力细丝是细胞骨架的重要成分。

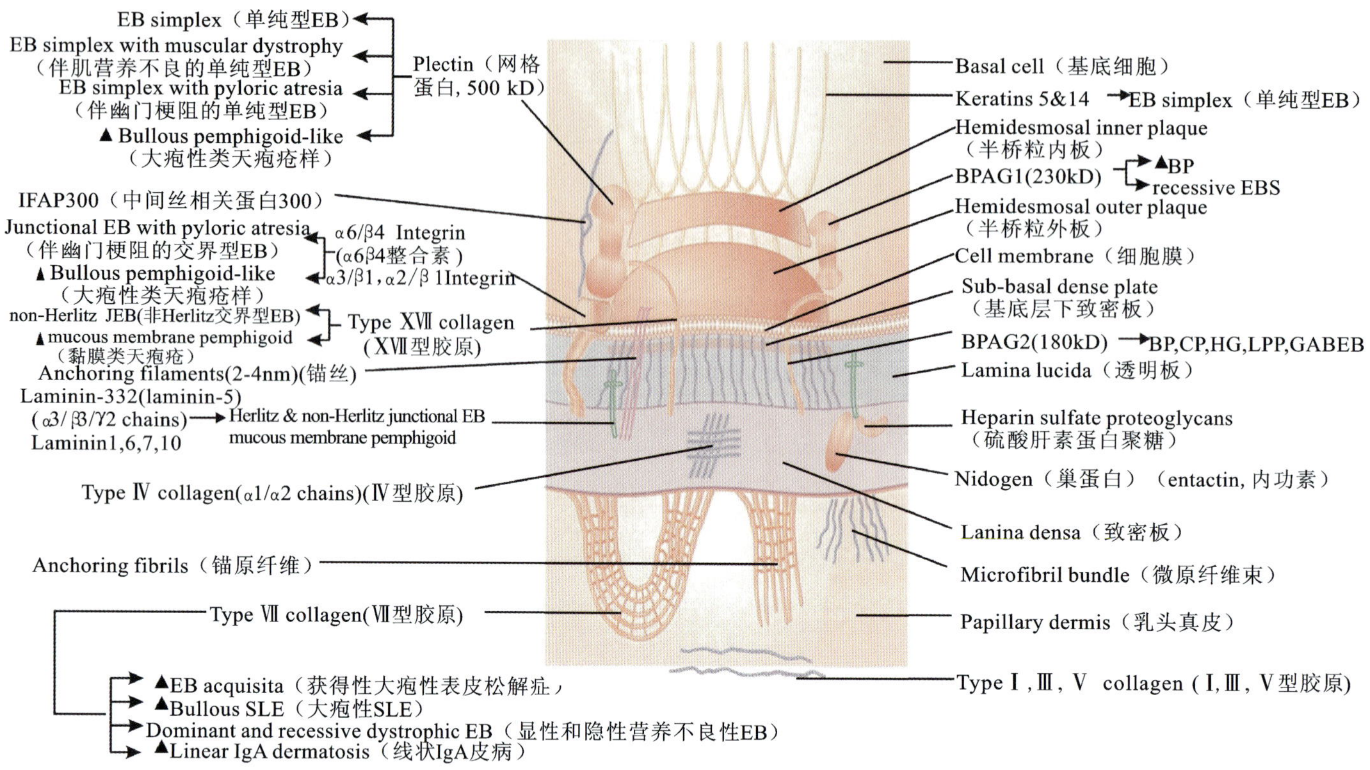

Figs. 1-7　Illustration the important structural molecules in the epidermis, hemidesmosomes, BMZ, papillary dermis and the causes of diseases due to encoding gene mutations or autoantibody targeting these molecules

(图 1-7　表皮、半桥粒、基膜及乳头真皮的重要结构分子及编码这些结构分子的基因突变或存在针对这些结构分子的自身抗体(▲表示)时所导致的相应疾病示意图)

(BP 为大疱性类天疱疮;BPAG 为大疱性类天疱疮抗原;CP 为瘢痕性类天疱疮;EB 为大疱性表皮松解症;EBS 为单纯型大疱性表皮松解症;GABEB 为泛发性萎缩性良性大疱性表皮松解症;HG 为妊娠疱疹;JEB 为交界性 EB;LPP 为扁平苔藓样类天疱疮;SLE 为系统性红斑狼疮)

Tab. 1-1　The gene mutations of structural molecules of the skin or autoantibodies, their locations and diseases

(表 1-1　皮肤结构分子或自身抗体的基因突变、定位及其相关疾病)

Molecules(分子)	Locations(定位)	Diseases(基因突变相关的疾病)
Epidermis(表皮)		
Desmoglein-1(Dsg1)(桥粒芯蛋白-1,Dsg1)	Desmosomes of upper epidermal keratinocytes (表皮上部的角质形成细胞的桥粒)	Pemphigus foliaceus(落叶型天疱疮), endemic pemphigus (地方型天疱疮), striate palmoplantar keratoderma(线状掌跖角皮症)
Desmoglein-3(Dsg3)(桥粒芯蛋白-3,Dsg3)	Desmosomes of lowermost and basal epidermal cells (表皮最下部和基底层细胞的桥粒)	Pemphigus vulgaris (寻常型天疱疮)
Desmoglein-4(Dsg4)(桥粒芯蛋白-4,Dsg4)	Desmosomes(桥粒)	Localized recessive hypotrichosis(局限性隐性少毛症), recessive monilethrix (隐性念珠状发)
Plakophilin1(桥粒斑菲素蛋白 1)	Desmosomes(桥粒)	Ectodermal dysplasia(外胚叶发育不良)
Desmoplakin(桥粒斑蛋白)	Desmosomes(桥粒)	Woolly hair(羊毛状发), keratoderma(角皮症), striate palmoplantar keratoderma (线状掌跖角皮症)
Desmocollin (桥粒黏蛋白)	Desmosomes(桥粒)	Hypotrichosis with scalp vesicles (伴头皮水疱的少毛症)

续表

Molecules(分子)	Locations(定位)	Diseases(基因突变相关的疾病)
Desmocollin 1(桥粒黏蛋白 1)	Desmosomes(桥粒)	Atypical pemphigus (非典型性天疱疮),IgA pemphigus (sub-corneal type)(IgA 天疱疮,角质层下型)
Desmocollin 3(桥粒黏蛋白 3)	Desmosomes(桥粒)	Atypical pemphigus (非典型性天疱疮)
Comeodesmosin (角膜锁链蛋白)	Desmosomes(桥粒)	Hypotrichosis simplex (单纯性少毛症)
Connexin 26(连接蛋白 26)	Intercellular gap junction between adjacent keratinocytes(相邻的角质形成细胞间间隙连接)	Hystrix-like-ichthyosis deafness syndrome(高起鱼鳞病-耳聋综合征),keratitis-ichthyosis-deafness syndrome (角膜炎-鱼鳞病-耳聋综合征),palmoplantar keratoderma with deafness (伴有耳聋的掌跖角皮症),Vohwinkel's syndrome (Vohwinkel 综合征)
Connexin 30(连接蛋白 30)	Intercellular gap junction between adjacent keratinocytes(相邻的角质形成细胞间间隙连接)	Clouston's syndrome (Clouston 综合征)
Connexin 30.3(连接蛋白 30.3)	Intercellular gap junction between adjacent keratinocytes(相邻的角质形成细胞间间隙连接)	Erythro-keratoderma variabilis (可变性红斑角皮症)
Connexin 43(连接蛋白 43)	Intercellular gap junction between adjacent keratinocytes(相邻的角质形成细胞间间隙连接)	Oculodentodigital dysplasia (眼-牙-指(趾)发育不良)
Plectin(网格蛋白)	The innermost part of hemidesmosomes (半桥粒最内侧)	EB simplex(EBS,单纯性大疱性表皮松懈症),EBS with muscular dystrophy(伴肌营养不良的EBS),EBS with pyloric atresia(伴幽门梗阻的EBS)
K2e(角蛋白 K2e)	Superficial suprabasal epidermal cells (基底层上浅表表皮细胞)	Ichthyosis bullosa of Siemens (Siemens 大疱性鱼鳞病)
K6a,K16,K17 (角蛋白 K6a、K16、K17)	Mucous membranes and palmoplantar epidermis;and/or epidermis under hyperplastic conditions (黏膜和掌跖表皮;过度角化表皮)	Pachyonychia congenita(先天性厚甲症),palmoplantar keratoderma(掌跖角皮症)
K4,K13 (角蛋白 K4、K13)	Suprabasal mucous membrane(黏膜基底层上)	White spongy nevus(on tongue)(白色海绵痣(舌))
K9(角蛋白 K9)	Suprabasal palmoplantar epidermis(掌跖部基底上表皮)	Vörner type palmoplantar keratosis (epidermolytic palmar plantar keratoderma) (Vörner 掌跖角皮症(表皮松解性掌跖角皮症))
K3,K12(角蛋白 K3、K12)	Anterior epithelium of the cornea(角膜前上皮)	Juvenile epithelial corneal dystrophy(Meesman) (青少年上皮性角膜营养不良)
K5,K14(角蛋白 K5、K14)	Keratinocytes in the basal cell layer(基底细胞层角质形成细胞)	Epidermolysis bullosa simplex(单纯性大疱性表皮松解症)
K1,K10(角蛋白 K1、K10)	Suprabasal keratinocytes(基底层上角质形成细胞)	Epidermolytic hyperkeratosis (表皮松解性角化过度)/bullous ichthyosiform erythroderma (大疱性鱼鳞病样红皮病)

续表

Molecules(分子)	Locations(定位)	Diseases(基因突变相关的疾病)
Keratinocyte-specific transglutaminase (角质形成细胞特异性转谷氨酰胺酶)	Suprabasal epidermis (基底层上表皮)	Lamellar ichthyosis (板层状鱼鳞病)
Profilaggrin (丝聚蛋白原)	Keratohyaline,granular layer of epidermis (角质透明颗粒,表皮颗粒层)	Ichthyosis vulgaris(寻常型鱼鳞病), atopic dermatitis (特应性皮炎)
Basement membrane zone (基膜带)		
BPAG-1(BP230)(a desmoplakin homologue) (类天疱疮抗原-1(BP230),桥粒斑蛋白的类似物)	Inner plaque of basal cell hemidesmosomes (基底细胞半桥粒的内斑块)	Bullous pemphigoid (大疱性类天疱疮)
BPAG-2(collagen type ⅩⅦ BP-180) (类天疱疮抗原-2(ⅩⅦ型胶原 BP-180))	Transmembrane portion of basal cell hemidesmosome (基底细胞半桥粒的跨膜部分)	Generalized atrophic benign epidermolysis bullosa (泛发性萎缩性良性大疱性表皮松解症),bullous pemphigoid(大疱性类天疱疮),herpes gestationis (妊娠疱疹),cicatricial pemphigoid(瘢痕性类天疱疮)
Ladinin (97-Kd/120000, considered as a degradation product of the BPAG2,BP180) Ladinin (97-Kd/120000,认为是 BPAG2、BP180 的降解产物)	Lamina lucida (透明板)	Linear IgA bullous dermatoses (线状 IgA 大疱性皮病)
Uncein	Lamina lucida (透明板)	Recessive junctional type of epidermolysis bullosa(隐性交界性大疱性表皮松解症)
Collagen type ⅩⅦ (ⅩⅦ型胶原)	Lamina lucida(透明板),transmembrane portion of basal cell hemidesmosome (基底细胞半桥粒的跨膜部分)	Non-Herlitz junctional EB(非 Herlitz 型 EB), mucous membrane pemphigoid(黏膜类天疱疮)
Integrin $\alpha6/\beta4$ (整合素 $\alpha6/\beta4$)	Transmembrane and outer plaque of basal cell hemidesmosome (基底细胞半桥粒的跨膜和外斑块)	Junctional epidermolysis bullosa (交界性大疱性表皮松解症)
Laminin 5 (kalinin,epiligrin, nicein,BM600) (层粘连蛋白 5(缰蛋白,表皮整联配体蛋白,nicein 粘连蛋白,BM600))	Anchoring filaments of lamina lucida (透明板的锚丝)	Junctional epidermolysis bullosa (Herlitz's) (交界性大疱性表皮松解症(Herlitz's)), cicatricial pemphigoid(瘢痕性类天疱疮)
Dermis(真皮)		
Collagen type Ⅰ (Ⅰ型胶原)	Dermis (80% of reticular and papillary dermal collagen) (真皮(80%的网状和乳头真皮的胶原))	Ehlers-Danlos syndrome types 7A、7B (Ehlers-Danlos 综合征的 7A、7B 型)
Collagen type Ⅲ (Ⅲ型胶原)	Dermis (15% of reticular and papillary dermal collagen) (真皮(15%的网状和乳头真皮的胶原))	Ehlers-Danlos syndrome type 4 (Ehlers-Danlos 综合征的 4 型)

续表

Molecules(分子)	Locations(定位)	Diseases(基因突变相关的疾病)
Collagen type Ⅴ (Ⅴ型胶原)	Perivascular periadnexal dermis (血管和附属器周围的真皮)	Ehlers-Danlos syndrome type 2 (Ehlers-Danlos 综合征的 2 型)
Collagen type Ⅶ (Ⅶ型胶原)	Anchoring fibrils (锚纤维)	Epidermolysis bullosa dystrophica(营养不良性大疱性表皮松解症),EBA(获得性 EB),bullous SLE(大疱性 SLE),linear IgA dermatoses(线状 IgA 皮病)
Elastin (弹力蛋白)	Papillary and reticular dermis (乳头和网状真皮)	Pseudoxanthoma elasticum (弹力纤维性假黄瘤)
Fibrillin (原纤蛋白)	Elastic microfibrils beneath BMZ and dermis (基膜带下部和真皮的弹力微原纤维)	Marfan's syndrome (Marfan 综合征)
Appendages(附属器)		
CFTA(cystic fibrosis transmembrane conductance regulator) CFTA(囊性纤维化跨膜电导调节子)	Apical surface of cells lining the eccrine duct (外泌汗腺导管被膜细胞的顶面)	Cystic fibrosis (囊性纤维化)
EDA gene (无汗性外胚叶发育不良基因)	Epidermis or follicle ORS or follicle matrix or sebaceous glands or eccrine glands (表皮,毛囊外根鞘,毛囊基质,皮脂腺,外泌汗腺)	Anhidrotic ectodermal dysplasia (无汗性外胚叶发育不良)
Keratins Ha 1-4,Hb 1-4 (角蛋白 Ha1-4、Hb 1-4)	Hair shaft (毛干)	Monilethrix (Hb group keratin mutation) (念珠状发(Hb 组角蛋白突变))

(cited from Evan R. Farmer,Antoinette F. Hood. *Pathology of the Skin*. 2 nd ed. USA:McGraw-Hill Companies,Inc. 2000:91;Hiroshi Shimizu. *Shimizu's Textbook of Dermatology*. Japan:Sanbi Printing Co. ,Ltd. ,2007:7;Callonje E,Brenn T,Lazar A,et al. *Mckee's Pathology of the Skin with Clinical Correlations*. 4th ed. Philadelphia:Elsevier Limited. 2012:14)

The prickle cells are separated by intercelluar spaces and connected to each other by intercellular bridges named desmosomes. The intercellular spaces contain neutral mucopolysaccharides, acid mucopolysaccharides (glycosaminoglycans) and lipids. Hyaluronic acid is an important acid mucopolysaccharide and also a very important natural moisturizing factor which is mainly located in the matrix between keratinocytes, but also exists in the basal layer and the *stratum corneum*.

棘细胞之间有一定的间隙并由细胞间桥即桥粒连接。相邻的棘细胞之间的间隙内有中性和酸性黏多糖(糖胺聚糖)和脂质。透明质酸是一种重要的酸性黏多糖,也是一种非常重要的天然保湿因子,在棘细胞间极其丰富,但也见于基底层和角质层。

3) Granular cell layer (*stratum granulosum*)

This layer is composed of 2-3 layers of keratinocytes but can be 10 layers deep in the palms of the hands and soles of the feet and is characterized by basophilic keratohyaline granules in their cytoplasm. Keratohyaline granules are composed of profilaggrin (the precursor of filaggrin),loricrin and keratin filaments. Filaggrin is a 50 kD protein that is responsible for aggregation of keratin

(三) 颗粒细胞层(颗粒层)

由 2～3 层构成,但在掌跖部位可达 10 层,其特点是胞质内含有嗜碱性的角质透明颗粒。角质透明颗粒由丝聚蛋白原(丝聚蛋白的前体)、兜甲蛋白(loricrin)和角蛋白细丝构成。丝聚蛋白的分子量为 50 kD,其功能是聚集角蛋白

filaments in cytoplasm, whereas profilaggrin is a fairly large (600 kD) histidine-rich phosphorylated protein. Shortly after forming in the *stratum corneum*, filaggrin is apt to break down into amino acid residues that undergo further metabolic processes resulting finally in urocanic acid and pyrrolidone carboxylic acid. The urocanic acid acts as a blocker for ultraviolet light and the pyrrolidone carboxylic acid acts as a natural humectant, helping to maintain hydration of the cornified layer when the humidity of the environment is otherwise unfavorable for the human body. Filaggrin gene mutation has been found in some patients with atopic dermatitis (one of the clinical symptoms being skin dryness) and ichthyosis vulgaris.

丝，丝聚蛋白原为高分子量(600 kD)、富含组氨酸、磷酸化的蛋白。丝聚蛋白在其形成后的比较短的时间内即在角质层内分解为游离氨基酸，并进一步代谢形成尿刊酸(urocanic acid)和咯烷酮羧酸(pyrrolidone carboxylic acid)，尿刊酸可以阻断紫外线，咯烷酮羧酸则是一种天然保湿剂，在低湿度的环境中对角质层起水合作用。在一些特应性皮炎(其临床特点之一是皮肤干燥)和寻常型鱼鳞病患者中已发现有丝聚蛋白的基因突变。

Under electron microscopy, the lamellar bodies-known as Odland bodies-can be seen in the cytoplasm of granular cells. These membrane-coated granule structures are also called keratinosomes, which are synthesized primarily in the prickle cells and appear first near the perinuclear cytoplasm of granular cells. As keratinocytes move up to the top of the granular cell layer, the keratinosomes increase in both number and size, some can be discharged into the intercellular spaces. The intracellular keratinosomes are seen as round or oval bodies, 300-500 nm in diameter, containing glycolipids and sterols. In the granular cell layer, these keratinosomes fuse with the cytoplasmic membrane to release their contents into the intercellular spaces, where they form an adhesive substance to bind together the cornified cells, which act as a barrier against water loss. The second function of Odland bodies is to enhance the cross-linkage between cornified cells by means of filaggrins.

在电镜下，颗粒层内有板层颗粒即 Odland 小体，又称为膜被颗粒或角质体。板层颗粒主要在棘细胞内合成，并首先出现于棘细胞核周的胞质内，在表皮上部其数量迅速增多，体积增大，在颗粒层的细胞内和细胞外均有板层颗粒，为 300～500 nm 直径的圆形或椭圆形小体，Odland 小体与颗粒细胞的浆膜融合并将其内容物从颗粒层排出到细胞外间隙中，其主要成分为糖脂和固醇，Odland 小体有 2 个重要功能：一是起到屏障作用以防止水分丢失，二是与丝聚蛋白一起介导角质层细胞的黏附。

The granular cells are interconnected by tight junctions consisting of two transmembrane proteins, occludins and claudins, which serve as a barrier to prevent fluid loss.

颗粒细胞层细胞之间通过紧密连接相互联系，紧密连接的主要跨膜蛋白是封闭连接蛋白(occludin)和闭合蛋白(claudin)，其功能是防止体液的渗漏。

4) Horny cell layer (*stratum corneum*)

(四) 角质细胞层(角质层)

The *stratum corneum* is the outermost layer of the epidermis. Under normal conditions, it consists of flat, polyhedral, anucleate cornified cells. These cells contain abundant keratin to prevent skin dehydration. The cells have an eosinophilic appearance in hematoxylin-eosin stained sections. Furthermore, the lipids filling the intercellular space between the horny cells act to further strengthen this water impermeability. More than half of the lipids are ceramides, with cholesterols, free fatty acids and cholesterol sulfates making up most of the remaining lipids.

位于表皮的最外层，正常情况下，角质细胞层由扁平、多角形的、无核的角化细胞构成，其中含有大量的角蛋白，可以防止皮肤脱水。在苏木素-伊红染色切片中呈嗜酸性。角质层细胞间的脂质半数以上为神经酰胺(ceramides)，其他包括胆固醇、游离脂肪酸和胆固醇硫酸盐，这些脂质填充于角化细胞之间，在防止跨表皮水丢失中起重要作用。

5) *Stratum lucidum*

(五) 透明层

A thin homogeneous eosinophilic zone between the granular

在颗粒层和角质层之间有一狭窄的

layer and horny cell layer that is often found in the areas where the horny cell layer is thick, and is most prominently seen in the skin of the palms of the hands and the soles of the feet.

6) Mucosal epithelium

Unlike the keratinized epidermis, the mucosal epithelium lacks granular and horny cell layers. The prickle cells tend to be more vacuolated and lighter stained because of glycogens accumulation in their cytoplasm. As stated above, in keratinized epidermis, the cells of mucosal epithelium become smaller, shrinking and desquamating as they move outward to the surface of mucosa. In addition, the cells of mucosal epithelium have poorly developed tonofilaments, and fewer fully developed desmosomes. The oral mucosal epithelium contains numerous microvilli, which are fine, hair-like extensions of the apical membrane.

7) Keratin

A total of 54 functional keratin genes have been uncovered in the human genome, of which 21 are found to be associated with monogenic disorders. Keratins, synthesized by keratinocytes, constitute tonofilaments to serve as thc basis of thc cell cytoskeleton. Two types of keratin have been described: type Ⅰ is acidic and type Ⅱ is neutral to alkaline. The intermediate filaments are formed by a pair (one Type Ⅰ and one Type Ⅱ) of keratins, but the composition varies depending on the differential stages of the keratinocytes during its journey towards the surface. Keratins play roles not only in construction of the cytoskeleton but also in cell signaling, stress response and apoptosis. The different mutations derived from keratin types have been associated with some skin disorders, as shown in Tab. 1-1.

2. Langerhans cells

Langerhans cells are derived from bone marrow, and can be found in the epidermis by the 7th week of gestation. They are normally scattered in the *stratum spinosum* layer of the epidermis, accounting for 3%-5% of the cell mass in this layer. In general, the density of these cells is 460/mm^2 to 1000/mm^2 on average; however, the amount of Langerhans cells varies with skin regions, such as more cells are found in the extremities than in the trunk. The number of cells also varies with individuals. Finally, the number may be decreased or even go to zero under the effects of repeated exposure to UV light or the effects of topical application of potent steroids. On the other hand, the number of Langerhans cells can be increased in other skin diseases, such as mycosis fungoides (MF) and contact allergic reactions.

Langerhans cells are dendritic cells that also can be found in

嗜酸性均质区域，一般在角质较厚的部位均可能有此层存在，但以掌跖最为明显。

（六）黏膜上皮

与角化的表皮不同，黏膜上皮无颗粒层和角质层，棘细胞胞质内含有大量的糖原而染色淡，呈空泡化。与前述的角化表皮一样，黏膜上皮细胞在向黏膜表面移行时，棘细胞变小、皱缩，最终脱落。此外，黏膜上皮细胞的张力丝发育不良，仅有很少数发育良好的桥粒。口腔黏膜上皮在其顶部含有许多细小的如发一样伸展的微绒毛。

（七）角蛋白

人类染色体上有 54 种功能性角蛋白(keratin)基因，其中 21 种与单基因病相关联。角蛋白在角质形成细胞内合成并形成张力丝，起到细胞骨架的作用。角蛋白有两型：Ⅰ型为酸性，Ⅱ型为中性到碱性角蛋白。二者成对结合在一起形成中间丝，角蛋白在表皮的不同部位因角质形成细胞的分化不同而异。角蛋白不仅在细胞骨架中发挥作用，还在细胞信号、应急反应及凋亡中具有直接的作用。不同的角蛋白突变引起不同的皮肤病(表 1-1)。

二、朗格汉斯细胞

朗格汉斯细胞(Langerhans cells)来源于骨髓，在胚胎的第 7 周就可在表皮中发现它们，在正常情况下，它们位于表皮棘层，占该层的 3%～5%，密度为 460～1000 个/mm^2。其在肢端皮肤中多于躯干皮肤。它们在不同的个体中具有显著的部位差异性。朗格汉斯细胞的数量在反复的紫外线照射和长期局部使用强效糖皮质激素情况下会减少甚至耗竭。在蕈样霉菌病(MF)患者中其数量会增加，在接触性变态反应中其数量也会增加。

朗格汉斯细胞为树枝状细胞，也见

the oral mucosa, vagina, lymph nodes, thymus, and occasionally in the dermis.

In HE stained sections, Langerhans cells are present as clear cells in the suprabasal epidermis and are not distinguished from the keratinocytes nearby (Fig. 1-2). However, the dendritic characters can be clearly demonstrated in cross sections stained with gold chloride. Other positive markers for identification of these cells are adenosine triphosphatase (ATPase), aminopeptidase, HLA-DR antigen, S-100, and more specific CD1a monoclonal antibodies.

Langerhans cells are distinguished by markedly folded nuclei and a set of highly characteristic cytoplasmic organelles known as Birbeck granules under electron microscopy but having no tonofilaments or desmosomes. These rod or tennis racket-shaped bodies, which range in size from 0.1-1 μm, are distinctive for Langerhans cells. However, Birbeck granules can appear in the tumor cells of histiocytosis X and infantile self-healing reticulohistiocytosis.

Langerhans cells are one type of antigen presenting cells. Thus, their main functions are to recognize, uptake and process antigens prior to presenting antigen signals to T lymphocytes in the skin. They are not only important to maintain the epidermal homeostasis in the healthy skin, but play key roles in contact sensitization and immunosurveilances against viral infection or tumor pathogenesis.

3. α-dendritic cells

α-dendritic cells are also called indeterminate cells because their origin and function have not been well-defined. This group of cells resembles Langerhans cells in their ultrastructures and in their specific reaction with CD1a monoclonal antibodies, however no Birbeck granules and desmosomes have ever been found in α-dendritic cells. It is considered that α-dendritic cells are Langerhans cell-related, or are even precursors of Langerhans cells, to mediate the antigen-presenting in the skin.

4. Melanocytes

Melanocytes are dendritic cells that originate in the neural crest. In the skin, melanocytes are situated at the basal cell layer of the epidermis, appearing as small "clear cells" with round to oval, dark-stained nuclei in hematoxylin-eosin (HE) sections. The clear space in the cytoplasm is an artifact of fixation due to shrinkage of the melanocyte cytoplasm around the nucleus (Fig. 1-3). Although this group of cells is termed "clear cells", not every "clear-looking" cell in the basal cell layer is a melanocyte. For example, Langerhans cells (as described above in the section on the prickle cell layer) and even some keratinocytes with fixation artifacts may have a similar

于口腔黏膜、阴道、淋巴结、胸腺,偶见于真皮。

在常规 HE 切片中,朗格汉斯细胞位于表皮基底层上(图 1-2),表现为透亮的细胞,但难以辨认。在用氯化金染色的切片中表现为树枝状。朗格汉斯细胞可以被 ATP 酶(ATPase)、氨基肽酶、HLA-DR 抗原、S-100 及更特异的 CD1a 单克隆抗体标记阳性。

电镜下,朗格汉斯细胞的特征是具有显著折叠的核和胞质内有 Birbeck 颗粒(Birbeck granule),不含有张力丝和桥粒。Birbeck 颗粒大小为 0.1～1 μm,呈棒状或网球拍状,对其具有诊断意义。但这些颗粒也见于组织细胞增生症 X 的肿瘤细胞和婴儿自愈性组织细胞增生病。

朗格汉斯细胞作为抗原提呈细胞,其重要功能是识别、摄取、处理抗原,将抗原信号提呈给皮肤中的 T 细胞,并在正常皮肤的自稳中有着复杂的功能。朗格汉斯细胞在接触致敏、病毒感染和皮肤肿瘤的监视中起关键作用。

三、α-树枝状细胞

α-树枝状细胞也称为未定类细胞。其起源和功能尚不清楚。这些细胞类似于朗格汉斯细胞,因为其具有与朗格汉斯细胞类似的超微结构特征、能特异性与 CD1a 单克隆抗体反应,但缺乏 Birbeck 颗粒和桥粒。可能与朗格汉斯细胞相关或是后者的前体细胞,介导皮肤中的抗原提呈。

四、黑素细胞

黑素细胞(melanocyte)是来源于神经嵴的树枝状细胞。它们位于表皮基底层,在 HE 染色切片中,由于在制片过程中脱水和固定的关系它们表现为小的细胞,具有圆形到卵圆形深染的核,胞质透明,因而称为透明细胞(图 1-3)。但是,在表皮的基底层,并非所有的透明细胞均是黑素细胞,少数基底层角质形成细胞可以由于同样的人工收缩的原因而呈现同样的外观。上述棘层的朗格汉斯细

vacuolated appearance in the cytoplasm. Melanocytes can also be found in the hair bulb, outer root sheath of hair follicles, inner ear, choroid and iris of the eye and meninges. The dendritic feature of melanocytes can be highlighted with S100 protein immunohistochemistry.

Melanocytes are found in all body sites of the skin, but their concentration does vary. The density of melanocytes is similar to that of Langerhans cells in the skin. They are most abundant on the cheeks and male genitals at 2000/mm^2, compared to the lowest density on the trunk of 800/mm^2 in total, and the ratio of melanocytes to keratinocytes in the basal layer is 1∶10 on average.

Inside the cytoplasm of melanocytes we find special organelles called 'melanosomes', in which melanin is synthesized and packed (Fig. 1-8). The melanosomes are formed and assembled in the Golgi apparatus, which can be observed in the epidermis as early as the 8-10th week of fetal development. Melanosomes enclosed by a double-lipid membrane are divided into four stages (Ⅰ, Ⅱ, Ⅲ and Ⅳ) based upon the degree of melanin development inside.

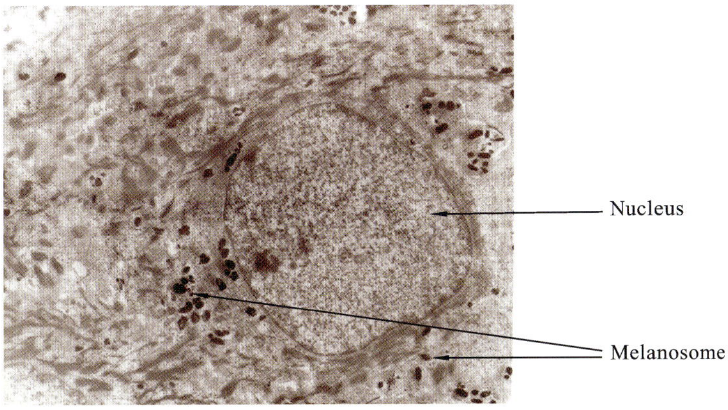

Fig. 1-8 Electron microscopy of melanosome(图 1-8 黑素小体的电镜照片)

For example, stage Ⅰ melanosomes measure around 0.3 μm in diameter and contain no melanin; whereas stage Ⅱ to Ⅳ melanosomes are 0.5 μm in diameter. The dendrites of melanocytes extend in all directions, to facilitate the transfer of melanin granules to the surrounding keratinocytes. On average, one melanocyte connects with 36 keratinocytes, forming an epidermal melanin unit. Melanocytes can be stained by S-100 and Melan-A. Melanin can be even better seen with DOPA (3, 4-dihydroxyphenylalanine) reaction, silver staining such as Masson-Fontana staining.

The differences in color among the human races result, not from differences in the number of melanocytes, but from their activity as measured by the number and size of the melanosomes.

胞也称为透明细胞。黑素细胞还见于毛球、毛囊外根鞘、内耳、眼的脉络膜和虹膜及脑膜。黑素细胞的树枝状特点可采用 S100 蛋白免疫组化的方法凸显出来。

黑素细胞见于身体各个部位，不同部位密度有所不同，其密度与皮肤中朗格汉斯细胞的密度类似，其中以面部和男性的生殖器部位密度最高，约为2000个/mm^2，而躯干部位最低，约为 800 个/mm^2。表皮基底层细胞的 10% 是黑素细胞。

黑素细胞的胞质内有黑素小体(图1-8)，后者是在高尔基体内合成和组装的。在妊娠 8～10 周的胚胎表皮中就可以发现黑素小体。黑素是经由酪氨酸在黑素小体内合成和包装的。黑素小体具有脂质双层膜，根据其含黑素的多少分为Ⅰ、Ⅱ、Ⅲ、Ⅳ四级。

Ⅰ级黑素小体的直径为 0.3 μm，不含黑素，Ⅱ到Ⅳ级黑素小体的直径为 0.5 μm。黑素细胞的树枝状突起向各个方向伸展，以向其周边的角质形成细胞输送黑素。平均每个黑素细胞为其周围约 36 个角质形成细胞提供黑素小体，称之为表皮黑素单位(epidermal melanin unit)。黑素细胞可被 S-100 及 Melan-A 阳性染色。黑素能通过 3,4-二羟基苯丙氨酸(DOPA)反应、银染色技术如 Masson-Fontana 反应而更好地显示。

不同的种族间黑素细胞的分布和密度并无差异。不同种族皮肤颜色的差异是由黑素小体的多少和大小决定的。反

However, repeated exposure to ultraviolet lights may cause increases in the number and size of melanocytes, and even an increase in activity.

复的紫外光的暴露能增加黑素细胞的数目、大小及其活性。

Electromicroscopically, melanocytes are distinguished by the presence of melanosomes in their cytoplasm and dendrites, and the absence of tonofilaments and desmosomes(Fig. 1-8).

电镜下,黑素细胞没有张力丝和桥粒。其胞质和树枝状突起中有丰富的黑素小体(图1-8)。

The tyrosine kinase receptor KIT and its ligand-stem cell factor are crucial for the migration of melanocytes from the neural crest to the skin, and the proliferation, differentiation, and maturation of melanocytes. Microphthalmia transcription factor (MITF)is closely related to the melanocytes and melanin synthesis during the embryonic development via regulation the transcription of tyrosinase.

酪氨酸激酶受体KIT及其配体干细胞因子在黑素细胞由神经嵴迁移到皮肤以及其增殖、分化和成熟中起至关重要的作用。小眼转录因子(MITF)与黑素细胞的胚胎发育密切相关,并通过调节酪氨酸酶的转录参与黑素的合成。

5. Merkel cells

五、Merkel细胞

Merkel cells are found in the basal cell layer of the epidermis and account for 0.2%-0.5% of the epidermal cells. They are mostly seen in the skin of the fingers, in oral mucosa and in the outer root sheath of the hair follicles. Usually they are not easily recognized in HE sections, but a special meniscoid structure called the Merkel disk (ending of a nerve fiber) can be observed with silver-impregnated staining. Presumably, these cells function as the tactile sensors that are particular to sense light touch. Merkel cells are connected with the adjacent keratinocytes through desmosomes as other epidermal cells do, but in the cytoplasm one can also see intermediate filaments and some membrane-bound, electron-densed neurosecretory-type granules 80-200 nm in diameter. Merkel cells also contain low-molecular weight cytokeratin (CKs) such as CK8, -18, -19, and -20 and express neuroendocrine markers such as chromogranin A and synaptophysin. CK20 and neuroendocrine markers are specific for the diagnosis of Merkel cell carcinoma.

Merkel细胞位于表皮的基底层,占表皮细胞的0.2%~0.5%,最多见于手指、口腔黏膜和毛囊的外根鞘。其在普通切片光学显微镜下不易辨认。在银浸染的切片中表现为半月形的盘状特征,称为Merkel盘,并有感觉神经末梢终止于此。因此,其可能是一种特殊的触觉感受器。Merkel细胞与其相邻的角质形成细胞如同其他表皮细胞一样通过桥粒相连。其胞质中含有中间丝以及直径为80~200 nm的电子致密的具有胞膜的神经分泌型颗粒。Merkel细胞含有低分子量的细胞角蛋白(CKs)如CK8、18、19、20,并表达神经内分泌标志如嗜铬素A和突触素。CK20和神经内分泌标志是诊断Merkel细胞癌的特异性标志。

Dermis

真　皮

The dermis is divided into two components: papillary dermis (the thin zone immediately below the epidermal rete ridges), and the thick reticular dermis that lies below the papillary dermis, accounting for the 2/3 of the dermis. The dermis is primarily composed of connective tissues that include collagen fibers, elastic fibers, reticular fibers and the extrafibrillar matrix, all of which are produced by fibroblasts.

真皮(dermis)可分为乳头真皮(位于表皮下)和网状真皮。网状真皮位于乳头真皮的下方,占真皮厚度的2/3。真皮中的主要成分是结缔组织,包括胶原纤维、弹力纤维、网状纤维和基质,它们都是由纤维母细胞产生的。

In addition to fibroblasts, there are other important cells involved in the skin's immune and inflammatory responses scattered throughout the dermis, especially in the papillary dermis layer. They are mast cells, macrophages and lymphocytes and even dendritic mesenchymal cells (dermal dendrocytes) that are

在真皮内特别是乳头真皮,除纤维母细胞外,还有一些其他的很重要的细胞参与皮肤的免疫和炎症反应,如肥大细胞、巨噬细胞、淋巴细胞以及真皮中的树突状间充质细胞(又称为真皮树突状

responsible for antigen presentation and play important roles in immune response of the skin. Along with the fibrous bundles and cells, the epidermal appendages, the smooth muscle cells such as arrector pili muscles, blood vessels and nerves complete the structure of the dermis.

细胞，具有提呈抗原的功能，在皮肤的免疫反应中起重要作用）。真皮中还有表皮附属器、平滑肌如立毛肌、血管和神经。

1. Collagen fibers

一、胶原纤维

Collagen fibers are the main constituents of connective tissue, making up about 70% of the dry weight of the dermis. There are at least 8 different collagens in human skin. The major types of collagens in the dermis are type Ⅰ (85%-90%), type Ⅲ (8%-11%), and type Ⅴ (2%-4%).

胶原纤维(collagen fibers)是真皮结缔组织中最丰富的成分，约占真皮干重的 70%。人类皮肤至少有 8 种不同的胶原纤维。真皮中的胶原主要是Ⅰ型(85%～90%)，Ⅲ型(8%～11%)和Ⅴ型(2%～4%)。

Whereas type Ⅰ collagen and type Ⅲ collagen and their corresponding precursors, type Ⅰ and type Ⅲ precollagens, are represented in all dermal layers, type Ⅴ collagens are also widespread in the dermis as well as in the lamina lucida. Other types of collagens that can be found in the dermis are type Ⅵ collagens that are mainly concentrated perivascularly or around nerves; types Ⅳ, Ⅶ and ⅩⅦ collagens are found in the BMZ. The major component of anchoring fibrils is type Ⅶ collagen.

除Ⅰ型和Ⅲ型胶原及其前体Ⅰ型和Ⅲ型原胶原分布于真皮全层外，Ⅴ型胶原在真皮内分布广泛而且在透明板内也有。Ⅵ型胶原主要位于真皮的血管和神经周围。Ⅳ型，Ⅶ型和ⅩⅦ型胶原主要是在基膜带。Ⅶ型胶原还是锚原纤维的主要成分。

Mature collagen fibers have a diameter of 2-15 μm, and appear red with hematoxylin-esosin (HE) stains. They wrap around each other to form a finely woven network in the papillary dermis and around the appendages. In contrast, they form thick collagen bundles in the reticular dermis. Collagens in the papillary dermis are mainly type Ⅲ and vertically orientated, whereas, type Ⅰ collages are dominant in the reticular dermis and parallel to the epidermis (Fig. 1-9).

成熟的胶原纤维的直径为 2～15 μm。在 HE 切片中胶原呈红色。其在真皮的乳头层和附属器周围表现为细小的网状分布，而在网状真皮则呈束状。乳头真皮内主要是Ⅲ型胶原，垂直走向，而网状真皮内的胶原主要是Ⅰ型胶原，与表皮平行(图 1-9)。

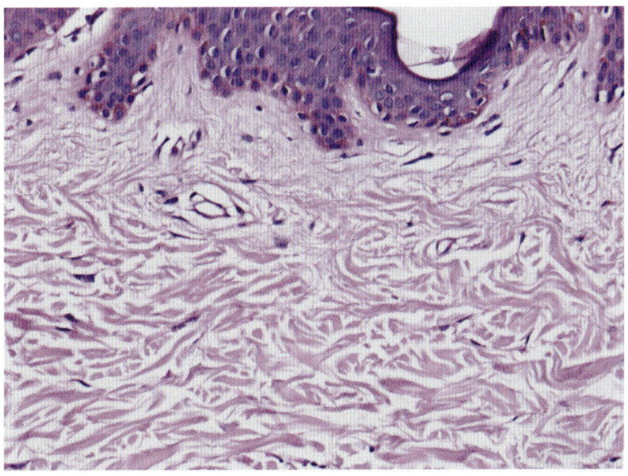

Fig. 1-9 A comparison of the collagens in the papillary and reticular dermis, HE staining

(图 1-9 胶原纤维在乳头真皮和网状真皮内的比较，HE 染色)

Electron microscopy discloses that the collagen fibrils are 100-500 nm long and 1. 5 nm wide with many distinct cross bands spaced about 68 nm apart.

电镜下，胶原纤维的长度为 100～500 nm，宽度为 1. 5 nm，其特征是每间隔 68 nm 有重复的横行的条纹。

2. Elastic fibers

The elastic fibers play an important role in maintaining the elasticity of the skin. These fibers are inconspicuous with HE stains, but are visualized as brownish black by orcein or as dark blue to black by Weigert resorcin fuchsin stains. They are 1-3 μm in diameter, consisting of elastin and microfibrillar proteins to entwine closely with collagen bundles to provide for the skin not only the necessary integrity and strength but elasticity as well. Such fibers extend from the dermal-epidermal basement membrane to the reticular dermis. In contrast to the coarsest and thickest bundles that run parallel to the surface of the skin in the deeper portion of dermis, the elastic fibers become progressively thinner towards the upper portion of the dermis until they get to the junction within the papillary dermis. The delicate elastic fibers are perpendicular to the dermal-epidermal junction and terminate at the BMZ.

3. Reticular fibers

The reticular fibers are not visible in HE stained tissue sections, but are blackened by silver stain (argyrophilic type Ⅲ collagen) measuring 0.2-1 μm in diameter. Under normal conditions, reticular fibers are prominent within and underneath the BMZ, around appendages, blood vessels and fat cells.

4. Ground substance

The ground substance is also known as the extracellular matrix of the dermis. It is an amorphous substance, composed of glycosaminoglycans or acid mucopolysaccharides and electrolytes. The major compositions of acid mucopolysaccharides are hyaluronic acid (nonsulfated acid mucopolysaccharides), chondroitin sulfate, dermatan sulfate and neutral mucopolysaccharides, which are deposited between collagen fibers and collagen bundles.

5. The cells in the dermis

1) Fibroblasts

The fibroblasts are derived from the mesenchymal cells. They are responsible for producing all three fibers (collagens, elastins and reticular fibers) and the base materials (glycosaminoglycans) in the dermis. As may be seen with light microscopy, the fibroblasts interspersed through the collagen fibers have bipolar spindle-shaped, elongated ovoid nuclei and indistinct cytoplasm. The fibroblasts in the dermis and in periadnexal areas express vimentin and CD34 respectively when stained with immunohistochemistry.

2) Mast cells

Mast cells are thought to originate from the bone marrow

二、弹力纤维

弹力纤维(elastic fibers)在使皮肤具有弹性上具有重要作用。在光镜下常规HE染色切片中辨认不清楚,用地衣红可染成棕黑色或Weigert雷琐辛品红染成深蓝色到黑色。弹力纤维的直径为1～3 μm,是由弹力蛋白和丝状蛋白组成的。弹力纤维呈波浪状并与胶原纤维束缠绕在一起,以保持皮肤的完整性、强度和弹性。这些纤维从表皮基膜伸向网状真皮。在真皮的下部弹力纤维比较粗而且最厚,并与表皮平行。从真皮的下部往真皮的上部弹力纤维越来越少。在乳头真皮内弹力纤维纤细,并与真皮-表皮交界垂直,并终止于基膜带。

三、网状纤维

网状纤维(reticular fibers)在常规HE切片中不能辨认,是一种具有嗜银性的Ⅲ型胶原,直径0.2～1 μm。正常情况下,它们见于基膜带、附属器、血管周围和每一脂肪细胞周围。

四、基质

基质(matrix)或细胞外基质(extracellular matrix)是一种无定型物质,是由糖胺聚糖或酸性黏多糖和电解质组成的,酸性黏多糖的主要成分包括透明质酸(一种非硫酸化的酸性黏多糖)、硫酸软骨素、硫酸皮肤素和中性黏多糖。这些成分位于胶原纤维和胶原束间。

五、真皮内的细胞

(一) 纤维母细胞(成纤维细胞)

纤维母细胞(fibroblasts)来源于间充质细胞,它们合成真皮中所有的三种纤维(胶原纤维、弹力蛋白、网状纤维)及碱性物质(糖胺聚糖)。纤维母细胞散在分布于胶原纤维间,光镜下呈双极梭形,长的卵圆形核,胞质不明显。免疫组化显示真皮内和附属器周围的纤维母细胞分别表达波形蛋白和CD34。

(二) 肥大细胞

肥大细胞(mast cells)来源于骨髓,

precursors. Usually they reside in the vicinity of blood vessels of the dermis, especially around the postcapillary venules. On average, the mast cells are about 10 μm in diameter, oval to spindle-shaped, with oval nuclei that may not be easily recognized in HE stained section. However, numerous red-violet granules can be revealed in its cytoplasm when exposed to Giemsa stains.

Mast cells synthesize and store certain allergenic mediators such as histamine, heparin, serine proteinases, and cytokines (e. g., tumor necrosis factor α) in these granules. They can be released into the extracellular spaces soon after the mast cells are stimulated by certain antigens, giving rise to an anaphylactic reaction. Except for allergic responses, mast cells also play an important role in inflammatory reactions by producing and releasing other inflammatory substances such as prostaglandins, leukotrienes, platelet activating factors, etc.

在正常真皮中可以发现它们，主要位于血管周围，特别是毛细血管后静脉周围。在常规 HE 染色中不容易发现它们。肥大细胞的直径平均约为 10 μm，呈圆形到梭形，核呈卵圆形，通过 Giemsa 染色可以看到，肥大细胞的胞质中有许多紫红色的颗粒。

肥大细胞在受到特定的抗原刺激后能释放其颗粒中原已合成和储存的介质，如组织胺、肝素、丝氨酸蛋白酶及某些细胞因子(如肿瘤坏死因子 α)到细胞外，并因此导致过敏反应。此外，肥大细胞还能产生和释放炎症物质，如前列腺素、白三烯、血小板活化因子等，在炎症反应中发挥重要作用。

3) Histiocytes

The histiocytes are tissue macrophages that originate in the bone marrow as monocytes. These monocytes migrate and circulate in the blood and are trapped in various organs where they undergo differentiation into the histiocytes under the influence of various environmental and growth factors. In the dermis, they are called macrophages, epithelioid histiocytes and foreign body giant cells depending on the types of stimuli. Primarily located in the perivascular space in dermis, they are highly variable in size and morphology; as macrophages they are 20-80 μm in diameter with circular nuclei, eosinophilic nucleoli, Golgi apparatus, smooth and rough endoplasmic reticuli, and lysosomes in their cytoplasm. These histiocytes also are characterized by their reaction to CD68 antibody and may be involved in antigen presentation to T-cells.

(三) 组织细胞

组织细胞(histiocytes)是一种源于骨髓单核细胞的组织巨噬细胞。单核细胞游走、循环于血液中，为各器官捕获，在不同环境与生长因素的影响下，分化为组织细胞。在真皮中，这些细胞依据刺激类型的不同称为巨噬细胞、上皮样组织细胞和异物巨细胞，主要位于真皮血管周围，其大小与形态各异。巨噬细胞的直径为 20～80 μm，其胞质中有圆形的核、嗜酸性核仁、高尔基体、光面内质网、粗面内质网与溶酶体。此种组织细胞还具有对抗体 CD68 反应的特点，并可能向 T 细胞提呈抗原。

4) Dermal dendrocytes

Dermal dendrocytes are groups of cells that reside in the perivascular areas of the upper dermis layer. Originating in bone marrow, they are clearly distinct from epidermal Langerhans cells and can be identified by the immunohistochemical expression of CD1c, factor ⅩⅢ a, CD34 and HLA-DR, and by the absence of Birbeck granules in the cytoplasm. Its phagocytic properties may be related to antigen presentation in the dermis.

(四) 真皮树突状细胞

真皮树突状细胞(dermal dendrocytes)来源于骨髓，主要位于上部真皮的血管周围，与表皮朗格汉斯细胞明显不同，其特征是表达 CD1c、因子ⅩⅢa、CD34 和 HLA-DR，不含 Birbeck 颗粒，具有吞噬特性并可能与真皮的抗原提呈有关。

5) Lymphocytes

The peripheral lymphocytes include T and B lymphocytes. Both of them are derived from bone marrow. The T lymphocytes are responsible for the cellular immunity, whereas the B lymphocytes mediate humoral immunity. Lymphocytes have round

(五) 淋巴细胞

外周淋巴细胞(lymphocytes)包括 T 细胞和 B 细胞，二者均来源于骨髓。T 细胞介导细胞免疫，B 细胞介导体液免疫。淋巴细胞具有圆形而深染的核和狭

deeply basophilic nuclei and a very narrow rim of cytoplasm. The average diameter of lymphocytes is 8 μm. It is impossible to distinguish T and B lymphocytes under light microscopy. However, the T lymphocytes can be detected by antibodies such as UCHL, CD45RO, CD2, CD3, and CD5. Furthermore the functional subsets of T lymphocytes (helper and suppressor subsets) can be identified by CD4 and CD8 respectively. The B lymphocytes are positive for CD20, CD79α, lambda or kappa immunoglobulin light chains.

窄的胞质,其平均直径为 8 μm。在光镜下无法区别 T 细胞和 B 细胞。T 细胞能通过 UCHL、CD45RO、CD2、CD3 和 CD5 进行标记,其功能亚群辅助 T 细胞和抑制性 T 细胞能分别被 CD4 和 CD8 标记,而 B 细胞能被 CD20、CD79α、lambda 或 kappa 免疫球蛋白轻链标记。

A small number of dermal T lymphocytes may be found near post-capillary venules in normal skin. These are primarily the T-helper cells that play an important role in immunity.

正常皮肤中的毛细血管后静脉周围有少量的 T 细胞,主要是辅助 T 细胞。它们是皮肤免疫系统的重要组成成分。

Regulatory T-cells (T_{reg}-cells) are a subtype of T lymphocytes that express CD25 (IL-2 receptor), FoxP3 and CD4. These T_{reg}-cells can limit/suppress the skin immunity via regulation of the resident memory T-cells in the skin. Natural killer (NK) cells belong to the lymphocytic lineage and express CD56, CD57, CD16 and CD3ε, but do not express CD3, CD4, CD8 (rarely positive) and B-cell markers.

调节性 T 细胞是 T 细胞一个亚群,能表达 CD25(白介素-2 受体)、FoxP3 和 CD4,能抑制或限制定居皮肤的记忆 T 细胞对皮肤免疫的调节。自然杀伤(NK)细胞属于淋巴细胞系,能表达 CD56、CD57、CD16 和 CD3ε,而不表达 CD3、CD4、CD8(偶有阳性者)和 B 细胞标记。

6) Emigrant inflammatory cells in dermis

(六)真皮移入的炎症细胞

(1) Lymphocytes: at the sensitization period of the inflammatory reactions, the naive T-cells of the dermis will undergo clonal expansion to become T memory cells after they receive the antigen signals from the Langerhans cells. Once the bodies encounter the same antigens during the challenge reaction period, those T memory cells will recognize the antigens, proliferate and result in a cascade of cytokines which further lead to the recruitment of secondary inflammatory cells. T lymphocytes play an important role in the normal skin immunosurveillance and in delayed hypersensitivity reactions. B lymphocytes differentiate into plasma cells that produce antibodies to mediate humoral reaction, which is also regulated by T helper/suppressor cells.

(1) 淋巴细胞　在皮肤炎症反应的致敏阶段,初始 T 细胞在接受朗格汉斯细胞传来的信息后经过克隆性增殖变为记忆 T 细胞。在致敏反应阶段,记忆 T 细胞能识别特异性抗原和增殖并引起细胞因子级联反应,从而导致继发的炎症细胞聚集。T 细胞在正常皮肤的免疫监视和迟发反应中起重要的作用。B 细胞分化为浆细胞并产生抗体参与体液免疫,并受到辅助和抑制性 T 细胞的调节。

(2) Neutrophilic granulocytes: these cells are also known as neutrophils. They are 10-15 μm in diameter, and possess lobulated nuclei and numerous neutrophilic to slightly eosinophilic granules, as well as lysosomal enzymes in their cytoplasm. They are rare in normal skin. Neutrophils migrate into skin only in certain skin inflammatory processes such as psoriasis, seborrheic dermatitis, pityriasis lichenoides *et* varioliformis acuta (PLEVA), vasculitis, skin infections and the so-called neutrophilic dermatoses such as Sweet's syndrome, pyoderma gangrenosum, etc.

(2) 中性粒细胞(neutrophilic granulocytes)　又称为中性白细胞,中性粒细胞的直径为 10～15 μm。其具有分叶核,胞质中含有中性到轻度嗜酸性的颗粒以及溶酶体酶。中性粒细胞在正常皮肤中不常见。其参与一些炎症性皮肤病,如银屑病、脂溢性皮炎、急性痘疮样苔藓状糠疹(PLEVA)、血管炎和皮肤感染及所谓的嗜中性皮病如 Sweet 综合征、坏疽性脓皮病等。

(3) Eosinophils: they are one of the immune system components responsible for combating infection and parasites. They

(3) 嗜酸性粒细胞(eosinophils)　免疫系统的成分之一,在对抗感染和寄

are 12-17 μm in diameter, and are characterized by bilobed nuclei and strong eosinophilic brick-red granules after staining with eosin within the cellular cytoplasm. Along with mast cells, they facilitate the mechanism associated with anaphylactic reactions by phagocytic events during the degranulation of mast cells. Also, they can be found in certain skin disorders with eosinophilia that were caused by antigen-antibody complex deposition in the skin, as antigen-antibody complex is also an attractive agent to be phagocytized by eosinophils. These include pemphigus vulgaris, pemphigus vegetans, bullous pemphigoid, and granuloma faciale. Finally, eosinophils serve as the effector cells for parasitic infections.

(4) Basophilic granulocytes: these cells develop during haematopoiesis in the bone marrow before migrating into the bloodstream. They have a similar function to mast cells and are rarely found in human dermatitis but actively participate in the dermatitis of rodents.

(5) Plasma cells: plasma cells are 10-20 μm in diameter. They have deeply basophilic homogeneous cytoplasm and eccentrically located nuclei with regularly arranged chromatin particles which give the nuclei a cartwheel appearance. Plasma cells have an abundance of ribosomes and highly developed endoplasmic reticuli responsible for the synthesis of immunoglobulins. They come from B lymphocytes and gradually mature in the dermis. They are mainly found in certain infectious diseases such as early syphilis, rhinoscleroma, granuloma inguinale, and some deep fungal infections.

生虫感染中发挥作用。嗜酸性粒细胞的直径为 12～17 μm。HE 切片中其含有特征性的双叶核，胞质中有强嗜酸性、砖红色的颗粒。因为嗜酸性粒细胞能吞噬肥大细胞释放的颗粒而与肥大细胞一道参与变态反应。嗜酸性粒细胞也能吞噬抗原-抗体复合物，因此它们也见于那些抗原-抗体复合物的沉积导致嗜酸性粒细胞增多的一类皮肤病，如寻常型天疱疮、增殖型天疱疮、类天疱疮和面部肉芽肿。它们是寄生虫感染的效应细胞。

(4) 嗜碱性粒细胞（basophilic granulocytes）　来源于骨髓，在外周血中循环，其功能与肥大细胞类似，在人类皮炎中很少见，但却积极参与啮齿动物性皮炎。

(5) 浆细胞(plasma cells)　浆细胞的直径为 10～20 μm，具有深嗜碱性均一性的胞质，细胞核呈偏心性，具有规则排列的染色质颗粒，因而使细胞核呈车轮样外观。浆细胞有丰富的核糖体和高度发达的内质网而有利于免疫球蛋白的合成。它们在真皮内由 B 细胞发育而来。它们主要见于某些感染性疾病如早期梅毒、鼻硬结病、腹股沟肉芽肿和某些深部真菌感染。

6. Blood vessels

The cutaneous blood vessels supply nutrition to the skin and also have a thermoregulatory function. The dermal vasculature has two major horizontal plexuses which are connected to each other by vertically oriented reticular dermal blood vessels (Fig. 1-10). The first is the superficial or subpapillary plexus, and is located at the papillary-reticular dermal junction, from where the ascending arterial vessels form arterioles and supply the capillary loops in the dermal papillae. Such capillary loops project into every dermal papilla and supply nutrition to the epidermis. From these points they become descending venous limbs and then go on to merge with the venous channels of the superficial plexus.

The other horizontal plexus is the deep vascular plexus which is located at the dermal-subcutis junction. The blood vessels here usually have a larger diameter and connect with the branches in the fibrous septum of the subcutis.

The appendages are also exclusively surrounded by the characteristic plexuses. The blood supplies of the adnexa are from

六、血管

皮肤的血管为皮肤提供营养并具有调节体温的功能。真皮内血管系统有两个主要的水平方向的血管丛，二者之间通过垂直走行的起源于网状真皮血管的血管相连(图 1-10)。其中一个是浅层血管丛，或乳头下丛，位于乳头真皮-网状真皮交界处。从浅层血管丛分支而来的上升的动脉血管逐渐形成微动脉，进而在每一个真皮乳头内形成毛细血管袢为表皮提供营养，并从那里形成静脉下降支而加入到浅层血管丛的静脉血管系统。

另外一个水平丛是深层血管丛，位于真皮-皮下交界处。这里的血管通常管腔比较大，并与皮下的纤维间隔中的血管分支相连。

附属器也有特异的血管丛包绕。供应附属器的血液来自于连接浅层和深层

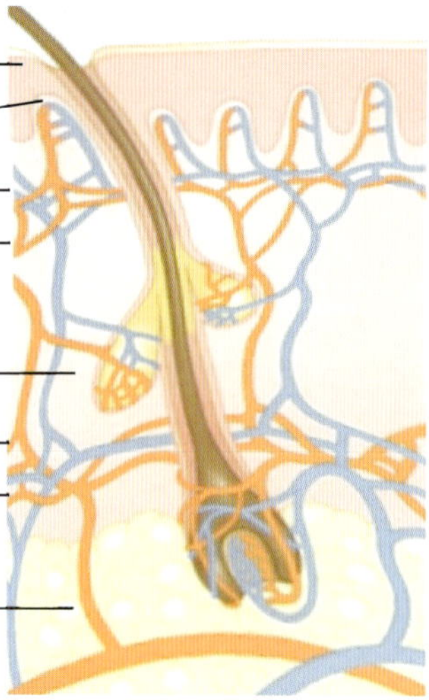

Fig. 1-10 Illustration the superficial and deep vascular plexus in the dermis

(图 1-10 真皮浅层和深层血管丛示意图)

the side branches of the vertical communicating vessels between the superficial and deep plexuses.

血管丛的垂直血管的侧支。

The vascular walls of the small arteries of the deep vascular plexus and the arterioles of the dermis both comprise three layers: the intima, the media, and the adventitia of connective tissue. The intima is composed of endothelial cells and an internal elastic lamina. The media of the small arteries usually has two to several layers of muscle cells.

深部血管丛的小动脉和真皮的微动脉有三层:内层、中层和结缔组织外膜。内层由内皮细胞和内弹力膜构成,小动脉的中层常有两层到几层肌细胞。

The capillaries are covered by a layer of endothelial cells and an incomplete layer of perivascular pericytes. The PAS-positive basement membrane surrounds the endothelial cells and pericytes. Characteristic Weibel-Palade bodies can be found in the cytoplasm of the endothelial cell. Endothelial cells of blood capillaries express factor Ⅷ and CD31.

毛细血管是由一层内皮细胞和位于周边不连续的周细胞构成。内皮细胞和周细胞有 PAS 阳性的基膜。内皮细胞的胞质内有特征性的 Weibel-Palade 小体。毛细血管内皮细胞表达Ⅷ因子和 CD31。

The venules of the deep plexus have valves, but the venules of the superficial plexus do not.

深部血管网的静脉有瓣膜,但浅层的静脉则没有。

The arteriovenous anastomosis, or glomus apparatus, is a special vascular structure of the skin. An arteriole and a venule are directly connected by the glomus instead of by the usual capillaries. The glomus apparatus is composed of a modified arterial segment (the Sucquet-Hoyer canal), a venous segment, and, in some areas, an intermediate segment.

动静脉吻合或球器官是一种特殊的皮肤血管结构。动脉与静脉通过血管球相连而不是像通常的通过毛细血管相连。球器官有变异的动脉段(Sucquet-Hoyer 管)、静脉段,在有的区域还有中间段。

In the fully developed anastomosis such as in the acral skin, the intermediate segment is quite tortuous and the glomus body is then found to be composed of 4-6 layers of glomus cells interleaved with loose connective tissue. These glomus cells that are regarded as smooth muscle cells tend to resemble epithelioid cells.

在充分发育的吻合处,如肢端皮肤,其中间段高度扭曲,并可见血管球小体,是由 4～6 层球细胞和周围疏松的结缔组织构成的。这些球细胞类似上皮样细胞,并被认为是平滑肌细胞。

A large number of filaments (5 nm in diameter) and dense bodies of the myofilaments (300 nm to 400 nm in diameter) can be visualized in the cytoplasm of the glomus cells. The arteriovenous anastomosis or arteriovenous shunt controls the dermal blood flow and thus regulate body temperature. This shunt is innervated by the sympathetic nerves-that is evidenced by nerve fibers extending into the glomus cells.

在这些球细胞的胞质内有丰富的直径为5 nm的细丝和直径为300～400 nm的肌丝致密小体。动静脉短路控制真皮的血流并具有调节体温的功能。它们受交感神经的支配。有神经纤维伸入到球细胞内。

The glomus is most abundant in the pads, nail beds of the fingers and toes. Other areas such as the volar aspect of the palms and soles, the skin of the ears and the center of the face also have glomus.

血管球在指(趾)球部、甲床最为丰富,其他部位如掌跖面、耳部皮肤及面中部也有血管球。

7. Lymphatic vessels

The lymphatic vessels are usually inconspicuous in normal skin and lined by a layer of flattened endothelial cells. The endothelial cells of the lymphatics have no pericytes or Weibel-Palade bodies or basement membrane. The capillary lymphatics are oriented from the dermal papillae and fuse into the postcapillary lymph vessels and then into the dermal and subcutaneous lymph vessels. Valves can be observed in some of the endothelial cells of the lymphatic vessels. Lymphatic vessels can be visualized by the positive expression of D2-40, LYVE-1, Prox-1 and podoplanin in their endothelial cells.

七、淋巴管

淋巴管在正常皮肤常不明显,覆盖有单层扁平的细胞。淋巴管的内皮细胞没有周细胞、Weibel-Palade小体和基膜。毛细淋巴管起源于真皮乳头且并入到毛细后淋巴管,然后并入真皮及皮下淋巴管。有的淋巴管的内皮细胞可以观察到瓣膜。淋巴管能通过内皮细胞阳性表达D2-40、LYVE-1、Prox-1和podoplanin得以识别。

8. Nerves

The nerves in the normal skin are usually invisible in the routine HE stained sections except for the large myelinated nerve bundles, the Meissner and Vater-Pacini corpuscles. However, they can be revealed by special stains such as S-100.

八、神经

除大的有髓鞘的神经束、Meissner和Vater-Pacini小体外,正常皮肤在常规HE染色切片中常不容易看到神经。然而,用特殊染色法(如S-100)则能显示。

The nerves in the skin can be divided into two kinds: the myelinated nerves (the sensory nerves) and the unmyelinated nerves (the autonomic nerves). The former include free nerve endings, and some special nerve end organs of the skin such as the Meissner end corpuscles, Vater-Pacini corpuscles, mucocutaneous end organs, and Ruffini corpuscles. The latter innervates the arrector pili muscles, blood vessels, glomus apparatuses, apocrine and eccrine glands and controls their functions (Fig. 1-11). The sebaceous glands are not supplied by the autonomic nerves and their functions are regulated by the endocrine stimuli.

皮肤的神经分为两种:有髓神经(感觉神经)和无髓神经(植物神经)。前者包括游离神经末梢和一些特殊的皮肤神经末梢器(special nerve end organs of the skin),如Meissner终末小体、Vater-Pacini小体、皮肤黏膜终末器和Ruffini小体。后者支配立毛肌、血管、血管球器、顶泌汗腺和外泌汗腺并控制其功能(图1-11)。皮脂腺则不受植物神经支配,其功能由内分泌调节。

1) Free nerve endings

Free nerve endings can be found at all levels of the dermis, but they are most widespread in the papillary dermis. The free nerve endings can be penicillate fibers, papillary nerve endings, hair follicle-associated free nerve receptors, or associated with Merkel cells.

(一) 游离神经末梢

可见于真皮各层,但在真皮乳头最为丰富。游离神经末梢可以是点状纤维、乳头状神经末梢、毛囊相关游离神经受体,或与Merkel细胞相关。

Penicillate fibers make up the greater part of the subepidermal

点状纤维在有毛皮肤构成表皮下神

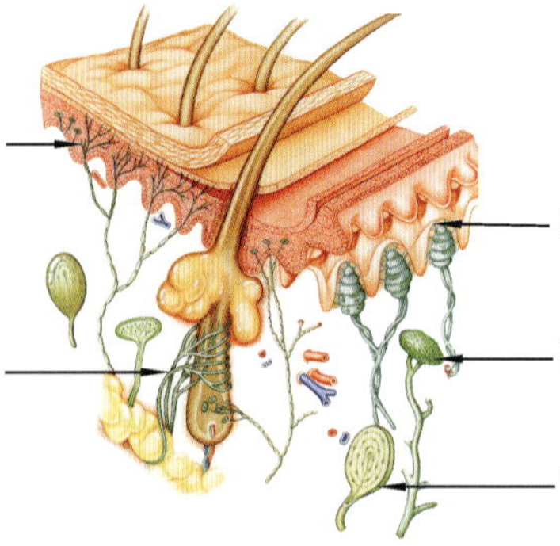

Fig. 1-11　Illustration of the nerves in the skin(图 1-11　皮肤中的神经示意图)

neural network in hairy skin. Their main functions are to conduct the perceptions of touch, temperature, pain, and itching. The papillary nerve endings are located at the orifice of the follicles. Hair follicle-associated free nerve receptors encircle the hair follicle about the level of the sebaceous gland and are involved in the bending and movement of hairs. The Merkel cells have been found to be associated with the intraepidermal free nerve endings according to the neurosecretory granules found in their cytoplasm.

经网的主体。其主要功能是感受触觉、温度觉、痛觉和痒觉。乳头状神经末梢位于毛囊的开口。毛囊相关游离神经受体在大约皮脂腺的水平包绕毛囊,并与毛发的弯曲和移动有关。Merkel 细胞与表皮内的游离神经末梢相关,其胞质内有神经内分泌颗粒。

2) Meissner end corpuscle

Meissner corpuscles are a type of nerve endings in the skin that are responsible for touch sensation. They are distributed throughout the skin, but are concentrated in areas especially sensitive to light touch, such as the fingertips, palms, soles, lips, tongue, face and the male prepuce. Situated just beneath the epidermis within the dermal papillae, the size of Meissner corpuscles is 30 μm by 80 μm, pinecone-shaped under light microscopy (Fig. 1-11, Fig. 1-12). Electron microscopy reveals that Meissner corpuscles are primarily composed of irregular layers of flattened, largely elongated laminar cells which are atypical Schwann cells.

(二) Meissner 终末小体

Meissner 小体(Meissner corpuscles)是一种皮肤的神经终末器,其功能是介导触觉。广泛分布于皮肤,特别是手指端、掌跖、唇、舌、面部以及男性的包皮等对轻触觉很敏感的部位。这些小体位于真皮乳头,其大小为 30 μm×80 μm,类似松果,在光镜下即可看到(图1-11,图 1-12)。电镜研究显示 Meissner 小体主要由数层不规则的扁平的显著伸长的层状细胞构成,这些细胞是变异的 Schwann 细胞。

3) Vater-Pacini corpuscle (or lamellated corpuscle)

Vater-Pacini corpuscles are oval to round nerve endings located in the subcutis mainly in the volar aspects of the palms and soles, and especially in the tips of fingers and toes. On some occasions, they can be found in the subcutis of the nipple and of the anogenital areas. They are as large as 1 mm in diameter, so they can be easily found by light microscopy (Fig. 1-13). They are also called lamellated corpuscles because they have a symmetrical lamellated inner core. They transmit the sense of pressure.

(三) Vater-Pacini 小体(环层小体)

Vater-Pacini 小体(Vater-Pacini corpuscles)是卵圆形或圆形神经末梢,位于皮下,主要是掌跖面,特别是手指和足趾端。少数也位于乳头和肛门生殖器的皮下。其直径大到 1 mm,因而在光镜下就很容易看到(图 1-13)。因其具有对称的层状内核,所以也称为环层小体。其功能是介导压觉。

4) Mucocutaneous end organs

They are found in the papillary dermis at the mucocutaneous junctions such as the glans, prepuce, clitoris, labia minora, perianal region, and vermilion border of the lip. They are averagely 50 μm in

(四) 皮肤黏膜终末器

皮肤黏膜终末器位于皮肤黏膜交界处的乳头真皮层,如龟头、包皮、阴蒂、小阴唇、肛周、唇红缘等处。其直径平均为

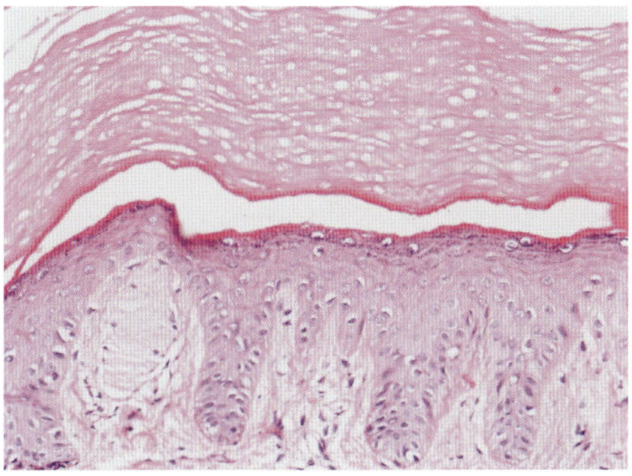

Fig. 1-12　Meissner end corpuscle, HE staining
（图 1-12　Meissner 终末小体，HE 染色）

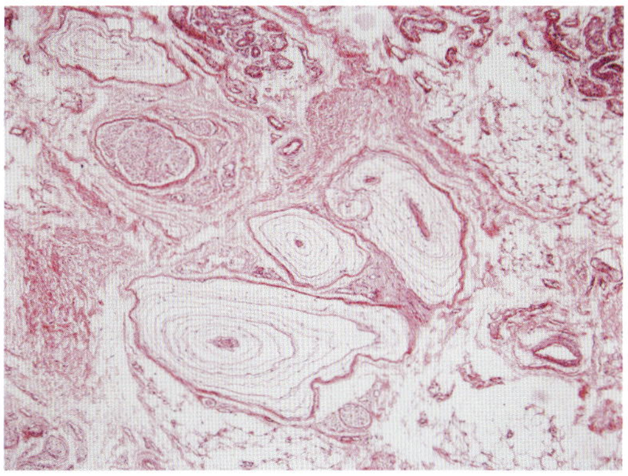

Fig. 1-13　Vater-Pacini corpuscle, HE staining
（图 1-13　Vater-Pacini 小体，HE 染色）

diameter and are similar to the Meissner corpuscles, but cannot be recognized in the routine stained sections under light microscopy.

50 μm，类似于 Meissner 小体，但在常规切片光镜下不能看到。

5) Ruffini corpuscles

Ruffini corpuscles are rare and mainly located in the subcutis of acral skin. These oval or spindle shaped bodies take charge of conducting the sense of temperature.

（五）Ruffini 小体

Ruffini 小体比较少，位于肢端皮肤的皮下。其为卵圆形或梭形，介导温度觉。

9. Muscles

The muscles in the skin can be divided into two kinds: smooth muscle and striated muscle. Smooth muscles are involuntary muscles including arrector pili muscles, the smooth muscles in the tunica dartos of the external genitals, in the areola of the nipples, and in the wall of blood vessels. The smooth muscles have characteristic "cigar-shaped" nuclei located in the center of the muscle cells. In addition, there are plenty of 5 nm in diameter myofilaments in their cytoplasm.

Striated muscles are voluntary muscles occurring in the platysma and the muscles of expression on the face. They have characteristic cytoplasmic cross-striations. Their nuclei are peripherally located just beneath the sarcolemma.

九、肌肉

皮肤的肌肉可分为两种：平滑肌和横纹肌。平滑肌是不随意肌，如立毛肌、外生殖器肉膜和乳晕区的平滑肌及血管壁的肌层。平滑肌具有特征性的"雪茄"样位于肌细胞中央的核。胞质内具有丰富的直径为 5 nm 的肌丝。

横纹肌是随意肌，见于颈阔肌和面部的表情肌。胞质具有特征性的横纹，细胞核边聚于肌纤维膜下。

10. Appendages

1) Hair and hair follicles

(1) Hair or hair shaft: the cylindrical part of a single hair above the skin is called the hair shaft, and is made up of dead cells that have turned into keratin and arisen at a certain angle to the skin surface. It has three components: an inner medulla, a cortex, and an outer cuticle.

①Medulla: the medullary cells are loosely arranged 2-3 layers in the core of hair shaft which are pale staining cuboidal cells with melanin granules in their cytoplasm. The medulla in human hair gradually disappears as hair grows.

十、附属器

（一）毛发和毛囊

(1) 毛发(hair)或毛干(hair shaft)单根毛发的皮肤以上部分呈圆柱形称之为毛干，由已转化为角蛋白的死亡的细胞构成。毛发与皮肤表面呈一定角度。毛发由内向外分为三层：毛髓质、毛皮质和毛小皮。

①毛髓质位于毛发中央，由 2～3 层着色淡的立方形细胞构成，胞质内含有黑素颗粒。随着毛根的上长，髓质逐渐消失。

②Cortex: being the main component of hair, cortex surrounds the hair medulla and makes up several layers of the fusiform, tightly packed keratinized cells. These cortex cells are aligned with their long axis parallel to the direction of the hair. The color of hair depends primarily upon the amount, the size and distribution of melanosomes within it. In contrast to the"soft keratins" found in the epidermis, the keratins isolated in hair are hard keratins which are very resistant to degradation and characterized by high concentrations of cystine, glycine and tyrosine.

②毛皮质为毛发的主体，位于髓质外，由数层梭形、排列紧密的角化细胞组成。这些毛皮质细胞的长轴与毛发的长轴相平行。毛发的颜色与毛皮质中黑素小体的多少和大小及分布有关。与表皮中的"软角蛋白"不同，毛皮质的角化是形成所谓的硬角蛋白，这些硬角蛋白不易降解，富含胱氨酸、甘氨酸和酪氨酸。

③Cuticles: the cuticle, located peripheral to the hair cortex, is composed of a layer of transparent overlapping flattened cells arranged like shingles and pointing upward with their distal portion. The cuticle surrounds the hair cortex and interlocks tightly with the cells of the inner root sheath cuticle which acts as a protective barrier for the softer inner structure.

③毛小皮位于毛皮质的外层，由一层透明状、排列成叠瓦状的扁平细胞组成，并指向毛干的上方。毛小皮包绕在毛皮质外，并与内根鞘小皮交错紧密咬合从而对内层的软性结构起保护层的作用。

(2) Hair follicles: the hair follicle is composed of several cylindrical layers of cells and connective tissue that enclose the hair. The three bulges under the surface of the epidermis develop during the maturation of the follicle. The uppermost bulge can become an apocrine gland, but only in certain regions. The middle bulge turns out to be the sebaceous gland and the lowermost one develops into the attachment point for the arrector pili muscle. The arrector pili muscle originates in the upper dermis and terminates at this lowermost bulge (the follicular bulge, the site where the follicular stem cells are located) (Fig. 1-14). When the body is chilled or under emotional stress, the skin would give a gooseflesh-like appearance at the perifollicular areas and the hair would erect due to the contraction of the arrector pili muscle.

(2) 毛囊(hair follicles)　毛囊由几层呈圆柱形排列的细胞及结缔组织组成，并包绕毛发。毛囊在其成熟过程中在其下侧形成三个隆突。最上端的一个形成顶泌汗腺，但仅仅限于某些区域。中间的一个形成皮脂腺，最下面的一个形成立毛肌的附着处。立毛肌起源于真皮上部，而止于毛囊最下面的隆突(毛囊隆突，该处为毛囊干细胞所在)(图 1-14)，在遇到冷和情绪紧张时，立毛肌收缩并引起毛发垂直竖起及毛囊周围像鸡皮疙瘩样外观。

The expanded lower terminus of the follicle is the hair bulb, which encloses an ovoid-shaped papilla of capillaries, nerves and connective tissue (Fig. 1-15). The hair matrix cells are a pool of undifferentiated cells that produce the hair and the inner root sheath with large vesicular nuclei and a deeply basophilic cytoplasm. Melanocytes can be found mainly among the basal cells of the hair matrix lying on top of the dermal hair papilla but rarely appear between the basal cells of the hair matrix on the lateral side of the hair papilla.

毛囊的下部末端膨大形成毛球，呈卵圆形的毛乳头由富于血管和神经的结缔组织构成并突入到毛球的底部内(图 1-15)。毛母质细胞为一群未分化的细胞，能产生毛发和内根鞘。毛母质细胞具有大的泡状核和深嗜碱性的胞质。黑素细胞主要位于真皮毛乳头顶部的毛母质的基底细胞之间，少数见于毛乳头侧面的毛母质的基底细胞之间。

In longitudinal sections, the hair follicle is seen to be anatomically divided into three segments. From the uppermost to the lowermost these are as follows: the upper portion or the so called follicular infundibulum, which extends from the pilar orifice above to the entrance of the sebaceous duct below, is lined continuously with epidermis on top and even undergoes keratinization just as the epidermis does. CD1a positive Langerhans

纵切面上，可见毛囊分为三个部分，从上到下，最上面的部分称为毛囊漏斗部(follicular infundibulum)，是从毛囊的开口到皮脂腺导管的入口，被覆的是表皮，以类似表皮的方式角化，正常的毛囊漏斗部含有 CD1a 阳性的朗格汉斯细胞，可能与毛囊免疫有关，在慢性 UV 暴露

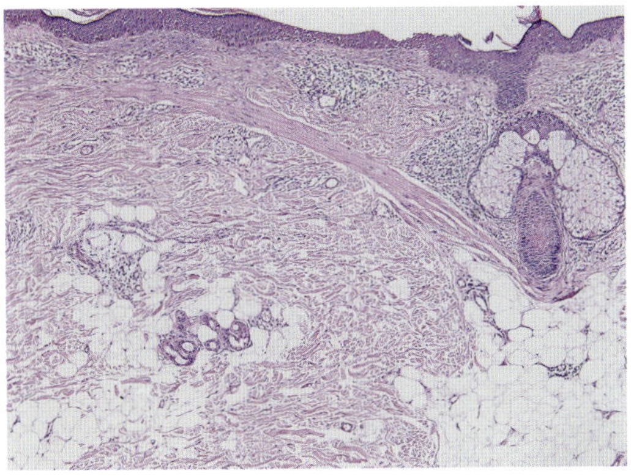

Fig. 1-14　The arrector pili muscle, HE staining
(图 1-14　立毛肌, HE 染色)

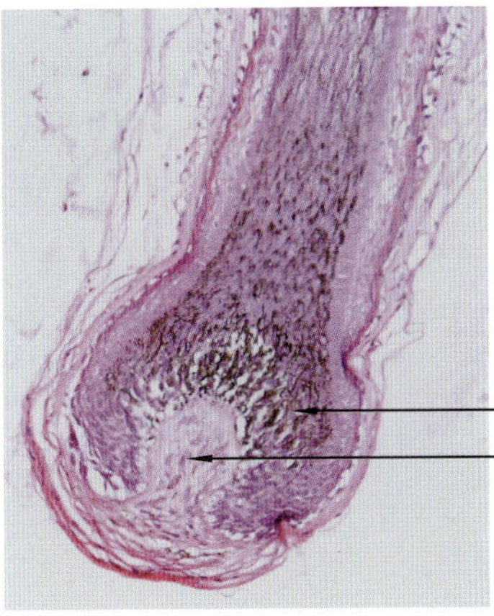

Fig. 1-15　Hair bulb and dermal hair papilla, HE staining
(图 1-15　毛球和真皮毛乳头, HE 染色)

cells in the follicular infundibula may reflect their important roles in follicular immunity. However, with chronic UV exposure the Langerhans cells in the follicular infundibula remain intact while those in the epidermis deplete; the middle portion or the so-called isthmus is the short midsection of the follicle bounded above by the entrance of the sebaceous duct to the attachment point of the arrector muscle; the lowest portion stretches from the insertion point of the arrector muscle to the base of the follicle (Fig. 1-1). The hair follicle is composed of three layers from innermost to outermost: inner root sheath, outer root sheath, and connective tissue sheath (Fig. 1-16, Fig. 1-17, Fig. 1-18).

中表皮的朗格汉斯细胞可能被耗竭，而毛囊漏斗部的朗格汉斯细胞却能保持完整；中部称为峡部(isthmus)，是从皮脂腺导管的入口到立毛肌附着处；下部是从立毛肌的附着处到毛囊底部(图 1-1)。毛囊从内到外由内毛根鞘、外毛根鞘及结缔组织鞘组成(图 1-16，图 1-17，图 1-18)。

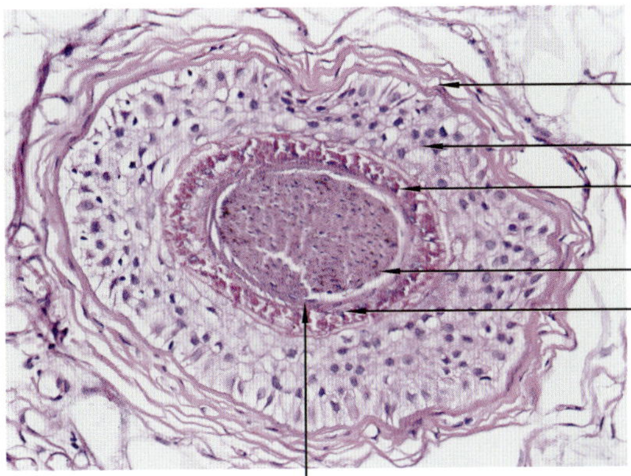

Fig. 1-16　Cross section of the hair follicle, HE staining(图 1-16　毛囊结构横断面, HE 染色)

①Inner root sheath: it consists of three distinct layers, known (from inside out) as the inner root sheath cuticle, Huxley's layer, and Henle's layer. Melanin pigment is absent in the cytoplasm of the cells from all three layers. Instead the large eosinophilic cytoplasmic inclusions called trichohyalin granules, or soft keratins are typically seen in each layer of inner root sheath. Such trichohyalin is also a structural protein similar to that produced and retained in the keratohyaline granules in the granular layer of

①内毛根鞘(inner root sheath)：由内向外分为内根鞘小皮、赫胥黎层(Huxley's layer)、亨勒层(Henle's layer)三层。三层均不含色素。特点为三层细胞的胞质内均含有嗜酸性小体即毛透明蛋白颗粒(即所谓的软角蛋白)，这些毛透明蛋白是一种结构蛋白，类似于表皮颗粒层中产生和储存的角质透明

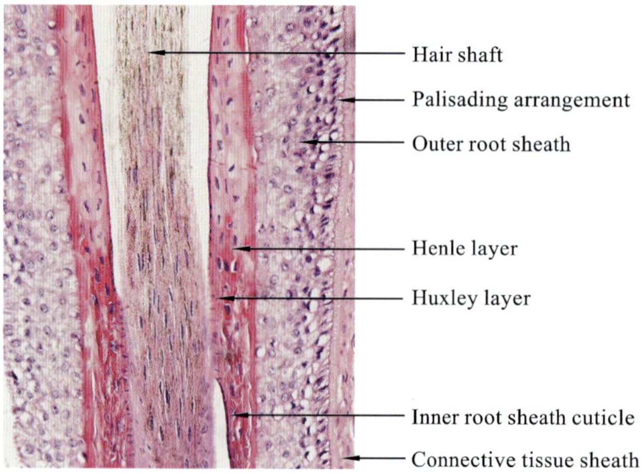

Fig. 1-17 Longitudinal section of the hair follicle, HE staining
(图 1-17 毛囊的结构纵切面,HE 染色)

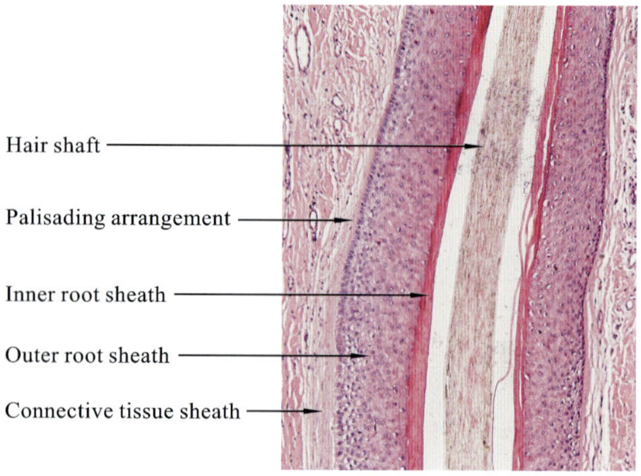

Fig. 1-18 The middle part of the hair follicle (longitudinal section), HE staining
(图 1-18 毛囊中部(纵切面),HE 染色)

epidermis(Fig. 1-16, Fig. 1-17).

颗粒(图 1-16,图 1-17)。

a. Inner root sheath cuticle: this layer is one cell thick and somewhat flattened; the proximal edges of the individual cells become slightly dislocated axially so that they overlap with the distal ends of the cells below. This allows a tight interlock to be formed with the cells of the cuticle of the hair shaft that are oriented upwards.

a. 内根鞘小皮:为单排竖列的扁平细胞,呈重叠状排列,并指向下方,与指向上方的毛小皮细胞相重叠,紧密相连接。

b. Huxley's layer: this layer is composed of two layers of oval cells. These cells move upward along the inner side of the Henle's layer. In the cells of Huxley's layer, numerous intracytoplasmic trichohyalin granules can be found at the level of the keratogenous zone of the hair from where the cells begin keratinization; and later on to serve as the molds for the hair shaft development.

b. 赫胥黎层:一般为两排类椭圆形细胞组成。沿着亨勒层内侧向上移行。这些细胞在毛发的角质生长区水平胞质内含有大量的毛透明蛋白颗粒并角化,从而为毛干提供铸型。

c. Henle's layer: this layer of oval cells is also one cell thick and is connected with the outer root sheath through the desmosomes. The cells of Henle's layer are the first cell line to cornify in the follicle, laying a foundation for the formation of hair shaft. As with Huxley's layer, the cells of Henle's layer acquire trichohyalin granules immediately after they have arisen from the matrix.

c. 亨勒层:由单排卵圆形细胞构成并通过桥粒与外根鞘连接。亨勒层细胞在毛囊中首先发生角化,并为毛干的形成提供铸型。如同赫胥黎层,亨勒层在其由毛母质形成后即有毛透明蛋白颗粒。

The three layers of the inner root sheath disappear once they reach the level of the isthmus of the hair follicle.

内根鞘的三层在达到毛囊的峡部时消失。

② Outer root sheath: this layer is at the same level as the *stratum spinosum* of the epidermis, and surrounds the inner root sheath of hair follicles like a sleeve all the way to the bulb. It is composed of several layers of flattened cells with clear vacuolated cytoplasm that presumably possesses abundant glycogens. Histologically these cells are large and the outermost layer of the cells arranges in a palisading fashion (Fig. 1-17, Fig. 1-18). In

②外毛根鞘犹如表皮的棘细胞层,位于内毛根鞘的外侧,由几层扁平细胞构成,这些细胞因为胞质中含有糖原而呈透明空泡样。这些细胞较大,其最外一层细胞常呈栅栏状排列(图 1-17,图 1-18)。与内毛根鞘不同,外毛根鞘在峡部以下水平不发生角化。外毛根鞘在峡

contrast to the inner root sheath, the outer root sheath does not keratinize below the level of the isthmus. However, at the level of the isthmus (from the attachment of the arrector pili muscle to the entrance of the sebaceous duct) where the inner root sheath disintegrates, the outer root sheath is no longer covered by the inner root sheath and undergoes the type of homogeneous cornification called trichilemmal keratinization (Fig. 1-19). The upper portion of the outer root sheath expresses K5/14, K1/10, K6/16; while the deeper one expresses K5/14/17. There are some inactive, amelanotic melanocytes in the basal layer of the outer root sheath that can convert to melanin-producing cells after skin injuries such as dermabrasion.

部(从立毛肌的附着处到皮脂腺导管入口)与内毛根鞘分离不再被覆有内根鞘，并进行均质性角化，即外毛根鞘式角化(图 1-19)。在外毛根鞘的上部表达角蛋白 K5/14、K1/10、K6/16 而深部则表达 K5/14/17。在外毛根鞘的基底细胞间有一些非活化的无黑素的黑素细胞(amelanotic melanocyte)，这些黑素细胞在皮肤受到损伤(如皮肤磨削)时则能活跃起来，并成为能产生黑素的细胞。

③Connective tissue sheath: this is located on the outside of the outer root sheath (Fig. 1-16, Fig. 1-17, Fig. 1-18). The concentric circular and longitudinal layers of collagens and elastic fibers become contiguous with the adjacent connective tissue of the dermis that envelops the entire hair follicle. It includes glassy or vitreous layer and fibrous root sheath. The former is a homogeneous eosinophilic zone similar to the epidermal basement zone located in the outside of the outer root sheath and the latter is located at the outermost layer that is composed of thick collagen bundles.

③结缔组织鞘位于外毛根鞘的外侧(图 1-16，图 1-17，图 1-18)，含有同心圆和纵向排列的胶原和弹力纤维，并与真皮的结缔组织连接，包绕整个毛囊。包括玻璃层和纤维根鞘，前者位于外毛根鞘的外面，为均质嗜酸性区域，类似表皮的基膜，后者位于最外层，由厚的胶原束构成。

(3) Cycles of hair growth: human hair follicles operate independently from one to another. It is normal to find adjacent follicles in different phases of hair growth. The life cycle of each hair passes through three stages: anagen (growth stage), catagen (regression stage), and telogen (resting stage). On average the duration of these three stages in adult scalp hair is, respectively, about 3 years (2-6 years), 3 weeks (4-6 weeks), and 3 months (3-4 months).

At any time, approximately 84%, 2%, 14% of scalp hairs are in the anagen, catagen and telogen stage respectively in normal humans. A small population of cells in the lowermost bulge area of the follicle works as the stem cells to start differentiation at the end of the telogen phase. Once a signal is received from the follicular papilla, these progenitor cells descend into the dermis to form a solid core and then develop a tapered hair shaft that grows upward toward the surface of the epidermis, and a new cycle of hair growth begins.

On average 70-100 hairs at telogen stage are shed every day and usually the same number of hairs begins in the scalp. Humans are born with a certain number of follicles that remains unchanged throughout life.

Scalp hair grows at a speed of 0. 27-0. 4 mm per day. The growth rate of hair is influenced by a number of factors such as genetics, hormone, health and nutrition status, pregnancy, drugs

(3) 毛发生长周期　人类毛囊的发育彼此独立，相邻的正常毛囊可以处于不同的毛发生长周期。毛发生长周期可分为三个时期：生长期(anagen)、退化期(catagen)、休止期(telogen)。成人头发的这三个时期分别为 3 年(2～6 年)、3 周(4～6 周)、3 个月(3～4 个月)。

正常人的头发大约有 84%、2%、14%分别处于生长期、退化期和休止期。在毛囊最下面的一个隆突中(干细胞位于毛囊隆突区)有一小群细胞具有干细胞特性，在休止期末，干细胞在收到来自毛乳头的刺激信号后进行分裂，并向真皮内生长形成实体性核心，进而形成指向皮肤表面的逐渐变细的毛发，即新一轮的周期就开始了。

正常人每日可脱落 70～100 根头发，同时也有等量的头发生长。人类皮肤的毛囊从出生后其数量似乎不再变化。

头发每日生长 0. 27～0. 4 mm，毛发的生长受到许多因素的影响，如遗传、激素水平、健康和营养状况、妊娠、药物(特

(especially chemotherapeutic drugs), etc.

别是化疗药物)等。

2) Sebaceous gland

(二) 皮脂腺

This is a holocrine gland that usually consists of a single lobule or a collection of lobules that open into a system of ducts (Fig. 1-1, Fig. 1-19). The stratified squamous epithelium completely lines the sebaceous duct and extends into the epithelium of the pilary canal. Usually several lobules share a common excretory duct. Each lobule comprises a layer of small cuboidal or flattened basophilic basaloid cells (germinative cells) in the periphery and some pale staining cells with fully laden lipids in the center. The sebaceous cells express high level of EMA (epidermal membrane antigen) but none of CEA, CAM5.2 and S100.

皮脂腺(sebaceous gland)是一种全浆分泌腺,由皮脂腺导管和一个或几个皮脂腺小叶构成(图 1-1,图 1-19)。皮脂腺导管由复层鳞状上皮构成,并伸入毛管的上皮内。多个皮脂腺小叶常共一个分泌导管。皮脂腺小叶由位于周边称为生发细胞的一层小的立方形或扁平的嗜碱性基底样细胞和位于中央富含脂质的淡染细胞构成。免疫组化显示皮脂腺细胞强表达 EMA,而不表达 CEA、CAM 5.2和 S100。

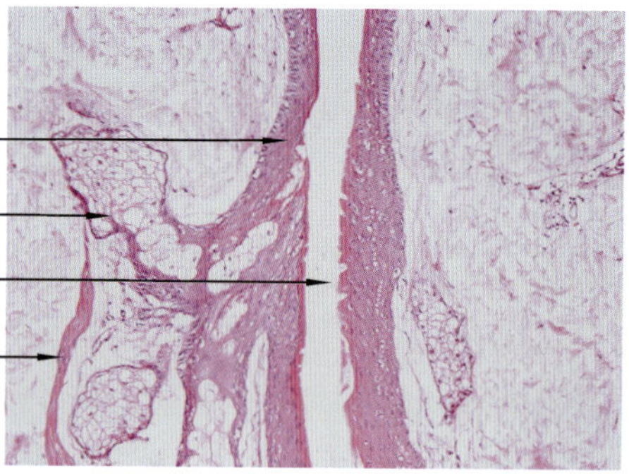

Fig. 1-19 The opening of the sebaceous gland to the hair follicle and trichilemmal keratinization
(图 1-19 皮脂腺的毛囊入口及外毛根鞘式角化)

The cells in the core of the sebaceous glands are small, with intact nuclei in their centers. With the accumulation of sebum, the cell becomes bigger while its nuclei condense, and with the cell's gradual displacement into the hair follicle near the opening of the gland, the shape of its nuclei becomes irregular as well. In routine HE sections, this accumulation of lipids in the cytoplasm causes the appearance of a delicate network caused by lipid lysing during the preparation of the slide (Fig. 1-20). The majority of the sebum released by the sebaceous glands is glycerides and free fatty acids (57.5%), wax esters (26%), squalene (12%), cholesterol, and cholesterol esters. The oily secretion of the sebaceous glands serve multiple functions in the body such as keeping the hair and skin surfaces moist, controlling water evaporation through the skin, and preventing invasion and infection by environmental pathogens.

在皮脂腺的深部细胞较小,中央具有较完整的核,随着皮脂的聚集,细胞逐渐增大,而核则相应地浓缩,随着细胞逐渐向毛囊的皮脂腺开口临近,其形态也变得不规则。在常规 HE 染色切片中,这些淡染的皮脂腺细胞的细胞核位于中央,其胞质因为胞质中的脂质在切片处理过程中被溶解而呈细网状外观(图 1-20)。皮脂腺通过皮脂腺导管向毛囊中排出由甘油酯和游离脂肪酸(57.5%)、蜡脂类(26%)、角鲨烯(12%)、胆固醇和胆固醇酯构成的皮脂。皮脂的功能是润泽毛发和皮肤表面、控制皮肤水分的丢失以及防止某些病原体的侵袭和感染。

The sex hormones such as testosterone in men, adrenal androgens in women, or hormones in infants from the mother, are the best known stimulators of sebaceous glands and are probably responsible for the development and enlargement of the glands at puberty.

已知性激素是皮脂腺最主要的刺激因子,青春期皮脂腺的生长和发育主要受到性激素的控制:在男性是睾酮,在女性是肾上腺皮质雄激素,在新生儿是来自母亲的激素。

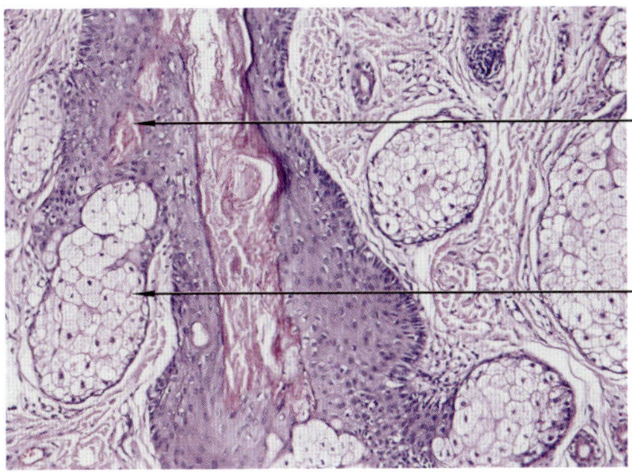

Fig. 1-20　Sebaceous gland(图 1-20　皮脂腺)

With the exception of the palms and soles, sebaceous glands are generally found everywhere on the body. In humans they are especially abundant in areas such as the face, scalp and midline of the back, and also maintain high numbers in the sternal regions, armpits, perianal areas and external genitals.

皮脂腺除掌跖外分布于全身皮肤，而以面部和头皮及背中线最丰富。胸骨区、腋窝、肛门周围及外生殖器也富于皮脂腺。

Most sebaceous glands are associated with hair follicles. In this case, the sebaceous glands are called pilosebaceous glands. However, in some cases, sebaceous glands are not associated with hair follicles but open directly onto the skin's surface, which are termed free sebaceous glands. These are particularly prevalent in hairless areas such as the nipples and areola of both male and female breasts (Montgomery's tubercles in female), the vermilion border of the lips and buccal mucosa (Fordyce's spot), the vagina, the labia minora, the inner aspect of the prepuce, the coronal sulcus of the penis (Tyson's glands), and in rare cases the glans of the penis. The Meibomian glands of the eyelids are modified free sebaceous glands.

大多数皮脂腺与毛囊相关联，称为毛囊性皮脂腺，但有少数不与毛囊相连，而是直接开口于皮肤表面，称为游离皮脂腺，它们见于无毛区，如男性和女性的乳头和乳晕（在女性 Montgomery's 结节）、口唇的唇红缘和颊黏膜（Fordyce 点）、阴道、小阴唇、包皮的内侧面及阴茎冠状沟（Tyson's 腺），偶见于龟头。眼睑的 Meibomian 腺是变异的游离皮脂腺。

3) Apocrine gland

（三）顶泌汗腺

The predominant secretion mode of the apocrine gland is decapitation, a process whereby the apical portion of the secretory cell cytoplasm pinches off and enters the lumen of the gland (Fig. 1-21). It consists of a straight duct and a coiled secretory portion deep in the dermis. Since the apocrine ducts run from the coiled gland to the infundibulum part of the hair follicle above the entrance of the sebaceous gland, it can be further classified into the intraepidermal duct and the intradermal duct. However, the apocrine duct occasionally opens directly on the skin surface close to a pilosebaceous follicle.

顶泌汗腺（apocrine gland）的主要分泌模式是断头分泌，即分泌时分泌细胞将其胞质的顶端一起排入到腺体腔内（图 1-21）。顶泌汗腺由直行导管和真皮深部的盘曲分泌部构成。顶泌汗腺的导管在皮脂腺导管的入口上方进入毛囊，因此，其导管可分为表皮内导管和真皮内导管。偶尔顶泌汗腺导管直接开口在某个毛囊皮脂腺邻近的皮肤表面。

The ductal portion of the apocrine glands comprises the periluminal cuticles and two layers of basophilic cuboidal cells. No myoepithelial cells enclose the ducts. The secretory portion of the apocrine gland has one layer of secretory cells which are surrounded by discontinuous myoepithelial cells with no duct cell types.

顶泌汗腺的导管部由围绕腔面的嗜酸性小皮和两层嗜碱性立方状细胞构成，不含肌上皮细胞。顶泌汗腺的分泌部为一层分泌细胞，其周围包绕有不连续的肌上皮细胞，不含导管细胞。

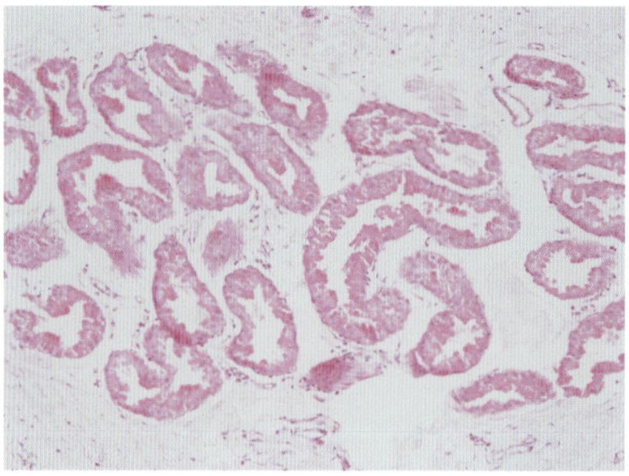

Fig. 1-21 Apocrine gland(图 1-21 顶泌汗腺)

Some very large PAS-positive, diastase-resistant granules can be found in the eosinophilic cytoplasm of the secretory cells. The height of these secretory cells significantly varies with the secretion stages.

分泌细胞在其嗜酸性的胞质内有许多非常大的、PAS 染色阳性、耐淀粉酶的颗粒。分泌细胞的高度依据其分泌期的不同而有显著的变化。

The lumen of the secretory portion of apocrine gland is usually slightly irregular and is 200 μm in diameter, in contrast to the smaller size (20 μm in diameter) of the eccrine gland.

顶泌汗腺的分泌部常呈轻度不规则,直径为 200 μm,与外泌汗腺 20 μm 较小的腔形成明显的对比。

Apocrine glands are predominantly distributed in the axilla and anogenital regions. The ceruminous glands of the external ear canals, Moll glands of the eyelids and the mammary glands within the areola (Montgomery areolar tubercles in female) are modified apocrine sweat glands.

顶泌汗腺主要分布于腋窝和肛门生殖器区。外耳道的耵聍腺、眼睑的 Moll 腺及乳晕的乳腺(女性的 Montgomery 乳晕结节)属于变异的大汗腺。

The secretions of the apocrine glands can be different in color and also odorless at first, but as the glycoproteins or fat in the secretions are broken down by the microbes on the skin's surface, a special odor is developed. Apocrine glands are active during puberty and controlled by adrenergic or even emotional stimuli.

顶泌汗腺的分泌物可呈不同的颜色,最初也是无异味的。当分泌物中的糖蛋白和脂肪被皮肤表面的微生物分解后则产生异味。顶泌汗腺的活动只有在青春期才活跃起来,并受到肾上腺素的支配,特别是情绪的刺激。

4) Eccrine gland

(四) 外泌汗腺

This gland opens directly to the skin's surface and is composed of a ductal and a secretory portion. The eccrine gland duct can be divided into intraepidermal and intradermal segments. The former is also called the acrosyringium or epidermal sweat duct unit, and it enters from the base of the rete ridge and goes upward to the surface of the skin in a spiral course. The latter (intradermal) duct consists of a straight duct and a coiled duct (Fig. 1-1, Fig. 1-22).

外泌汗腺(eccrine gland)直接开口于皮肤表面。外泌汗腺由导管部和分泌部组成。其导管可分为表皮内段和真皮内段,前者又称为末端汗管或表皮内汗腺导管单位,是从表皮嵴的底部进入,并螺旋上升到皮肤表面,后者(真皮内导管)由真皮内垂直导管和盘曲导管构成(图 1-1,图 1-22)。

Intraepidermal eccrine ducts derive from dermal duct cells, and are composed of 2-3 layers of outer cells and an inner layer of cells whose luminal surface forms an eosinophilic cuticle before cornification. The intraepidermal eccrine ducts start to keratinize at the level in the middle squamous layer and are completely keratinized at

表皮内外泌汗腺导管来源于真皮导管细胞,是由一层腔细胞和 2～3 层外层细胞构成。表皮内外泌汗腺导管在角化前其腔侧覆盖有一层嗜酸性的小皮。表皮内外泌汗腺汗管在鳞状细胞的中部开

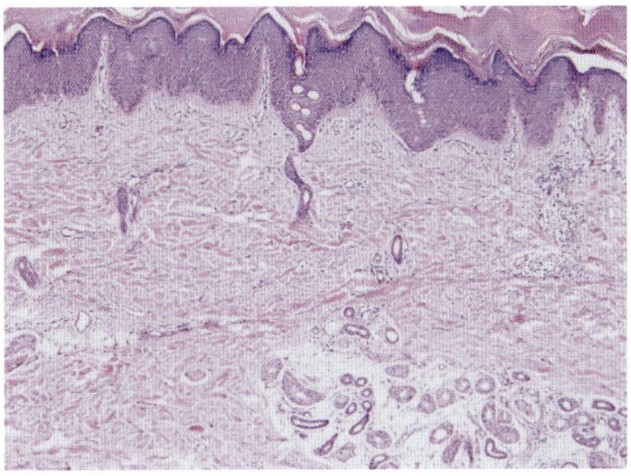

Fig. 1-22　Eccrine gland and its duct(图 1-22　外泌汗腺和汗管)

the level of the *stratum granulosum* of the surrounding epidermis.

Intradermal straight eccrine duct consists of two layers of small, cuboidal, deeply basophilic cells connected by desmosomes. The lumen of the duct is also covered by the PAS-positive, diastase-resistant eosinophilic cuticle.

The intradermal coiled duct has one layer of luminal cells and one layer of basal cells. It is the transitional portion between the intradermal straight duct and the secretory portion of the eccrine gland. The main function of this portion is to reabsorb sodium ions from the sweat.

The secretory portion of the eccrine gland is composed of one layer of secretory cells. The secretory cells can be divided into two types: clear cells and dark cells. The clear cells are larger than the dark cells and have a wider base and a relatively narrow top facing the lumen. This gives rise to a pyramidal appearance. The clear cells contain PAS-positive, diastase-labile glycogen and secrete large amounts of aqueous material. In contrast to the clear cells, the dark cells have a broader top facing the lumen and abundant basophilic granules in their cytoplasm. The dark cells contain PAS-positive, diastase-resistant mucopolysaccharides and secrete sialomucin. The secretory cells are surrounded by the myoepithelial cells containing fibrils and by a hyaline BMZ containing collagen fibers.

The eccrine gland can be found in any part of the human skin except the vermilion border of the lips, the nail beds, the labia minora, the clitoris, the glans of the penis, or the inner aspect of the prepuce. However, they present mostly at the palms, soles and axillae.

The function of the eccrine gland is to regulate body temperature and to maintain general cutaneous homeostasis.

Eccrine glands can be highlighted by positive staining with S-100 and carcinoembryonic antigen (CEA). Other staining markers such as CK7 and CAM5.2 are expressed only in the secretory

始角化，在其周围表皮的颗粒层水平完全角化。

真皮内直行导管由两层小的、立方状、深嗜碱性的细胞构成，并通过桥粒连接。导管腔覆盖有 PAS 阳性耐淀粉酶的嗜酸性小皮。

真皮内盘曲导管由一层腔细胞和一层基底细胞构成，是外泌汗腺真皮内垂直部与分泌部之间的过渡部分。其主要功能是从最初形成的汗液中重吸收钠离子。

外泌汗腺的分泌部是由一层分泌细胞构成的。分泌细胞可分为两种：一种是透明细胞，另一种是暗细胞。透明细胞比暗细胞大，具有较宽的底部和面向腔面相对较窄的顶部，像金字塔，含有 PAS 阳性、淀粉酶易分解的糖蛋白及分泌大量的水状物质；而暗细胞则与明细胞相反，具有面向腔面较宽的顶部，并含有较多嗜碱性颗粒及 PAS 阳性、耐淀粉酶的黏多糖和分泌唾液黏蛋白。围绕分泌细胞的是含有原纤维的肌上皮细胞和含有胶原纤维的透明基膜带。

除唇红缘、甲床、小阴唇、阴蒂、龟头、包皮内侧面外，外泌汗腺遍布全身。而以掌跖和腋窝最多。

外泌汗腺的功能是调节体温和维持皮肤的生理平衡。

外泌汗腺可以通过 S-100 和癌胚抗原(CEA)阳性染色而凸现出来。外泌汗腺和顶泌汗腺只有其分泌部表达 CK7、

portion of both eccrine and apocrine glands but not among the ductal cells.

CAM5.2,而导管部不表达。

5) The nail units

The nail units are made up of several components which form, support, protect and frame the nail itself. These include the nail plate, the cuticle and hyponychium, nail folds, the nail matrix and nail bed (Fig. 1-23, Fig. 1-24).

(五) 甲单位

甲单位(nail units)是由甲板、甲小皮和甲下皮、甲皱襞、甲母质及甲床构成,并对甲的形成、支撑、保护和塑形起重要作用(图1-23,图1-24)。

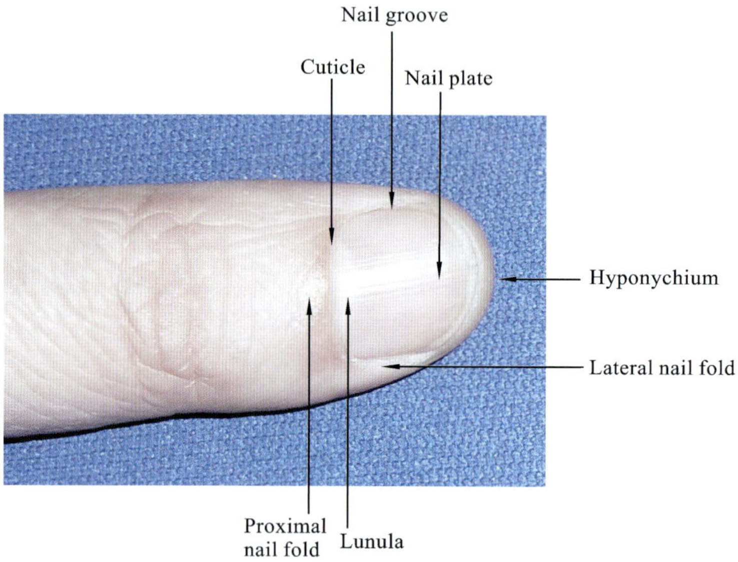

Fig. 1-23　Nail unit(图1-23　甲单位)

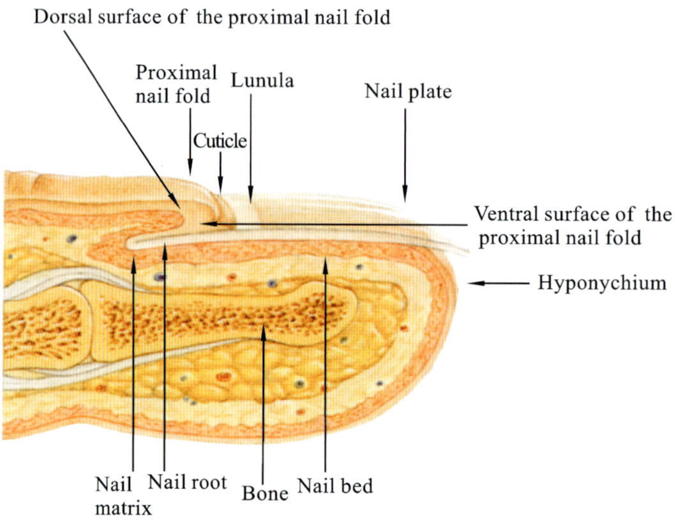

Fig. 1-24　Illustration the structure of finger nail(图1-24　手指甲结构示意图)

The epithelium in the nail plate is different from that found at other body sites in terms of clinical and histological appearance. It is composed of hard keratins. The skin tissues that encircle the proximal portion, sides and the distal portion of the nail plate are termed the proximal, lateral and distal folds, respectively. The nail grooves are on the sides of the nail between the nail plate and the skin.

从临床上和组织学上,甲板的上皮与身体其他部位者不同,是一种硬角蛋白,围绕甲板的近端、两侧以及远端的皮肤分别称为近端甲皱襞、侧甲皱襞和远端甲皱襞。在甲皱襞与甲板之间是甲沟。

The proximal nail fold is composed of two layers of epidermis, the dorsal surface and ventral surface of the proximal nail fold, both of which contain granular layer. The former contains eccrine sweat glands but no pilosebaceous units. The latter is also called eponychium and has no rete ridges and appendages but contains keratohyalin granules. The ventral surface of the proximal nail fold and the nail matrix form the roof and floor of the proximal nail groove respectively and nail plate lies between them.

近端甲皱襞含有两层表皮，背侧面和腹侧面，均含有颗粒层。前者含有小汗腺而无毛皮脂腺单位，后者又称为甲上皮，没有表皮突和附属器，含有角质透明颗粒。近端甲皱襞腹侧与甲母质分别为近端甲沟的顶部和底部，二者之间是甲板。

The overlapping skin surrounding the nail plate that extends from horny layer of the proximal fold is called the cuticle. The name hyponychium is given to the portion of skin at the end of finger beneath the free edge of the nail. In the proximal portion of the nail plate, there is a pale white crescent-shaped area, called the lunula. It is the softest part of the nail due to its incomplete cornification.

甲小皮是近端甲皱襞延伸的一层角质层并部分覆盖甲板。甲下皮位于远端甲皱襞的下方。在甲板的近端有一淡白色、半月形区域，称为甲半月。甲半月是甲最软的部分，其形成的原因是因为未充分角化。

The nail root is at the base of the nail and is protected by a set of proximal folds in which the matrix of nail is embedded. Being the only living part of the nail, the matrix produces the keratin cells that ultimately form nail plate by a process similar to the trichilemmal keratinization in hair development. It has been shown that the distal region of the nail matrix produces the ventral portion of the nail plate (lunula is the clinical name) containing melanocytes, Langerhans cells and Merkel cells. By contrast, the proximal region of the nail matrix is only responsible for the dorsal portion of nail development.

位于甲的底部，由近端甲皱襞覆盖和保护的甲板称为甲根。甲母质即位于甲根的下方，且是甲唯一活跃的地方，甲母质产生角蛋白细胞并最后以类似毛发生长的外毛根鞘角化的方式通过甲角化而产生甲板。甲母质的远端区域产生甲板的腹侧且形成临床可见的甲半月，并含有黑素细胞、朗格汉斯细胞和 Merkel 细胞。甲母质的近端区则产生甲板的背侧面。

The nail bed lies underneath the nail plate and extends from the edges of the germinal matrix (lunula) to the hyponychium. The epithelial structure of the nail bed differs from the epidermis of the skin in that it carries out an onycholemmal type of keratinization during the nail formation.

甲床位于甲板的下方，从生发区甲母质的边缘(甲半月)延伸至甲下皮。甲床的结构类似于表皮，但与之不同的是通过甲根鞘式角化。

Although no real subcutis and pilosebaceous structures are present in the nail bed, elastic fibers, fat tissue, blood vessels, lymphatics and myelinated—and even encapsulated—nerve endings can sometimes be found.

甲床皮肤没有真正的皮下组织和毛皮脂腺结构，但含有弹力纤维、脂肪组织、血管、淋巴管和有髓鞘的及有包囊的神经末梢。

The nail growth rate varies from person to person; on the average, the daily growth rate is about 0.1 mm for the fingernails and the toenail growth rate is only 1/3-1/2 of that of fingernails.

每个人的指甲生长速度不同，指甲的平均生长速度约为每日 0.1 mm，趾甲生长的速度为指甲的 1/3～1/2。

Subcutaneous Tissue (Fat)

皮下组织(脂肪)

Beneath the dermis, the connective tissue forms the fat layer, known as subcutaneous tissue in which the fat cells (adipocytes) manufacture fat in their cytoplasm. The strands of collagen divide the population of fat cells into lobules. These fibrous septae accommodate the major blood vessels, lymphatics and nerves (Fig. 1-1).

真皮下方的结缔组织为脂肪层，即皮下脂肪层，其中的脂肪细胞胞质内有脂肪。胶原束将这些脂肪细胞分为小叶，小叶之间有纤维间隔，间隔中有血管、淋巴管和神经(图 1-1)。

Chang-zheng HUANG(黄长征)

Section Two　Function of the Skin

The skin is the largest and the most visible organ of the human body. It provides the first protective barrier between the body and the environment and serves a variety of functions. The main functions of the skin are to act as a barrier to the penetration of microorganisms or harmful chemicals, to shield the body from the sun's radiation, to prevent the loss of fluids, to help regulate the body's temperature, and to provide resistance to mechanical forces. The skin also plays an important immunological role, involving cells located both in the epidermis and the dermis. Furthermore, a variety of sensory receptors in the skin enable the human body to sense incoming stimuli such as touch, pain, vibration, pressure, warmth, cold, and itching. The aim of this chapter is to correlate skin functions with specific structures.

1. The skin as a barrier

(1) The epidermis and *stratum corneum*: the mechanical barrier between the body and the outside world.

Throughout our lives, our bodies lose water by evaporation via the skin. Some evaporation is normal and necessary, but preventing excessive water loss is exceptionally important both to the skin itself and to the body as a whole. Water makes up 70%-75% of the weight of the basal layer, but only 10%-15% of the weight of the *stratum corneum*.

The skin acts as a two-way barrier to prevent the inward and outward passage of water and electrolytes. The barrier function is largely dependent on the epidermis. In fact, a flap of epidermis is almost impermeable as an intact piece of skin, whereas the residual dermis without the epidermis is almost completely permeable.

The *stratum corneum* is a particularly important epidermal component for the prevention of water loss. The barrier depends on both the cornified material of the keratinocytes and the intercellular material, particularly the lipids. This highly effective barrier is tough but flexible when well hydrated. However, as soon as the water content falls below 10% it becomes dry, less flexible, and prone to damage.

(2) Microorganisms and destructive chemicals: the uppermost layer of the skin is covered by the acidic mantle (pH between 4 and 5.5). This is the hydrolipidic film which inhibits replication of non-resident bacteria, and serves as a barrier for the skin. It is composed of a mixture of sweat, sebum, lipids, and antibiotic peptides. The *stratum corneum* is not a sterile place, and many resident bacteria

第二节　皮肤的功能

皮肤是人体最大的可见的器官。皮肤是人体抵御外界有害物质侵入的第一道防线，并具有多种功能，包括阻止微生物或有害化学物质进入、吸收日光中的辐射、防止水分的流失、调节体温和对抗机械外力等。皮肤具有重要的免疫功能，这依赖于表皮层和真皮层的细胞成分。此外，皮肤中有几种不同类型的感受器，能够感受触觉、痛觉、震颤、压力、冷热和瘙痒等刺激。本节主要介绍皮肤的功能及其与皮肤结构的关系。

一、皮肤的屏障功能

(1) 表皮和角质层　机体与外界的机械性屏障。

在生活中，我们的身体持续不断地通过皮肤缓慢地蒸发丢失水分，不论对皮肤本身还是对整个身体，防止过度的水分丢失都是极其重要的。水分占基底层重量的 70%～75%，而只占角质层的 10%～15%。

皮肤是一个双向的屏障，能够阻止水和电解质的出入。屏障主要位于表皮层，离体的表皮层和完整的皮肤一样是没有通透性的，但当表皮层被剥离，残留的真皮层几乎是完全可通透的。

在表皮层中，角质层在控制水分丢失的过程中起着尤其重要的作用。屏障功能主要依赖于角质形成细胞的角质成分和细胞间质，尤其是脂质。角质层如果有一定的含水量时是强韧而有弹性的。如果含水量低于 10%，皮肤就变得干燥，弹性下降，抵抗外来伤害的能力也会减弱。

(2) 微生物和有害化学物质　在皮肤的表层覆盖着一层 pH 值在 4～5.5 的酸性膜。这是一层具有抑制细菌繁殖和保护皮肤的屏障功能的水脂膜。它是由汗液、皮脂、脂质、抗菌肽等组成的混合物。角质层中并不是无菌的，存在着大

(10^{12} bacteria/m^2) inhabit it. Three species of bacteria are particularly well adapted to withstand the acidic environment and the antibiotic peptides: *Staphylococcus*, *Propionibacterium*, and *Corynebacterium*. They feed on cornified cell debris or sebum, and inhibit the growth of other less desirable bacteria. Therefore, maintaining the physiological pH of the skin is essential to avoid the proliferation of pathogens. The over-or underperformance of personal hygiene may disturb the equilibrium of these cutaneous floras.

量的常驻菌群(10^{12}个/m^2)。有三种细菌能够抵抗酸性环境和抗菌肽:葡萄球菌、丙酸杆菌和棒状杆菌。它们以角质细胞的碎屑或脂质为食,并且能够抑制其他有害菌的生长。保持皮肤生理的 pH 值对抑制病原体的增殖起着重要作用。过度清洁和清洁不够都会使皮肤菌群失衡。

An intact *stratum corneum* creates an impermeable layer that insulates one's body from bacterial invasions (either by normal skin flora or by pathogenic microorganisms). Therefore, a break in the skin barrier produced by a minor injury or disease will provide paths of entry for microbes, among which *Streptococci* and *Staphylococci* are of significance. It is noted that a single organism may give rise to different manifestations of infection, depending in part on the nature of the injury. For example, cellulitis, a dermal and subcutaneous inflammation, may follow a minor abrasion of the skin, but impaired skin barrier function even though involving large area, as one sees in the lesions of atopic dermatitis, tends to be associated with more superficial infections. In addition, the appendages of the skin (e. g., hair, sweat or sebaceous glands) can provide routes for infection by organisms such as *Staphylococcus aureus* or fungi. Regarding bacterial physiological features, it is easy to imagine that microbes are more readily colonized or grown in moist areas (i. e., flexural sites), while the dryness or continuous shedding of corneal cells from the skin surface will produce unfavorable conditions for bacterial colonization and growth.

完整的皮肤角质层能抵挡皮肤正常菌群和病原微生物的入侵。但是皮肤轻度的损伤和皮肤病能为病原微生物提供入口,尤其是链球菌和葡萄球菌。相同的病原体可能在皮肤上产生不同的感染模式,这与皮肤损伤的状态有关。例如,蜂窝织炎是位于真皮和皮下组织的炎症,可由皮肤上的小擦伤引起。而一些较大面积的皮肤屏障功能受损,如特异性皮炎的皮损,则与浅表的感染有关。除此之外,皮肤附属器如毛发、汗腺和皮脂腺,也为一些微生物的入侵提供了通道,如金黄色葡萄球菌和真菌。从细菌的生理特性上,潮湿部位(皱褶部位)更容易引起微生物的定植,而干燥的皮肤表面和角质细胞的不断脱落能抑制病原微生物的生长。

As previously mentioned, the *stratum corneum* acts as a two-way barrier, which prevents both excessive water loss from the body and the influx of polar molecules from the environment. However, in cases dealing with non-polar chemicals, the skin only impede penetration rather than completely preventing it.

皮肤的角质层能阻止过多的水分流失以及防止极性分子的进入,是一道良好的双向屏障。然而,一些潜在的有害的化学物质是非极性的,皮肤的屏障功能不能完全阻止这些物质的渗透,只能减少它们的渗透量。

Other groups of chemicals of concern here are ones that may cause allergic skin reactions. Good examples are metals such as nickel, which are constantly absorbed through the skin. The Langerhans cells in the skin will take the metal up first, then T lymphocytes will produce specific antibodies against it. As a result, an allergic skin reaction will take place when the T lymphocytes migrate to the source of the stimulus.

另一类需要防御的是能引起皮肤过敏反应的化学物质。如果一种化学物质(如镍)不断地被皮肤吸收,它会被朗格汉斯细胞摄取,随后 T 细胞产生针对这种物质的特异性抗体。当 T 细胞移行至入侵的化学物质处时,皮肤就会立刻产生过敏反应。

(3) UV Radiation: various kinds of radiation (e. g., infrared, visible, ultraviolet) are found in sunlight, of which ultraviolet (UV) radiation affects the skin the most. Exposure to the short-

(3) 紫外线辐射 日光辐射由红外线、可见光和紫外线组成,紫外线是影响皮肤的主要成分。例如,短时间暴露于

wavelength UVB (290-320 nm) in particular may cause sunburn over a short period of time, or may promote skin cancer over a prolonged period of time. Because UVB usually targets the upper layer of the skin, it is also partially responsible for premature aging of the skin. Longer-wavelength UVA (320-400 nm) affects the deeper layer of the skin (dermis), and is considered to play a major role in photoaging. However, UVA radiation is also primarily responsible for production of the various types of vitamin D.

短波紫外线 UVB (290～320 nm)会引起皮肤晒伤，长时间的接触甚至可以引起皮肤癌。UVB 常作用于皮肤的上层，因此对引起皮肤老化起重要作用。长波紫外线 UVA (320～400 nm)穿透皮肤更深，目前认为它的主要作用是导致皮肤老化。UVA 对产生各种维生素 D 也具有重要作用。

The skin has two barriers to defend against UV radiation: a melanin barrier in the epidermis; and a protein barrier concentrated in the *stratum corneum*. Both of them can absorb radiation efficiently, thereby minimizing the effects of radiation on DNA and other cellular constituents. Melanin is synthesized by melanocytes in the basal layer of the epidermis and is transferred to surrounding keratinocytes via melanosomes. The partially protective mechanism of delayed tanning (which occurs 2-3 days after exposure to either UVA or UVB) is associated with an increase in the number of functional melanocytes, an increase in the number of synthesized melanosomes, and an increased rate of transfer of melanosomes to the keratinocytes. However, repeated exposure to ultraviolet radiation over the long term will eventually cause epidermal thickening and damage that will increase the chance of developing skin cancer. The evidence shows that the more sun exposure people undergo, the higher their risks of skin cancer are, such as squamous cell carcinoma, basal cell carcinoma, and malignant melanoma.

皮肤有两道屏障抵御紫外线辐射：表皮的黑素屏障和角质层中的蛋白屏障。两道屏障都能吸收辐射，从而减少 DNA 和其他细胞成分对紫外线的吸收。黑素由表皮基底层的黑素细胞合成，再以黑素小体的形式运输到周围的角质形成细胞中。延缓型皮肤晒黑(发生于暴露在 UVA 或 UVB 下 2～3 天后)能提供部分的保护功能，是通过增加有功能的黑素细胞，能更多地合成黑素小体，并更快地运输到角质形成细胞中来达到目的的。而长期慢性的日光暴露会导致表皮层增厚以及损伤而产生皮肤癌。日光照射越多，皮肤癌的危险性就越大，包括鳞状细胞癌、基底细胞癌和恶性黑素瘤。

Absorption of radiation by epidermal lipids and low molecular weight degradation products of epidermal proteins may contribute to protection from UV radiation. One example is urocanic acid, which is a product of histidine deamination, and a normal constituent of the epidermis that undergoes a chemical reaction in response to the incoming radiation. The role of UV-induced cytokines on the regulation of melanin production has not yet been determined.

表皮层的脂质能够吸收紫外线辐射而起防护作用，皮肤表面的一些低分子量的自然降解产物也可以起到同样的作用，如尿刊酸是组氨酸受辐射作用后的脱氨产物，具有微弱的抗辐射作用。紫外线诱导的细胞因子在黑素产生中的作用目前还不清楚。

2. Percutaneous absorption

二、经皮吸收

Percutaneous absorption is defined as the passive process of absorption, whereby drugs, allergens, and other substances pass through intact skin into the body.

经皮吸收是指通过完整未受损的皮肤被动吸收药物、变应原以及其他物质的过程。

Oxygen, nitrogen, and carbon dioxide can diffuse into the epidermis in small amounts; indeed some animals (insects in particular) use their skin as their sole organ of respiration. However, we are more interested in the process of absorption through the skin of topically applied substances such as medication in the form of ointments or adhesive patches.

氧气、氮气和二氧化碳能够少量地弥散进入表皮层，一些动物(特别是昆虫)使用皮肤作为它们唯一的呼吸器官。然而，我们更感兴趣的是局部应用药物(如软膏或贴片)被皮肤吸收的过程。

The skin is considered to be a composite membrane, with three

皮肤被认为是由角质层(10 μm)、有

anatomically distinct layers: the *stratum corneum* (10 μm thick), the viable epidermis (100 μm), and the uppermost papillary layer of the dermis (100-200 μm), each having a different diffusion constant. The *stratum corneum* plays the most important role in limiting percutaneous absorption, acting as a composite semipermeable membrane. Healthy adult human skin allows some perfusion of almost any substance, and rates of penetration for different substances may differ by factors of ten thousand.

活力的表皮层(100 μm)以及真皮乳头的上层(100～200 μm)组成的复合膜结构，每层都有不同的扩散常数。表皮层中角质层是控制经皮吸收功能最重要的一层，它表现出一种复合的半透膜的特性。正常的成年人皮肤对几乎所有的物质都有一定的通透性，而不同物质的通透率的差别可以有 10000 倍。

The efficiency of the barrier varies from site to site even in the same individual. For instance, the skin of the scrotum is particularly permeable, and the skin of the face, forehead and dorsa of the hands may be more permeable to water than areas on the trunk, arms or legs. The palms and soles of the feet are particularly impermeable to nearly all molecules except water.

身体不同部位的皮肤的屏障功能也是不同的。阴囊的通透力最强，面部、前额和手背的皮肤对水的通透性比躯干四肢的皮肤强。掌跖部位的皮肤几乎对除水以外所有的分子都是不可通透的。

The barrier's function is also affected by other factors, such as age, environmental conditions and physical trauma. Any of these conditions may result in enhanced permeability and accelerate the uptake of medications administrated topically.

许多因素可以影响皮肤的屏障功能，如年龄、环境、外伤等，而增强皮肤的通透性能够使皮肤吸收更多的局部用药。

3. Temperature regulation

三、温度调节

The skin provides sensory input for the temperature control center and balances the body's temperature by allowing heat loss or conservation.

皮肤能向体温调节中枢提供信息，是体温调节的感受器，并能调节热量的散失和守恒。

The thermoreceptor cells are distributed irregularly in the skin. These include both warm-and cold-sensitive receptors, as well as receptors that detect extreme temperatures without distinguishing between hot and cold. Any stimulus in response to temperature changes on the skin will be sent to the hypothalamus (the central control center), leading either to sweating or shivering, or the cessation thereof. However, the skin thermoreceptors play a relatively minor role in regulating core temperature. Skin temperature changes are greatly associated with human behaviors.

皮肤的温度感受器细胞不规则地分布在皮肤里，包括热和冷敏感的感受器，也有仅能识别温度剧烈变化的感受器，而不能区分热和冷。温度改变引起的刺激信号的改变被传输到下丘脑(控制中心)，导致出汗或发生寒战。但是，皮肤的温度感受器在调节深部体温中的作用相对很小，而皮肤的温度变化与人的行为息息相关。

From an effector standpoint, the skin plays a major role in the regulation of body temperature. Heat can be lost through the skin's surface by radiation, convection, conduction, and evaporation. Of great importance for these mechanisms is the rich blood supply of the dermis, which is much greater than simple nutritional requirements would dictate. In addition, this blood supply features a system of arteriovenous shunts, particularly abundant in the feet, hands, lips, nose and ears, which can divert the blood flow to an extensive and more superficial venous plexus. Dilated blood vessels in the venous plexus increase perfusion and heat loss while constricting those same vessels greatly reduces cutaneous blood flow and conserves heat.

从效应器的角度来说，皮肤在人体的体温调节方面起着重要的作用。热量可以通过辐射、对流、传导、蒸发的方式从皮肤表面散失。真皮层丰富的血供在散热方面比提供营养起着更重要的作用。在手足、嘴唇、鼻子和耳朵存在着丰富的动静脉网，能使血液流向周边和更表浅的静脉丛。扩张的血管增加血液灌流量使热量丧失，收缩的血管减少皮肤的血流量从而保存热量。

4. Mechanical properties

A number of studies have shown exactly how the skin provides both a rigid framework to support the contents of the body and a flexible covering allowing the body to change its shape during movement. The epidermis is designed to respond to mechanical forces to some extent and also has the ability to repair itself if damaged. The dermis in particular provides the necessary elasticity to cope with such mechanical forces, and in general, the mechanical properties of the skin depend on the dermis.

Due to its protein and lipid constituents, the *stratum corneum* is a relatively strong and elastic tissue. The network of the structural proteins allows the energy of exogenous forces to be dissipated within the tissue and away from the point of impact. The elasticity of the *stratum corneum* can be influenced by the degree of hydration of the corneal cell proteins, which in turn depends on the water content of the tissue and the humidity of the surrounding environment. *Stratum corneum* proteins, lipids, and low molecular weight byproducts of keratohyalin breakdown-referred to as natural moisturizing factors-will bind and retain water in the *stratum corneum*, thus maintaining its elasticity.

The epidermis itself is relatively strong and holds together even under pressure of blister fluids. On the other hand, the dermal-epidermal interface in human skin is relatively weak. The collagens in the papillary layer are usually very weak, and many blistering agents appear to act on this layer.

Skin is elastic to some extent and can, for a few seconds at a time, be reversibly stretched by 10%-50%. The initial response appears to involve a reorientation of collagen fibers along the load axis and a decrease in their degree of convolution. The tone of the skin is probably maintained by elastic fibers, and it seems likely that these fibers also provide the small forces that restore slack skin to its original dimensions.

From these considerations it is clear that disorders in which the skin is hyperelastic, such as Ehlers-Danlos syndrome, must involve a breakdown of the collagen mechanism. The striae distensae seen in adolescence, pregnancy and in situations of excessive systemic glucocorticoids (whether administered or as part of Cushing's syndrome) are thought to be associated with a breakdown of the fibril overlap, so that there is no restoring force to limit further slip.

A further property of the skin is that it can be compressed. If a small object is pressed onto the skin, a depression is formed which remains until the object is removed; thus, skin molds itself around the object exerting the force, and the pressure on any one point is

四、机械性能

研究表明，皮肤不仅是身体坚固的支持框架，也为移动和运动引起的形状改变提供一个弹性包被。表皮层具有一定程度的抵挡机械性损害的能力，并且具有损伤后自我修复的能力。真皮对于机械力则提供弹性保护。皮肤的机械性能主要依赖于真皮层。

由于角质层的主要成分是蛋白质和脂质，因此是相对坚固的有弹性的组织。蛋白质形成的网络结构使外力通过组织分散了。角质层的弹性也受到角质细胞蛋白水化度的影响，而水化度又依赖于组织含水量和周围环境的湿度。角质层的蛋白、脂质和透明角质分解的低分子量产物，是一种天然的保湿因子，连接并保持角质层中的水分，因此也能保持弹性。

即使在疱液的压力下表皮本身也是相对坚固并紧密连接在一起的。另一方面，人皮肤真皮和表皮交接处是相对薄弱的。乳头层的胶原特别薄弱，因此许多发疱剂是作用于这一层的。

皮肤有一定的弹性，可在数秒钟内被牵拉10%～50%。皮肤最初的反应是胶原纤维向负重轴方向的重排以及螺旋减少。皮肤的紧张度主要通过弹力纤维维持，弹力纤维也为松弛的皮肤提供一定的回缩力。

因此，我们认为与皮肤弹性过度有关的疾病，如Ehlers-Danlos综合征，与胶原纤维系统的降解有关。在青春期、孕期和系统大量使用糖皮质激素或作为Cushing综合征的部分表现的时候，皮肤上可出现膨胀纹，这是因为皮肤的弹力纤维降解，导致皮肤失去了限制滑动的黏合力。

皮肤的另一个特性是能受压。如果在皮肤上放置一个小的物体，被压出的凹陷在物体被移走后即可恢复。物体周围的皮肤通过重新塑形而使物体施加的

reduced. This displacement morphological change of the skin is thought to be due to the flow of some ground substance through the dermis between the collagen fibers.

作用力在每个点都得以减轻。这种形态学改变主要是由于真皮胶原纤维之间的基质物质的流动所导致。

5. Sensory functions

五、感觉功能

Nerves in the skin direct the sensations of touch (including vibration and pressure), pain, temperature, and itching. Nerve endings either exist freely in the skin or are encapsulated as specialized sensory receptors such as Meissner and Pacinian corpuscles. The sensory nerves are myelinated (A fibers) or non-myelinated (C fibers). The speed of transmission of a nerve impulse is faster in myelinated fibers than in non-myelinated fibers.

皮肤中的感觉神经能传导皮肤的触觉(包括振动觉和压觉)、痛觉、冷热觉和痒感。神经末梢一部分游离存在于皮肤内,一部分以特异性的感受器形式存在,如 Meissner 小体和 Pacinian 小体。感觉神经分为有髓鞘(A 纤维)和无髓鞘(C 纤维)。前者的神经脉冲的传导速度比后者快。

The touch sensation is mediated by mechanoreceptors in the skin, which include two main functional groups according to the way they respond to constant or persistent stimuli. Slowly adapting mechanoreceptors respond continuously to a persistent stimulus, whereas rapidly adapting mechanoreceptors respond either to the initial or terminal onset of a frequently applied stimulus, but not throughout the whole stimulating process.

触觉是由皮肤的机械感受器介导的,依据其对短暂和持续刺激的反应方式的不同而分为两类,慢适应机械感受器感应持续刺激,而快适应机械感受器感应初始的或者终末的频繁刺激,它不能感受整个刺激过程。

Hairy and glabrous skins have different types of mechanoreceptors. The predominant mechanoreceptors in hairy skin are the hair follicle receptors. Glabrous skin (e. g. , the hairless skin of the palms and soles) has two main types of superficial mechanoreceptors: a rapidly adapting receptor (i. e. , the Meissner corpuscle) and a slowly adapting receptor (i. e. , the Merkel's cell).

有毛和无毛的皮肤中的机械感受器也不相同。有毛皮肤中主要的机械感受器是毛囊感受器,无毛皮肤(如掌跖部位)中有两种浅表机械感受器:快适应的 Meissner 小体和慢适应的 Merkel 细胞。

The subcutaneous tissue and the deeper dermis beneath both hairy and glabrous skin also contain two types of mechanoreceptors: the Pacinian corpuscle, which is a rapidly adapting receptor; and Ruffini's corpuscle, a slowly adapting one. These mechanoreceptors differ from the receptors in the epidermis primarily in the area over which impulses are picked up and transmitted to a particular corpuscle. In contrast to the small receptive-field size of Meissner corpuscles and Merkel's cells in the upper dermis, the receptive fields of Pacinian and Ruffini's corpuscles are larger.

有毛皮肤和无毛皮肤的皮下组织和深层的真皮内有两种机械感受器:快适应的 Pacinian 小体和慢适应的 Ruffini 小体。这些与表皮的感受器不同,主要位于感觉被传送到特殊的小体的一些区域。相对于真皮浅层的 Meissner 小体和 Merkel 细胞的感受范围,Pacinian 和 Ruffini 小体的感受范围要大得多。

Pain is mediated by nociceptors, which are receptors that respond selectively to stimuli that can damage tissue. Three types of nociceptor can be identified. Mechanical nociceptors are activated by strong mechanical stimulation, such as sharp objects. Pricking of the skin gives rise to two kinds of sensation. The initially felt "pricking" or "fast" pain is punctate, superficial and local, and this is followed by a more diffuse "burning" or "slow" pain. Thermal nociceptors respond to cold or heat. In humans, heat nociceptors respond when the temperature of their receptive field exceeds

痛觉是由一种伤害性感受器介导的,这种感受器选择性地感受能导致组织损伤的刺激。伤害性的感受器包括三种。机械性伤害感受器由强烈的机械刺激活化,如锐器。皮肤穿刺能够引起两种皮肤感觉。最初的锐痛感或快痛感是具体、表浅和局限的,然后就能感受到更弥漫的烧灼感或慢痛。温度性伤害感受器感应冷和热。在人体,热伤害感受器

45 ℃, the heat pain threshold, and cold nociceptors respond to cold noxious stimuli.

感应它的感受野内超过 45 ℃的高温,这是热引起疼痛的阈值。冷伤害感受器感应寒冷的伤害性刺激。

Itching can be defined subjectively as a poorly localized, non-adapting, usually unpleasant sensation which elicits a desire to scratch. Itching as a symptom of skin disease is generally independent of external stimulation. Teleologically speaking, itching, together with the resultant scratching, may be of some biological value in combating parasitic infestations.

瘙痒被认为是一种主观上的局部不舒适感和不适应感,这种不愉快的感觉通常会引起搔抓的欲望。瘙痒作为一种皮肤病的症状通常不依赖于外来的刺激。从某种角度来说,瘙痒能导致搔抓,可能在防止寄生虫感染中有一定的生理价值。

The theory that pain and itching are transmitted along the same nerve pathways proposed by Rothman and others has been the prevailing view until recently. According to this interpretation, low intensity stimulation of unmyelinated polymodal C fibers results in the sensation of itching, whereas high intensity stimulation causes pain. However, a number of features of pain and itch argue against this interpretation, for example, the difference in motor responses (itch induces scratching whereas pain evokes withdrawal). Also, morphine would then appear to act on the two sets of nerves differently (it relieves pain but makes itching worse), which is incompatible with current models for how morphine is thought to operate in the nervous system.

Rothman 等提出,疼痛和瘙痒是通过相同的神经通路传导的,这种理论在目前也是主流的。根据这种解释,对无髓鞘的 C 纤维的低密度刺激能引起瘙痒感,而高密度刺激引起疼痛感。然而,关于疼痛和瘙痒的一些特性有悖于这种解释。例如,运动反应的不同,瘙痒引起搔抓动作,疼痛引起缩回动作。吗啡有两种不同的神经反应:它缓解疼痛却加重痒感,这与吗啡作用于神经系统的现有模式相矛盾。

Warmth and cold are mediated by thermal receptors. Such fibers show a steady discharge dependent on temperature, but no response to non-painful intensities of mechanical stimulation. Temperature sensitivity is punctate, each afferent fiber being connected to a few receptive spots with a diameter in hairy skin of less than 1 mm.

温度感受器感受冷和热。这种神经纤维依赖于温度,但不能感应非疼痛的强烈机械刺激。温度敏感性是有具体的点的,每个传入纤维与数个接收点连接,而在有毛皮肤上每个接收点的直径不到 1 mm。

Neuropeptides are released from nerve terminals following depolarization, and play a role in regulating synaptic transmission. A number of neuropeptides have been identified in human skin, including substance P, vasoactive intestinal peptide (VIP), somatostatin, calcitonin-gene related peptide (CGRP), neuropeptide Y, and bombesin. In addition to acting as neurotransmitters, neuropeptides play a role in the mediation of inflammation in the skin.

神经肽是由神经末梢在去极化后释放的,在调节突触传递方面起着重要作用。现已经证实在皮肤中存在着大量的神经肽,包括 P 物质、血管活性肠肽(VIP)、生长抑素、降钙素基因相关肽(CGRP)、神经肽 Y 和蛙皮素。神经肽除了是神经递质,也可介导皮肤的炎症反应。

6. Immunological function

六、免疫功能

The skin has a very complicated defense system, which involves different types of cells and their interactions with each other. It is therefore no surprise that the skin has an immune function. The first line of defense relies on the Langerhans cells, which are dendritic cells originating in the bone marrow. The defense is then taken over by T lymphocytes and macrophages.

皮肤具有非常复杂的防御系统,涉及多种不同类型的细胞相互作用。因此可以说皮肤也是具有免疫功能的。皮肤的免疫功能首先是通过朗格汉斯细胞实现的,它是骨髓来源的树突状细胞,继而 T 细胞和巨噬细胞参与后续过程。

Langerhans cells make up about 2% of the epidermal cells and

朗格汉斯细胞的数量大约占表皮层

are responsible for an immune response against antigens applied locally to the skin. If an antigen penetrates and crosses the horny layer, these cells will capture it and leave the epidermis. Within 6 hours they may be found in dermal lymphatic vessels where they pass the antigen to T lymphocytes, and the T lymphocytes initiate the immunological cascade reaction to eliminate the antigen and keep it in the "immunological memory". If the same antigen again penetrates the epidermis, even years later, it will be immediately recognized and the immunological reaction will be rapid and effective.

细胞的2%，对位于皮肤内的抗原产生免疫应答。如果抗原穿透并通过角质层，朗格汉斯细胞能捕获这些抗原并离开表皮层。不到6 h就能到达皮肤的淋巴管，在淋巴管，朗格汉斯细胞将抗原递呈给T细胞，继而T细胞释放免疫级联反应从而清除抗原并产生"免疫记忆"。如果相同的抗原再次进入表皮层，甚至是多年以后，它也能立即被识别，免疫反应也将更快速和有效。

If the antigen however manages to cross this first line of defense, the macrophages of the dermis will entrap it and eliminate it. Furthermore, the skin's immunological function may also be complemented by the keratinocytes which, in the case of an infection, produce more IL-1, which stimulates T lymphocytes activity.

如果抗原直接通过了第一道屏障，真皮内的巨噬细胞能够识别它并清除。角质形成细胞在皮肤感染的免疫反应中也起了一定作用，它能产生IL-1，刺激T细胞的活化。

7. Excretory and endocrine function

七、排泄和内分泌功能

The skin excretes sweat and other substances from the body, through the eccrine glands, sebaceous glands, and apocrine glands. The clear secretion produced by eccrine glands is the main source of human sweat. Sweat is formed of water (99%), less than 1% of solid ingredients, mostly sodium chloride, a small amount of potassium chloride, urea, etc. Eccrine glands produce sweat in response to emotional tension, heat and pain. Sweat aids the control of body temperature and serves to expel waste materials such as salt and urea.

皮肤的排泄功能主要通过汗腺和皮脂腺完成。小汗腺分泌稀薄的汗液，是人汗的主要来源。汗液中水占99%以上，固体成分不足1%，大部分为氯化钠，还有少量的氯化钾、尿素等。汗液的产生受情绪、高温和疼痛的影响，汗液能够帮助控制体温和排出盐、尿素等代谢产物。

The sebum secreted by sebaceous glands can keep skin supple and waterproof and hair soft. Sebum has bactericidal effect and forms part of the acid mantle to protect skin from microorganism colonization. The glands are stimulated by hormonal action, especially androgens.

皮脂腺分泌的皮脂能够滋润皮肤和毛发，防止水分蒸发，皮脂呈弱酸性，可以抑制和杀灭皮肤表面的细菌。皮脂腺的分泌受内分泌影响较大，尤其是雄激素的作用。

Apocrine glands produce a much thicker secretion than eccrine glands, containing protein, carbohydrates, and lipids. The substance secreted provides nutrients for bacteria on the skin. However, the bacteria's decomposition of sweat is what creates the characteristic acrid odor. Before puberty, the apocrine glands are inactive; hormonal changes in puberty cause the glands to increase in size and begin functioning.

顶泌汗腺分泌物为较黏稠的乳状液，含蛋白质、碳水化合物和脂类等，为皮肤上的细菌提供营养，分泌物被细菌分解后产生特别的气味。这种腺体在青春期前呈静止状态，青春期后由于受性激素的刺激，分泌活跃，分泌物的作用尚未知。

Recently attention has been focused on identifying and understanding the complex endocrine properties of human skin, such as expression and function of specific hormone receptors; synthesis of hormones from major classes of compounds used by the body for other purposes; metabolism, activation, inactivation, and elimination of the hormones in specialized cells of the tissue; and exertion of biological activity and release of tissue hormones in

近年来的研究格外关注如何了解皮肤的内分泌功能，例如特异性激素受体的表达和功能，利用体内一些化合物合成所需激素，在组织的特殊细胞里调节激素的新陈代谢、激活、失活和清除，发挥生物活性并将组织激素释放到循环中。

the circulation.

Specifically, hormones exert their biological effects on the skin through interaction with high-affinity receptors, such as several receptors for peptide hormones and neurotransmitters, steroid, and thyroid hormones. Hormones that exhibit a wide range of biological activities on the skin with distinct effects are growth hormone/insulin-like growth factor-I, neuropeptides, sex steroids, glucocorticoids, retinoids, vitamin D, peroxisome proliferator-activated receptor ligands, eicosanoids, melatonin, and serotonin.

具体来说，激素是通过与高亲和性受体的相互作用在皮肤上发挥生物效应，如肽激素和神经递质，类固醇和甲状腺激素。能在皮肤上表现出广泛生物活性的激素包括生长激素/胰岛素样生长因素Ⅰ、神经肽、性类固醇、糖皮质激素、维 A 酸、维生素 D、过氧物酶体增生物激活受体配体、二十烷类、褪黑激素和血清素。

Human skin produces, activates, or inactivates metabolically numerous hormones which are probably important for skin functions but also for functions of the entire human body, such as sex hormones (especially in aged individuals), insulin-like growth factor and binding proteins, neuropeptides, prolactin, catecholamines, retinoids, steroids, vitamin D, and eicosanoids. These functions are undertaken in most cases by different skin cell populations in a coordinated way, indicating the endocrine autonomy of the skin. Characteristic examples are the metabolic pathways of the corticotropin-releasing hormone/propiomelanocortin axis, steroidogenesis, vitamin D, and retinoids. The human skin is thus the largest peripheral endocrine organ.

皮肤也能产生、激活或灭活大量对皮肤功能以及人体机能起重要作用的激素，如性激素(尤其是老年人)、胰岛素样生长因子及其结合蛋白、神经肽、催乳素、儿茶酚胺、维 A 酸、类固醇、维生素 D 和类花生酸。在大多数情况下，不同的皮肤细胞能非常协调地控制这些功能，说明皮肤能够自主分泌。典型的例子就是促肾上腺皮质激素/阿片促黑素细胞皮质素原释放轴，类固醇的生成，维生素 D 和维 A 酸的合成代谢途径。因此皮肤被认为是最大的外周内分泌器官。

8. Bioengineering and the skin

To date, there are various bioengineering parameters and techniques that have been used in the studies, which include the measurements of transepidermal water loss (TEWL), *stratum corneum* hydration, cutaneous blood flow, skin color, skin surface pH, and combining bioengineering techniques in contact dermatitis.

TEWL measurement has been designed to assess the barrier function of the *stratum corneum*. If the skin barrier function is damaged by irritants or by any inflammatory process, there will be a corresponding increase in TEWL. Formerly, TEWL was taken to measure only the water vapour passing through the *stratum corneum* by passive diffusion, but TEWL today refers to the total amount of water loss through the skin, including sweating. Many irritants damage the skin by impairing the barrier function of the *stratum corneum*, and TEWL measurement has been reported to be more sensitive in assessing such irritancy effects than visual scoring, laser Doppler flowmetry, colourimetry, and skin thickening by ultrasound A-scan. TEWL measurements are also applied to detect subclinical eczema, to predict its progress, and to assess therapeutic effects.

TEWL levels decrease with age, especially becoming apparent after the fifth decade. The decrease in TEWL with age is considered

八、生物工程学和皮肤

目前有很多种生物工程学测量参数和技术正在研究中，如经表皮水分丢失(TEWL)、角质层含水量、皮肤血流、皮肤颜色测量、皮肤表皮 pH 值以及多种生物工程技术在接触性皮炎中的研究。

TEWL 的检测被用来评价角质层的屏障功能。如果皮肤屏障功能受到刺激物或炎症反应的破坏，TEWL 值就会增加。在过去，TEWL 值用来提示通过角质层被动扩散的水分蒸发，在现在 TEWL 值指的是通过皮肤的水分丢失的总量，包括排汗。许多刺激物能够削弱角质层的屏障功能从而使皮肤受损，在评价这种刺激效应方面，TEWL 值检测相对于视觉评分、激光多普勒血流仪、比色法和 A 型超声检测皮肤厚度等方法，更加敏感。TEWL 值的检测可以用来发现亚临床状态的湿疹，预测湿疹的危险性以及评价治疗效果。

TEWL 值随年龄增大而降低，尤其在 50 岁以后更加明显。这种随年龄的

to be partly due to an increased size of cornified cells and increased thickness of the *stratum corneum* that results from an accumulation of cornified cells. *Stratum corneum* hydration is also dramatically decreased in elderly persons; the "dryness" of the skin in the elderly differs from pathologically dry skin, in which barrier function is impaired.

TEWL 值变化可能与角质细胞的体积增大和角质细胞堆积引起角质层厚度的增加有关。角质层的水合作用也随着年龄增大而减弱，老年人干燥的皮肤和病理性的干燥皮肤也有不同，它不存在皮肤屏障功能的受损。

Yan LI(李延), Juan TAO(陶娟)

Chapter Two Basic Knowledge of Dermatopathology

第二章 皮肤组织病理学的基本知识

Section One The Role of Dermatopathologic Examination and Skin Biopsy Techniques

第一节 皮肤病理检查的作用和皮肤组织活检技术

1. The role of dermatopathologic examination

Dermatopathologic examination is a very important diagnostic aid for skin dermatoses, particularly for skin tumors and viral dermatoses such as molluscum contagiosum. It is also very useful in identifying the etiological agents in infectious diseases such as fungal infections. A close clinical and pathologic correlation can clarify or exclude a diagnosis for some dermatoses such as bullous disorders, pustular skin diseases, metabolic disease, connective tissue diseases, and some skin granulomas. Even though the histological changes may not be characteristic of certain skin diseases, it may still provide a valuable data point in a differential diagnosis. Therefore, it is important to correlate pathological findings with clinical observations throughout the diagnostic process.

一、皮肤病理检查的作用

皮肤病理检查在皮肤病的诊断中具有非常重要的作用，特别是皮肤肿瘤、病毒性皮肤病（如传染性软疣）等可凭借皮肤组织病理检查而确诊；有些皮肤病（如真菌感染）可通过皮肤组织病理检查找到病原菌从而明确疾病的病因；有些皮肤病（如水疱、脓疱性皮肤病、代谢障碍性皮肤病、结缔组织病及某些肉芽肿性皮肤病等）在临床和病理的密切配合下常可得出诊断或可排除可疑的诊断。而一些皮肤病为非特异性病理改变，仅能作为临床的参考以及在鉴别诊断上具有一定的意义。在进行皮肤病理诊断中必须强调临床和病理的密切结合和联系。

2. The skin biopsy techniques

Skin biopsy is one of the most important and most widely used techniques in dermatological clinical practice, and helps dermatopathologists to make a straightforward diagnosis when properly carried out. Currently, the skin biopsy techniques used in clinical practice are punch biopsy, shave biopsy, incisional biopsy, complete excisional biopsy, and curettage biopsy.

(1) Punch biopsy: this is performed with a cylindrical knife ranging from 2-6 mm in diameter. Ideal samples from the punch biopsy include the full thickness of the skin including subcutaneous fat. It is often used to diagnose inflammatory skin conditions and skin tumors.

(2) Shave biopsy: the technique requires a razor to scrape off a portion of affected tissue and is therefore somewhat dependent on the skill of the user. Superficial shave biopsies are only used for lesions in which the characteristic histological changes are mainly located in the epidermis or the superficial dermis such as seborrheic keratosis, actinic keratosis, verruca, nevocytic nevus, and basal cell carcinoma, etc. On some occasions, saucerization is used in deep shave biopsy procedures to obtain larger samples as desired.

二、皮肤组织活检技术

皮肤活检术是皮肤科日常工作中最重要和最常用的操作之一，对皮肤病理医师的正确诊断往往起到非常重要乃至决定性的作用。皮肤活检术的方法包括：环钻活检术、削切活检术、皮损内楔形切除活检术、全皮损切除活检术和刮取活检术。

（1）环钻或钻孔活检术　采用2～6 mm 环钻取材，可以用来取小范围的全层皮片，应深达皮下脂肪层，主要用于炎症性皮肤病，也用于肿瘤损害取材。

（2）削切活检术　术者需要一定的技巧，采用刀片削切部分皮损组织。浅表削切活检术仅用于损害的组织病理学特征主要位于表皮或真皮浅层者，如脂溢性角化病、日光性角化病、疣、痣细胞痣、基底细胞癌等。深层削切活检术是一种蝶形手术，能取得更多的组织。

(3) Incisional biopsy: this is the most frequently used technique in routine dermatological practice. The advantage of an incisional biopsy is that the size and depth of the wedge-shaped incision can be controlled more easily.

(4) Complete excisional biopsy: this is essentially the same as incisional biopsy, except the entire lesion or tumor is removed. It is often done in cases of small and easily excisable lesions; it is also done when the patient specifically asks for the procedure, in which case the borders of the lesion or atypical pigmented lesions need to be evaluated further by the physicians.

(5) Curettage biopsy: this is occasionally used for biopsy purpose, and the lesion is removed by curettage. It is not the preferred biopsy technique as the procedure can cause damage to the architecture of the skin tissues.

3. The processing of the skin samples

The biopsied samples should be fixed immediately to prevent autolysis. 10% formaldehyde fixation is used for routine hematoxylin-eosin (HE) staining, or 2% glutaraldehyde fixation is used for immunofluorescence testing or electron microscopic examination. Some tissue components such as elastic fibers, reticular fibers, nerves, and melanocytes can be better seen with special staining methods.

(3) 皮损内楔形切除活检术　皮肤科最常用的技术。其优点是能根据临床需要从损害内楔形切取不同大小和深度的组织。

(4) 全皮损切除活检术　与皮损内楔形切除活检术基本相似，所不同者是前者切除全部损害或肿瘤。其可用于损害比较小、能全切除或患者要求切除的损害、需要评估边缘的损害以及某些非典型性色素性损害。

(5) 刮取活检术　一种仅偶尔使用的皮肤活检的方法。它是用刮勺器刮取损害，由于在操作过程中对组织结构的破坏，一般不采用。

三、皮肤组织标本的处理

组织取材后应立即置于10%甲醛液中固定以免组织降解，并用于常规苏木素-伊红(HE)染色或置于2%戊二醛中固定以用于免疫荧光或电镜检查。有的组织，如弹力纤维、网织纤维、神经、黑素细胞等，尚需用特殊染色才能显示良好。

Section Two　Dermatopathology Glossary of Terms

(1) Hyperkeratosis: abnormally increased thickness of the horny cell layer (Fig. 2-1).

(2) Horny plug or follicular plug: the thickened keratins plugging the orifice of hair follicles or sweat pores (Fig. 2-2). It is seen in lupus erythematosus, lichen sclerosis *et* atrophicus, pityriasis rubra pilaris, porokeratosis, lichen pilaris, lichen spinulosis, etc.

第二节　皮肤组织病理学基本术语

(1) 角化过度(hyperkeratosis)　角质层异常地增厚称为角化过度(图 2-1)。

(2) 角质栓(horny plug)或毛囊角栓(follicular plug)　指角质增厚，在毛囊口或汗孔口形成栓塞状(图 2-2)，见于红斑狼疮、硬化性萎缩性苔藓、毛发红糠疹、汗孔角化症、毛发苔藓、小棘苔藓等。

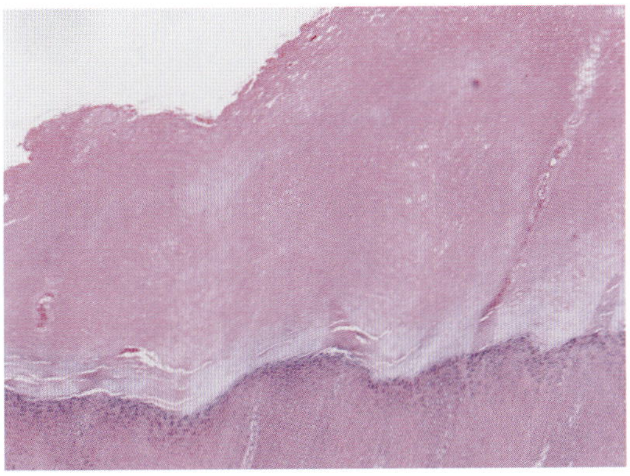

Fig. 2-1　Hyperkeratosis(图 2-1　角化过度)

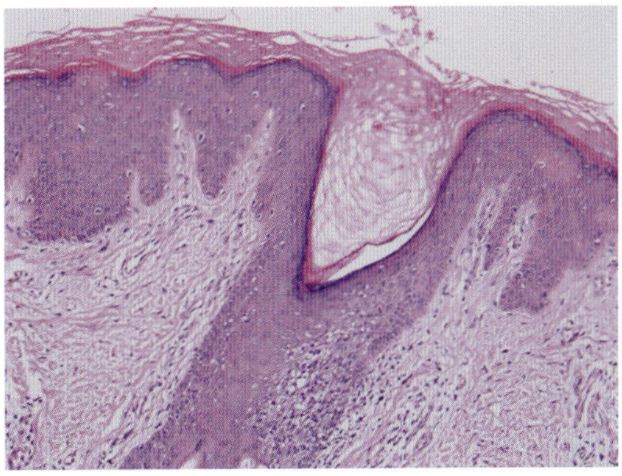

Fig. 2-2　Follicular plug(图 2-2　毛囊角栓)

(3) Parakeratosis: the nuclei remain in the cells of the horny

(3) 角化不全(parakeratosis)　由于

cell layer due to incomplete keratinization of the keratinocytes, usually accompanied by hyperkeratosis and hypogranulosis (Fig. 2-3).

(4) Cornoid lamella: a wedge-shaped or columnar parakeratosis arising from epidermal invagination (Fig. 2-4), a characteristic of porokeratosis.

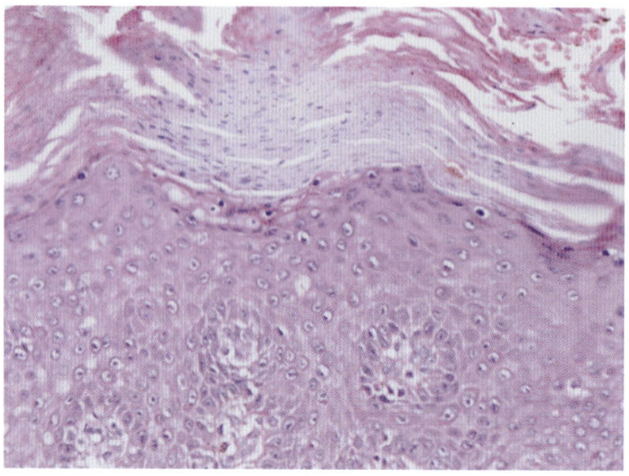

Fig. 2-3　Parakeratosis(图 2-3　角化不全)

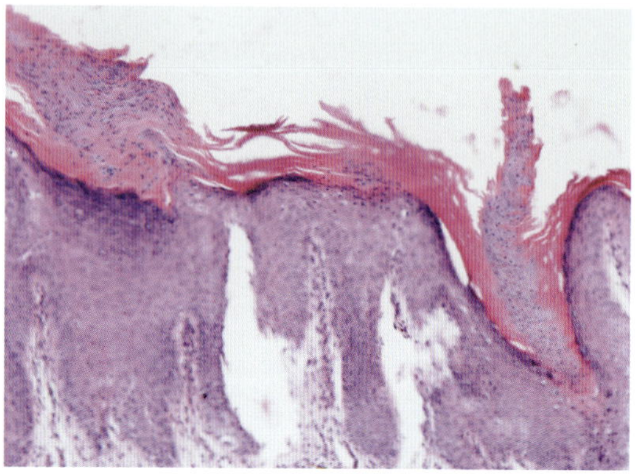

Fig. 2-4　Cornoid lamella(图 2-4　柱状板层)

(5) Dyskeratosis: the abnormally premature keratinization of individual keratinocytes in the epidermis or adnexa. The dyskeratotic cells are apoptotic cells characterized by shrunken nuclei with homogenous eosinophilic cytoplasm. It can manifest as corps ronds, corps grains, keratin pearls, colloid body, viral inclusion body, etc.

① Corps ronds: usually found in the horny layer, granular layer, and in the upper part of the spinous layer. These dyskeratotic cells are characterized by large, round, basophilic, pyknotic nuclei in the center with a perinuclear halo and outermost basophilic cytoplasm (Fig. 2-5). These changes are seen mainly in keratosis follicularis (Darier's disease), warty dyskeratoma, transient acantholytic dermatosis (Grover's disease), and focal acantholytic dyskeratoma.

② Corps grains: found in the horny layer, corps grains may resemble parakeratosis. However, they are differentiated by larger cells, clear nuclei with surrounding dyskeratotic materials (either basophilic or eosinophilic) and sometimes accompanied by a perinuclear halo (Fig. 2-6). They are seen in keratosis follicularis (Darier's disease) and warty dyskeratoma.

③Keratin pearls: a group of concentric or laminated keratinocytes. The center is gradually or fully keratinized with homogenous eosinophilic apoptotic cells (Fig. 2-7). Keratin pearls are commonly seen in well-differentiated squamous cell carcinomas.

④Colloid body: also called Civatte body. These often appear as

不完全角化，导致细胞核滞留于角质层内，常伴角化过度和颗粒层减少(图2-3)。

(4) 柱状板层(cornoid lamella)　起源于表皮凹陷的楔形或柱状的角化不全称为柱状板层(图 2-4)，是汗孔角化症的特点。

(5) 角化不良(dyskeratosis)　表皮或附属器的单个角质形成细胞提前不成熟的角化，称为角化不良。角化不良细胞出现细胞凋亡现象，表现为细胞核固缩、胞质均质红染。表现形式可以是圆体、谷粒、角珠、胶样小体、病毒包涵体等。

①圆体(corps ronds)：见于角质层、颗粒层和棘层上部，这些角化不良细胞表现为中心是一大而圆的均匀的嗜碱性固缩的核，周围绕有透亮的晕，晕的周围有一嗜碱性胞质(图 2-5)。圆体主要见于毛囊角化病(Darier's 病)、疣状角化不良瘤、暂时性棘层松解性皮病(Grover's 病)、局灶性棘层松解性角化不良瘤。

②谷粒(corps grains)：见于角质层内，似角化不全细胞而略大，但核清晰，状如谷粒，周围绕有嗜碱性的也可呈嗜酸性的角化不良的物质或核周晕，见于毛囊角化病(Darier's 病)和疣状角化不良瘤(图 2-6)。

③角珠(keratin pearls)：表现为呈同心圆或层状排列的鳞状细胞团，其中央为逐渐或完全角化的均质红染的凋亡细胞(图 2-7)，常见于高分化的鳞癌。

④胶样小体(colloid body)：也称为

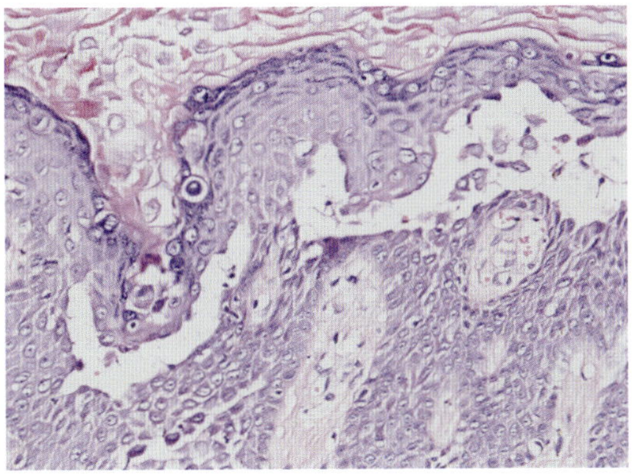

Fig. 2-5　Corps ronds(图 2-5　圆体)

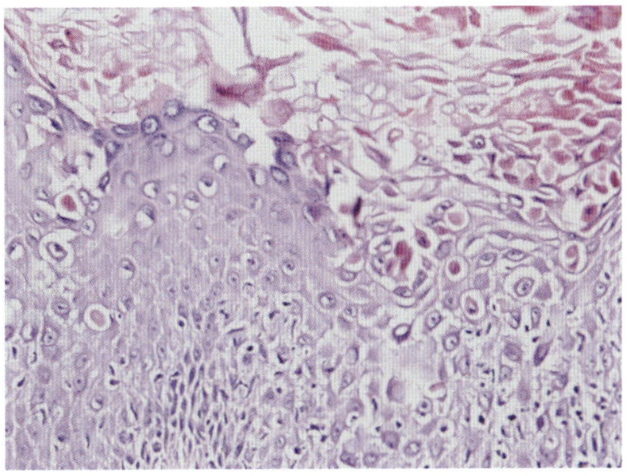

Fig. 2-6　Corps grains(图 2-6　谷粒)

single or multiple bodies that are composed of homogenous, eosinophilic, round, degenerated keratinocytes with or without shrunken nuclei in the basal cell layer, the prickle layer, and the papillary dermis (Fig. 2-8). These bodies are seen primarily in lichen planus, lupus erythematosus, erythema multiforme, and graft-versus-host disease, as well as other conditions.

Civatte 小体。在靠近基底层和棘层或真皮乳头层内出现单个或数个均质红染的、嗜酸性、圆的、变性的角质形成细胞，可有或无皱缩的细胞核(图 2-8)，主要见于扁平苔藓、红斑狼疮、多形红斑、移植物抗宿主病等。

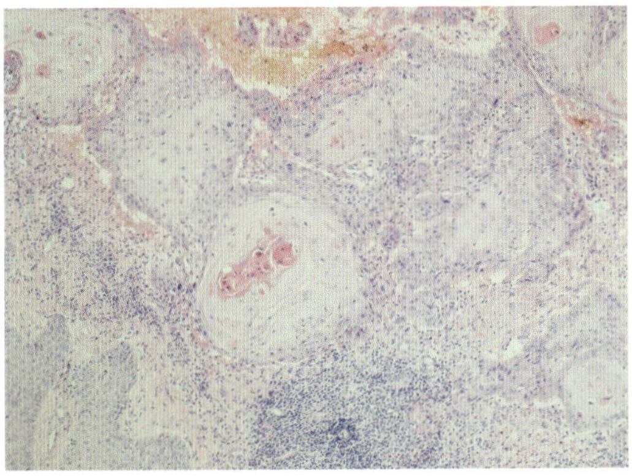

Fig. 2-7　Keratin pearls(图 2-7　角珠)

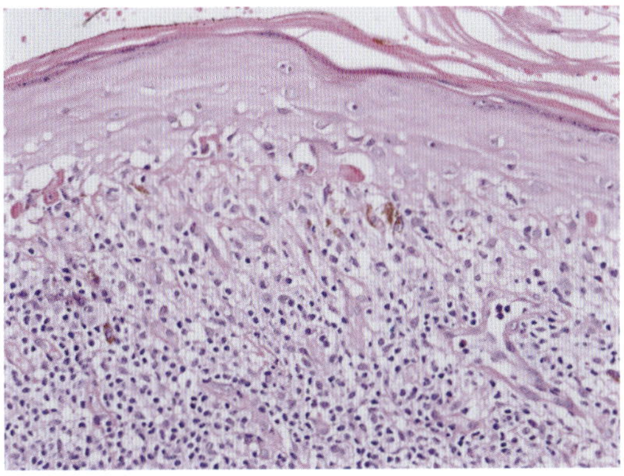

Fig. 2-8　Colloid body(图 2-8　胶样小体)

⑤ Viral inclusion body: these are homogeneous, eosinophilic bodies in virus-infected keratinocytes (Fig. 2-9). They are easily seen in herpes simplex, herpes zoster, molluscum contagiosum, orf, milker's nodules, etc.

⑤ 病毒包涵体(viral inclusion body):病毒在感染的角质形成细胞内形成均质嗜酸性的小体(图 2-9)，常见于单纯疱疹、带状疱疹、传染性软疣、羊痘、挤奶人结节等。

(6) Hypogranulosis: a decreased thickness of the granular layer, frequently accompanied by parakeratosis (Fig. 2-10). It often occurs in psoriasis, ichthyosis vulgaris, etc.

(6) 颗粒层减少(hypogranulosis) 颗粒层数目减少，常伴有角化不全(图 2-10)，常见于银屑病、寻常型鱼鳞病等。

(7) Hypergranulosis: normally the granular layer is composed of 1-3 rows of spinous keratinocytes. An abnormally increased thickness of granular layer is called hypergranulosis, and is usually accompanied by hyperkeratosis (Fig. 2-11). It is found in hyperkeratotic dermatoses such as lichen planus, verruca vulgaris, verruca plana, lichen simplex chronicus, primary cutaneous amyloidosis, etc.

(7) 颗粒层增厚(hypergranulosis) 正常颗粒层通常由 1～3 排细胞组成，如果厚度异常增加，谓之颗粒层增厚(图 2-11)，常与角化过度相伴随，因此见于角化过度性疾病，如扁平苔藓、寻常疣、扁平疣、慢性单纯性苔藓、原发性皮肤淀粉样变等。

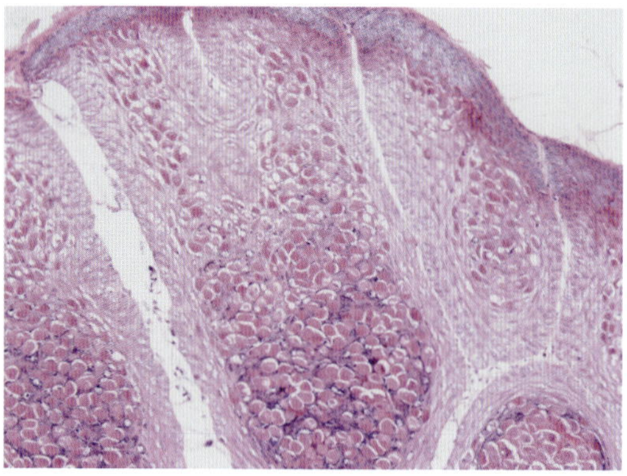

Fig. 2-9　Viral inclusion body(图 2-9　病毒包涵体)

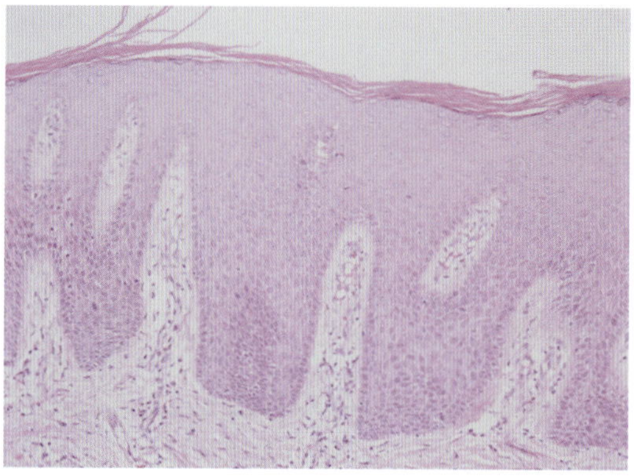

Fig. 2-10　Hypogranulosis(图 2-10　颗粒层减少)

(8) Acanthosis: prominent increased thickness of the prickle cell layer of the epidermis (Fig. 2-12).

(8) 棘层增厚(acanthosis)　棘细胞层的厚度显著增加，称为棘层增厚(图 2-12)。

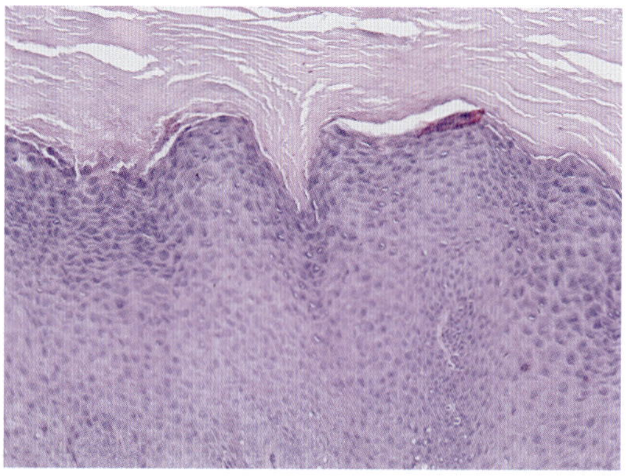

Fig. 2-11　Hypergranulosis(图 2-11　颗粒层增厚)

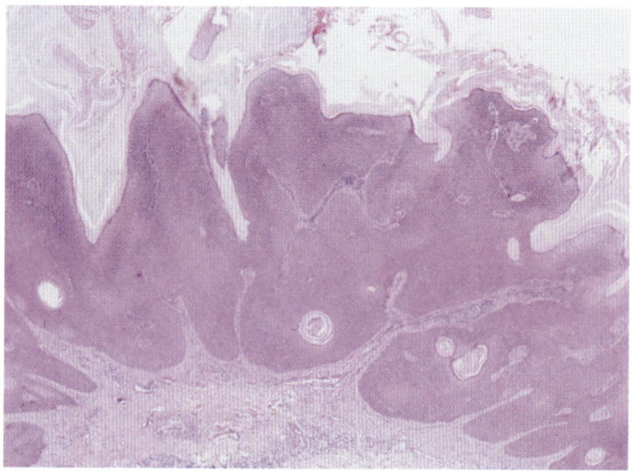

Fig. 2-12　Acanthosis(图 2-12　棘层增厚)

(9) Papillomatosis: the upward projection of the dermal papilla, frequently accompanied by hyperkeratosis and elongation of the rete ridges, resulting in an uneven morphology of the epidermis (Fig. 2-13). These patterns are seen in verruca vulgaris, condyloma accuminatum, seborrheic keratosis, sebaceous nevus, acanthosis nigricans, etc.

(10) Verrucous hyperplasia: a condition coexisting with hyperkeratosis, hypergranulosis, acanthosis, and papillomatosis (Fig. 2-14). It is found in verruca vulgaris, verrucous tuberculosis cutis, verrucous nevus, etc.

(11) Pseudoepitheliomatous hyperplasia: this is the irregular downward growth of the epidermis, with prominent acanthosis, accompanied by elongation and/or widening of the rete ridges that may reach below the level of the sweat glands. It is quite similar under microscopy to squamous cell carcinomas, but the cells are well differentiated and are never atypical in comparison to the latter (Fig. 2-15). This pattern is associated with chronic inflammatory

(9) 乳头瘤样增生(papillomatosis)　真皮乳头不规则向上延伸使得表皮呈凹凸不平的波浪起伏，常伴有角化过度和表皮突向下延伸(图 2-13)，见于寻常疣、尖锐湿疣、脂溢性角化病、皮脂腺痣和黑棘皮病等。

(10) 疣状增生(verrucous hyperplasia)　表皮角化过度、颗粒层增厚、棘层增厚以及乳头瘤样增生同时存在(图 2-14)，见于寻常疣、疣状皮肤结核、疣状痣等。

(11) 假上皮瘤样增生(pseudoepitheliomatous hyperplasia)　表皮不规则地向真皮内增生，棘层显著增厚，表皮突延长增宽，增生的表皮可达汗腺以下水平，颇似鳞癌，但细胞分化良好，无异型性(图 2-15)，见于慢性炎症反应如疣状皮肤结核、深部真菌感染、慢性皮肤溃疡边

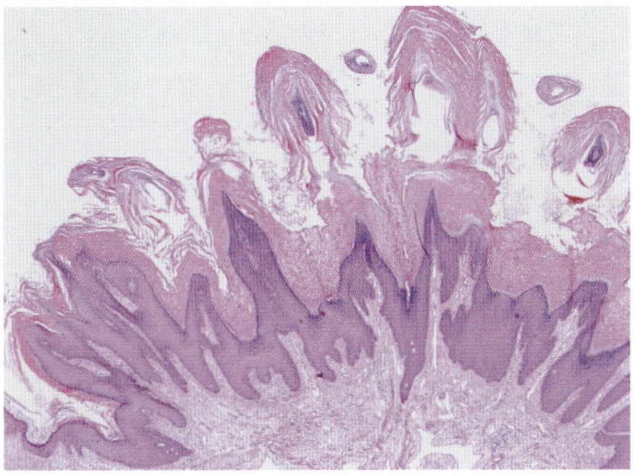

Fig. 2-13　Papillomatosis(图 2-13　乳头瘤样增生)

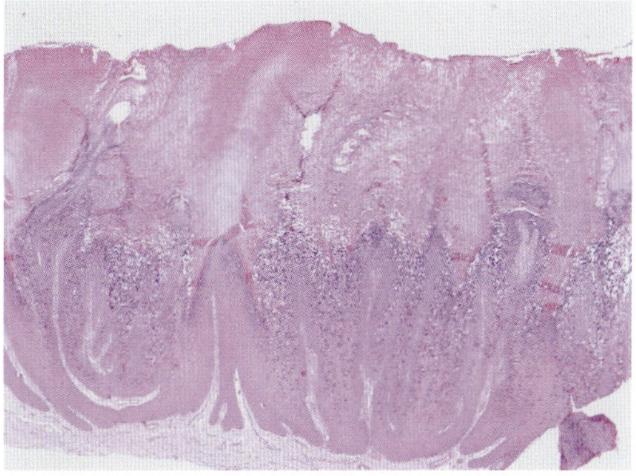

Fig. 2-14　Verrucous hyperplasia(图 2-14　疣状增生)

responses such as verrucous tuberculosis cutis, deep fungal infection, the borders of the chronic cutaneous ulcers, etc.

(12) Epidermal atrophy: the prominent thinning of the epidermis and disappearance of rete ridges give rise to a smudged appearance for the dermoepidermal junction that the epidermis can eventually become a very thin line (Fig. 2-16). It is most common in atrophic dermatoses, lichen sclerosis *et* atrophicus, scleroderma, etc.

缘等。

(12) 表皮萎缩(epidermal atrophy)　表皮明显变薄、表皮突消失致使表皮和真皮交界处波浪起伏的形态消失，甚至形成一条直线(图 2-16)，见于萎缩性皮肤病、硬化性萎缩性苔藓、硬皮病等。

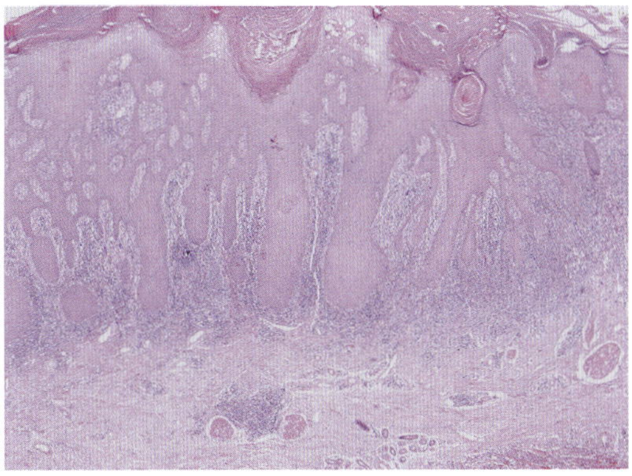

Fig. 2-15　Pseudoepitheliomatous hyperplasia
(图 2-15　假上皮瘤样增生)

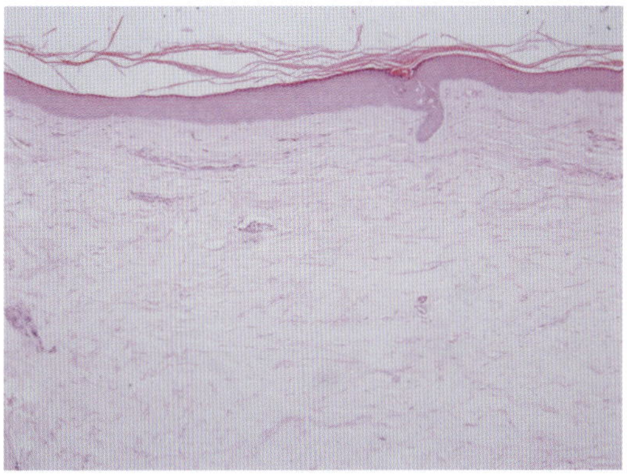

Fig. 2-16　Epidermal atrophy
(图 2-16　表皮萎缩)

(13) Epidermal edema: this includes intercellular and intracellular edema. In most cases, intercellular and intracellular edema coexists. The manifestations vary with the severity of the edema as follows.

① Spongiosis: this condition describes the widening of the intercellular spaces due to intercellular edema, in the course of which the intercellular bridge becomes clear, like a sponge (Fig. 2-17). It is commonly seen in dermatitides such as eczema, contact dermatitis, etc.

②Ballooning degeneration: under this condition the intracellular edema is so conspicuous that the cells are expanding and the intercellular bridges disappear, which result in an acantholysis and the eventual formation of intraepidermal vesicles

(13) 表皮水肿(epidermal edema)　表皮水肿分细胞间和细胞内水肿。通常两者同时存在。根据水肿的程度不同而有以下的表现。

①海绵形成(spongiosis)：细胞间水肿导致细胞彼此的间隙增宽，细胞间桥拉长清晰可见，似海绵状(图 2-17)，常见于皮肤的炎症，特别是湿疹、接触性皮炎等。

②气球变性(ballooning degeneration)：显著的细胞内水肿而使细胞肿胀、细胞间桥消失，导致棘层松解和表皮内水疱、大疱的形成，松解的棘细胞状如圆球飘

or bullae. The acantholytic spinous cells are round like a balloon floating in the vesicles or bullae, and are thus called ballooning cells (Fig. 2-18). These cells are diagnostic for cutaneous viral infections and the process is termed ballooning degeneration.

荡于疱中,貌似气球,称为气球细胞(图 2-18),这一过程称为气球变性。气球变性见于病毒性水疱,具有诊断意义。

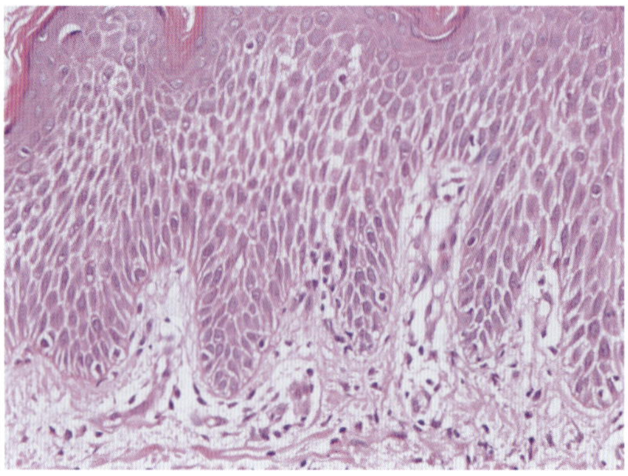

Fig. 2-17 Spongiosis(图 2-17 海绵形成)

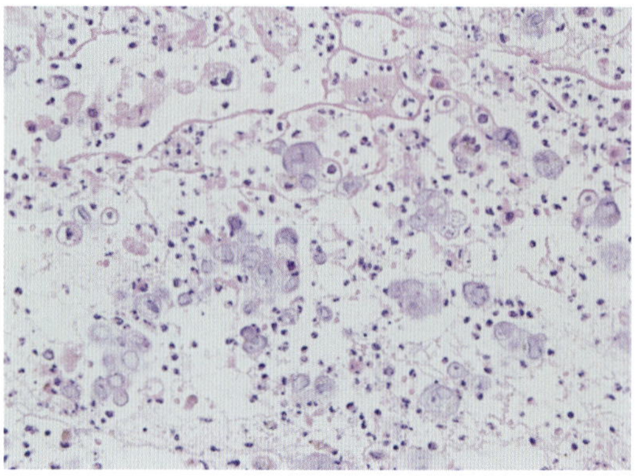

Fig. 2-18 Ballooning degeneration(图 2-18 气球变性)

③ Reticular degeneration: with the increase of intracellular edema, the keratinocytes eventually break down to form a multilocular blister, in which the remnants of cell membrane that survive partial rupture become the septate of a set of blisters, giving rise to a weblike appearance (Fig. 2-19). This phenomenon can be seen in eczema, irritant contact dermatitis, erythema multiforme, viral infections, etc.

(14) Granular degeneration: this is also called epidermolytic hyperkeratosis, and is characterized by the accumulation of vacuolated cells containing basophilic keratohyaline granules in the cytoplasm of the granular and suprabasal cell layers, usually accompanied by hyperkeratosis and acanthosis (Fig. 2-20). It is typically seen in congenital bullous ichthyosiform erythroderma (epidermatolytic hyperkeratotic ichthyosis), epidermolytic palmoplantar keratoderma, and systemic epidermal nevus.

③网状变性(reticular degeneration):严重的细胞内水肿使角质形成细胞破裂,但部分细胞膜依然存留,形成多房性水疱,房间隔由毗邻残留的细胞壁构成,呈网状,此种情况称为网状变性(图 2-19),见于湿疹、刺激性接触性皮炎、多形红斑和病毒感染等。

(14) 颗粒变性(granular degeneration) 又称为表皮松解性角化过度,在颗粒层和基底层上的棘层内有大量含有嗜碱性的透明角质颗粒、胞质空淡的细胞,常伴有角化过度和棘层增厚(图 2-20)。特征性地见于先天性大疱性鱼鳞病样红皮病(表皮松解性角化过度性鱼鳞病)、表皮松解性掌跖角皮症、系统性表皮痣。

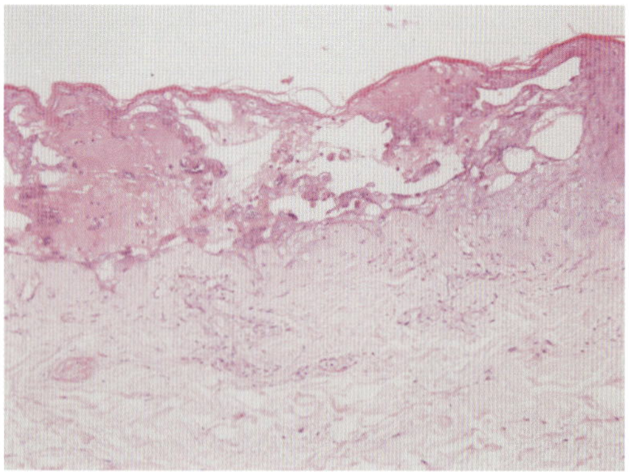

Fig. 2-19 Reticular degeneration(图 2-19 网状变性)

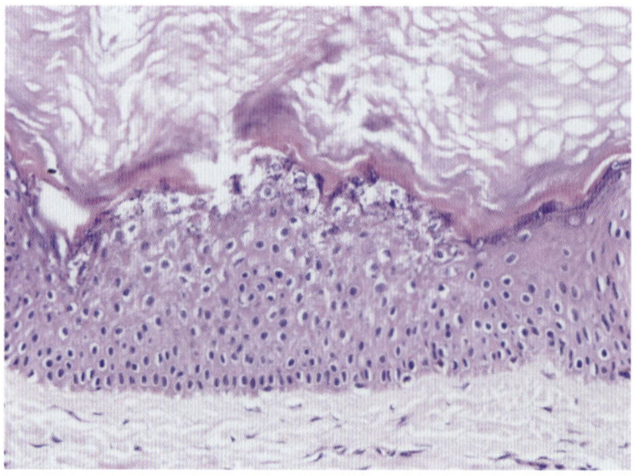

Fig. 2-20 Granular degeneration(图 2-20 颗粒变性)

(15) Koilocyte: koilocytes are found in the granular layer or

(15) 空泡细胞(koilocyte)(或凹空

the upper or middle parts of the spinous layer of the epidermis. These cells are variable sized vacuolated keratinocytes with pale cytoplasm, and possess shrunken nuclei surrounded by perinuclear halos as seen physiologically in lips and vulva mucosa and pathologically in papillomavirus infection such as condyloma acuminatum, verruca plana, etc (Fig. 2-21).

(16) Acantholysis: the formation of intraepidermal clefts, vesicles, or bullae due to dissolution or separation of the desmosomes between spinous cells is called acantholysis. It usually occurs in pemphigus vulgaris, familial benign chronic pemphigus, keratosis follicularis (Darier's disease), etc. Isolated or even clusters of acantholysed spinous cells (which are usually large and round with oval nuclei surrounded by condensed eosinophilic cytoplasm) now float in cavities termed acantholytic cells (Fig. 2-22). This set of circumstances is seen in all types of pemphigus, viral bullae, keratosis follicularis, and actinic keratosis, etc.

细胞）在颗粒层、棘层的中上部有细胞大小不一、胞质比较透明、嗜碱性皱缩的细胞核、核周围有空晕的细胞，称为空泡细胞。生理情况见于口唇、外阴黏膜。病理情况下见于乳头瘤病毒感染，如尖锐湿疣、扁平疣等(图 2-21)。

(16) 棘层松解(acantholysis)　由于棘细胞层的细胞间桥粒溶解或分离，导致在表皮内形成裂隙、水疱或大疱，见于寻常型天疱疮、家族性良性慢性天疱疮、毛囊角化病(Darier's 病)等。松解的棘细胞单个或聚集成簇游离于大疱之中，细胞胞体较大而圆，核呈圆形，其周围常绕以浓缩的嗜酸性胞质，称为棘层松解细胞(图 2-22)，见于各型天疱疮、病毒性大疱、毛囊角化病和日光性角化病等。

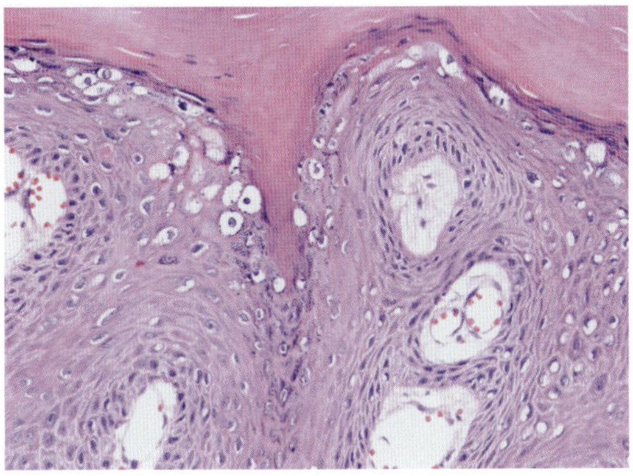

Fig. 2-21　Koilocyte(图 2-21　空泡细胞)

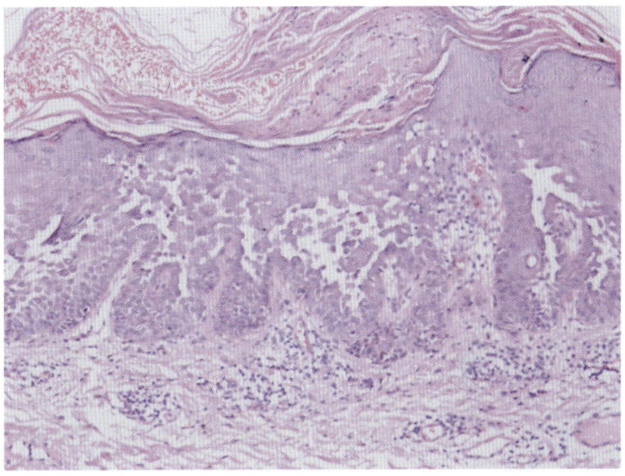

Fig. 2-22　Acantholysis(图 2-22　棘层松解)

(17) Villus: dermal papillae are covered by a single layer of basal cells or a few layers of epidermal cells protruding into the epidermal clefts or cavities formed by acantholysis in the course of certain diseases (Fig. 2-23).

(18) Vesicle and bulla: they are fluid-filled cavities. Clinically, a blister less than 1 cm in diameter is referred to as a vesicle, whereas those with diameters greater than 1 cm are denoted as bullae. Pathologically, these are further categorized as intraepidermal (Fig. 2-24) or subepidermal (Fig. 2-25) bullae, according to the respective location of the bullae. Intraepidermal bullae may be caused by acantholysis as seen in pemphigus, keratosis follicularis, familial benign chronic pemphigus, viral infection, allergic dermatoses (e. g., contact dermatitis), erythema multiforme, toxic bullous epidermolysis, etc. Subepidermal bullae are commonly seen in bullous pemphigoid, dermatitis herpetiformis, epidermolysis bullosa, bullous systemic lupus

(17) 绒毛(villus)　真皮乳头上覆盖一层基底细胞或几层表皮细胞，其呈指状突出到疾病过程中因棘层松解而形成的裂隙或大疱内，称为绒毛(图 2-23)。

(18) 水疱(vesicle)和大疱(bulla)　含有液体的空腔，临床上将疱的直径小于 1 cm 者称为水疱，而大于 1 cm 者称为大疱。病理上将位于表皮内和表皮下的疱分别称之为表皮内疱(图 2-24)和表皮下疱(图 2-25)。表皮内疱可因棘层松解所致如天疱疮、毛囊角化病、家族性良性慢性天疱疮、疱疹病毒感染、变态反应性皮肤病如接触性皮炎、多形红斑、中毒大疱性表皮松解症等。表皮下疱常见于类天疱疮、疱疹样皮炎、大疱性表皮松解症、大疱性系统性红斑狼疮、线状 IgA 大

erythematosus, linear IgA bullous dermatosis, etc.

疱性皮病等。

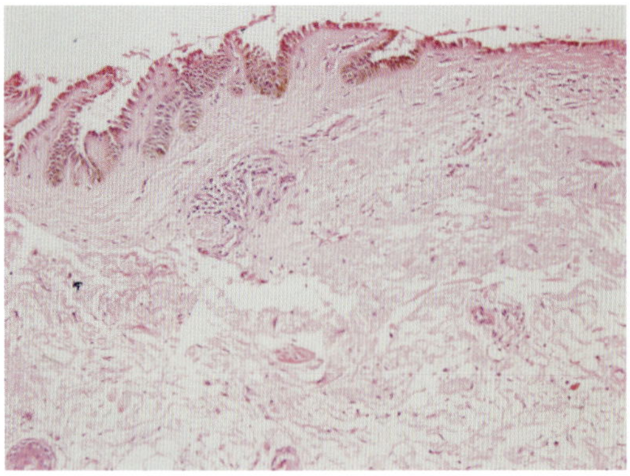

Fig. 2-23　Villus(图 2-23　绒毛)

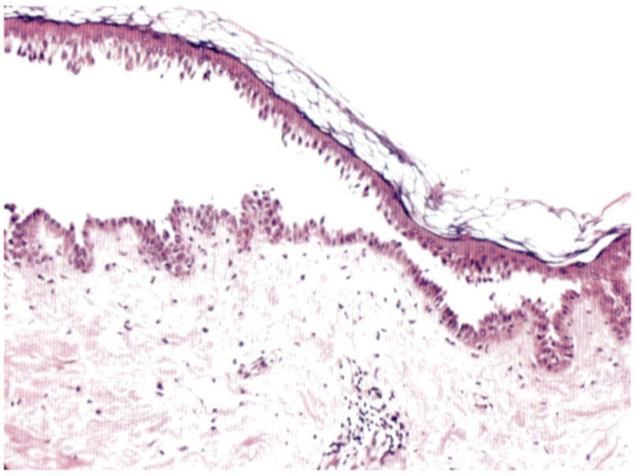

Fig. 2-24　An intraepidermal bulla(图 2-24　表皮内疱)

(19) Munro's microabscess: aggregation of neutrophils in the parakeratotic *stratum corneum* (Fig. 2-26). It is characteristic of psoriasis vulgaris. However, it is also seen in impetigo, Reiter's syndrome, and seborrheic dermatitis.

(19) Munro 微脓肿(Munro's microabscess)　位于角质层的角化不全区域内，由中性粒细胞聚集而成(图 2-26)，是寻常型银屑病的特点，但也见于脓疱疮、Reiter 综合征和脂溢性皮炎。

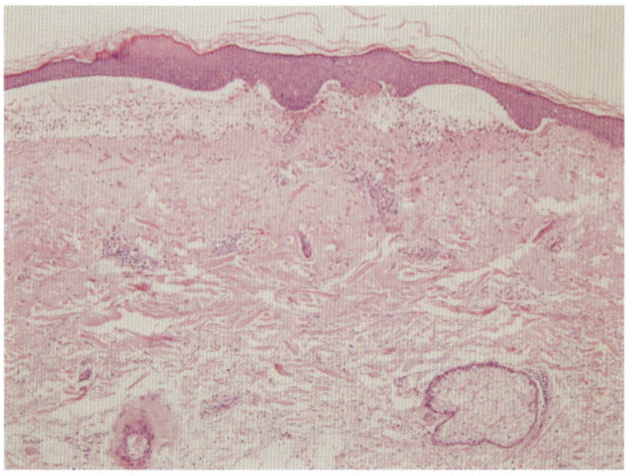

Fig. 2-25　A subepidermal bulla(图 2-25　表皮下疱)

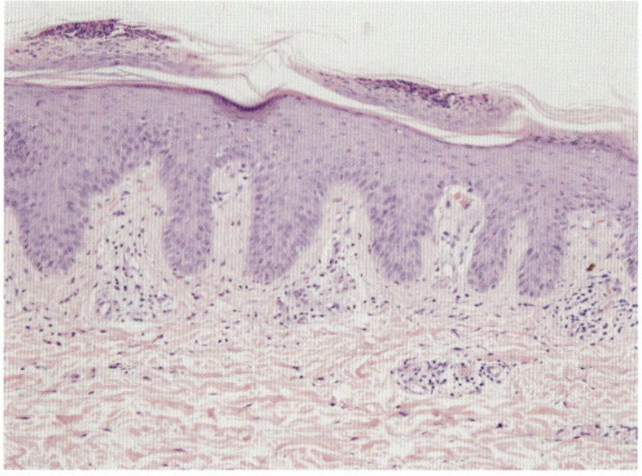

Fig. 2-26　Munro's microabscess(图 2-26　Munro 微脓肿)

(20) Kogoj spongiotic abscess: aggregation of neutrophils in the sponge-like areas of the granular layer and/or in the upper parts of the spinous layer (Fig. 2-27). It is seen in pustular psoriasis, palmoplantar pustulosis, impetigo herpetiformis, and Reiter's syndrome.

(20) Kogoj 海绵状脓肿(Kogoj spongiotic abscess)　在颗粒层和/或棘细胞层上部的海绵形成区的网络中，有中性粒细胞的聚集(图 2-27)，见于脓疱型银屑病、掌跖脓疱病、疱疹样脓疱病、Reiter 综合征。

(21) Pautrier's microabscess: clusters of atypical lymphocytes in the spinous layer, usually surrounded by a clear space, as seen in mycosis fungoides (Fig. 2-28).

(21) Pautrier 微脓肿(Pautrier's microabscess)　在棘细胞层内有异型的淋巴细胞聚集，其周围常有透亮区(图 2-28)，见于蕈样肉芽肿。

(22) Liquefaction degeneration of basal cell layer: also called vacuolar degeneration or hydropic degeneration. It manifests as the formation of vacuoles or spaces beneath the basal cell layer due to the degeneration of the basal cells, which leads to the disappearance of the basal cell layer. As a result, the epidermis contacts the dermis

(22) 基底细胞液化变性(liquefaction degeneration of basal cell layer)　也称为空泡变性或水变性，基底细胞变性在基底层下形成空泡或空隙，基底层完全消失，使表皮和真皮直接接触，二者的界限

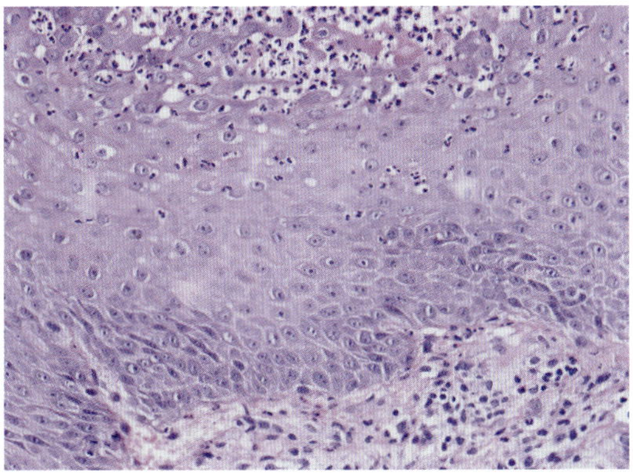

Fig. 2-27 Kogoj spongiotic abscess
(图 2-27 Kogoj 海绵状脓肿)

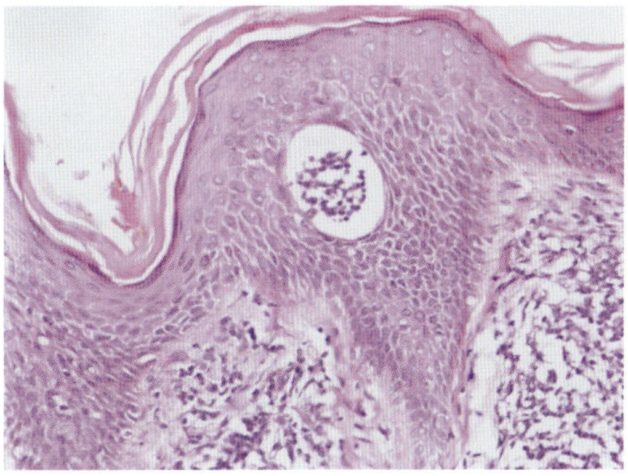

Fig. 2-28 Pautrier's microabscess
(图 2-28 Pautrier 微脓肿)

directly and the dermo-epidermal junction is ill-defined. Finally, the subepidermal clefts or bullae are formed, frequently accompanied by perfusion of melanin into the dermis (Fig. 2-29). It is found in quite a few inflammatory dermatoses that possess interface changes such as lichen planus, lichen striatus, lichen nitidus, lichen sclerosus *et* atrophicus, lupus erythematosus, dermatomyositis, erythema multiforme, fixed drug eruption, primary cutaneous amyloidosis, etc.

模糊，甚至导致表皮下裂隙或大疱，常伴有黑素游离于真皮(图2-29)，见于许多具有界面改变的炎症性皮肤病，如扁平苔藓、线状苔藓、光泽苔藓、硬化性萎缩性苔藓、红斑狼疮、皮肌炎、多形红斑、固定型药疹、原发性皮肤淀粉样变等。

(23) Hyperpigmentation: a melanin increase in the basal cell layer (Fig. 2-30). It is seen in seborrheic keratosis, dermatofibroma, acanthosis nigricans, Addison's disease, post-inflammatory hyperpigmentation, etc.

(23) 色素增加(hyperpigmentation)

表皮基底层黑色素增多(图 2-30)，见于脂溢性角化病、皮肤纤维瘤、黑棘皮病、阿狄森病和炎症后色素沉着等。

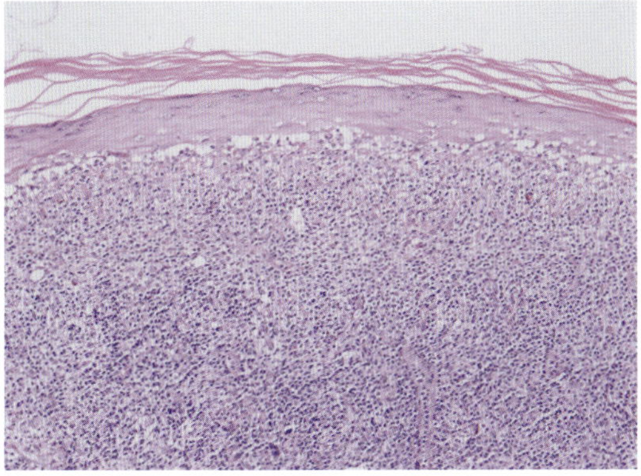

Fig. 2-29 Liquefaction degeneration of basal cell layer
(图 2-29 基底细胞液化变性)

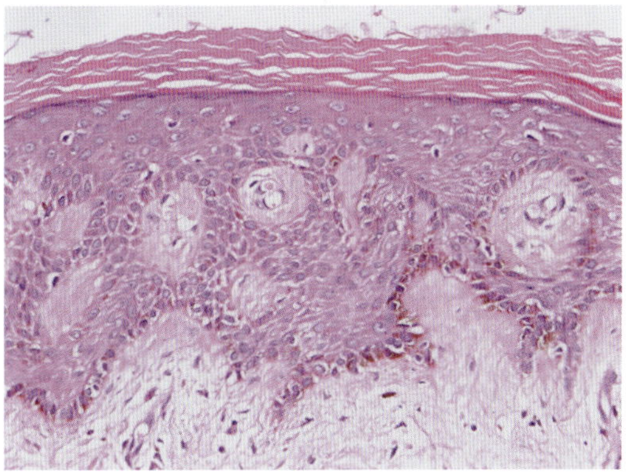

Fig. 2-30 Hyperpigmentation
(图 2-30 色素增加)

(24) Hypopigmentation: decreased or absence of melanin in the basal cell layer, such as in vitiligo.

(24) 色素减少(hypopigmentation)

基底层内色素减少或缺如，见于白癜风。

(25) Pigment incontinence: this is caused by damage to the basal cell layer which results in the deposition of melanin in the superficial dermis. The melanin is phagocytosed by macrophages or dissociated in the dermis (Fig. 2-31). Cells that have phagocytosed melanin are called melanophages. Pigment incontinence occurs in incontinentia pigmenti, lichen planus, lupus erythematosus, fixed

(25) 色素失禁(pigment incontinence)

在病理过程中，基底细胞受损，导致黑素逸聚在真皮的浅层，或被吞噬细胞吞噬，或游离在组织间隙中，这种色素游离的现象，称为色素失禁(图2-31)。吞噬了黑素的吞噬细胞称为噬黑素细胞，见于

drug eruption, etc.

色素失禁症、扁平苔藓、红斑狼疮、固定型药物疹等。

(26) Retraction space: the clefts commonly seen between the tumor mass of basal cell carcinoma and the surrounding interstitial tissue caused by the disappearance of the mucinous protein during sample preparation (Fig. 2-32).

(26) 收缩间隙(retraction space) 通常指基底细胞癌的肿瘤团块与其周围的间质之间由于其间的黏蛋白在切片的制作过程中脱失形成的裂隙(图 2-32)。

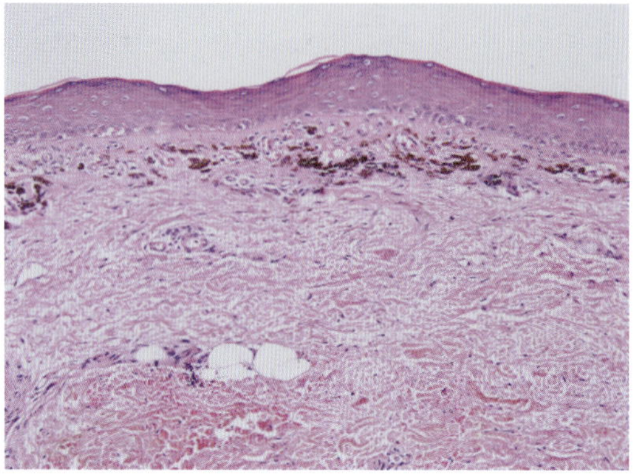

Fig. 2-31 Pigment incontinence(图 2-31 色素失禁)

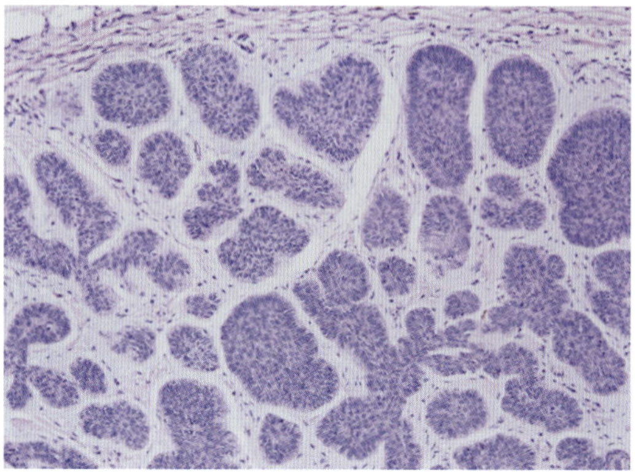

Fig. 2-32 Retraction space(图 2-32 收缩间隙)

(27) Anaplasia: refers to the loss of differentiation in normal cells and is characteristic of tumor cells. The anaplastic cells are characterized by large, polymorphic nuclei with hyperchromasia and distinctly atypical mitoses (Fig. 2-7). It occurs in malignant tumors.

(27) 间变(anaplasia) 间变即去分化,是肿瘤细胞的异型表现,细胞常具有大的、深染、多形性的核,且伴有异型核分裂现象(图 2-7),见于恶性肿瘤。

(28) Squamous eddies: these consist of keratinocytes arranged in concentric circles or whorls. Those keratinocytes possess eosinophilic and pale cytoplasm without dyskeratotic or atypical mitoses (Fig. 2-33). These eddies can be found in inverted follicular keratosis, irritating seborrheic keratosis and squamous cell carcinoma.

(28) 鳞状涡(squamous eddies) 角质形成细胞呈同心圆状排列或呈漩涡状,中央的细胞胞质淡红染、透明,但无角化不良或不典型性细胞(图 2-33),见于倒置性毛囊角化病、刺激性脂溢性角化病和鳞状细胞癌。

(29) Granulomas and naked tubercles: nodular proliferations arising from variable proportions of epithelioid cells, histiocytes, and multinucleated giant cells that also contain some lymphocytes, neutrophils, eosinophils, and plasma cells (Fig. 2-34). They can be classified as infectious granulomas in tuberculosis, leprosy, deep fungi infection, etc and also as noninfectious granulomas in sarcoidosis, granuloma annulare, necrobiosis lipoidica, foreign body granuloma, etc. A granuloma with few or no lymphocyte infiltrations or surrounded by fibrous tissues is called a naked tubercle as seen in sarcoidosis (Fig. 2-35).

(29) 肉芽肿(granuloma)及裸结节(naked tubercle) 由上皮样细胞、组织细胞和多核巨细胞组成的结节状增生,其各自的比例多少不同,可伴有淋巴细胞、中性粒细胞、嗜酸性粒细胞及浆细胞(图 2-34)。可分为感染性肉芽肿(见于结核病、麻风病、深部真菌病等)和非感染性肉芽肿(见于结节病、环状肉芽肿、类脂质渐进性坏死、异物肉芽肿等)。肉芽肿周边很少或无淋巴细胞浸润,有时有纤维组织包绕称为裸结节,见于结节病(图2-35)。

(30) Palisading: this usually refers to granulomata, where the degenerated collagen or necrobiotic tissue in the central area is surrounded by a mass of cells in a palisade arrangement. These cells are epithelioid cells, histiocytes, lymphocytes, and giant cells (Fig.

(30) 栅栏状(palisading) 通常指肉芽肿,其中央为变性的胶原或渐进性坏死组织,周边由呈栅栏状排列的上皮样细胞、组织细胞、淋巴细胞和巨细胞所

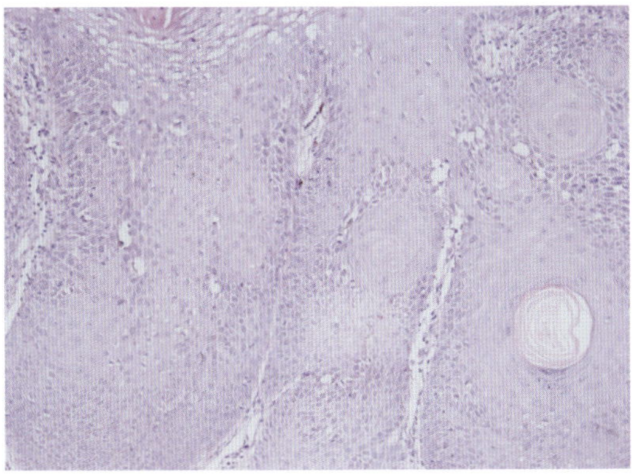

Fig. 2-33　Squamous eddies(图 2-33　鳞状涡)

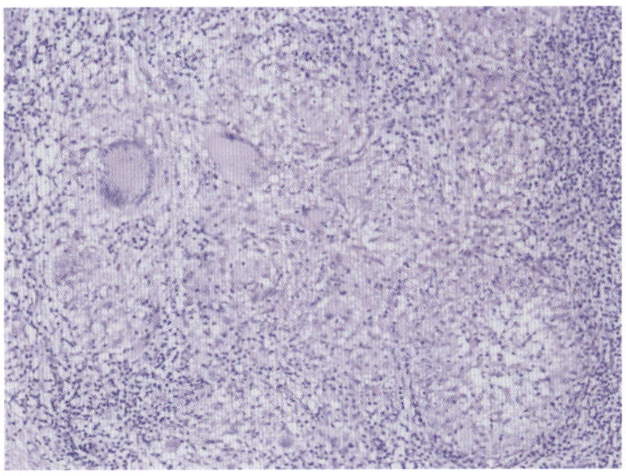

Fig. 2-34　Granuloma(图 2-34　肉芽肿)

2-36). The typical palisading granuloma is seen in granuloma annulare, necrobiosis lipoidica, rheumatoid nodule, and gout.

围绕(图 2-36)。典型的栅栏状肉芽肿见于环状肉芽肿、类脂质渐进性坏死、类风湿结节和痛风。

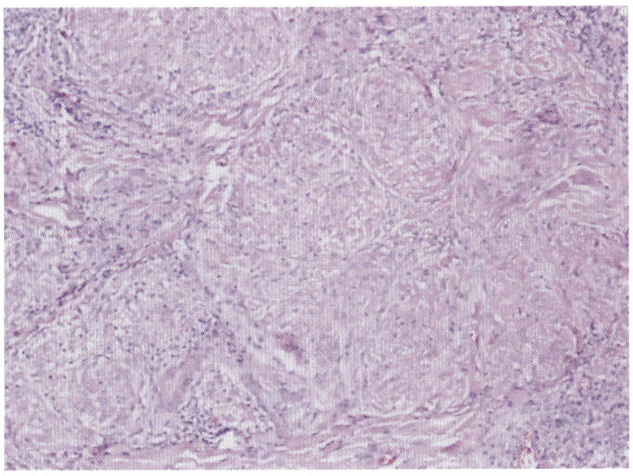

Fig. 2-35　Naked tubercle(图 2-35　裸结节)

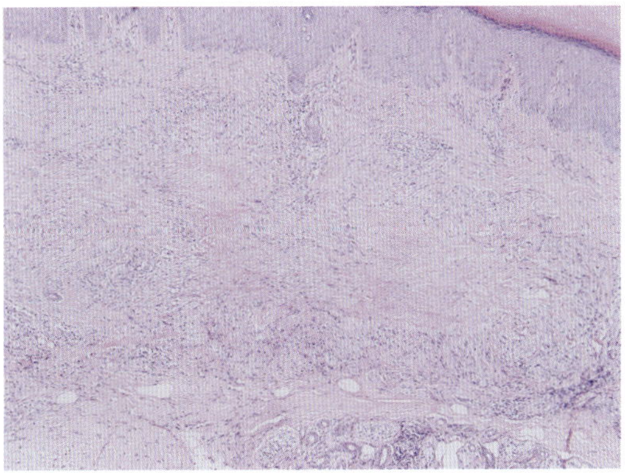

Fig. 2-36　Palisading(图 2-36　栅栏状)

(31) Caseous necrosis: this is a special coagulative necrosis in which the original structures in the necrotic tissue are completely destroyed, leaving pink-colored amorphous granular materials under HE staining (Fig. 2-37). It is commonly seen in tuberculosis cutis, late syphilis, and in the nerve damage associated with tuberous leprosy.

(32) Necrobiosis: in contrast to caseous necrosis, the tissue necrosis is incomplete. The outline of the normal structure remains but resists staining. Degenerate tissue may be surrounded by palisading arrangements of cells composed of histiocytes, fibroblasts, foreign giant cells, or epithelioid cells. This condition is seen in granuloma annulare (Fig. 2-36), necrobiosis lipoidica (Fig. 2-38), rheumatoid nodule, etc.

(33) Homogenization: the dermal connective tissues manifest as an amorphous homogenous eosinophilic appearance (Fig. 2-39). It is seen in lichen sclerosus *et* atrophicus, and in scleroderma.

(31) 干酪样坏死(caseous necrosis)　一种特殊的凝固性坏死，坏死组织被完全破坏而失去其原有结构形成无定形的颗粒状物质，在 HE 切片中呈淡红色(图 2-37)，常见于皮肤结核、晚期梅毒和结核样型麻风的神经损害。

(32) 渐进性坏死(necrobiosis)　由于组织坏死不完全失去其正常的着色但保留正常结构的轮廓，周边可见组织细胞、成纤维细胞、异物巨细胞或上皮样细胞呈栅状围绕，见于环状肉芽肿(图 2-36)、类脂质渐进性坏死(图 2-38)、类风湿结节等。

(33) 均质化(homogenization)　真皮结缔组织的一种无定形均质一致的变化(图 2-39)，此种变化的组织染色嗜酸性，表现为暗淡不透光，见于硬化性萎缩性苔藓和硬皮病。

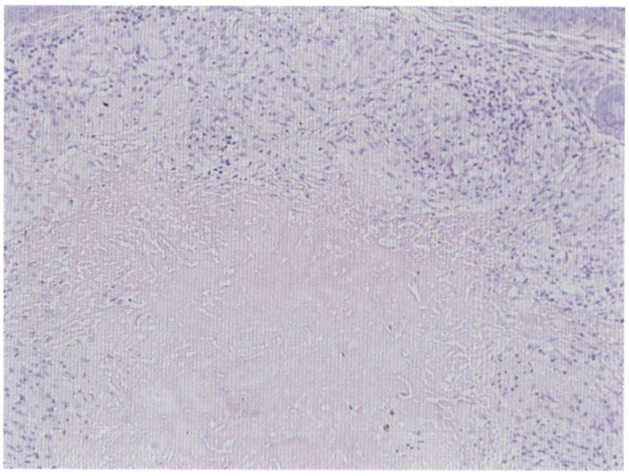

Fig. 2-37 Caseous necrosis(图 2-37 干酪样坏死)

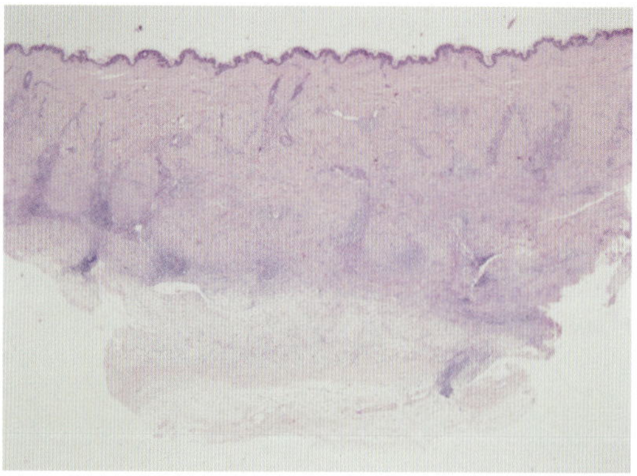

Fig. 2-38 Necrobiosis lipoidica(图 2-38 类脂质渐进性坏死)

(34) Hyaline degeneration: this condition manifests as a glassy semi-translucent material found in tissues or in cells. This hyaline material appears as a light red homogenous refringent substance when stained with hematoxylin-eosin (HE), as in the case of keloid (Fig. 2-40). In some cases, such hyalines can be found in plasma cells, for example in leprosy and rhinoscleroma, where they are known as Russell bodies.

(34) 玻璃样变性(hyaline degeneration)(或透明变性) 在组织内或细胞内出现玻璃样半透明的均质性物质,即所谓透明蛋白。在 HE 染色时呈均一淡红色,具有折光性,见于瘢痕疙瘩(图 2-40)。如发生于浆细胞内,则称为 Russell 小体(Russell bodies),见于麻风、鼻硬结病。

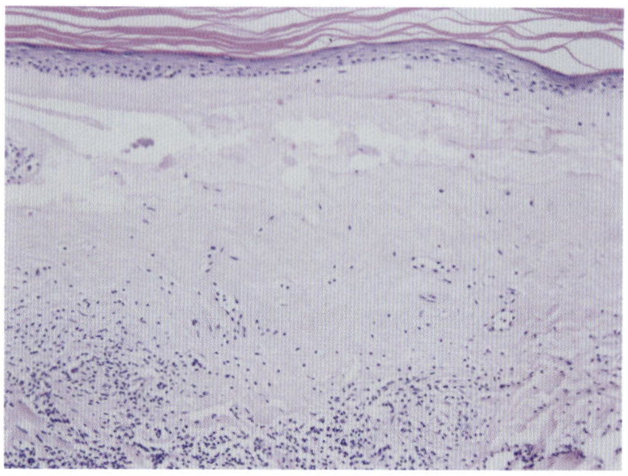

Fig. 2-39 Homogenization(图 2-39 均质化)

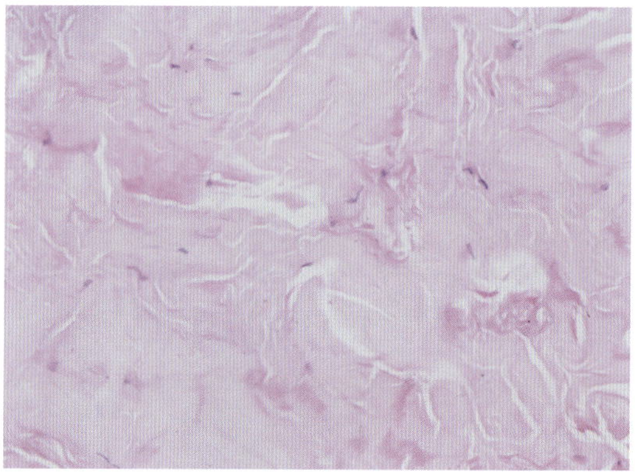

Fig. 2-40 Hyaline degeneration(图 2-40 玻璃样变性)

(35) Fibrinoid degeneration: in this case the fibrinoid substance is widespread among the degenerated collogenous fibers or around the damaged vessel walls, which manifests as refringent, eosinophilic, and homogenous appearance, as seen in rheumatoid nodules, lupus erythematosus, and leukocytoclastic vasculitis (Fig. 2-41).

(36) Degeneration of elastic fibers: this refers to the fractured, twisted, basophilic appearance of the elastic fibers (Fig. 2-42). It is seen in pseudoxanthoma elasticum, acrokeratoelastoidosis, etc.

(37) Basophilic degeneration: the normal eosinophilic appearance of the collagens in the superficial dermis is replaced with gray-blue

(35) 纤维蛋白样变性(fibrinoid degeneration) 纤维蛋白沉积在通常伴有变性改变的胶原纤维或受损伤的血管壁,使其呈现折光嗜酸性均质的外观,称为纤维蛋白样变性,见于类风湿结节、红斑狼疮、白细胞碎裂性血管炎(图 2-41)。

(36) 弹力纤维变性(degeneration of elastic fibers) 通常需弹力纤维染色方能证实,显示弹力纤维断裂、破裂,聚集成团或粗细不均呈卷曲状,呈嗜碱性变(图 2-42),见于弹力纤维性假黄瘤、肢端角化性类弹力纤维病等。

(37) 嗜碱性变性(basophilic degeneration) 真皮浅层胶原纤维失去其正

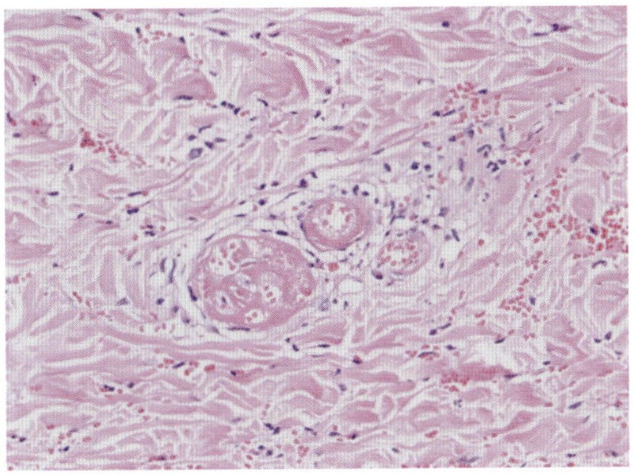

Fig. 2-41　Fibrinoid degeneration
(图 2-41　纤维蛋白样变性)

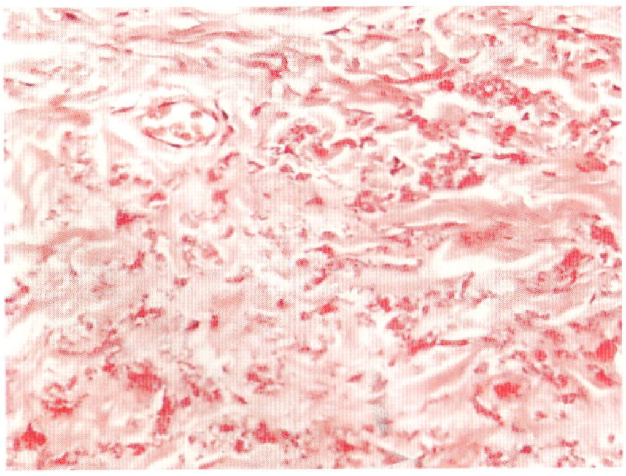

Fig. 2-42　Degeneration of elastic fibers
(图 2-42　弹力纤维变性)

amorphous or granular materials (Fig. 2-43). It is seen in actinic keratosis, discoid lupus erythematosus, solar elastoidosis, etc.

常特点而呈淡蓝灰色无定形或颗粒状(图 2-43),见于日光性角化病、盘状红斑狼疮、日光性弹性纤维病等。

(38) Colloid degeneration: this appears as a mass of weak eosinophilic, sometimes basophilic, amorphous, homogenous colloidal substances with prominent peripheral clefts, in which the remnants of nuclei can sometimes be seen (Fig. 2-44). It is found in colloid milium, etc.

(38) 胶样变性(colloid degeneration)　组织中有弱嗜酸性,有时轻度嗜碱性,无结构的,均一性胶样物质沉积,周围常有明显的裂隙,并有残留的细胞核(图 2-44),见于胶样粟丘疹等。

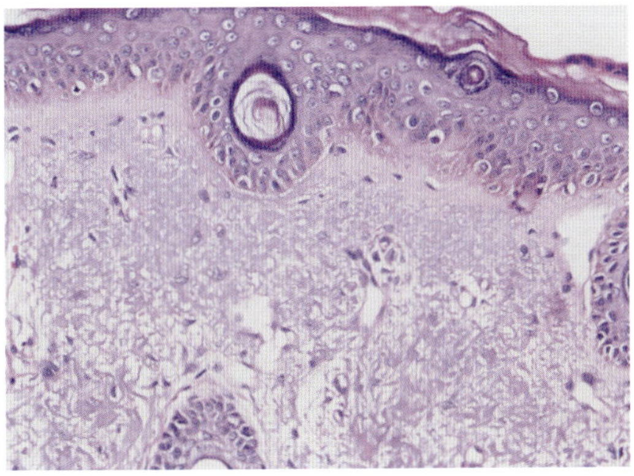

Fig. 2-43　Basophilic degeneration(图 2-43　嗜碱性变性)

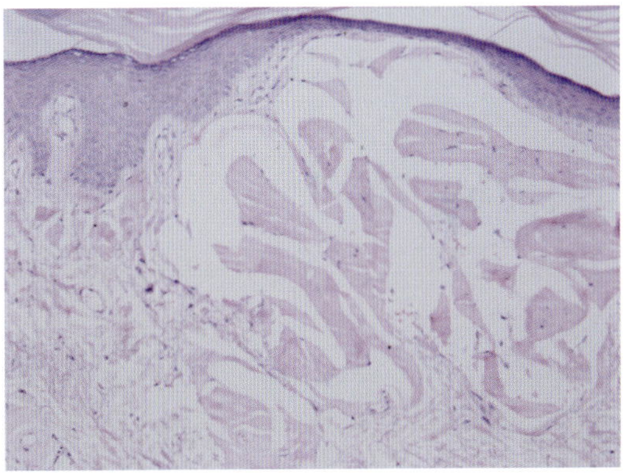

Fig. 2-44　Colloid degeneration(图 2-44　胶样变性)

(39) Amyloid degeneration: this term refers to the deposition of light red, homogenous amyloid substances in the dermal papilla or the walls of small blood vessels. A cleft can always be seen because of the retraction of the amyloid substances during the process of tissue fixation and dehydration. The amyloid substances are metachromasic and purple when stained with crystal violet. They are yellow when stained with Van Gieson. This degeneration is seen in cutaneous amyloidosis (Fig. 2-45).

(39) 淀粉样变性(amyloid degeneration)　真皮乳头内或小血管壁有淡红色、均匀一致的团块即淀粉样物质的沉积,由于固定脱水时淀粉样物质收缩,可发生裂隙,对结晶紫呈异染现象并呈紫红色,Van Gieson 染色呈黄色,见于皮肤淀粉样变(图 2-45)。

(40) Mucinous degeneration: this condition is characterized by the deposition of mucin among the dermal collagens, results in the splitting up of collagen bundles into fibers and also results in the widening of spaces between the fibers. The main components of mucin are acid mucopolysaccharide and proteins. They appear pale

(40) 黏液变性(mucinous degeneration)　在真皮纤维束间有黏液物质聚积,导致胶原纤维束的分隔和间隙增宽,主要成分为酸性黏多糖和蛋白质。HE 染色呈淡蓝色,阿新兰染色呈蓝色(图 2-46),

blue when stained with hematoxylin-eosin (HE) and blue with Asian blue (Fig. 2-46). These occur in pretibial myxedema, lichen myxedematosus, etc.

见于胫前黏液性水肿、黏液水肿性苔藓等。

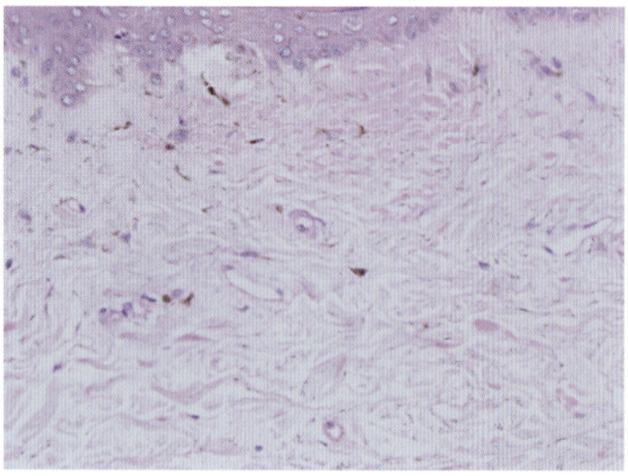

Fig. 2-45　Amyloid degeneration(图 2-45　淀粉样变性)

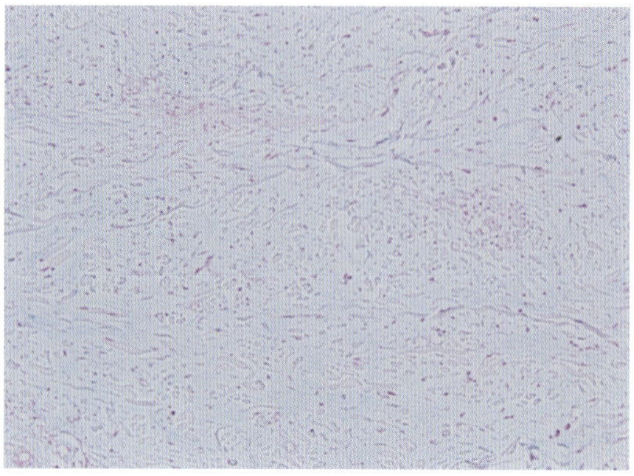

Fig. 2-46　Mucinous degeneration(图 2-46　黏液变性)

(41) Dermal atrophy: the thickness of the dermis is decreased due to attenuation of the collagen and/or elastic fibers. It is frequently accompanied by the atrophy or disappearance of the hair follicles and sebaceous glands. Good examples are macular atrophy and linear atrophy.

(41) 真皮萎缩(dermal atrophy)　整个真皮厚度减少，由于胶原纤维或弹力纤维或二者均减少所致，常伴有毛囊及皮脂腺萎缩或消失，见于斑状萎缩或线状萎缩。

(42) Panniculitis: it refers to the inflammatory cell infiltration, edema, degeneration, or necrosis in the subcutaneous tissue caused by different etiologies. Fibrosis may occur in the late stages of the lesion. The histiocytes that have phagocytosed the lipids, which are released by degenerated or necrotic fat cells, are termed foam cells. The pathologic changes mainly located in the septa of the fat are called septal panniculitis (Fig. 2-47), and is typically seen in erythema nodosum, whereas those mainly in the lobules are named lobular panniculitis (Fig. 2-48) as seen in nodular vasculitis. The term mixed panniculitis may be used when both septa and lobules are involved.

(42) 脂膜炎(panniculitis)　不同原因引起的皮下脂肪组织炎症细胞浸润、水肿、变性或坏死，晚期病变者可发生纤维化，组织细胞吞噬变性坏死的脂肪细胞释放的脂质，称为泡沫细胞。病变以脂肪间隔为主者称为间隔性脂膜炎(septal panniculitis)(图 2-47)，典型代表为结节性红斑；以脂肪小叶内为主者称为小叶性脂膜炎(lobular panniculitis)(图2-48)，如结节性血管炎；二者均累及者称为混合性脂膜炎。

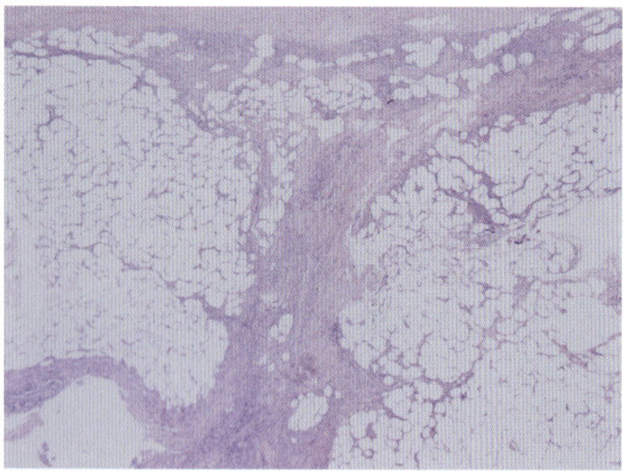

Fig. 2-47　Septal panniculitis(图 2-47　间隔性脂膜炎)

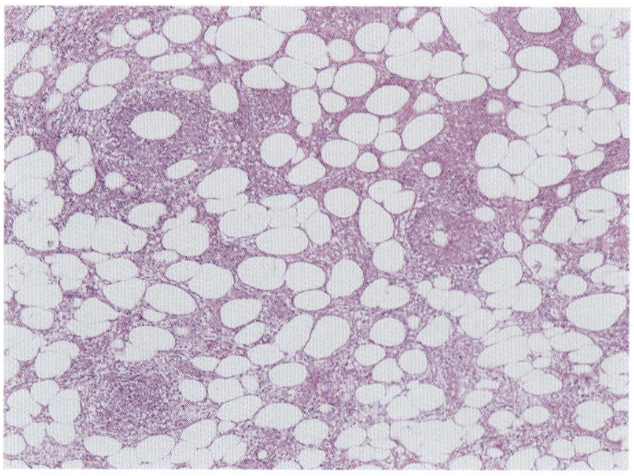

Fig. 2-48　Lobular panniculitis(图 2-48　小叶性脂膜炎)

Chang-zheng HUANG(黄长征), Ming WANG(王明), Bao CHAI(柴宝)

Chapter Three　Symptoms, Signs and Basic Diagnostic Techniques for Dermatoses

In general, the symptoms of skin diseases can be divided into subjective symptoms and objective symptoms (signs). These symptoms form the foundation of dermatologic diagnosis.

【Symptoms】

Subjective symptoms are the "feelings" of the patients, often taking the form of complaints of conditions such as pruritus (itching), pain, burning, formication or numbness. In certain circumstances, there are constitutional reactions such as fever, arthralgia, weight loss, general malaise, etc.

Among all the subjective symptoms related to skin diseases, the most common and distressful one is itching, which is defined in Dorland's Medical Dictionary as an unpleasant cutaneous sensation which provokes the desire to scratch or rub the skin. It can variously be described as prickling, tingling numbness, formication and even "intolerable" feelings. The degree of itching depends on the affected skin regions, and varies with individual patients. This diversity of feelings may somehow reflect the roles of psychological influence and nerve sensation on the subjective symptoms. A large number of skin diseases will provoke itching, including contact dermatitis, eczema, urticaria, drug eruptions, scabies, lichen planus, mycosis fungoides, pediculosis, xerosis, etc.

Besides skin disease, pruritus can be concomitant with underlying conditions such as hepatobiliary abnormalities (especially biliary obstructive disease), severe renal insufficiency, iron-deficiency anemia, endocrine disorders (such as hypothyroidism, diabetes), or internal malignancy (especially lymphoma), etc. Furthermore, certain drugs can make the skin itch; these include antidepressants, belladonna alkaloids, opiates, and oral contraceptives.

The skin can be painful in some skin disorders. Pain is one of the common subjective symptoms. The following medical conditions are possible causes of skin pain: herpes zoster, furuncles, carbuncles, cellulitis, and vasculitis. The phrases often used to describe pain are drilling pain, burning pain, and lancing or radiating pains.

Other subjective symptoms relating to skin disorders are abnormal skin sensations, e. g., hypoesthesia or hyperesthesia. One of the hallmarks of leprosy is a lack of skin sensation.

第三章　皮肤病的症状、体征和基本诊断方法

皮肤病的症状可分为主观症状和客观症状(体征)。患者特有的症状是皮肤病诊断的基础。

【症状】

主观症状即患者的"感觉",多是关于下述情况的主诉,如瘙痒、疼痛、烧灼感、蚁行感、麻木感等。某些患者会出现发热、关节疼痛、体重减轻、乏力等全身症状。

瘙痒是皮肤病最常见和令人苦恼的主观症状。Dorland 医学词典将其定义为"一种产生搔抓或摩擦欲望的不舒服的皮肤感觉"。不同患者对瘙痒的描述不一致,有的是刺痛、麻感或蚁行感,有的是无法忍受的感觉。瘙痒的反应程度也有部位和个体差异,可能与心理状态和主观的神经敏感有关。瘙痒常见于接触性皮炎、湿疹、荨麻疹、药疹、疥疮、扁平苔藓、蕈样霉菌病、虱病、皮肤干燥症等。

某些系统性疾病也可以引起瘙痒,包括肝胆疾病(特别是胆管阻塞性疾病)、重度肾功能不全、缺铁性贫血、内分泌疾病(甲状腺功能低下、糖尿病)和内脏肿瘤(特别是淋巴瘤)等。抗抑郁药、颠茄生物碱、阿片制剂、口服避孕药等药物会引起皮肤瘙痒。

许多皮肤疾病可表现为皮肤疼痛。疼痛是另一种常见的主观症状,常发生在带状疱疹、疖、痈、蜂窝织炎或血管炎。疼痛的性质可以是钻痛、烧灼痛、刀割样痛或放射样疼痛。

其他主观症状有感觉异常,包括感觉减退或感觉过敏。麻风的特点之一就是皮肤感觉丧失。

【Signs】

Signs (or objective symptoms): any changes caused by the skin disorders itself that can be seen or palpated by doctors. They are of paramount importance for diagnosis since the characterized signs are more or less restricted to certain diseases. The skin areas showing these signs are usually called lesions, which can be classified as primary or secondary lesions. The primary lesions are the "original" lesion(s), and identification of such lesions is the most important aspect of dermatologic examination. However, these lesions may continue to develop or be modified by aggravating trauma, extensive scratching, or other external factors, thereby producing secondary lesions.

(1) Primary lesions: the characteristic primary lesions result from the initial pathologic changes, and are the ones with true diagnostic value.

① Macule: this is simply a flat circumscribed change in the color or texture of the skin, without elevation or depression. The term is usually applied to the lesions of relatively small size, up to 1 cm; larger than this, the changes are referred to as patches. Macules may manifest in a variety of ways as: erythema as seen in drug eruptions (Fig. 3-1), hypopigmented macules as is the case for pityriasis versicolor (Fig. 3-2), hyperpigmented macules as seen in fixed drug eruptions (Fig. 3-3), depigmented macules in vitiligo (Fig. 3-4), petechia in allergic purpura (Fig. 3-5), or ecchymosis in allergic cutaneous vasculitis (Fig. 3-6), etc.

Purpura is usually considered to be one type of macules resulting from the extravasation of the red blood cells into skin or mucous membranes, resulting from either coagulopathy or capillary dysfunction. When the hemorrhagic area is greater than 2 mm in diameter, it is referred to as ecchymosis (Fig. 3-6). Petechia is a hemorrhagic macule less than 2 mm in diameter (Fig. 3-5).

【体征】

体征(或客观症状)是皮肤病本身导致的、医师可见或触摸到的改变。由于这些改变或多或少仅限于某些特定的皮肤病,因而对诊断至关重要。皮肤发病部位的这些改变也称为皮损。皮损有原发性和继发性两种类型,原发性损害是疾病的初发损害,辨别原发性损害是诊断皮肤病的重要依据;继发性损害是由原发性损害演变而来,或因损伤、过度搔抓、外在因素引起。

(1) 原发性损害(primary lesions)皮肤病理变化直接形成的损害,具有诊断价值。

①斑疹(macule):斑疹只是皮肤颜色或表面质地的改变,皮面不隆起或凹陷。直径通常小于 1 cm。斑片(patch)是指直径大于 1 cm 的斑疹。斑疹有多种形式,包括红斑如药疹(图 3-1)、色素减退斑如花斑糠疹(图 3-2)、色素沉着斑如固定型药疹(图 3-3)、色素脱失斑如白癜风(图 3-4)、瘀点如过敏性紫癜(图 3-5)、瘀斑如变应性皮肤血管炎(图 3-6)等。

紫癜也是斑疹的一种类型,是红细胞外溢于血管到皮肤或黏膜所致。紫癜意味着凝血障碍或毛细血管功能异常。大面积紫癜(直径大于 2 mm)称为瘀斑(图 3-6),小于 2 mm 者为瘀点(图 3-5)。

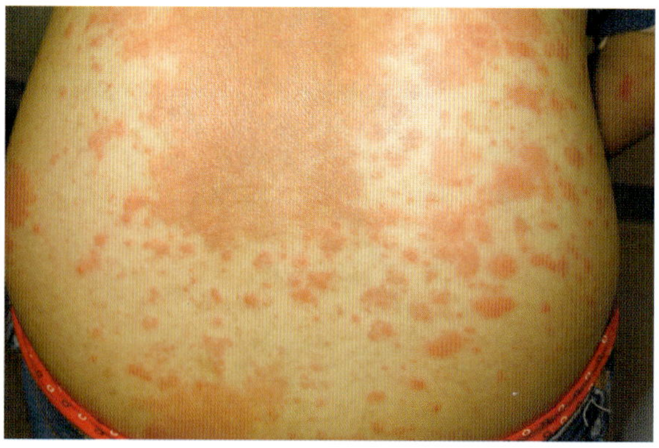

Fig. 3-1　Erythema(图 3-1　红斑)

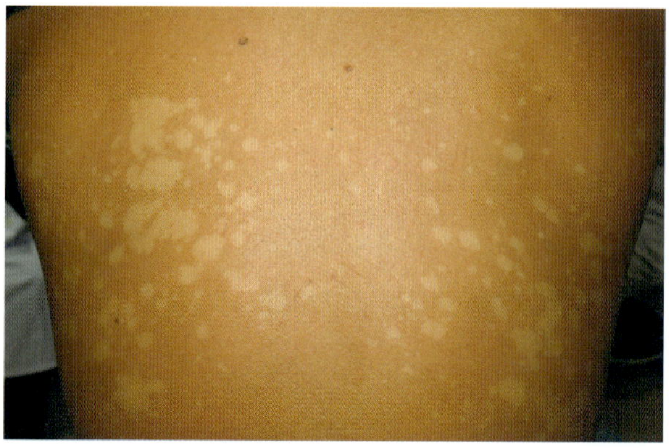

Fig. 3-2　Hypopigmented macule(图 3-2　色素减退斑)

② Papules: these are solid, palpable, and elevated lesions less

②丘疹(papules):可触及的直径小

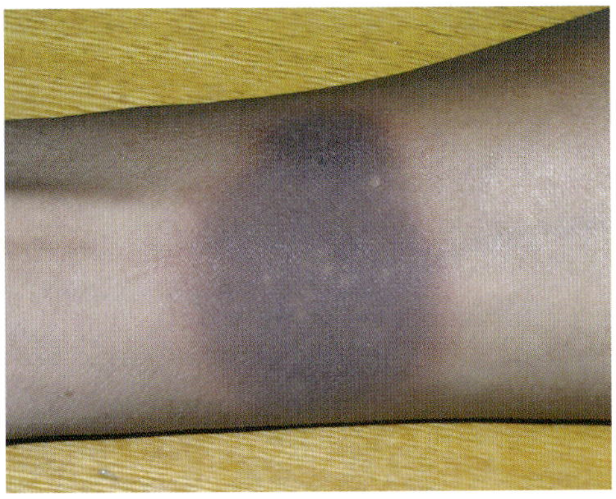

Fig. 3-3　Hyperpigmented macule(图 3-3　色素沉着斑)

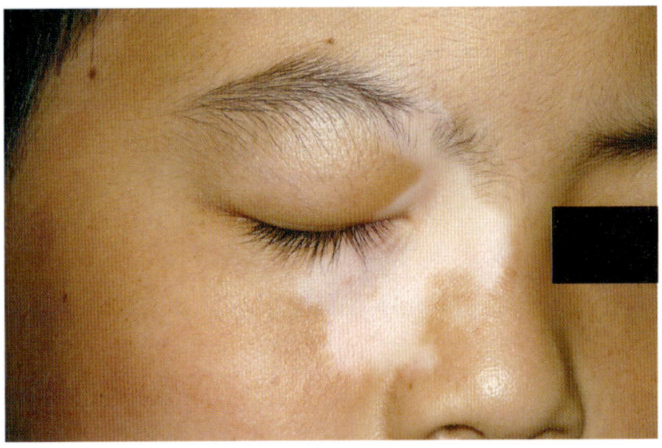

Fig. 3-4　Depigmented macule(图 3-4　色素脱失斑)

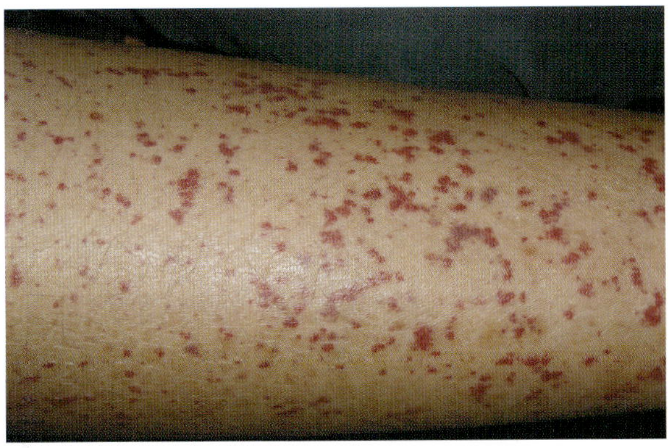

Fig. 3-5　Petechia(图 3-5　瘀点)

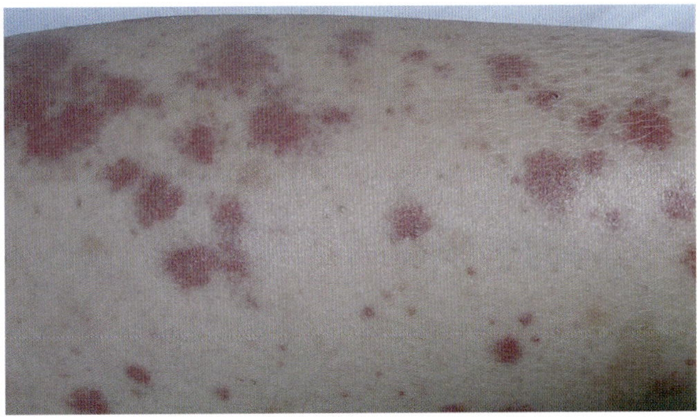

Fig. 3-6　Ecchymosis(图 3-6　瘀斑)

than 1 cm in diameter (Fig. 3-7). They appear in the following skin diseases: contact dermatitis, eczema, insect bites, lichen planus, nevi, warts, seborrheic keratosis, actinic keratosis, acne, skin cancers, etc.

③Plaques: these are palpable and elevated lesions more than 1 cm in size (Fig. 3-8) that are common in psoriasis, leprosy, mycosis fungoides, granuloma annulare, etc.

于 1 cm 的隆起皮面的实质性损害(图 3-7)。见于接触性皮炎、湿疹、虫咬皮炎、扁平苔藓、痣、疣、脂溢性角化病、日光性角化病、痤疮、皮肤癌等。

③斑块：可触及的隆起性损害，直径大于 1 cm(图 3-8)。银屑病、麻风、蕈样霉菌病、环状肉芽肿等常会形成斑块。

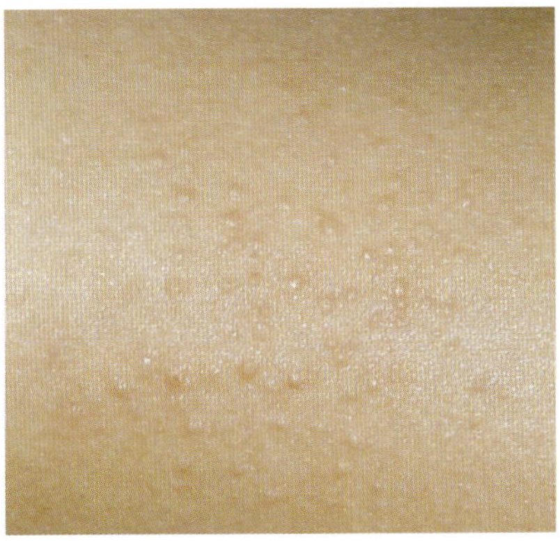

Fig. 3-7　Papule(图 3-7　丘疹)

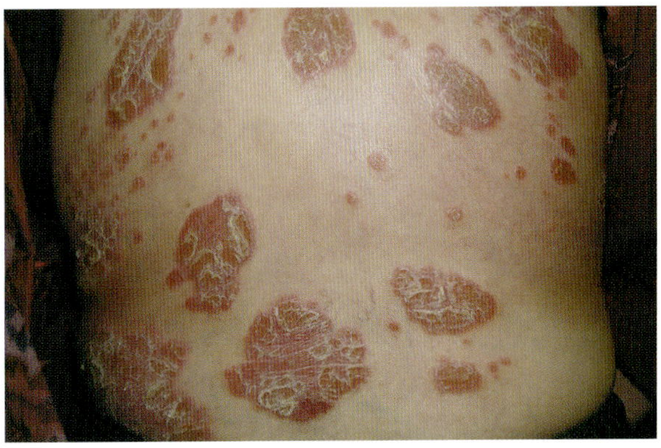

Fig. 3-8　Plaque(图 3-8　斑块)

④ Nodules: they are circumscribed, solid and deeply seated lesions which usually affect the deep dermis or subcutaneous tissues (Fig. 3-9). They are often seen in tumors such as lipomas,

④结节：一种局限性、实质性、深在性的皮损，位于真皮深层或皮下组织中(图 3-9)，常指肿瘤如脂肪瘤、淋巴瘤、纤

lymphoma, and fibromas, etc.

⑤ Vesicles: these are sharply circumscribed, elevated, clear fluid-containing cavities less than 1 cm in diameter (Fig. 3-10). Vesicles are commonly found in herpes, acute contact dermatitis, eczema, and autoimmune blistering disorders.

维瘤等。

⑤水疱:境界清楚、高出皮肤、直径小于 1 cm、内含液体的腔隙性损害(图 3-10)。水疱可以是疱疹病毒感染、急性接触性皮炎、湿疹或某些自身免疫性疱病的表现。

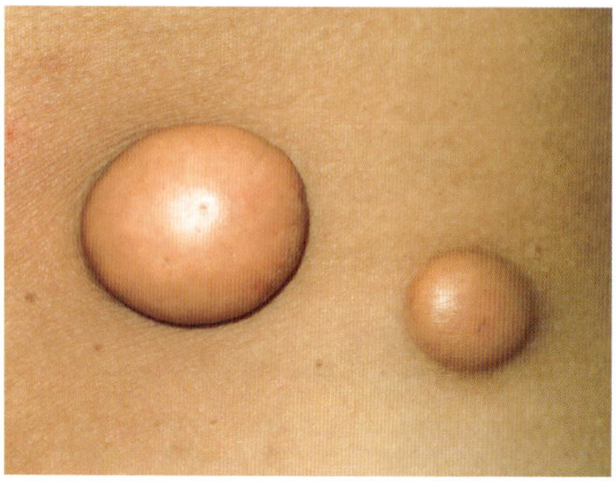

Fig. 3-9　Nodule(图 3-9　结节)

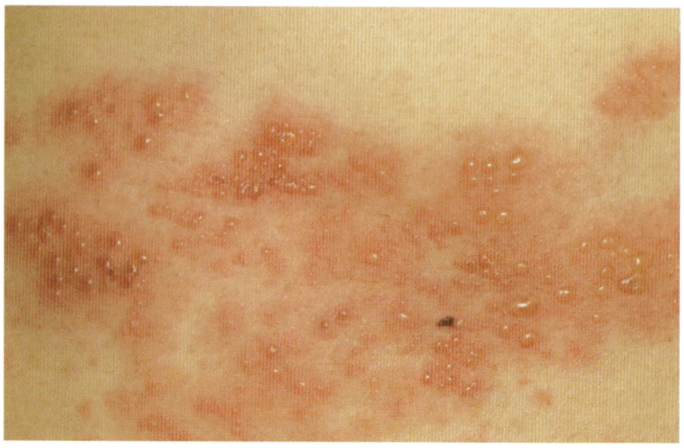

Fig. 3-10　Vesicle(图 3-10　水疱)

⑥ Bullae: vesicles greater than 1 cm in diameter are called bullae (Fig. 3-11). These may be caused by burns, insect bites, irritant contact dermatitis, drug reactions, or classic bullous skin disorders such as pemphigus or bullous pemphigoid.

⑦Pustules: these are elevated and circumscribed collections of pus (Fig. 3-12). Vesiculopustule is a term used to describe a vesicle containing pus. Pustules are most common in bacterial infections (impetigo, folliculitis), but may also occur in other inflammatory skin conditions such as pustular psoriasis.

⑥大疱:直径大于 1 cm 的水疱(图 3-11)。烧伤、昆虫叮咬、刺激性接触性皮炎、药疹可以出现大疱,天疱疮和大疱性类天疱疮是典型的大疱性疾病。

⑦脓疱:含有脓液的隆起的局限性皮损(图 3-12)。水疱含有脓液时,称为水疱脓疱疹。脓疱常见于细菌感染(脓疱疮、毛囊炎),也可见于一些炎症性疾病,如脓疱型银屑病。

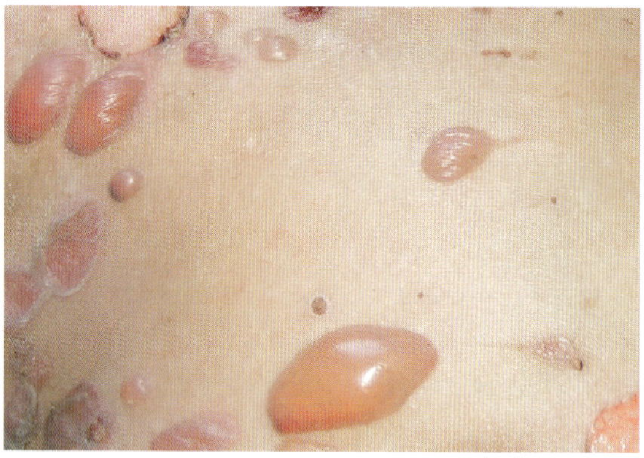

Fig. 3-11　Bullae(图 3-11　大疱)

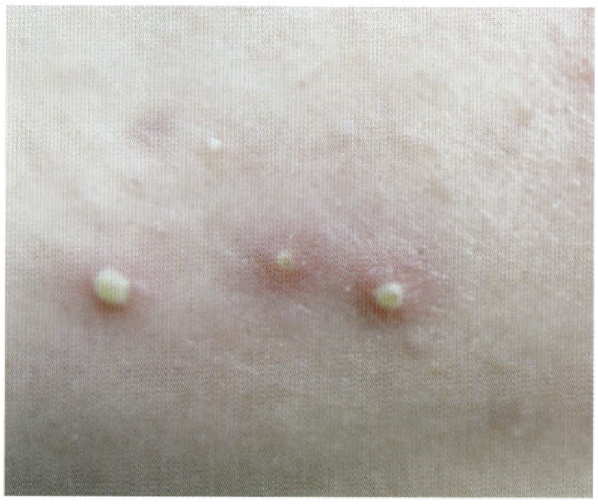

Fig. 3-12　Pustule(图 3-12　脓疱)

⑧ Wheals: these are transient, well demarcated and elevated swellings of the skin (Fig. 3-13). Although these are most commonly a sign of urticaria, it has been noted that other allergic causes for example, drugs, foods, or material consumed or contacted by sensitive humans, or even physical stimuli such as temperature, pressure and sunlight can be a trigger for wheal development.

⑧风团:暂时性、局限性、隆起性、水肿性皮损(图 3-13)。风团最常见于荨麻疹,也可以由药物、食物、接触物等变应原引起,温度、压力、阳光等物理性刺激也可以引起风团。

⑨Cysts: closed sacs containing fluids or semi-solid materials with a distinct membrane that separates the cysts from the nearby tissue (Fig. 3-14). It can be manifested in acne, epidermal cysts and sebaceous cysts.

⑨囊肿：内含液体或半固体的密闭的囊性损害（图 3-14），囊肿与周围组织由囊壁分开。见于痤疮、表皮囊肿、皮脂腺囊肿。

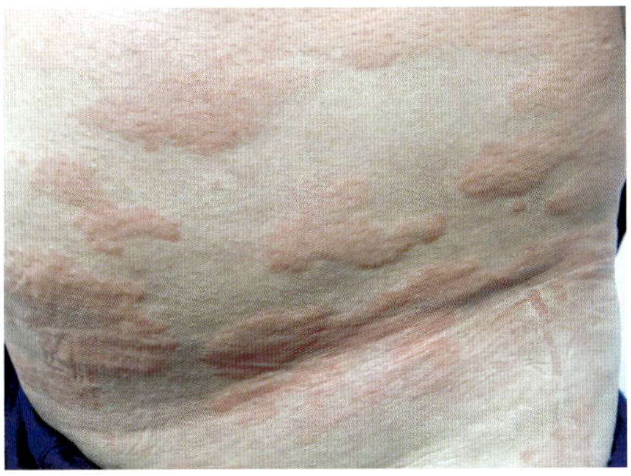

Fig. 3-13　Wheal(图 3-13　风团)

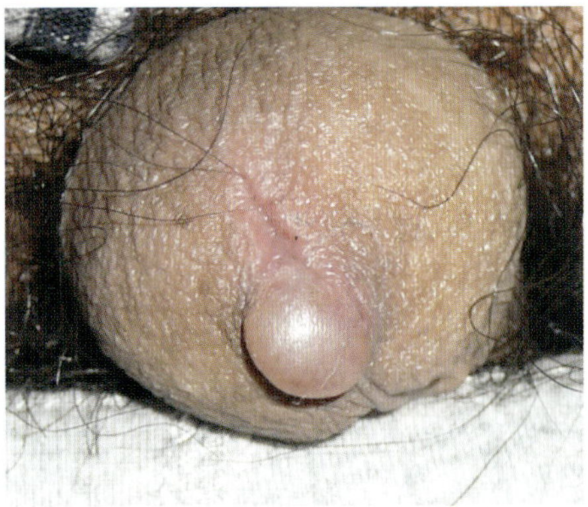

Fig. 3-14　Cyst(图 3-14　囊肿)

(2) Secondary lesions: these skin lesions represent evolutionary or complication-related changes, produced by scratching, stimulants, or infections over the course of the dermatoses. It should not be considered distinct from the primary lesions, but rather as an aid in interpreting the "dynamic" pathological process of the disease.

(2) 继发性损害(secondary lesions)由原发性损害演变而来，或因为搔抓、刺激、感染等因素形成。不能视其为与原发损害不同的损害，而应该理解为是对疾病的动态发展过程的一种阐释。

①Scales: these are dry or greasy laminated masses of keratin, which are shed from the *stratum corneum* (Fig. 3-15). Scaling often appears in psoriasis, exfoliative dermatitis, seborrheic dermatitis, pityriasis rosea, and pityriasis versicolor.

①鳞屑(scales)：干燥或油腻的薄片层状的角质片，为已经脱落或即将脱落的角质形成细胞（图 3-15）。鳞屑可见于银屑病、剥脱性皮炎、脂溢性皮炎、玫瑰糠疹、花斑糠疹等。

②Erosions: these are small discontinuities of the epidermis or mucous membrane that heal without scar formation (Fig. 3-16). The causes of the erosions can be due to trauma, inflammation or infectious diseases. In essence, erosions are formed in places where the vesicles or pustules rupture and a linear erosion is likely to be associated with scratching or rubbing.

②糜烂(erosions)：表皮或黏膜上皮的局限性缺损，愈合后不形成瘢痕（图 3-16）。糜烂可以是外伤性或是发生于各种炎症性或感染性疾病。水疱或脓疱破溃后常形成糜烂，搔抓、摩擦也可以引起线状糜烂。

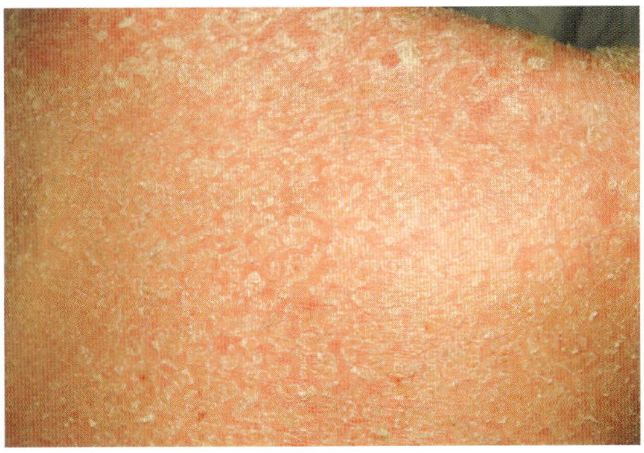

Fig. 3-15　Scale(图 3-15　鳞屑)

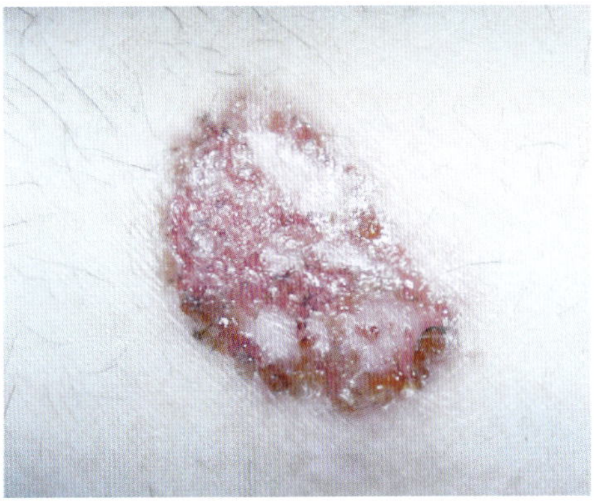

Fig. 3-16　Erosion(图 3-16　糜烂)

③ Ulcers: the occurrence of ulcers represents a destructive process which involves the deep epidermis or mucosa and extends into the dermis and even into the subcutaneous layer. In contrast to erosions, ulcers always heal with scar formation (Fig. 3-17). The cause of the ulcer is at times readily apparent, but in some instances the related factors may be multiple and obscure. These factors include infection, trauma, and vascular diseases (e. g., vasculitis, stasis dermatitis, peripheral arterial diseases, etc.).

③溃疡(ulcers):皮肤或黏膜较深的局限性缺损,病变深达真皮,甚至皮下组织,与糜烂不同,溃疡愈合后常有瘢痕形成(图 3-17)。溃疡形成的原因可以很明确,但也可以是多种因素或不明确,包括感染、外伤、血管性疾病(血管炎、郁积性皮炎、外周动脉性疾病等)。

④ Crusts (Scabs): crusts are the dried remains of exudates from erosive or ulcerated skin lesions. They may consist of dried serum, blood, or pus and dead cells (Fig. 3-18). It is particularly common in the skin following an inflammatory reaction or infection, as in the case of impetigo.

④痂(crusts):糜烂或溃疡皮损分泌物干涸后的残余物,由干涸的血清、血液、脓液、死亡的细胞组成(图 3-18)。痂可发生于皮肤炎症或感染性疾病,如脓疱疮。

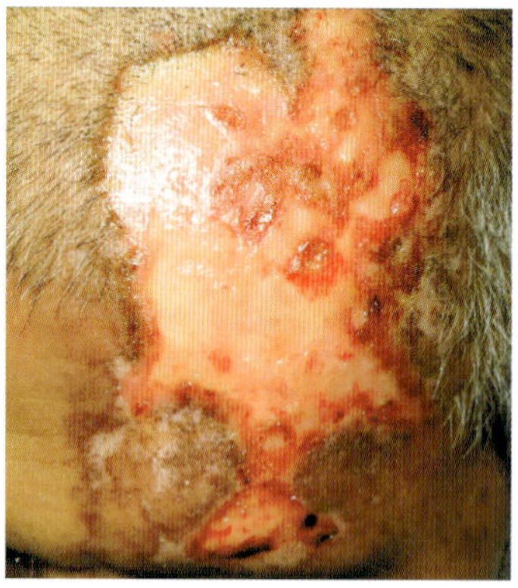

Fig. 3-17　Ulcer(图 3-17　溃疡)

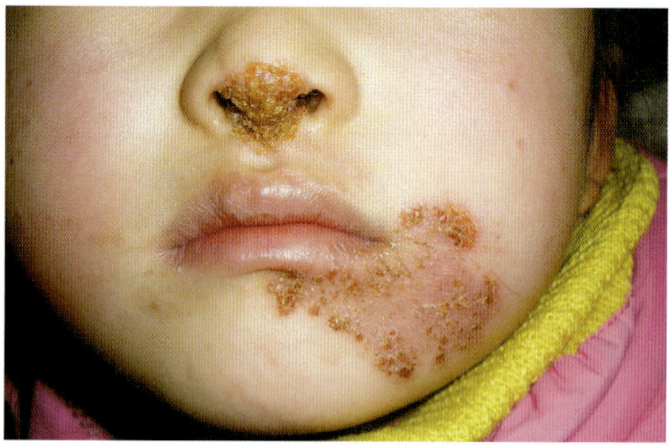

Fig. 3-18　Crust(图 3-18　痂)

⑤ Atrophy: this is the partial or complete diminution of the skin, involving the epidermis, dermis and subcutaneous tissue (Fig. 3-19). Epidermal atrophy manifests as dry, wrinkled, and cigarette paper-like skin. Severe atrophy affecting the dermis and subcutaneous tissue may result in a depression on the surface of the skin. Repeated exposure to sunlight, aging, inflammatory or neoplastic skin disorders (e. g., cutaneous T-cell lymphoma), and lupus erythematosus are often associated with skin atrophy. Long-term use of topical potent glucocorticoids also causes the skin to lose elasticity and become thinner.

⑤萎缩(atrophy):局部或全部皮肤变薄,可发生于表皮、真皮及皮下组织(图 3-19)。表皮萎缩表现为皮肤干燥、皱纹,像是卷烟纸。真皮及皮下组织萎缩表现为局部皮肤凹陷。萎缩可由慢性日光照射、老化、某些炎症性或肿瘤性皮肤病(如皮肤 T 细胞淋巴瘤)引起。红斑狼疮与皮肤萎缩关系密切。局部长期使用强效糖皮质激素也会引起皮肤弹性丧失及变薄。

⑥ Scars: scars are composed of new connective tissue that replaced the lost normal structure in the dermis or deeper parts after an injury or disease. Thus, scarring is a natural part of the healing process. Exuberant growth will lead to a thickened and raised scar, known as a hypertrophic scar (Fig. 3-20). Poor growth may form a thin, atrophic scar(Fig. 3-21). Keloids are hypertrophic scars that grow progressively beyond the area of the original wound (Fig. 3-22).

⑥瘢痕(scars):真皮或深部组织外伤或病变后,由新生结缔组织取代正常的皮肤结构形成的损害。瘢痕的形成是愈合过程中的自然进程。瘢痕可以增厚而高出皮面形成增生性瘢痕(图 3-20);瘢痕也可以萎缩凹陷,形成萎缩性瘢痕(图 3-21)。瘢痕疙瘩是一种增生性瘢痕,它可以超出损伤部位(图 3-22)。

⑦ Excoriations: these are punctuated or linear abrasions produced by mechanical means such as scratching (Fig. 3-23). It is

⑦抓痕(excoriations):由机械性方式(如搔抓)引起的点状或线状皮肤缺损

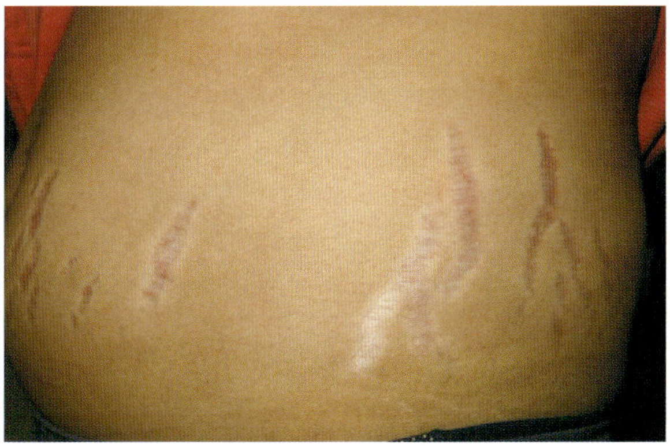

Fig. 3-19　Atrophy(图 3-19　萎缩)

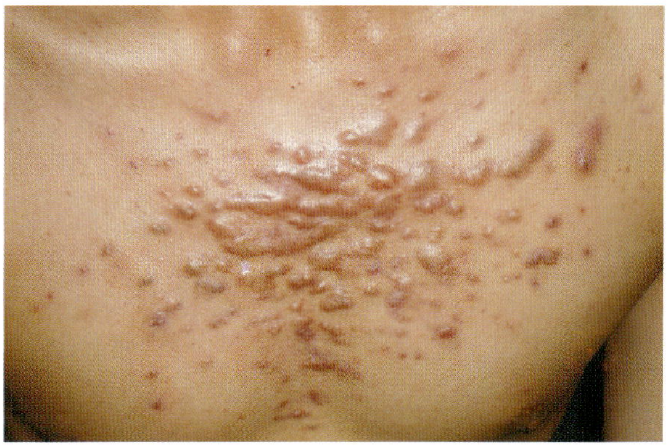

Fig. 3-20　Hypertrophic scar(图 3-20　增生性瘢痕)

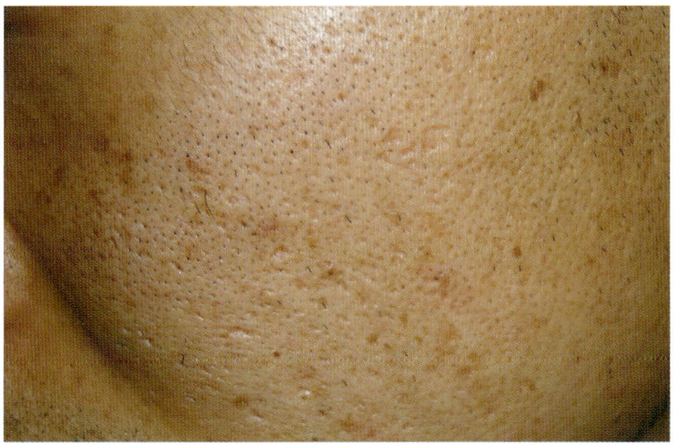

Fig. 3-21　Atrophic scar(图 3-21　萎缩性瘢痕)

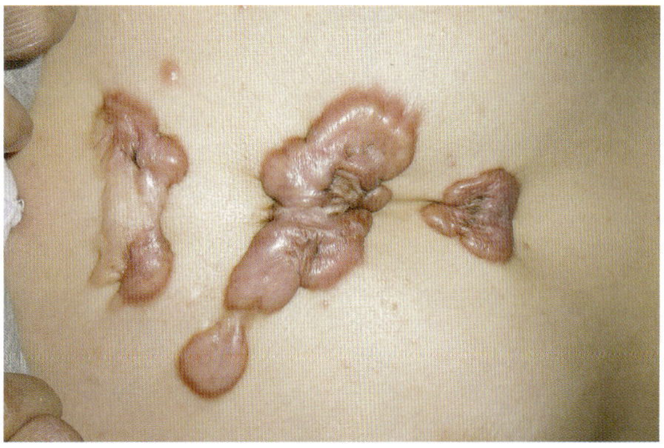

Fig. 3-22　Keloid(图 3-22　瘢痕疙瘩)

not uncommon to see the inflammatory reaction around the excoriation or crusts covering the lesion. They are often shown in pruritic and neurocutaneous dermatoses.

⑧Fissures: these are linear clefts through the epidermis or into the dermis (Fig. 3-24). They occur frequently in thickened skin disorders that result from inflammation and dryness on the skin surface. Afterwards the skin loses its elasticity. Fissures are easily found in fingers and toes, palms and heels, corners of the mouth, lips, etc.

(图 3-23)。在抓痕的周围常有炎症或表面覆盖痂。抓痕常见于瘙痒性皮肤病或神经功能障碍性皮肤病。

⑧皲裂(fissures):指发生在表皮或真皮的线状裂口(图 3-24)。它常因皮肤炎症、干燥引起皮肤肥厚、失去弹性而产生。皲裂常发生在指趾、掌跖、口角、唇等部位。

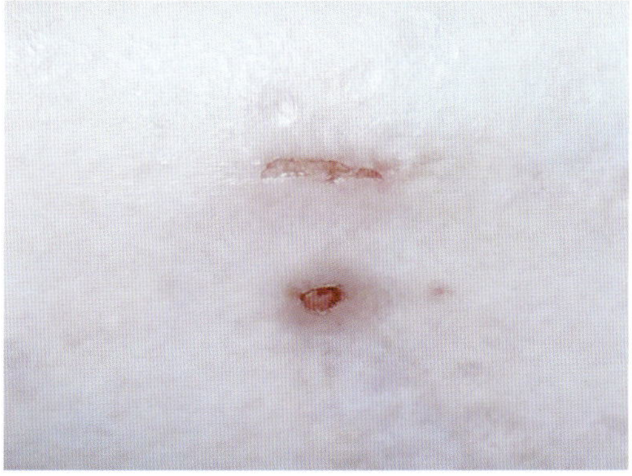

Fig. 3-23　Excoriation(图 3-23　抓痕)

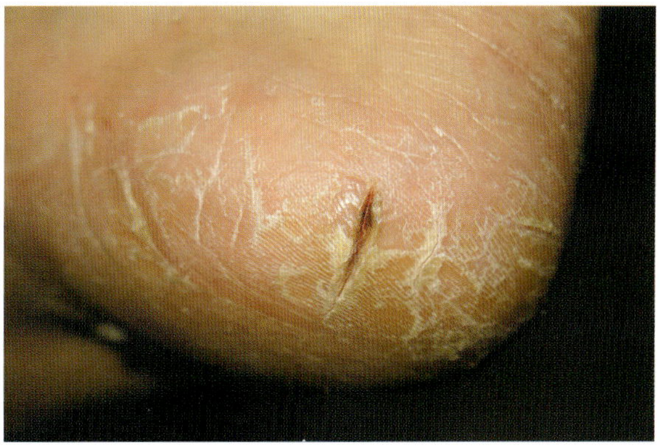

Fig. 3-24　Fissure(图 3-24　皲裂)

⑨Telangiectasias: telangiectasias are persistent dilated small

⑨毛细血管扩张(telangiectasias):

blood vessels in the superficial dermis (Fig. 3-25). They can develop anywhere on the body but are commonly seen on the face around the nose, cheeks and chin (e. g. , in rosacea). Scleroderma and the long-term use of topical fluorinated glucocorticoids are often accompanied by telangiectasia. It is also known that numerous inherited or idiopathic conditions display cutaneous telangiectasia.

指皮肤真皮浅层小血管持久性扩张(图 3-25)。其可发生于皮肤任何部位,常见于鼻周、颊部和颏(如酒糟鼻)。硬皮病或长期局部使用含氟糖皮质激素者常伴发毛细血管扩张。毛细血管扩张也可发生在一些遗传性疾病或特发性疾病。

⑩Maceration: this refers to the softening and whitening of the *stratum corneum* when it is kept wet for long period of time (Fig. 3-26). It often affects interdigital areas as well as the pads of the fingers and toes. As a result of this, the skin involved can easily get infected or torn apart.

⑩浸渍(maceration):因长时间处于潮湿环境而使皮肤角质层变软、变白(图 3-26),常见于指、趾间,浸渍部位的皮肤易发生感染或被撕脱。

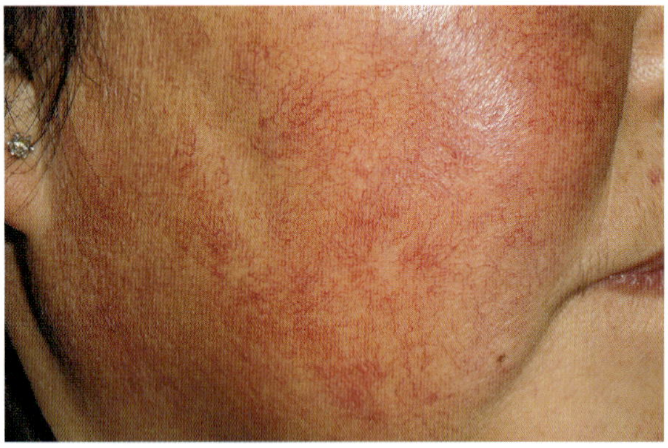

Fig. 3-25 Telangiectasia(图 3-25 毛细血管扩张)

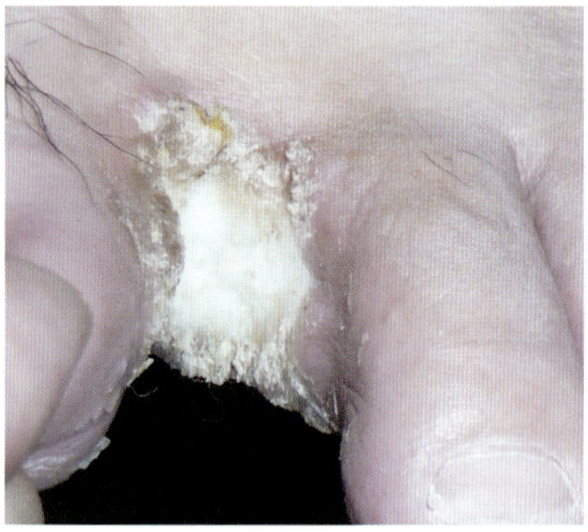

Fig. 3-26 Maceration(图 3-26 浸渍)

⑪Lichenification: this term refers to the thickening of the skin as a result of constant scratching or rubbing. The skin markings become gradually more pronounced, ultimately resulting in a leathery or bark-like appearance (Fig. 3-27). It is so named because of the similarity of the presentation to that of lichens growing on rocks. Lichenification is a characteristic lesion in lichen simplex chronicus, atopic dermatitis, chronic eczema and other disorders characterized by constant itching.

⑪苔藓样变(lichenification):在长期的搔抓和摩擦等刺激下,皮肤粗糙增厚,纹理加深,外观似皮革或树皮样(图 3-27),因类似石上生长之苔藓而得名。其常见于慢性单纯性苔藓、特应性皮炎、慢性湿疹和其他瘙痒性疾病。

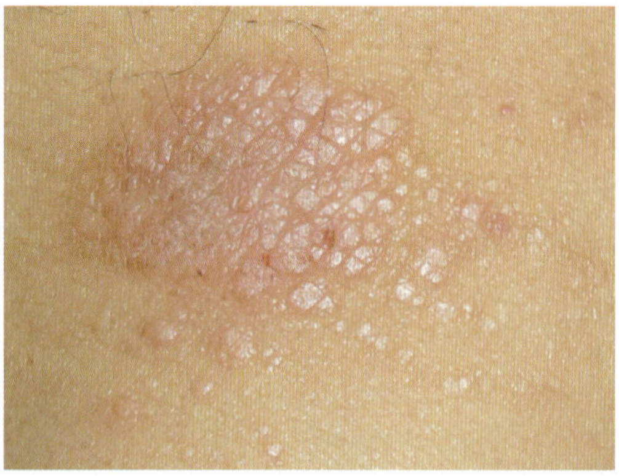

Fig. 3-27 Lichenification(图 3-27 苔藓样变)

【Basic Diagnostic Techniques of Dermatoses】

【皮肤病的基本诊断方法】

The principles of diagnosis of skin diseases are dependent not

不同的皮肤病可以表现出相同的症

only upon the subjective symptoms, but also and more importantly on an accurate inspection of the individual skin lesions, since similar symptoms and signs can easily appear in different skin diseases. In many cases, the appearance of skin lesions is distinctive enough for a definite diagnosis. Occasionally, symptoms and signs in some patients are inadequate, and a complete history and laboratory tests are essential to establish the diagnosis.

状和体征。掌握症状和特别的体征是诊断皮肤病的关键。在许多情况下，有的皮肤损害很特殊，视诊即可确立诊断。而在某些患者，单靠症状和体征是不够的，为了得到正确的诊断，还必须有完整的病史和实验室检查。

【Medical History】

General information: the medical history in a patient with a skin disease should be obtained with the same care that is exercised in a patient with any medical illness. The patient's age, gender, race, health status, occupation, hobbies, and living conditions are all important clues. It is also important to trace the development of the disease as accurately as possible by inquiring about the onset and course of the disease, and whether it is intermittent, constant, or progressive.

Chief complaint: this is the main symptom or reason for which the patient has sought treatment. It should include the lesions, location, the subjective symptoms, and the duration.

History of the present illness (HPI): refers to a detailed interview prompted by the chief complaint. The questionnaire should cover the course of the disease from the beginning of symptoms and should include the following: ①onset of the illness; ②the morphologic features of lesions such as shape, location, color; ③severity and frequency; ④precipitating and palliating factors that affect symptoms including food, drug and contact substances; ⑤progression: whether the patient is exhibiting systemic symptoms (fever, weight loss) or not, itching or pain sensation; ⑥ detailed previous treatment, such as medication, dosage, whether given by systemic or topical means, and the response to it. It is also particularly important to state if any glucocorticoids or immunosuppressive drugs have been used.

History of past illnesses: an inquiry with regard to all illnesses and medications of the patient in the past.

Personal history: there are few skin diseases in which environmental factors require no consideration. A variety of physical, chemical, or microbiological mechanisms are likely related to the presenting problem, so it is important to note any environmental factors such as travel history or living and working conditions (temperature, humidity, occupational factors), seasonal factors, etc. Habitation in certain parts of the world predisposes one to distinctive diseases for that particular geographic location, such as leprosy, leishmaniasis, and histoplasmosis. Sexual orientation and practices are also useful for diagnosis in genital ulcer diseases, HIV

【病史】

一般资料：皮肤病的病史如同其他疾病一样必须仔细询问，患者的年龄、性别、种族、健康状况、职业、爱好、居住环境都是重要线索，还必须描述疾病的发生和发展过程，是间歇性还是持续性发作，是否进行性加重。

主诉：患者就诊的主要症状和原因。其包括皮损及其部位、主观症状和持续的时间。

现病史：详细记录患者的主诉和发病到就诊的全过程，包括最初发病的时间；皮疹的形态、部位、颜色；疾病的严重程度及发生频率；询问疾病的影响因素，如食物、药物、接触物等；还要描述皮肤病的局部症状（如瘙痒、疼痛）和全身症状（如发热或体重减轻等）；了解治疗经过有助于疾病的诊断和治疗，包括特殊药物及使用剂量、系统或局部用药及治疗效果，有无使用糖皮质激素或免疫抑制剂。

既往史：患者曾经患过何种疾病及诊疗情况。

个人史：皮肤病常需要考虑环境因素。许多物理的、化学的或微生物因素与皮肤病相关。了解旅居外地史，工作和家庭生活环境的温度、湿度和气候，职业，好发季节等都非常重要。某些疾病有特定的地理分布，如麻风、利什曼病、组织胞质菌病等。性生活史是诊断性病的重要依据，如生殖器溃疡、HIV 感染和其他性病。

infections, and other sexually transmitted diseases.

Family history: family history should be questioned if genetically influenced disease is considered and also if an infectious disease is suspected.

家族史：家族中有无同类疾病，特别是有关遗传病或感染性疾病时。

【Physical Examination】

【体格检查】

Examination should be conducted in a well-lit room; natural sunlight is the ideal illumination. In addition to a careful history and physical examination, some simple diagnostic tools can be helpful for the diagnosis. For example, Wood's light (wavelength 365 nm) has been used in the diagnosis of tinea capitis, tinea versicolor, and erythrasma. It also aids in identifying hypo-and hyper-pigmented areas in vitiligo and melasma. A magnifying lens is also of importance in inspecting tiny lesions. It is important to feel (palpate) the lesions for firmness or fluctuation, to scratch any scales for their characteristics, and to scrape the crust away in order to see the base of lesion.

体格检查必须有充足的光线，自然光是最理想的光源。除仔细询问病史和体格检查外，有些简易设备可以辅助诊断，如 Wood 光(波长 365 nm)常用在帮助诊断头癣、花斑癣、红癣。也用于辅助诊断色减或色沉性皮肤病，如白癜风或黄褐斑。放大镜可以帮助观察一些小的皮损。触诊可用以了解皮疹的质地、有无波动感；摩擦可以发现鳞屑的特性；刮除痂可以观察皮损的基底状况。

The dermatologic examination should ideally include an inspection of the entire body surface, especially when skin lesions are widespread. In such cases the distribution and configuration of skin lesions can be better evaluated. This is optimally done by having the patient undress completely and viewing all affected areas closely. In particular, primary lesions and secondary lesions should be identified.

全身发疹的患者要了解皮疹的分布和排列，全身皮疹要充分暴露，并在一定距离对其进行全面观察。然后，辨别疹形，确定是原发损害还是继发损害。

The location of eruptions may be an important diagnostic clue because some skin diseases tend to affect particular parts of the body. For example, acne is easily found in those parts of the skin that contain the highest concentration of sebaceous glands; sunlight-related skin diseases (sun burn, lupus erythematosus, and actinic dermatitis) appear predominantly in sun-exposed areas.

皮损的分布能为皮肤病的诊断提供重要线索，因为许多皮肤病常常影响身体的特定部位。例如，痤疮好发于皮脂腺密集区域，日光相关疾病(如日晒伤、红斑狼疮、光化性皮炎)多发生于曝光部位。

In some cases, the pattern or distribution of skin lesion is consistent with its pathogenesis, and this is extremely helpful for diagnosis. For example, psoriasis often symmetrically affects the scalp, extensor arms, and legs. On the other hand, atopic dermatitis typically often involves the flexor arms and legs.

在某些情况下，皮疹的分布与疾病的发病机制有一定关系。皮疹的分布也有助于皮肤病的诊断。银屑病常对称分布于头皮、四肢伸侧。特应性皮炎常累及四肢的屈侧。

The arrangement of lesions can also provide very valuable diagnostic information. Terms that are commonly used to describe the relationship among neighboring lesions are clustered, grouped, linear, zosteriform, annular, confluent, etc. When vesicular lesions are clustered on an erythematous base, this is the classical appearance of herpes simplex. Linear lesions are frequently seen in plant contact dermatitis. Annular lesions, which consist of many small lesions on an active border arranged in a round to oval shape with an area of central clearing, are typically seen in tinea corporis.

皮疹的排列对确立诊断很有价值。常用来描述皮疹排列的术语有簇集性、群集性、线状、带状、环状、融合等。红斑基础上出现簇集性水疱是单纯疱疹的特征表现。线状皮疹在植物接触性皮炎中常见。环状皮疹多呈圆形或卵圆形，中央无皮疹，边缘常由小皮疹组成，如体癣。

The concentration of melanin, hemoglobin, and carotene all

皮肤的颜色由黑素、血红蛋白、胡萝

affect the color of the skin; thus the color of lesions aids in diagnosis. Red skin can occur in inflammatory or infectious diseases. Superficial vascular lesions such as port-wine stains may also appear red. Orange skin is most often seen in hypercarotenemia. Yellow is the typical color for jaundice, xanthelasmas and xanthomas, and for pseudoxanthoma elasticum. Violet skin may result from cutaneous hemorrhage or vasculitis. A light violet color of the eyelids is characteristic of dermatomyositis. Black skin lesions are more likely relevant to melanin either due to an increased number of melanocytes or to excessive production of melanin in the skin, as in nevi and melanoma.

卜素决定。皮疹颜色对诊断有帮助。炎症性或感染性皮肤病表现为红色；表浅的血管瘤如葡萄酒色痣也是红色的；橙色的皮肤常见于高胡萝卜素血症；黄色是黄疸、睑黄瘤和黄瘤、弹力纤维假黄瘤的特点；紫红色皮肤是皮肤出血或血管炎的结果；眼睑淡紫色皮疹是皮肌炎的特有表现；黑色皮疹常与黑素相关，包括黑素细胞或黑素增多，如痣和黑素瘤。

【Special Clinical Signs】

Dermatographism is the appearance of linear wheals in the distribution of the skin after stroking the skin with a blunt object. It is a common form of physical urticaria.

Darier's sign refers to blistering of a lesion when stroked. It occurs in patients with urticaria pigmentosa or other types of mastocytosis.

Nikolsky's sign is a skin condition in which the top layers of the skin slip free from the lower layers when slightly rubbed. A positive result may be present in patients with toxic epidermal necrolysis or with certain autoimmune bullous diseases.

Auspitz' sign is the appearance of pinpoint bleeding after removal of scale from plaques in psoriasis.

Koebner's phenomenon refers to the skin lesions appearing on lines of trauma (scratching, rubbing and injury). This is most often seen in psoriasis and lichen planus.

【特殊临床表现】

皮肤划痕症(dermatographism)：皮肤用钝器划过后在划痕部位产生条索状风团。这也是物理性荨麻疹的表现。

Darier 征(Darier's sign)：阳性表现为划痕处出现水疱，常见于色素性荨麻疹或其他类型的肥大细胞增生症。

尼氏征(Nikolsky's sign)：轻擦患者皮肤出现表皮剥脱，见于中毒性表皮坏死松解症和某些自身免疫性大疱病。

奥氏征(Auspitz's sign)：银屑病患者的斑块去掉鳞屑后出现点状出血的表现。

同形反应(Koebner's phenomenon)：指在外伤(如搔抓、摩擦、损伤)的部位发生皮疹。银屑病、扁平苔藓常有这种表现。

Bo CHENG(程波), Guan-nan ZHU(朱冠男)

Chapter Four　Topical and Physical Treatment of Skin Diseases

第四章　皮肤病的外用药治疗和物理治疗

Section One　Topical Treatment of Skin Diseases

第一节　皮肤病的外用药治疗

An ideal topical agent may be defined as one which maintains high concentrations locally with little systemic absorption. In other words, it has high efficacy and minimal side effects.

外用药物治疗时皮损局部药物浓度高、系统吸收少，因而具有疗效高和不良反应少的特点。

1. Types, functions and representative drugs of topical medications (as shown in Tab. 4-1)

一、常用外用药物的种类、作用及其代表性药物(表 4-1)

Tab. 4-1　Types, functions, and representative drugs of topical medications

(表 4-1　外用药物的种类、作用及代表药物)

Types(种类)	Functions(作用)	Representative drugs(代表药物)
clearing agents (清洁剂)	removal of exudates, scales, crusts and medicinal residues (清除渗出物、鳞屑、痂和残留药物)	saline, 3% boric acid, etc. (生理盐水、3%硼酸溶液等)
protective agents (保护剂)	protect skin, reduce friction and alleviate irritation(保护皮肤、减少摩擦和缓解刺激)	calamine lotion, zinc oxide powder, etc. (炉甘石、氧化锌粉等)
antipruritic agents (止痒剂)	reduce itching and scratching (减少瘙痒和搔抓)	various tar preparations, glucocorticoids, etc. (各种焦油制剂、糖皮质激素等)
keratoplastics (角质促成剂)	promote keratinization of *stratum corneum* and vasoconstriction, decrease exudation and infiltration(促进表皮角质层正常化、收缩血管、减轻渗出和浸润)	salicylic acid (3%), calcipotriol ointment, etc. (3%水杨酸、钙泊三醇软膏等)
keratolytics (角质剥脱剂)	increase shedding of dead keratinocytes in the *stratum corneum*(使过度角化的角质层细胞松解脱落)	salicylic acid (5%-10%), retinoic acid (0.01%-0.1%), etc. (5%～10%水杨酸、0.01%～0.1%维 A 酸等)
astringents (收敛剂)	precipitate proteins to seal moist surface, arrest exudation, inhibit secretion and inflammation(凝固蛋白质、减少渗出、抑制分泌、促进炎症消退)	silver nitrate, 2% aluminium acetate, 5% formaldehyde, etc. (硝酸银、2%醋酸铝和 5%甲醛等)
corrosives (腐蚀剂)	demolition and removal of proliferative granulomatous growths or neoplasms(破坏和去除增生的肉芽组织或赘生物)	30%-50% trichloroacetic acid, 5%-20% lactic acid, etc. (30%～50%三氯醋酸、5%～20%乳酸等)
antiseptics (抗菌剂)	bactericidal or bacteriostatic (杀灭或抑制细菌)	5%-10% benzoyl peroxide, 2% mupirocin, etc. (5%～10%过氧化苯甲酰、2%莫匹罗星等)
antifungals (抗真菌剂)	fungicidal or fungistatic (杀灭和抑制真菌)	2% ketoconazole, 1% terbinafine, etc. (2%酮康唑、1%特比萘芬等)
antivirals (抗病毒剂)	inhibit viral duplication or cytotoxic(抑制病毒复制或细胞毒性)	3%-5% acyclovir, 10%-40% podophyllin, etc. (3%～5%无环鸟苷、10%～40%足叶草酯等)

续表

Types(种类)	Functions(作用)	Representative drugs(代表药物)
pesticides (杀虫剂)	kill sarcoptic mite, lice, demodex (杀灭疥螨、虱、蠕形螨)	5% permethrin, 5%-10% sulfur ointment, 1% gamma benzene hexachloride cream, etc. (5%苄氯菊酯、5%～10%硫黄软膏、1%γ-666 霜等)
sunscreen agents (遮光剂)	absorb or block UV rays from penetrating the skin(吸收或阻止紫外线穿透皮肤)	5% titanium dioxide, 10% zinc oxide, etc. (5%二氧化钛、10%氧化锌等)
depigmenting agents (脱色剂)	reduce pigmentation by inhibiting tyrosinase activity (通过抑制酪氨酸酶的活性减轻色素沉着)	3% hydroquinone, 20% azelaic acid, kojic acid, glycolic acid, etc. (3%氢醌、20%壬二酸、曲酸、乙醇酸等)
retinoids (维 A 酸类)	regulate epidermal keratinization and inhibit epidermal proliferation via keratoplastic and keratolytic effects; regulate melanin metabolism (通过角质促进和角质松解效应调节表皮角化和抑制表皮增生；调节黑素代谢等)	0.025%-0.05% all TRANS retinoic acid cream, 0.1% tazarotene gel, 0.1% adapalene gel (0.025%～0.05%全反式维 A 酸霜、0.1%他扎罗汀凝胶、0.1%阿达帕林凝胶)
glucocorticoids (糖皮质激素)	"three anti" effects (anti-inflammatory, anti-proliferative, anti-pruritic) plus immunosuppressive effect(三抗效应：抗炎、抗增生、止痒；免疫抑制作用)	0.05% clobetasol dipropionate ointment, 0.1% mometasone furoate cream, etc. (0.05%丙酸氯倍他索软膏、0.1%糠酸莫米松乳膏等)

2. Formulas of topical agents

(1) Solution: a homogeneous mixture of one or more solutes (i. e., active agents) dissolved in a solvent (usually water). These drugs have cleaning and convergent effects mostly in wet compresses. Solutions containing 3% boric acid are most commonly used for skin diseases.

(2) Tincture or spiritus: also a drug solution or infusion but using ethanol as the solvent. A tincture is a non-volatile drug in an ethanol solution and a spiritus is a volatile drug in an ethanol solution. Commonly used agents are 2.5% tincture iodine, 3% salicylic acid spiritus, etc.

(3) Powder: it has a dry, protective and cooling effect and is mainly used for acute dermatitis with no erosion and exudation. It is particularly suitable against lesions in fold areas. Commonly used active agents are talc and calamine powder, etc.

(4) Lotion: also known as oscillating agent, it is a mixture of powder (30%-50%) with water. However, unlike the solution described above, the two are not mutually soluble. The main effects of lotion are anti-itching, cooling, drying and protection. Calamine lotion is most commonly used in clinical settings.

(5) Oil: has a vegetable oil base. Oil-based topical agents have the functions of cleaning, protection and lubrication. It is mainly used for subacute dermatitis and eczema with 25%-40% zinc oxide oil used most commonly.

(6) Emulsion: is an oil and water mixture. There are two

二、外用药物的剂型

(1) 溶液 药物的水溶液，具有清洁、收敛作用，主要用于湿敷。常用的有3%硼酸溶液等。

(2) 酊剂和醑剂 药物的乙醇溶液或浸液。酊剂是非挥发性药物的乙醇溶液，醑剂是挥发性药物的乙醇溶液。常用的有 2.5%碘酊、3%水杨酸醑等。

(3) 粉剂 有干燥、保护和散热作用。主要用于急性皮炎无糜烂和渗出的皮损，特别适用于间擦部位。常用的有滑石粉、炉甘石粉等。

(4) 洗剂 也称振荡剂，是粉剂(30%～50%)与水的混合物，两者互不相溶。有止痒、散热、干燥及保护作用。常用的有炉甘石洗剂等。

(5) 油剂 用植物油溶解药物或与药物混合。有清洁、保护和润滑作用，主要用于亚急性皮炎和湿疹。常用的有25%～40%氧化锌油。

(6) 乳剂 油和水经乳化而成的剂

types: one is water in oil (W/O) and the other one is oil in water (O/W, also referred to as cream). Emulsions can be used for both water-soluble and fat-soluble drugs. Emulsions have protective and moisturizing effects and good permeability, and are mainly used for subacute and chronic dermatitis.

(7) Ointment: uses vaseline, vegetable oil mixed with beeswax, or animal fats as a matrix for the active agent. Ointments protect wounds and prevent fissures, making them especially beneficial in treating chronic eczema and lichen simplex chronicus.

(8) Paste: similar to ointment formulation but contains 25% to 50% solids, mostly used in mild exudate conditions from subacute eczema and dermatitis. However, the use of pastes should be avoided on the hair.

(9) Plaster: a semi-solid matrix containing the active agent is attached to a hard backing material. Plaster can be firmly attached to the surface of the skin, thereby prolonging the effect. Meanwhile, it will prevent moisture loss, soften the skin and promote long-term perfusion of the active agent.

(10) Film: is made of a volatile solvent with the active agent. The active agent is first dissolved into the solvent. A thin layer of the mixture is applied to the skin, after which the solvent quickly evaporates, leaving a film. This formula is commonly used for chronic dermatitis but it is also useful for occupational disease prevention.

(11) Gel: is a topical application of a polymer compound mixed in an organic solvent such as propylene glycol or polyethylene glycol. Gel can form a thin layer to provide cool lubrication with no irritant effect. It can be used for acute and chronic dermatitis.

(12) Aerosol: is made of the drug, polymer film material and liquefied gas. The preparation promotes an even distribution of drug on the surface of the skin, which is useful for treatment of acute and chronic dermatitis or infectious skin diseases.

(13) Others: dimethyl sulfoxide (DMSO) is a potent solvent for many water soluble and liposoluble drugs. DMSO has the added advantage of being able to carry the drug or other active agents with it as it perfuses through the epidermis.

3. Principles of topical therapy in dermatology

(1) The first consideration for the appropriate selection of topical medication is the etiology and pathogenesis of the skin disease. For example, antimicrobials will be chosen for infectious diseases of the skin, while corticosteroids and anti-histamines are the appropriate choices for treatment of conditions involving

型。有两种类型,一种为油包水(W/O),另一种为水包油(O/W),也称为霜剂(cream),水溶性和脂溶性药物均可配成乳剂,具有保护、润泽作用,渗透性较好,主要用于亚急性、慢性皮炎。

(7) 软膏　用凡士林、植物油加蜂蜡、动物脂肪等作为基质的剂型。具有保护创面、防止干裂的作用,主要用于慢性湿疹、慢性单纯性苔藓等疾病。

(8) 糊剂　含有 25%～50%固体粉末成分的软膏。多用于有轻度渗出的亚急性皮炎、湿疹等。毛发部位不宜用糊剂。

(9) 硬膏　由半固体基质贴附于裱褙材料上。硬膏可牢固地黏着于皮肤表面,作用持久,可阻止水分散失、软化皮肤和增强药物渗透性。

(10) 涂膜剂　将药物和成膜材料溶于挥发性溶剂中制成。外用后溶剂迅速蒸发,在皮肤上形成一均匀薄膜,常用于治疗慢性皮炎,也可以用于职业病防护。

(11) 凝胶　以高分子化合物和有机溶剂如丙二醇、聚乙二醇为基质配成的外用药物。凝胶外用后可形成一薄层,凉爽润滑,无刺激性,急、慢性皮炎均可使用。

(12) 气雾剂　由药物与高分子成膜材料和液化气体混合制成。喷涂后药物均匀分布于皮肤表面,可用于治疗急、慢性皮炎或感染性皮肤病。

(13) 其他　二甲基亚砜(dimethyl sulfoxide, DMSO)可溶解多种水溶性和脂溶性药物,药物的 DMSO 剂型往往具有良好的透皮吸收性。

三、皮肤科外用药物的治疗原则

(1) 正确选用外用药物的种类　应根据皮肤病的病因与发病机制等进行选择,如感染性皮肤病宜选抗感染药物,过敏反应性疾病选择糖皮质激素或抗组胺药。

hypersensitivity.

(2) The second principle is the clinical presentation or types of lesions. For instance, when acute dermatitis presents as erythema and papules without any exudation, one can select powder or lotion, whereas when inflammation leads to erosion or exudation, then one can select solutions for wet dressings. Finally, when erosion does appear but with minimal exudation, pastes can be applied.

In cases of subacute dermatitis without significant exudation, either paste or oil-based formulas may be used, and again, when no erosions are involved, then creams or pastes will be appropriate.

In cases of chronic dermatitis, all creams, ointments, plaster, tinctures and films should be effective.

Finally, for pruritus without any lesions, creams or tinctures can be useful alternatives.

(3) Patient age, gender, and clinical condition are the final factors when determining an appropriate therapy. Patients (or parents) should be given clear instructions regarding all medications they are expected to apply, and these should include the frequency and timing over the course of the day, the duration, the dosage, the precise area(s) where the drug should be applied, cautions against probable adverse reactions, and simple instructions for the management for such side effects.

(2) 根据皮损的表现或类型正确选用外用药物的剂型　原则为：①急性皮炎仅有红斑、丘疹而无渗液时可选用粉剂或洗剂，炎症较重，糜烂、渗出较多时宜用溶液湿敷，有糜烂但渗出不多时则用糊剂；②亚急性皮炎渗出不多者宜用糊剂或油剂，如无糜烂宜用乳剂或糊剂；③慢性皮炎可选用乳剂、软膏、硬膏、酊剂、涂膜剂等；④单纯瘙痒无皮损者可选用乳剂、酊剂等。

(3) 详细向患者解释用法和注意事项　应当针对患者的个体情况如年龄、性别、既往用药反应等向患者详细解释使用方法、使用时间、部位、次数和可能出现的不良反应及其处理方法等。

Dan LUO(骆丹), Bing-rong ZHOU(周炳荣)

Section Two　Physical Treatment for Skin Diseases

第二节　皮肤病的物理治疗

Dermatology has become a diverse field. It is one of the few areas of medicine in which a specialist can be both physician and surgeon, treating malignant and non-malignant diseases. Furthermore, many physical therapeutic methods are used in clinical practice.

皮肤病学具有多元化的特色，它是医学中较为少有的内外科兼有、恶性和非恶性疾病兼治的学科之一。物理治疗是临床工作中的重要方法。

1. Cryotherapy

一、冷冻治疗

Using liquid nitrogen (temperature: −196 ℃), applications for cryotherapy by cryospray, cryoprobe or a cotton-tipped applicator have been widely used for treatment of skin diseases. The nitrogen is applied to skin lesions for a few seconds or more depending on the area and depth of the lesion. The treatment can be repeated in some cases after each thawing cycle is completed. Indications for cryotherapy include warts, seborrhoeic keratoses, solar keratoses, and some skin cancers or precancerous lesions.

冷冻治疗(cryotherapy)是借助喷枪、探针、棉签等使用液态氮(温度：−196 ℃)进行皮肤病治疗的方法。液氮接触皮肤数秒，时间长短可根据预期治疗范围直径和深度而定，可根据需要重复数次治疗。临床可用于疣、脂溢性角化病、日光性角化病以及一些皮肤癌及癌前病变的治疗。

The treated area is likely to form a blister within a few hours that gradually dries up in a scabby appearance a few days later.

治疗区域通常在治疗后数小时内起疱，眶周治疗可能引起眼睑水肿，数天后

Treatment near the eye may result in a puffy eyelid, but the swelling will settle in a few days as well. Usually no special management is needed during the healing. The scab peels off after 5-10 days on the face and after 3 weeks on the hand. A sore or scab on the lower leg may persist as long as 3 months, as healing is often slow in this site.

消退。冷冻治疗几天后水疱干涸结痂，期间通常无需特别处理。面部痂一般5～10天后脱落，手部脱痂需要3周左右，而下肢由于愈合较慢可能时间更久，最长可达3个月。

2. Narrowband ultraviolet B

While treatment with narrowband ultraviolet B (NB-UVB) induces longer remissions than broadband ultraviolet B, it is still favored in clinical practice due to the lower risk of burns. NB-UVB, the emission spectrum is predominantly 311-313 nm, was proved to be safer and also more effective than broadband UVB for some skin conditions.

NB-UVB has been clinically used for psoriasis, atopic dermatitis (AD), seborrheic dermatitis, vitiligo, and mycosis fungoides (MF). It is also used for the treatment of photodermatoses, especially in UVA-sensitive patients. Other indications for NB-UVB treatment include actinic prurigo, hydroa vacciniforme, idiopathic solar urticaria, and polymorphic light eruption.

二、窄谱中波紫外线

窄谱中波紫外线(NB-UVB)即指波长为311～313 nm的紫外线，治疗后缓解期长、局部灼伤少，更有效、安全，临床使用已经超越了宽谱紫外线。

NB-UVB临床适应证包括银屑病、特应性皮炎(AD)、脂溢性皮炎、白癜风以及蕈样肉芽肿(MF)。NB-UVB还可以用于治疗日光性皮肤病，尤其UVA敏感的患者，适应证包括光化性痒疹、种痘样水疱病、特发性日光性荨麻疹以及多形性日光疹。

3. Laser

When lasers are used in surgery and medicine, especially for the removal of any kind of pigment, the approach is based on a theory proposed by Anderson and Parrish, also known as "selective photothermolysis". In this theory, the maximal effectiveness can be achieved with minimal damage on the surrounding tissue if the optimal parameters (laser wavelength, impulse time and energy) are chosen based upon the tissue's biological properties. Three key conditions must be met to achieve this goal: ① The target must contain chromophores that absorb a specific laser wavelength; ②These chromophores should not be present in the surrounding healthy tissue; ③ Laser energy should be delivered in high peak powers and short pulse widths of nano-to millisecond domains, achievable by using Q-switched lasers.

The main biological targets of lasers are hemoglobin, melanin and water, all of which absorb light energy very differently and have optimum absorption spectra depending on the wavelength of the incident photon energy. For visible light lasers and some near-infrared lasers, the main chromophore targets are hemoglobin and melanin. For the CO_2 laser at 10600 nm and the Er:YAG laser at 2940 nm, the only chromophore is water.

Many skin disorders can be treated by CO_2 laser, including seborrheic keratosis, warts and aging. Furthermore, the addition of fractional technology to the CO_2 laser has opened up more choices

三、激光

激光(laser)治疗皮肤病的主要依据是Anderson和Parrish提出的选择性光热作用(selective photothermolysis)理论，即根据不同组织的生物学特性，只要选择合适的激光参数(波长、脉冲持续时间、能量)，就可以保证最有效治疗病变部位的同时，对周围正常组织的损伤最小。要实现选择性光热作用，则必须满足三个条件：①靶组织中含有相应色基，可吸收相应波长的激光；②周边组织不含有对应色基；③高峰值能量和毫秒、微秒或纳秒级的短脉宽可减少对周边组织的损伤，通常通过调Q激光实现。

激光的生物学靶色基主要是血红蛋白、黑素和水。靶色基对不同波长的激光具有选择性吸收，对于可见光和近红外光，靶色基主要是血红蛋白和黑素，而10600 nm的CO_2激光及2940 nm的Er:YAG激光，靶色基均只有水。

CO_2激光治疗主要的适应证包括脂溢性角化、疣和嫩肤。此外，点阵CO_2激光拓宽了皮肤美容方面的应用，可用于

for aesthetic dermatological indications such as rejuvenation of photoaged skin and scar removal-a technique that is especially effective for acne scars.

嫩肤及瘢痕修复尤其痤疮瘢痕。

Pulsed-dye laser (PDL)at 585 or 595-nm is non-ablative (does not remove tissue) and targets oxyhemoglobin. Therefore, it is useful for vascular abnormality treatment and produces minimal damage to the surrounding tissue. Vascular skin diseases including port wine stains, infantile hemangiomas, telangiectasia, and scars are all treatable with PDL.

585 或 595 nm 脉冲染料激光(pulsed-dye laser,PDL)为非剥脱性激光,靶色基主要是氧合血红蛋白,可用于治疗血管性疾病,而对周边组织损伤较小,适应证为血管性皮肤病,包括鲜红斑痣、婴幼儿血管瘤、毛细血管扩张以及瘢痕。

Several short pulsed lasers, including pulsed dye, Q-switched ruby, Nd:YAG, and alexandrite lasers are now the preferred means for tattoo removal due to their selective photothermolysis. These lasers have also been used for cutaneous pigmentation disorders such as solar lentigines, café-au-lait macules, post-inflammatory pigmentation, melasma, and naevus of Ota.

短脉冲激光(包括脉冲染料、调 Q 红宝石、Nd:YAG 激光、紫翠宝石激光)对不同靶色基的选择性光热作用可以用于去除文身,调 Q 红宝石、Nd:YAG 激光、紫翠宝石激光还可以治疗皮肤色素沉着性疾病如日光性黑子、咖啡斑、炎症后色素沉着、黄褐斑和太田痣。

Lasers with wavelengths of 600-1100 nm (such as the ruby, alexandrite, Nd:YAG, and diode) penetrate deeply in the tissue and can be absorbed by eumelanin in the hair shaft and follicle, which is thought to be the target chromophore. Relatively long pulses are used to create sufficient damage to the follicles and can be used for hair removal clinically. These lasers work best on pale skin with pigmented hairs.

波长范围在 600～1100 nm 的激光,如红宝石、紫翠宝石、Nd:YAG 及半导体激光,穿透较深,可被毛鞘和毛囊中靶色基黑素吸收,较长的脉宽可破坏毛囊,故临床可用于脱毛,并且对于浅肤色皮肤的黑色毛发效果较好。

4. Photodynamic therapy (PDT)

四、光动力治疗

PDT requires application of a photosensitizer, commonly 5-aminolevulinic acid (5-ALA), which is preferentially absorbed by highly vascularized or metabolically active tissues and converted to protoporphyrin Ⅸ (PpⅨ). Upon exposure to light, PpⅨ causes the generation of reactive oxygen species that provoke significant cytotoxic effects. PDT may also interfere with synthesis and degradation of extracellular matrix, and may also modulate cytokine and growth factor expression.

光动力治疗(PDT)中需要使用光敏剂,常用的是 5-氨基酮戊酸(5-ALA),外源性的 ALA 进入体内后,可被增生活跃的细胞或血管化组织吸收,在细胞内转化为原卟啉Ⅸ,原卟啉Ⅸ经特定波长的光照射后产生活性氧,具有细胞毒作用。PDT 也可能改变细胞外基质合成和降解过程,并且参与调节细胞因子和生长因子的表达。

Besides its main application in condyloma acuminatum and acne, PDT is reported to be effective for the treatment of solar keratoses, superficial basal cell carcinoma, nodular basal cell carcinoma, Bowen's disease, squamous cell carcinoma, mycosis fungoides, and Kaposi's sarcoma.

光动力治疗除了用于治疗尖锐湿疣、痤疮外,还可治疗日光性角化病、浅表性基底细胞癌、结节性基底细胞癌、鲍温病、鳞状细胞癌、蕈样肉芽肿、卡波氏肉瘤等。

5. Intense pulsed light

五、强脉冲光

Intense pulsed light (IPL) devices emit polychromatic incoherent high-intensity pulsed light using a combination of flash lamps and bandpass filters. As with other lasers, IPL devices can lead to more or less selective thermal damage on the target

强脉冲光(intense pulsed light,IPL)是一种连续的多波长的非相干性光,强脉冲光治疗仪可以通过滤光片选择特定波长、能量和脉宽的光,IPL 作用机理和

depending on the wavelength spectrum, energy fluence, and pulse duration.

As IPL devices emit a spectrum of wavelengths, the three key chromophores melanin, hemoglobin, and water can be activated with a single light exposure. As with laser devices, pulse duration should be lower than the thermal relaxation time of the target structure to prevent unselective damage to the surrounding tissue. The combination of particular wavelengths, pulse durations, pulse intervals, and energy fluence facilitates the treatment of a wide spectrum of skin conditions, such as acne vulgaris, pigmented lesions, vascular lesions, unwanted hair growth, photodamaged skin, scars, and skin rejuvenation.

激光类似,通过选择性光热作用来破坏靶色基。

由于 IPL 可发射一段波长范围内的光,单次治疗可涵盖常见的三个主要作用色基即黑素、血红蛋白和水,和激光类似,脉宽需短于靶物质的热弛豫时间,从而减轻对周边组织的损伤。波长、脉宽、脉冲间歇和能量的合理选择可有效将 IPL 用以治疗痤疮、色素性疾病、血管病变、脱毛、皮肤光老化、瘢痕和嫩肤。

6. Botulinum toxin

Botulinum toxin (BTX) is a neurotoxic protein produced by the bacterium *Clostridium botulinum* and related species. It is also produced commercially for medical, cosmetic, and research use. In the current worldwide market, there are two major types of BTX: botulinum toxin type A (BoNT/A) and botulinum toxin type B (BoNT/B).

Botulinum neurotoxin type A (BoNT/A), when injected locally, effectively diminishes rhytides of the upper and lower face by inhibiting hyperdynamic musculature that can lead to wrinkle and line formation. A number of BoNT/A preparations are available for aesthetic use on the international market, all of which differ in manufacturing process, composition, potency, and approved indications. For cosmetic use, BTX is indicated for hyperkinetic facial lines (glabellar frown lines, crow's feet) and hypertrophic masseter muscle. In addition, BTX has been used successfully for some sweating and salivary disorders including axillary and palmar hyperhidrosis.

六、肉毒毒素

肉毒毒素(botulinum toxin,BTX)是由细菌肉毒梭菌和相关菌种产生的神经毒性的蛋白质,广泛用于医疗、化妆品和研究领域。市面可见两种类型的 BTX,即 A 型肉毒毒素(BoNT/A)和 B 型肉毒毒素(BoNT/B)。

BoNT/A 局部注射后能抑制肌肉高动力状态,最终达到减少面部皱纹的治疗目的。目前国际市场已经有了美容用的多种品牌 BoNT/A,各品牌之间的生产工艺、组成、作用效果和适应证不尽相同。皮肤美容方面,BTX 的适应证为动力性面部皱纹(眉间纹、鱼尾纹)和咬肌肥厚。BTX 也可用于汗腺、唾液腺疾病包括腋下和手足多汗症。

7. Soft tissue augmentation

The field of soft tissue augmentation has had a rapid growth over the past several years, mainly due to the development of the hyaluronic acid (HA) fillers and other related fillers which are now widely applied for rejuvenation of the skin.

HA or hyaluronan is a glycosaminoglycan, which consists of repeating non-sulphated disaccharide units of glucuronic acid and N-acetylglucosamine. Due to its highly hydrophilic nature, HA has the potential to greatly expand beyond the initial volume as it can draw and hold water from surrounding tissues. Other chemical properties of HA are beneficial in cosmetic use, such as formation of gel at even low concentration. Most importantly, HA is also a part of the natural extracellular matrix in all animal tissues. As such, it does not exhibit tissue or species specificity for potential

七、组织填充剂

近些年由于透明质酸(hyaluronic acid,HA)及其他填充剂被常规用于皮肤的年轻化治疗,组织填充治疗领域在过去数年中飞速发展。

HA 是一种高分子的聚合物,是由单位 D-葡萄糖醛酸及 N-乙酰葡糖胺组成的高级多糖。HA 高度亲水,可吸水,达到容量扩增作用,较低浓度即可形成凝胶。HA 天然存在,是细胞外基质中的重要的组成,没有物种或组织特异性,这也就减轻了潜在的免疫反应,使得 HA 广泛用于临床注射治疗,通过容量填充来改善各种皱纹。

immunological reactions, and has lower risk for body rejection-make HA fillers more popular than other filler material. When injected locally, HA filler is able to smooth out fine lines and wrinkles due to volume enhancement.

Other tissue filler products for augmentation in clinical settings are collagen, calcium hydroxylapetite, poly-L-lactic acid, etc.

其他用于组织填充的还包括胶原蛋白、羟基磷灰石、多聚-L-乳酸等。

Dan LUO(骆丹), Yang XU(许阳)

Part Two 第二部分

Chapter Five Dermatoses Caused by Viral Infection

第五章 病毒感染性皮肤病

Section One Herpes Simplex

第一节 单纯疱疹

Herpes simplex is a viral dermatosis caused by herpes simplex virus (HSV) infection, which is characterized by painful clustered vesicles on the skin and mucous membranes. The disease is self-limiting, but tends to recur.

单纯疱疹(herpes simplex)是单纯疱疹病毒(HSV)感染引起的病毒性皮肤病,以皮肤黏膜疼痛性成簇水疱为特征,有自限性,但常复发。

【Etiology and Pathogenesis】

【病因及发病机制】

Herpes simplex virus (HSV), a member of the alpha subfamily of human herpesvirus (HHV), is a double-stranded DNA virus that affects human beings only. It is sub-classified into type 1 (HSV-1, or HHV-1) and type 2 (HSV-2, or HHV-2) according to differences in their transmission modes and clinical features. These two subtypes share only approximately 50% homology in their genomes but can induce cross-reactive immunity to each other. HSV-1 primarily affects skin and mucous membranes in the extra genital regions (e. g., oral cavity, cornea) and the organs (e. g., brain), whereas HSV-2 primarily causes infections of skin and mucous membrane in the genital regions of adults and infections of the newborns.

HSV 属人类疱疹病毒(HHV)α 亚科,为双链 DNA 病毒,人是唯一宿主。根据其传染方式和临床特点的不同分为 1 型(HSV-1,或 HHV-1)和 2 型(HSV-2,或 HHV-2),两型基因组间约 50%同源,也存在交叉免疫。HSV-1 原发感染主要引起生殖器外皮肤黏膜(如口腔、角膜)和器官(如脑)的感染,HSV-2 原发感染主要引起生殖器部位皮肤黏膜和新生儿感染。

An important biological property of the alpha subfamily of HHV is to establish latent infections in neurons. When HSV enters injured skin or mucous membrane, the virus replicates first at the sites of entry and initiates a primary infection. The virus then invades local nerve endings and is transported through the retrograde axonal flow to the dorsal root ganglia where the virus establishes latency after further replication. In the latent stage, the virus resides in infected ganglia in a non-replicating state and may persist for a lifelong time in the host. A transient immunosuppression of the host triggered by fever, gastrointestinal disturbance, menstruation, or stress may reactivate the latent virus. The reactivated virus travels to the skin or mucous membranes along the peripheral nerve endings, where the virus replicates and manifests as recurrent herpes simplex.

HHV α 亚科的重要生物学特性之一是能在神经元中形成潜伏感染。HSV 通过破损的皮肤或黏膜后,首先在侵入部位复制,形成原发感染。以后,沿神经末梢上行至背根感觉神经节,并进一步复制而长期潜伏。在潜伏期,病毒在感染的神经节内处于非复制状态,并伴随宿主终生。当机体遇发热、胃肠紊乱、月经、过度疲劳等因素,导致抵抗力降低时,病毒被重新激活,并沿神经末梢移行至皮肤或黏膜内复制,表现为复发性单纯疱疹。

【Clinical Manifestations】

【临床表现】

HSV infection can cause many clinical forms, which are classified into primary and recurrent infections.

HSV 感染能引起多个临床病种,分原发型感染和复发型感染两种类型。

(1) Primary infections: the primary HSV infection occurs in individuals who are exposed to HSV at the first time. The incubation period generally ranges from 3 to 12 days, and the natural course is from 1 week to 3 weeks.

(1) 原发型　指首次感染 HSV 者。潜伏期 3～12 天，自然病程 1～3 周。

①Subclinical infections: approximately 90% of the primarily-infected individuals are asymptomatic. However, 40%-50% of them have serum antibodies against HSV.

①亚临床感染：约 90%原发感染者无临床症状，但其中 40%～50%可检出血清抗 HSV 抗体。

② Herpes gingivostomatitis: herpes gingivostomatitis is the most common manifestation of primary HSV infection. It most frequently affects children of 1-5 years old. The typical skin lesions are painful grouped vesicles on the lips, gingiva, palate, or tongue, which usually appear on an erythematous base, and the vesicles may soon become pustular or ulcerated, but eventually crust. The affected individual may exhibit fever, sore throat, and regional lymphadenopathy. The natural course of the disease is about 2 weeks.

②疱疹性龈口炎：原发型感染中最常见的表现。多见于 1～5 岁儿童。在唇、牙龈、腭、舌等部位发生成簇疼痛性水疱，水疱常发生在红斑基础上，很快转为脓疱或溃疡，进而结痂。常伴发热、咽痛、局部淋巴结肿大等。自然病程约 2 周。

③ Neonatal HSV infection: about 75% of neonatal HSV infections are caused by HSV-2, and the most common transmission route is by contact with herpetic lesions in the maternal genital tract during childbirth. The infection often appears within the first week of life. The clinical presentation varies with each individual. For subtle cases, vesicles or erosions are mostly restricted to the skin, mucosa, or eyes. In severe cases, encephalitis, pneumonia, dyspnea, jaundice, seizures, disseminated infection, or even death may occur. Many survivors from severe neonatal HSV infections may have permanent impairment of the nervous system.

③新生儿单纯疱疹：约 75%的新生儿单纯疱疹是 HSV-2 感染引起的，多因经产道娩出时与疱疹性损害接触而感染，出生 1 周后发病。临床表现轻重不等，轻者仅皮肤、黏膜、眼等部位出现水疱、糜烂，重者发生脑炎、肺炎、呼吸困难、黄疸、惊厥、播散性感染，甚至死亡。幸存者常遗留严重的神经系统后遗症。

④ Eczema herpeticum: eczema herpeticum, also known as Kaposi's varicelliform eruption, occurs when an HSV-1 infection in patients who concurrently suffer from eczema, atopic dermatitis, burns, or other inflammatory dermatoses. Children are most frequently affected. The disease is characterized by hundreds of umbilicated vesicles surrounded by a red halo, which are often overlaid on the top of currently existing skin lesions and are accompanied by fever and regional lymphadenopathy.

④疱疹性湿疹：又称 Kaposi 水痘样疹，常由 HSV-1 感染引起，常发生于湿疹、特应性皮炎、烧伤或其他炎症性皮肤病患者，多见于儿童。在原皮损基础上出现密集的脐凹状水疱，周围红晕，伴发热和淋巴结肿大。

⑤ Inoculation herpes: inoculation herpes is also known as herpetic whitlow. The characteristic skin lesions are vesicles of sudden onset with severe pain, which most commonly affect the paronychial area.

⑤接种性单纯疱疹：又称疱疹性瘭疽，以突发水疱伴局部剧烈疼痛为特征，常见于甲沟。

⑥Herpetic keratoconjunctivitis: herpetic keratoconjunctivitis, a HSV infection of the cornea, may lead to deep round or dendritic ulcers. Cornea perforations may occur in severe cases, causing blindness, and are often accompanied with conjunctival congestion and edema.

⑥疱疹性角膜结膜炎：角膜感染 HSV 后可形成深在圆板状或树枝状溃疡，重者可致角膜穿孔，甚至失明，常伴结膜充血和水肿。

(2) Recurrent infections: recurrent HSV infection tends to

(2) 复发型　常在同一部位反复发

occur repeatedly at the same mucocutaneous junction areas, such as perioral (Fig. 5-1), labial, and ocular mucosa. There may be pain, a burning sensation, itching, or paraesthesia before the rise of the typical clustered vesicles on an erythematous base (Fig. 5-2). The vesicles may soon become erosive and finally crusted. The nature course of the disease is around one week if not accompanied by secondary infections.

作。皮损好发于口周(图 5-1)、唇部、眼部等皮肤黏膜交界部位。复发时局部常先出现疼痛、灼热、瘙痒或感觉异常,继而出现成簇水疱(图 5-2),破溃后可形成糜烂、结痂。如无继发感染,自然病程约 1 周。

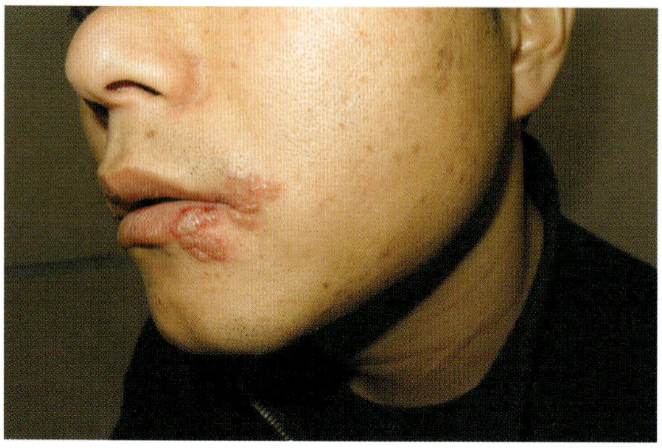

Fig. 5-1 Herpes simplex-perioral clustered vesicles
(图 5-1 单纯疱疹-口周成簇水疱)

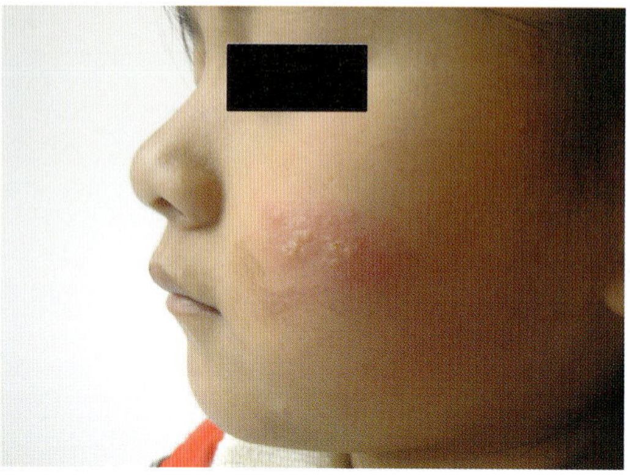

Fig. 5-2 Herpes simplex-facial clustered vesicles
(图 5-2 单纯疱疹-面部成簇水疱)

【Laboratory Findings】

In cytological smear (Tzanck's smear) tests, the presence of multinucleated giant cells or nuclear eosinophilic inclusion bodies in the specimen from ground base of herpetic lesions is of indicative value for HSV infection. Confirmation of HSV infection by polymerase chain reaction test for virus DNA or virus isolation in cell culture from vesicular fluid remains the definitive diagnostic approach. However, the virus is sometimes difficult to be detected especially when the disease is in the latent stage. The serum IgM antibodies against HSV are of diagnostic value for HSV infections in the central nervous system, whereas the IgG antibodies are useful only for epidemiology surveys.

【实验室检查】

用刮片或拭子从疱疹性损害的基底部取材,采用细胞学涂片(Tzanck's 涂片)检查见到多核巨细胞和核内嗜酸性包涵体可提示 HSV 感染,特殊病例可通过 PCR 法检测 HSV DNA、疱液病毒分离培养和鉴定等确诊,有的患者因潜伏感染可能找不到病原体。血清抗 HSV IgM 抗体对神经系统感染有一定诊断价值,IgG 抗体多用于流行病学调查。

【Diagnosis and Differential Diagnosis】

Herpes simplex is not difficult to be diagnosed, according to its typical characterizations of grouped vesicles at mucocutaneous junction sites and its tendency to recur, but it may sometimes require differentiation from herpes zoster, impetigo, or fixed drug eruptions.

【诊断与鉴别诊断】

根据皮肤黏膜交界处的成簇水疱和易于复发的特点,诊断不难。本病需与带状疱疹、脓疱疮和固定型药疹鉴别。

【Treatment】

The goals of treatments are to shorten the current attack, to prevent from secondary bacterial infections, and to avoid or postpone recurrence.

(1) Antiviral drugs: several antiviral drugs are effective for HSV infections, among which nucleoside analogs remain the most effective.

【治疗】

治疗目的为缩短病程,防止继发细菌感染,避免或减少复发。

(1) 抗病毒药 多种抗病毒药物均有效,但核苷类抗病毒药物仍为最有效

①Primary infection: recommended antiviral drugs include acyclovir 200 mg 5 times daily (or 400 mg 3 times daily), valacyclovir 1000 mg twice daily, or famciclovir 250 mg 3 times daily for 7-10 days.

② Recurrent infection: one of the following antiviral drugs should be given within 24 hours after onset and maintained for 5 days, acyclovir 200 mg 5 times daily (or 400 mg 3 times daily), valacyclovir 500 mg, once to twice daily, or famciclovir 125 mg twice daily.

For patients with frequent recurrences (more than 6 in a year), a modified regimen is recommended. Acyclovir 400 mg 3 times daily, valacyclovir 500 mg once daily, or famciclovir 250 mg twice daily, should be administered for a total of 6-12 months.

In severe cases, intravenous acyclovir (5-10) mg/(kg · d) in 3 divided doses may be administered for 5-7 days.

的药物。

①原发型：阿昔洛韦 200 mg/次，5 次/天，或 400 mg/次，3 次/天；伐昔洛韦 1000 mg/次，2 次/天；泛昔洛韦 250 mg/次，3 次/天。连用 7～10 天。

②复发型：皮损出现 24 h 内，阿昔洛韦 200 mg/次，5 次/天，或 400 mg/次，3 次/天；伐昔洛韦 500 mg/次，1～2 次/天；泛昔洛韦 125 mg/次，2 次/天。连用 5 天。

对频繁复发者（每年复发超过 6 次），阿昔洛韦 400 mg/次，3 次/天；伐昔洛韦 500 mg/次，1 次/天；泛昔洛韦 250 mg/次，2 次/天。连用 6～12 个月。

皮损广泛或症状严重者：阿昔洛韦 (5～10) mg/(kg · d)，分 3 次静脉滴注，连用 5～7 天。

(2) Topical therapy: the aims of topical treatments are to astringe the affected area and prevent from secondary bacterial infection. Commonly used agents include 3% acyclovir ointment, 1% penciclovir cream, and calamine lotion. A benzalkonium chloride solution (1 : 1000) or a Kangfuxin solution may be used for oral ulcers. Topical antibiotics such as 2.5% mupirocin ointment, 2% fusidic acid cream are used for secondary bacterial infections.

(2) 局部治疗　目的是保护和收敛皮损、防止继发细菌感染。可外搽 3%阿昔洛韦软膏、1%喷昔洛韦霜，或炉甘石洗剂，伴口腔溃疡者以 1 : 1000 新洁尔灭漱口或外搽康复新液，继发细菌感染时可外搽 2.5%莫匹罗星软膏、2%夫西地酸乳膏等抗生素制剂。

Section Two　Varicella and Herpes Zoster

Varicella (chickenpox) and herpes zoster (shingles) are two distinct clinical entities caused by the same varicella-zoster virus (VZV). Varicella is caused by a primary infection of VZV, characterized by widespread umbilicated vesicles accompanied by fever; herpes zoster is caused by reactivation of the latent VZV, characterized by grouped vesicles unilaterally distributed along a peripheral nerve accompanied with intense neuralgia.

第二节　水痘和带状疱疹

水痘（varicella）和带状疱疹（herpes zoster）是水痘-带状疱疹病毒（VZV）引起的但临床表现不同的两种病毒性皮肤病。水痘为 VZV 的原发感染所致，以皮肤黏膜泛发性脐凹状小水疱伴发热为特征。带状疱疹为潜伏 VZV 再激活所致，以沿周围神经支配区呈单侧分布带状排列的成簇水疱伴明显神经痛为特征。

【Etiology and Pathogenesis】

VZV is the third member of alpha subfamily of human herpesvirus (HHV) and currently known as HHV-3. It is morphologically identical to herpes simplex virus as described in the first section, i. e., a prickly enveloped DNA virus of 150-200 nm in diameter, a double-stranded DNA in the core enclosed by an icosahedral capsid, and a double-layered lipid envelope. Like the other two viruses in this subfamily, VZV affects human beings only.

【病因及发病机制】

VZV 属人类疱疹病毒（HHV）α 亚科的第 3 个成员，现称 HHV-3 型。其形态与 HSV 相同，为砖形囊膜病毒，直径为 150～200 nm，中心为双链 DNA，其外为 20 面体核衣壳，衣壳表面为一双层脂质囊膜。与 α 亚科其他两种病毒一样，人类是其唯一宿主。

VZV invades human body through mucous membrane of the upper respiratory tract and replicates first in the mucous epithelia at the site of entry. The virus then enters the blood stream to form a viremia, and eventually spreads to the whole body, which clinically manifests as varicella. Varicella mostly affects the skin and may occasionally affect other organs. After clinical resolution of the primary infection, some viruses migrate to the sensory ganglia through the sensory nerve fibers and establish a lifelong latent infection. A decline in the immunity of the host triggered by fever, stress, menstruation, or malignancy allows the virus to reactivate and replicate in the ganglia, and then migrate to the skin through the nerve endings, leading to intense neuralgia and grouped vesicles in the involved skin, which clinically manifests as herpes zoster.

VZV 经上呼吸道黏膜侵入后在黏膜上皮内生长繁殖，后进入血液引起病毒血症，病毒随血液循环播散全身，临床表现为水痘，以皮肤黏膜损害为主，偶尔引起其他器官损害。水痘痊愈后，部分病毒沿感觉神经末梢移行至脊神经后根神经节等处，形成慢性潜伏感染。当机体抵抗力下降时（如发热、疲劳、紧张、月经、恶性肿瘤等），潜伏病毒被激活，沿周围神经下行至相应节段皮肤内复制，引起神经痛和成簇水疱，临床表现为带状疱疹。

【Clinical Manifestations】

【临床表现】

(1) Varicella: varicella, or chickenpox, often occurs in winter and spring. It most commonly affects children of 2-10 years old. Varicella is a mild but highly contagious disease, which may sometimes cause an endemic outbreak in kindergartens or schools. Patients with varicella are the major source of transmission and the virus is transmitted by respiratory droplets, direct skin-to-skin contact, or indirect contact with the contaminated subjects. Children who have contact with patients with zoster may develop varicella. Human beings are quite susceptible to VZV infection, but a lifelong immunity against varicella may develop after an attack of varicella.

(1) 水痘　好发于冬春季，主要累及 2～10 岁儿童。该病一般症状不重，但传染性强，容易在幼儿园、学校等人群集中地传播甚至暴发流行。患者为主要传染源，主要经呼吸道飞沫、直接接触水疱液、间接接触病毒污染的物品而传染，与带状疱疹患者接触的儿童也可发生水痘。人群普遍易感，但一次发病可获终身免疫。

The incubation period of varicella is 2-3 weeks. Varicella has an acute onset with prodromal symptoms including fever, headache, sore throat, and malaise. The initial skin lesions are small erythematous macules that appear on the trunk within 24 hours, and then spread to the scalp, face, and extremities. These erythematous macules quickly become oval, mung bean-sized, tense umbilicated vesicles surrounded by red halos (Fig. 5-3). These vesicles begin to dry up in 2-3 days with crust formation, even while other lesions are forming. The mucous membranes are always involved and vesicles and erosions may be found on the mucosa of the mouth, throat, eye, vulva, anus, etc. The natural course of varicella is 2-3 weeks without scar formation after the skin lesions have resolved, if not accompanied with secondary infections. In immunosuppressed patients, the skin lesions may be disseminated over the entire body.

潜伏期 2～3 周。起病急，发病前有发热、头痛、咽痛、全身倦怠等前驱症状。在发病 24 h 内先在躯干出现皮疹，后逐渐蔓延至头部、面部和四肢。皮疹初起为针头大小红斑，迅即变为绿豆大小的椭圆形紧张性水疱，中央呈脐凹状，周围红晕明显（图 5-3）。2～3 天后水疱开始干涸结痂，痂脱而愈。黏膜亦常受累，口、咽、眼、外阴、肛门等处可见水疱或糜烂面。自然病程 2～3 周，愈后不留瘢痕。若患儿抵抗力低下，皮损可全身播散形成播散性水痘。

In severe cases, atypical skin lesions such as bullous, hemorrhagic, or necrotic varicella may occur, which may sometimes be accompanied with pneumonia or encephalitis. Varicella may also affect both neonates (called neonatal varicella) and adults (called adult varicella). The symptoms in adult varicella are always more

水痘还可出现一些非典型表现，如大疱性、出血性和坏死性水痘，严重者可并发水痘性肺炎、脑炎等。水痘也可累及新生儿（称新生儿水痘）及成人（称成人水痘），成人水痘症状常较重。

severe than in neonates.

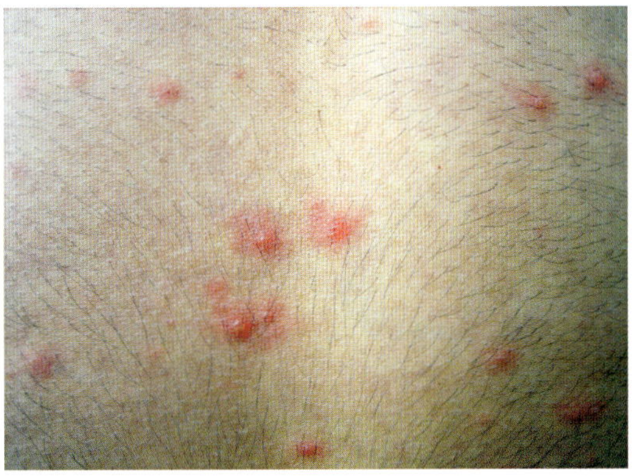

Fig. 5-3　Varicella-umbilicated vesicles on erythematous base

（图 5-3　水痘-红斑基础上脐凹状水疱）

（2）Herpes zoster: prior to the occurrence of herpes zoster (shingles), a mild prodrome including fever, anorexia, lassitude, regional neuralgia, or paraesthesia usually lasts for 1-3 days. Typical skin lesions often distribute unilaterally along the peripheral nerve-relevant dermatomes, in which the thoracic, trigeminal, lumbar, and sacral nerves are most frequently affected (Fig. 5-4). Rarely, two or more dermatomes or even bilateral involvement may be observed in immunosuppressed patients. The initial skin lesions are always erythema or papules over certain dermatomes relevant to the affected nerves, and quickly become a crop of vesicles with clear contents. The vesicles gradually dry up or rupture but eventually crust. The natural course is 2-3 weeks, or even 3-4 weeks in the elderly. However, in some rare cases, only linearly distributed erythemas and/or papules but without the typical clustered blisters may be seen, which are accordingly called abortive zoster (Fig. 5-5). Vesicles may turn to be hemorrhagic, necrotic, or bullous in severe cases (Fig. 5-6).

（2）带状疱疹　发疹前可有轻微的前驱症状，如发热、纳差、倦怠，局部皮肤可有疼痛或感觉异常，持续 1～3 天。皮损好发于胸、三叉神经、腰、骶部神经分布区域，通常呈单侧分布带状排列（图 5-4），但严重者可累及 2 个或 2 个以上神经节段，皮损可因此呈双侧分布。皮损初起为局限性红斑、丘疹，迅速变为成簇水疱，疱液澄清。水疱逐渐干涸，或破溃、结痂。自然病程 2～3 周，老年人可达 3～4 周。有时，皮疹仅有红斑、丘疹而无典型成簇水疱，称顿挫型（图 5-5）。严重者水疱可呈出血性、坏死性或大疱性（图 5-6）。

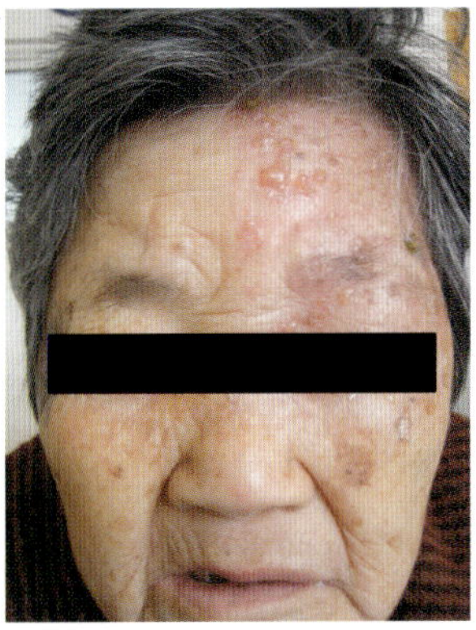

Fig. 5-4　Herpes zoster-on trigeminal nerve relevant dermatome

（图 5-4　带状疱疹-三叉神经分布区域）

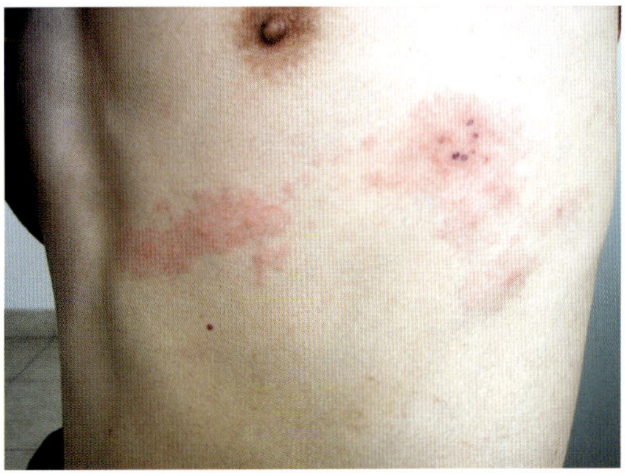

Fig. 5-5　Herpes zoster-thoracic, abortive

（图 5-5　带状疱疹-胸部，顿挫型）

Clinically, several uncommon presentations may be observed as follows.

临床上还可见一些特殊类型。

Herpes zoster ophthalmicus (HZO): the ophthalmic branch of the trigeminal nerve may be infected by the virus, leading to severe neuralgia, corneal ulceration, or even blindness in severe cases.

Herpes zoster oticus: When VZV spreads to the geniculate ganglion, both the facial and acoustic nerves may be involved, leading to otalgia, herpetiform vesicles on the external ear canal (Fig. 5-7), and facial paralysis (also called Ramsay-Hunt syndrome).

眼带状疱疹：病毒侵犯三叉神经节眼支所致，疼痛明显，严重者可致角膜溃疡，甚至失明。

耳带状疱疹：病毒侵犯膝状神经节使面神经和耳神经受累，出现耳痛、外耳道疱疹(图 5-7)和面瘫，又称 Ramsay-Hunt 综合征(Ramsay-Hunt syndrome)。

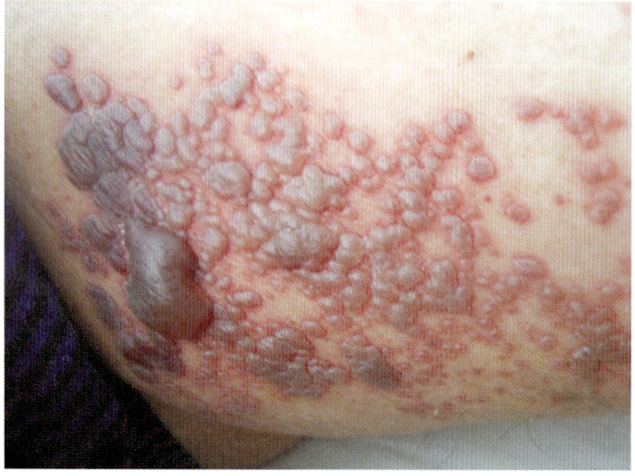

Fig. 5-6　Herpes zoster-bullous(图 5-6　带状疱疹-大疱性)

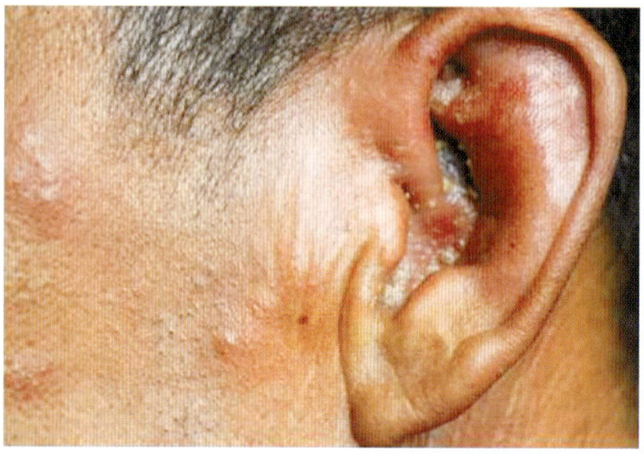

Fig. 5-7　Herpes zoster-oticus(图 5-7　带状疱疹-耳部)

Disseminated zoster: this unusual type most commonly affects immunosuppressed individuals with malignancies, or patients receiving radiation therapy, chemotherapy, or transplantation. Since the virus spreads throughout the whole body via blood stream, widespread varicella-like eruptions and impairment of lungs or brain may be observed.

Postherpetic neuralgia (PHN): this is the most common complication of herpes zoster in the elderly especially those elder than 60 years. The condition can persist for months or years after the skin lesions are recovered. It generally refers to neuralgia lasting for more than 90 days after appearance of skin lesions.

播散型带状疱疹：见于免疫功能低下者，如患恶性肿瘤、接受放化疗或器官移植等。病毒通过血液循环播散到全身，出现泛发性水痘样疹，并可侵犯肺和脑。

带状疱疹后遗神经痛：是老年带状疱疹患者的常见并发症，特别是 60 岁以上老年人，在皮损消退后疼痛仍可持续数月或数年。一般指带状疱疹皮疹发生后疼痛持续超过 3 个月。

【Laboratory Findings】

Cytological smears, virus isolation, direct immunofluorescence staining, and PCR tests for virus DNA are used to confirm VZV infection, especially in patients with atypical manifestations.

【实验室检查】

细胞学涂片、病毒分离培养、直接免疫荧光染色、PCR 法检测病毒 DNA 等方法可证实 VZV 感染，对不典型病例的诊断具有一定意义。

【Diagnosis and Differential Diagnosis】

(1) Varicella is readily diagnosed by its seasonal prevalence, predilection for children, typical umbilicated vesicles, and related systemic symptoms. However, it is necessary to differentiate it from impetigo or papular urticaria.

(2) Herpes zoster is also easily diagnosed on the basis of the unilaterally-distributed grouped vesicles with intense neuralgia. However, it should be differentiated from herpes simplex, contact dermatitis, acute appendicitis, or pleurisy.

【诊断与鉴别诊断】

(1) 水痘　根据发病季节、儿童好发、典型的脐凹状水疱及伴随症状，诊断不难。需与脓疱疮、丘疹性荨麻疹等鉴别。

(2) 带状疱疹　根据单侧分布带状排列的簇集性水疱伴明显神经痛等特点，诊断不难。需与单纯疱疹、接触性皮炎、急性阑尾炎、胸膜炎鉴别。

【Treatment】

(1) Varicella: the affected individual must be isolated until all blisters are crusted. Since varicella is usually self-limiting, symptomatic and supportive treatments are sufficient most of the time. Oral antihistamines and the topical use of calamine lotion may alleviate the symptoms. Antiviral drugs are used only in severe cases.

①Antiviral drugs: acyclovir is the most effective antiviral drug in current clinical practice. Oral acyclovir at 20 mg/kg 4 times daily for 5 days, or intravenous acyclovir at 8 mg/(kg · d) in 3 divided doses for 5-7 days may be administered. Other antiviral drugs such as interferon, vidarabine, and poly I : C may be good alternatives. Use of glucocorticoids should be avoided since they are likely to promote spread of the virus.

②Topical therapy: the purpose of topical treatment is to keep affected areas dry and to prevent from secondary infections. For intact vesicles, calamine lotion, acyclovir ointment, 3% ftibamzone lotion, idoxuridine lotion, or recombinant interferon alpha emulsion may be used. For ruptured lesions, 1% methyl violet solution or Kangfuxin solution may be a better choice. Topical antibiotics such as 2.5% mupirocin ointment or 2% fusidic acid cream may be used in cases with secondary bacterial infections. Alternate use of acyclovir eye drops and cortisone eye drops may alleviate inflammation of the affected eyes.

(2) Herpes zoster: since herpes zoster is generally a self-limiting disease, the treatment focuses on alleviating symptoms, shortening the clinical course, and preventing from postherpetic neuralgia. Ideally, treatments are initiated within 72 hours of onset, which include antiviral drugs, analgesics, neurotrophic drugs, immunomodulatory drugs, and glucocorticoids.

①Antiviral drugs: oral antiviral drugs such as acyclovir 800 mg 5 times daily for 5-10 days, valacyclovir 1000 mg 3 times daily for 7 days, or famciclovir 500 mg 3 times daily for 7 days, are recommended. In severe cases, intravenous acyclovir at 8 mg/(kg · d) in 3 divided doses may be administered for 5-7 days. Intramuscular injection of interferon α-2b 1-3 million IU once daily may inhibit viral replication.

② Glucocorticoids: early and short-term systemic use of glucocorticoids may decrease the incidence of PHN. For example, a substantial dose (e.g., 15-30 mg once in the morning) may be given for less than 1 week.

③ Analgesics: indomethacin 25 mg 3 times daily, or carbamazepine 0.1 g twice daily, or amitriptyline 25 mg 2-4 times

【治疗】

(1) 水痘　患者应隔离至水疱结痂干燥为止。因水痘为自限性疾病，只需采取对症支持治疗即可。口服抗组胺药物和外用炉甘石洗剂可减轻症状。重症者采用抗病毒药物治疗。

①抗病毒药物：阿昔洛韦仍是最有效的药物，口服每次 20 mg/kg，4 次/天，连续 5 天。严重者阿昔洛韦 8 mg/(kg · d)，分 3 次静脉滴注，连续 5～7 天。也可选择 α-2b 干扰素、阿糖腺苷、聚肌胞等。不宜使用糖皮质激素，以免引起病毒播散。

②局部治疗：主要目的是保护、干燥和预防继发感染。水疱未破溃者外用炉甘石洗剂，或阿昔洛韦软膏、3%酞丁胺搽剂、碘苷搽剂、重组 α 干扰素等。水疱破溃者外用 1%甲紫溶液或康复新液。继发感染时外用抗生素，如 2.5%莫匹罗星软膏、2%夫西地酸乳膏。无环鸟苷滴眼液和可的松滴眼液交替使用有助于减轻眼部炎症。

(2) 带状疱疹　因本病有自限性，治疗目的为减轻症状、缩短病程和预防后遗神经痛。最好在症状出现 72 h 内开始治疗。治疗药物包括抗病毒药物、止痛剂、神经营养剂、免疫调节剂和糖皮质激素。

①抗病毒药物：阿昔洛韦 800 mg/次，5 次/天，连续 5～10 天；伐昔洛韦 1000 mg/次，3 次/天，连用 7 天；泛昔洛韦 500 mg/次，3 次/天，连用 7 天。严重者，阿昔洛韦 8 mg/(kg · d)，分 3 次静脉滴注，连用 5～7 天。加用 α-2b 干扰素 100 万～300 万 IU，1 次/天，肌注，可有效抑制病毒复制。

②糖皮质激素：早期短程应用可减轻神经痛，如强的松 15～30 mg，晨服，连用不超过 1 周。

③止痛剂：吲哚美辛(消炎痛)25 mg/次，3 次/天；卡马西平 0.1 g/次，2

daily, may alleviate neuralgia. Cimetidine 0.2 g 3 times daily may be an alternative choice.

④ Neurotrophic drugs: intramuscular injection of vitamin B1 0.1 g plus vitamin B12 0.5 mg once daily or oral mecobalamin 0.5 mg twice daily or intramuscular mecobalamin 0.5 mg once daily is useful.

⑤Immunomodulator: subcutaneous injection of 2 mL of transfer factor twice a week, or intramuscular injection of gamma immunoglubin 3 ml once a week may be used.

⑥ Topical therapy: topical preparations for herpes zoster are the same as those for varicella. Physical modalities such as illumination with the infrared, ultraviolet, or microwave frequency bands, or by He-Ne laser, or high frequency radiation are effective for drying up vesicles and for alleviating neuralgia.

次/天;阿米替林 25 mg/次,2～4 次/天,可减轻疼痛。甲氰咪呱 0.2 g/次,3 次/天,也有一定疗效。

④神经营养剂:维生素 B1 0.1 g/次,1 次/天,肌注,维生素 B12 0.5 mg/次,1 次/天,肌注;或甲钴胺 0.5 mg/次,2 次/天,口服,或 0.5 mg/次,1 次/天,肌注。

⑤免疫调节剂:转移因子 2 mL,皮下注射,2 次/周;丙种球蛋白 3 mL,肌注,1 次/周。

⑥局部治疗:同水痘。物理治疗方法,如红外线、紫外线、微波、氦-氖激光、频谱等,对促进水疱干涸和减轻神经痛有效。

Section Three Warts

Verruca, commonly known as warts, are benign mucocutaneous hyperplasia caused by human papillomavirus (HPV) infections, which include verruca vulgaris, verruca plana, verruca plantaris, condyloma acuminatum, etc.

【Etiology and Pathogenesis】

HPV, belonging to genera *Papillomavirus* (family papovaviridae), is a 40-45 nm in diameter non-enveloped spherical virus enclosed in an icosahedral capsid comprising 72 capsomers. The virus genome comprises a double-stranded circular supercoiled DNA of 7.2-8.0 kb in size. More than 100 subtypes have been reported up to date, in which about 80 subtypes have been associated with human diseases. HPV may be transmitted by direct or indirect skin contact or autoinoculation. Usually, HPV enters an injured skin or mucous membrane and replicates at the entrance sites *in situ*, resulting in abnormal differentiation and proliferation of the infected epithelia. The infected epithelia eventually grow into a benign hyperplasia. The incubation period for HPV infection ranges from 1 month to 2 years.

【Clinical Manifestations】

(1) Verruca vulgaris: is also known as common warts. They are most commonly caused by HPV-2 infections. The disease may appear on the skin or mucous membranes of any sites, but is most frequently seen on the hands, especially around the fingers. The initial skin lesion is a pinhead-sized skin-colored translucent papule, which gradually becomes a larger, raised, skin-colored or brown, hyperkeratotic, and papillomatous papule (Fig. 5-8). The

第三节 疣

疣(verruca)是一种人乳头瘤病毒(HPV)感染引起的皮肤黏膜良性增生物,包括寻常疣、扁平疣、跖疣、尖锐湿疣等。

【病因及发病机制】

HPV 属乳头瘤病毒属乳多空病毒科,为球形无包膜病毒,直径为 40～45 mm,具有由 72 个病毒壳微粒组成的 20 面体衣壳。HPV 基因组长 7.2～8.0 kb,含双链环状超螺旋 DNA,多达 100 余种基因型,其中 80 余种与人类疾病有关。HPV 可经直接和间接接触,或自体接种方式传播。HPV 通过损伤的皮肤黏膜进入人体皮肤复制、增殖,致感染上皮细胞异常增生和分化,形成良性增生物。潜伏期 1 月至 2 年。

【临床表现】

(1) 寻常疣(verruca vulgaris) 多由 HPV-2 引起,可发生于皮肤黏膜任何部位,但好发于手部,尤其是手指。皮损最初为针头大小肤色半透明丘疹,数周至数月后体积逐渐增大,隆起,呈肤色或褐色的乳头瘤状角质性丘疹(图 5-8)。

entire process ranges from weeks to months.

Clinically, common warts around the eyelids or neck often present as slender, soft, filiform papules with a hyperkeratinized top surface and are therefore called verruca filliformis, while lesions on the scalp manifesting as finger-like pricks with a hyperkeratinized top surface are called digitate warts. Common warts on the periungual areas are called periungual warts, and those on the subungual areas are called subungual warts, regardless of their morphology. Nevertheless, no matter what type of common wart (s) the patient has, they are always asymptomatic.

发生于眼睑、颈部的细长、柔软、丝状突起伴顶端角化者称丝状疣，发生于头皮的单个或多个参差不齐的指状突起伴顶端角化者称指状疣，发生在甲周者称甲周疣，发生在甲床者称甲下疣。常无自觉症状。

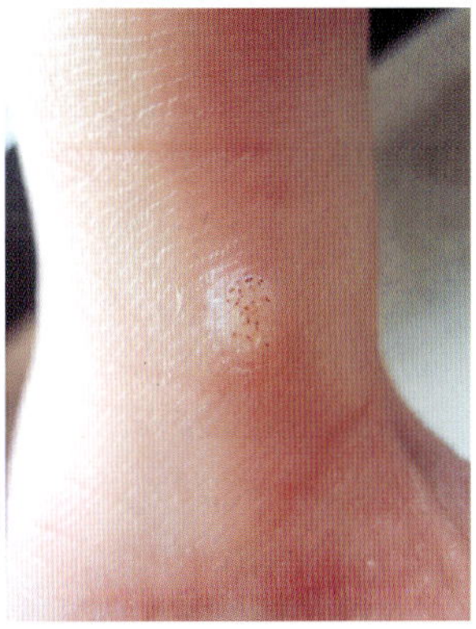

Fig. 5-8　Common warts-finger(图 5-8　寻常疣-手指)

(2) Verruca plana: is also known as flat warts. This type of warts is most commonly caused by HPV-3 infection. The face, forearms, and backs of the hands are most frequently affected. The typical skin lesions are flat or slightly elevated, brown or skin-colored papules of 1-5 mm in diameter (Fig. 5-9, Fig. 5-10). They may appear in a linear pattern due to scratching or trauma (Koebner's phenomenon). The skin lesions may regress spontaneously but may frequently recur.

(2) 扁平疣(verruca plana)　多由 HPV-3 引起。好发于颜面、手背和前臂。典型皮损为扁平或微隆起丘疹，肤色或褐色，直径为 1～5 mm(图 5-9，图 5-10)。搔抓或外伤可使皮损呈线状排列(Koebner 现象)。可自然消退，但常复发。

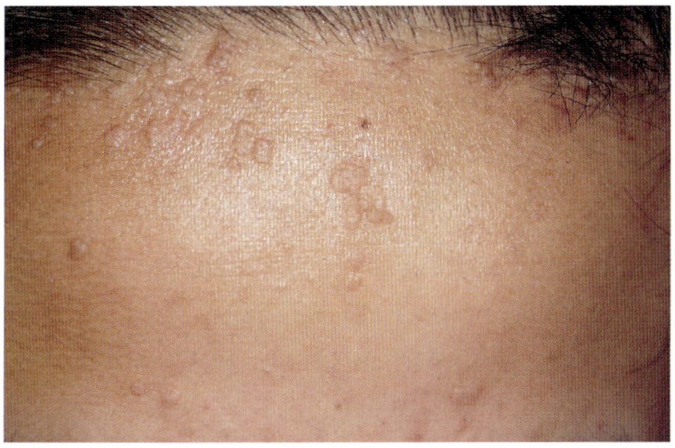

Fig. 5-9　Flat warts-forehead(图 5-9　扁平疣-额部)

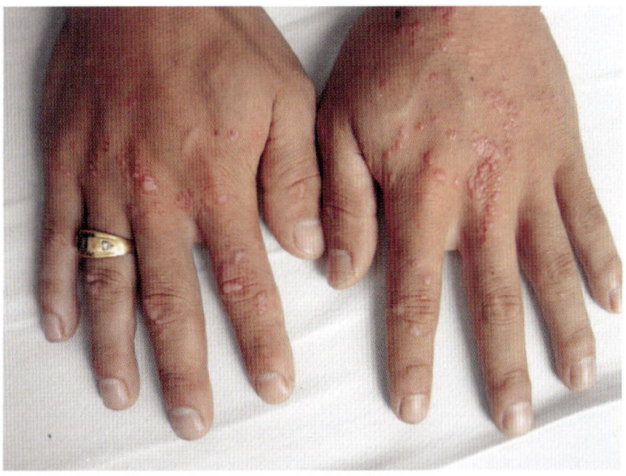

Fig. 5-10　Flat warts-dorsum of the hands(图 5-10　扁平疣-手背)

(3) Verruca plantaris: is also known as plantar warts. This is the most common warts on the soles. Most plantar warts are caused by HPV-1 infections. The typical skin lesions are firm

(3) 跖疣(verruca plantaris)　也称跖部疣，是一种发生于足底的寻常疣，多由 HPV-1 引起。典型皮损为坚硬的角

hyperkeratotic papules, which often have black speckling or bleeding spots on the top surface after mechanical removal of the horny layers due to rupture of the thrombosed capillaries. Multiple lesions may coalesce to form a "mosaic wart". Pain is always the predominant symptom of the disease.

质性丘疹,刮去角质层,可见因栓塞毛细血管破裂导致的黑色斑点和出血点。多个皮损可融合形成镶嵌疣。疼痛和压痛为主要症状。

【Diagnosis and Differential Diagnosis】

Diagnosis of warts is easily made based on the characteristic appearance and location of the skin lesions. Skin lesion biopsies or polymerase chain reaction tests for HPV DNA is necessary for confirming diagnosis in atypical cases. Plantar warts should be differentiated from corns or calluses. Corns and calluses have pain under direct pressure on the top of the skin lesion, whereas plantar warts have pain under lateral pressure. Warts occurring on the vulvar and genital areas should be differentiated from bowenoid papulosis, the later often manifests as multiple brown-colored papules and is commonly caused by HPV16 and shows similar features to Bowen's disease in histopathology.

【诊断与鉴别诊断】

根据发病部位和皮损形态即可诊断。不典型病例可通过病理活检或 PCR 法检测 HPV DNA 确诊。跖疣需与鸡眼和胼胝鉴别,鸡眼和胼胝在直接压迫时疼痛明显,而跖疣在侧面挤压时疼痛更明显。外阴和生殖器部位的疣还需与鲍温样丘疹病鉴别,后者多由 HPV16 引起,表现为多发褐色丘疹,组织病理上与鲍温病类似。

【Treatment】

The major therapies for warts include topical preparations and physical treatments.

(1) Topical therapy: topical preparations such as 0.05%-0.1% tretinoin cream or 0.1% adapalene gel once per evening along with recombinant interferon alpha-2b emulsion once to twice daily may be useful for flat warts. 5% 5-fluorouracil cream or 5-fluorouracil-dimethyl sulfoxide (DMSO) lotion, 3% ftibamzone cream or ftibamzone-DMSO lotion, once to twice daily may be useful for common warts. Pingyangmycin hydrochloride 10 mg in 20 mL of 1% procaine solution for intralesional injection once a week may be helpful for common warts and plantar warts as well. 5% imiquimod cream is an alternative choice for the treatment.

(2) Physical therapy: liquid nitrogen cryotherapy, electrodessication, CO_2 laser therapy, frequency bands or curettage can be used to remove the warts.

(3) Systemic therapy: to date, no oral antiviral drug has been shown to be definitely effective for warts. Retinoid, immunomodulatory medications (e. g., interferon or levamisole), and some Chinese herbs might be helpful for warts in a limited number.

【治疗】

以外用药物和物理治疗为主。

(1) 局部治疗　外搽 0.05%～0.1%维 A 酸霜或 0.1%阿达帕林凝胶,1 次/晚,联用重组 α-2b 干扰素乳膏,1～2 次/天,可试用于治疗扁平疣。5% 5-氟尿嘧啶霜或 5% 5-氟尿嘧啶-二甲基亚砜搽剂,3%酞丁胺霜或酞丁胺-二甲基亚砜搽剂,1～2 次/天,可试用于治疗寻常疣。盐酸平阳霉素 10 mg 溶于 1%普鲁卡因 20 mL 局部注射,1 次/周,可试用于治疗寻常疣和跖疣。5%咪喹莫特乳膏也可试用。

(2) 物理治疗　包括液氮冷冻、电灼、二氧化碳激光、微波、刮除术等。

(3) 系统治疗　目前尚缺乏确切有效的抗 HPV 药物,维 A 酸、免疫调节剂(干扰素、左旋咪唑等)和中药可试用。

Section Four　Molluscum Contagiosum

Molluscum contagiosum (MC) is a contagious dermatosis caused by molluscum contagiosum virus (MCV) and is characterized by umbilicus-shaped hemispherical papules.

第四节　传染性软疣

传染性软疣(molluscum contagiosum)是传染性软疣病毒(MCV)感染引起的传染性皮肤病,以脐凹状半球形丘疹为特征。

【Etiology and Pathogenesis】

MCV is a linear double-stranded DNA poxvirus. The virus has four subtypes, among which MCV-1 and MCV-2 are the most common. The MCV infection most frequently affects children, sexually-active adults, and immunocompromised individuals. The virus is likely to spread through direct skin-to-skin contact including sexual contact, or by sharing public showers or bathrooms, or by autoinoculation.

【病因及发病机制】

MCV 属痘病毒科，为线性双链 DNA 病毒。MCV 有四个亚型，其中 MCV-1 和 MCV-2 最为常见，主要感染儿童、性活跃的成年人和免疫功能低下者，可通过皮肤直接接触（含性接触）、共用物品、自体接种而传染。

【Clinical Manifestations】

The incubation period of molluscum contagiosum ranges from weeks to months. The skin lesions may develop anywhere. However, in children they are located predominantly on the face, trunk, and extremities. In adult patients, they are often located on the lower abdomen, inner thighs, pubic area, and genitalia. Typical skin lesions are dome-shaped, pearly, or skin-colored papules of 3-5 mm in diameter with a waxy appearance of the surface. The center of the lesion is umbilicated with a white curd-like core (called molluscum bodies) that can be easily squeezed out (Fig. 5-11). The skin lesions are generally self-limiting but can persist for years.

【临床表现】

潜伏期数周至数月。可见于任何部位，儿童好发于面部、躯干、四肢，成人则好发于下腹部、大腿内侧、耻骨部和外生殖器。典型皮损为直径 3～5 mm 的半球形丘疹，肤色或珍珠色，表面有蜡样光泽，中心有脐凹，内含白色乳酪样物质（称软疣小体），易挤出（图 5-11）。皮损有自限性，也可持续数年。

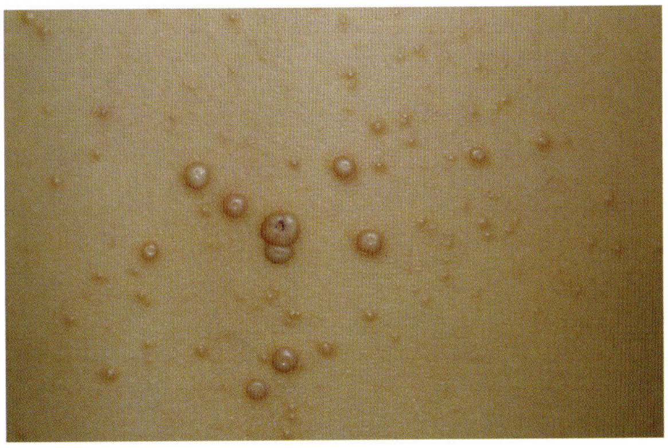

Fig. 5-11 Molluscum contagiosum-umbilicated lesions（图 5-11 传染性软疣-脐凹状皮损）

【Histopathology】

Acanthosis is presented in epidermis of the affected skin lesion. Molluscum bodies are always found in the infected cells of stratum malpighii, which are eosinophilic in lower parts of the epidermis but basophilic in the granular layer.

【组织病理】

表皮棘层增厚，马尔匹基层内可见软疣小体，在表皮下部呈嗜酸性，在颗粒层常呈嗜碱性。

【Diagnosis and Differential Diagnosis】

A diagnosis of molluscum contagiosum is made based on the typical skin lesions of dome-shaped papules with a central indentation and white curd-like suspension in the core. Histopathology of a biopsied lesion confirms the diagnosis. A single giant lesion of molluscum contagiosum should be differentiated

【诊断与鉴别诊断】

根据典型的半球形丘疹，中央有脐凹，内含白色乳酪样物质，诊断不难。组织病理可确诊。单个较大皮疹需与角化棘皮瘤和基底细胞上皮瘤鉴别。

from keratoacanthoma or basal cell epithelioma.

【Prevention and Treatment】

Scratching should be avoided to prevent from autoinoculation. A simple treatment for the skin lesion is squeezing out the curd-like core and then topically applying a tincture of iodine to prevent from secondary bacterial infection. Topical retinoid ointment or cantharidin tincture may also be beneficial. Cryotherapy, CO_2 laser, frequency bands, or high frequency electrodessication may be alternatives. Topical antibiotics should be applied in cases with secondary bacterial infections.

【预防和治疗】

避免搔抓，以防自体接种。可在消毒后挑破患处，挤出软疣小体，再外涂碘酒以防止继发细菌感染。也可外涂维A酸软膏、斑蝥素酊等，或用冷冻、二氧化碳激光、微波、高频电离子等物理治疗。继发细菌感染者外涂抗生素软膏。

Section Five　Hand-Foot-Mouth Disease

第五节　手足口病

Hand-foot-mouth disease is a contagious viral dermatosis characterized by painful vesicles on the hands, feet, as well as in and around the oral cavity.

手足口病(hand-foot-mouth disease)是一种以手部、足部和口腔疼痛性水疱为特征的传染性病毒性皮肤病。

【Etiology and Pathogenesis】

The disease is commonly caused by coxsackievirus type A16 or enterovirus type 71. However, other types of coxsackieviruses such as types A5, A7, A9, A19, B1 to B3, and B5 have also been implicated in the pathogenesis of this disease. The viruses reside not only in the rectum and nasopharynx, but also in the vesicle fluid of the lesions on the hands and feet. The etiological virus is transmitted by direct contact with nasopharyngeal or respiratory secretions, or with fecal matter.

【病因及发病机制】

病原体通常为柯萨奇病毒A16型和肠道病毒71型，也可为柯萨奇病毒A5、A7、A9、A19、B1、B2、B3或B5型。这些病毒存在于人的直肠、鼻咽部或手足部水疱液中，可经鼻咽部或呼吸道分泌物、粪便等途径传播。

【Clinical Manifestations】

Hand-foot-mouth disease may be endemic in the summer and autumn. The disease most commonly affects children under the age of five and may be endemic in kindergarten. The incubation period ranges from 3 to 7 days. The prodrome may include low fever, anorexia, abdominal pain, and often coughing.

The hands, feet and mouth are most frequently affected, whereas the buttocks are occasionally involved. The initial oral lesions are small painful vesicles surrounded by erythematous halos. These vesicles may soon become erosive or ulcerated. The papules on the palms and soles tend to form small vesicles with clear contents surrounded by erythematous halos (Fig. 5-12, Fig. 5-13, Fig. 5-14). The characteristic skin lesions are usually elliptical, with their long axis being parallel to the skin striae.

The disease may last for 7-10 days. Most patients have a good prognosis, and recurrence is rare. However, in a few cases, the patients suffering from enterovirus infections may be complicated by myocarditis, pneumonia, or meningoencephalitis, any of which

【临床表现】

手足口病多在夏秋季节流行。常见于5岁以下儿童，可在幼儿园中发生流行。潜伏期3～7天。前驱症状包括低热、纳差、腹痛、咳嗽等。

皮损可同时发生于手部、足部和口腔，偶见于臀部。也可表现为不全型，但以口腔损害为主。初发疹为口腔黏膜的疼痛性小水疱，绕以红晕，水疱破裂可很快形成糜烂、溃疡。掌跖部、指趾部初为红色斑疹或斑丘疹，很快变为小水疱，疱壁薄，内容澄清，绕以红晕(图5-12，图5-13，图5-14)。皮疹常呈椭圆形，与皮纹长轴平行。

本病经7～10天可自愈，预后良好，极少复发。由肠道病毒引起者可并发心肌炎、肺炎、脑膜脑炎，甚至死亡。

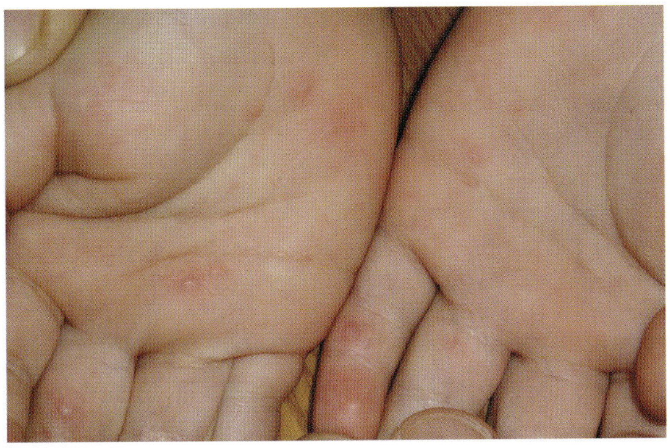

Fig. 5-12　Hand-foot-mouth disease-papules and vesicles on hands
（图 5-12　手足口病-手部丘疹和水疱皮损）

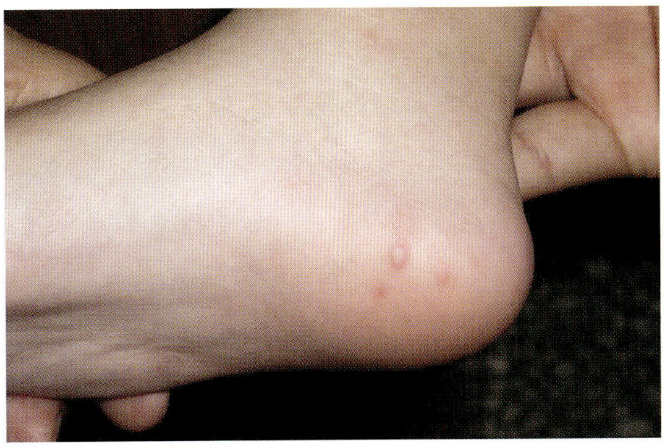

Fig. 5-13　Hand-foot-mouth disease-papules and vesicles on foot
（图 5-13　手足口病-足部丘疹和水疱皮损）

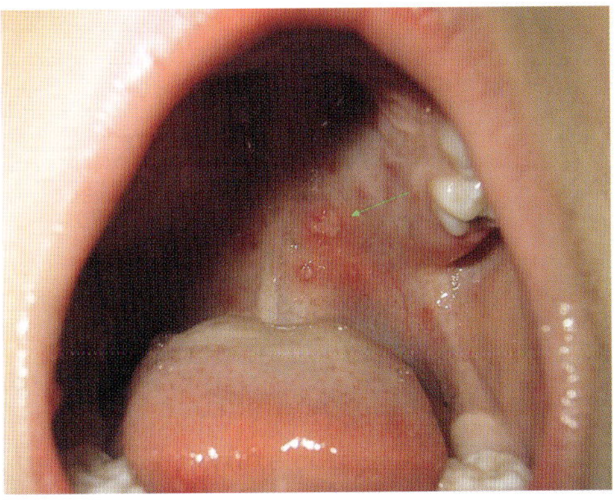

Fig. 5-14　Hand-foot-mouth disease-ulcers on oral cavity
（图 5-14　手足口病-口腔溃疡）

may lead to death.

【Diagnosis and Differential Diagnosis】

The diagnosis is easily made by time of the seasonal prevalence (in summer or autumn), and the typical vesicles on the hands, feet, and mouth. This condition should be differentiated from herpes simplex or erythema multiforme.

【诊断与鉴别诊断】

根据流行病学特点，及手部、足部和口腔皮疹特点容易诊断，需与单纯疱疹、多形红斑等鉴别。

【Treatment】

The affected children should be isolated as early as possible to prevent from transmission of the disease to others. Since the disease is self-limiting, only symptomatic and supportive treatments are necessary. For example, an oral ulceration gel or a Kangfuxin solution should be used for the oral ulcers to help recovery, and topical anesthetics may be used for relieving pain. A Chinese herb, *Radix isatidis*, is effective for shortening the duration of the disease.

【治疗】

患儿应尽早隔离，防止群体性传播。因本病有自限性，仅需对症和支持治疗。口腔溃疡贴膜、康复新液等可促进口腔溃疡愈合，口腔表面麻醉剂可减轻口腔溃疡引起的疼痛。口服板蓝根冲剂对缩短病程有一定效果。

Guan-qing WANG（王官清），Zhen-ling LU（卢珍玲）

Chapter Six　Dermatoses Caused by Bacterial Infections

第六章　细菌感染性皮肤病

Cutaneous bacterial infections are caused by resident or transient bacteria in the epidermis and mucosa. These bacteria invade the skin in places where barrier function is weak, such as hair follicles, sweat glands or trauma sites. The severity of the infection tends to depend on the amount of the invaded bacteria, the equilibrium between the bacterial virulence and the host's immune system.

细菌感染性皮肤病是由表皮或黏膜的常驻菌或暂驻菌引起的。这些细菌通过皮肤屏障功能较弱的部位(如毛囊、汗腺或皮肤小创伤处)侵入皮肤内部。感染的严重程度取决于细菌的数量、致病力以及和宿主抵抗力之间的平衡。

When a cutaneous bacterial infection is suspected, the causative bacteria should be identified by culture and their susceptibilities noted to available antibiotics.

当怀疑有细菌感染时,可通过细菌培养和微生物敏感性试验来确定致病菌,从而选用合适的抗生素。

This chapter will focus on four main subtypes of bacterial infections. These diseases are classified by their clinical features, which are: ① acute cutaneous infections (acute pyoderma); ②chronic cutaneous infections (chronic pyoderma); ③ systemic infections caused by toxin-producing bacteria; and ④ diseases with characteristic additional clinical features caused by specific bacteria.

本章介绍 4 种主要的细菌感染性疾病,这些疾病以临床特征分类:①急性皮肤感染(急性脓皮病);②慢性皮肤感染(慢性脓皮病);③产毒素菌引起的系统性皮肤感染;④特殊细菌引起具有特异临床特征的疾病。

Section One　Impetigo

第一节　脓　疱　疮

Impetigo, also called impetigo contagiosa, is a bacterial infection that occurs under the horny cell layer. The toxins produced by the bacteria cause blisters and crusts. The lesions are contagious and therefore the bacteria can spread by direct contact or autoinoculation.

脓疱疮(impetigo)又称为接触传染性脓疱疮,是由皮肤角质层下的细菌感染引起的,其产生的毒素造成皮肤大疱和痂,具有接触传染(自体接种)的特性。

Impetigo is most commonly seen in infants and can be divided into bullous and non-bullous impetigo depending on the infectious agents. Bullous impetigo is often caused by *Staphylococcus aureus* (*S. aureus*). Non-bullous impetigo usually manifests as crusts caused predominantly by group-A β-hemolytic *Streptococcus*. The main treatment of impetigo is to keep the skin clean and the use of effective antibiotics.

婴儿最易发生脓疱疮。根据致病菌的不同,脓疱疮可分为大疱性脓疱疮和非大疱性脓疱疮。大疱性脓疱疮由金黄色葡萄球菌引起;而非大疱性脓疱疮临床上主要表现为结痂,其主要是由于 A 组 β 溶血性链球菌感染引起。脓疱疮的主要治疗手段是使用抗生素和保持皮肤洁净。

1. Bullous impetigo

一、大疱性脓疱疮

【Etiology and Pathogenesis】

In the course of bullous impetigo, *Staphylococcus aureus* proliferates in the horny cell layer. The exfoliative toxins produced by *S. aureus* are serine proteases that can bind to and cleave the cell adhesion molecule desmoglein 1, which results in separation between the *stratum spinosum* and *granulosum* that eventually leads to blister formation.

【病因及发病机制】

金黄色葡萄球菌于角质层内繁殖,其产生的剥脱毒素是丝氨酸蛋白酶,后者能与细胞黏附分子桥粒芯蛋白 1 结合并将其裂解,在棘层和颗粒层间引起分离,临床上形成大疱。

【Clinical Manifestations】

Bullous impetigo occurs most commonly during summer in children under the age of three. It is highly contagious and tends to spread quickly in groups where a large number of young children are involved (e. g., daycare centers or nursery schools). The infection develops easily when there is a pre-existing wound on the skin, for example, a minor trauma or other skin disorders which produce persistent scratching such as eczema or atopic dermatitis.

Bullous impetigo begins with itching and slightly inflammatory vesicles that enlarge and later form flaccid bullae. Crescent-shaped accumulation of pus at the base of the bullae is a characteristic finding for this type of impetigo(Fig. 6-1). These blisters rupture easily and usually leave erosions. New blisters can be formed peripherally or spread to distant locations by autoinoculation through the purulent exudates. Nikolsky's sign may be positive. Bullous impetigo is transmitted primarily by contact with an infected person. It tends to heal without scarring; however, it may progress into staphylococcal scalded skin syndrome (abbreviated as SSSS; which is described in section 2 of this chapter) in some cases.

【临床表现】

大疱性脓疱疮(bullous impetigo)主要发生于夏季，常见于3岁以下的婴幼儿。因具有高度传染性，因而容易在小孩比较集中的场所(如日托所和托儿所)内造成大流行。大疱性脓疱疮首先发生于皮肤破损部位，如微小皮肤外伤、湿疹或特应性皮炎等常引起搔抓的疾病。

大疱性脓疱疮初为痒的轻度炎症性水疱，可增大并形成松弛的大疱，脓液沉积于疱底部呈半月形的积脓现象，是其特征(图6-1)。疱壁容易破裂，并形成糜烂面，分泌物向外流溢或通过搔抓不断将细菌带到其他部位，以致新的大疱不断产生。尼氏征可为阳性。大疱性脓疱疮通过接触感染者而传播。愈后不留瘢痕，但大疱性脓疱疮可进展成为葡萄球菌性烫伤样皮肤综合征(SSSS，见本章第二节)。

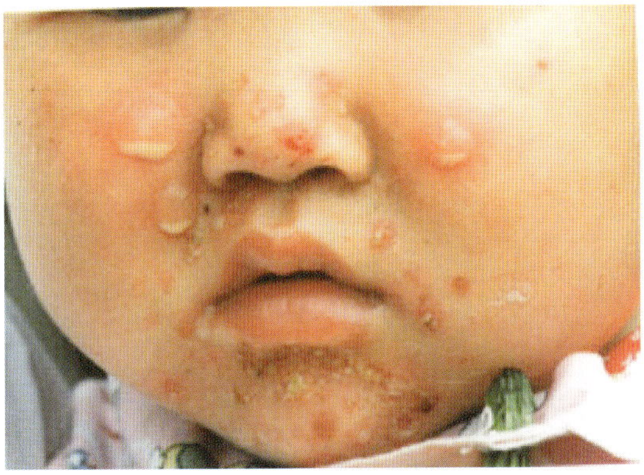

Fig. 6-1　Bullous impetigo(图6-1　大疱性脓疱疮)

【Diagnosis and Differential Diagnosis】

The diagnosis of bullous impetigo is based on bacterial culture and the features of the skin lesions. For example, blisters caused by insect bites are often severely inflamed but sterile, and this can be used to differentiate from bullous impetigo. In staphylococcal scalded skin syndrome, the characteristic features of the lesions around the eyes and mouth and usually a positive Nikolsky's sign will help to distinguish it from bullous impetigo. Adult onset cases should also be differentiated from pemphigus foliaceus.

【诊断与鉴别诊断】

根据临床皮损特点及细菌培养诊断。虫咬所致的大疱炎症较重，疱内液是无菌的。这与大疱性脓疱疮不一样。葡萄球菌性烫伤样皮肤综合征在眼周和口周会有特征性的皮损，尼氏征常阳性。成人发生的大疱性脓疱疮需与落叶性天疱疮区别。

【Treatment】

A person who has impetigo should be instructed in proper hygiene practices to prevent the spread of the infection (e. g.,

【治疗】

保持皮肤干燥。为预防传染，在皮损结痂之前，患者不可与他人共用毛巾。

keeping the lesion area dry and not sharing towels before crust formation). Topical application of antibiotic ointments and oral antibiotics are useful.

局部应用抗生素药膏和口服抗生素是有效的。

2. Non-bullous impetigo

【Etiology and Pathogenesis】

Streptococcus is mainly classified by its ability to hemolyze red blood cells. The group-A β-hemolytic *Streptococcus*, *Streptococcus pyogenes*, which hemolyzes red blood cells completely, accounts for most non-bullous impetigo. However, *Staphylococcus aureus* alone or mixed with *Streptococcus* spp. may also be seen in some cases.

【Clinical Manifestations】

Non-bullous impetigo, also known as streptococcal or crusted impetigo, begins as small erythematous patches that rapidly evolve into multiple pustules. The pustules break easily to release purulent exudates that dry and form thick and firmly adherent, yellowish-brown crusts(Fig. 6-2). The pus can be discharged when squeezing the crusts. Tender and swollen lymph nodes are commonly found in the affected regions as well. Often the patient has mild systemic complaints such as fever and sore throat. Compared with bullous impetigo, the onset of non-bullous impetigo is more acute and less dependent on age or seasons. The prevalence is greater among patients with atopic dermatitis.

二、非大疱性脓疱疮

【病因及发病机制】

链球菌根据其溶解红细胞的能力而进行大致分类。非大疱性脓疱疮主要由 A 组 β-溶血性链球菌(化脓性链球菌,能完全溶解红细胞)引起,也可由金黄色葡萄球菌或二者混合感染引起。

【临床表现】

非大疱性脓疱疮(non-bullous impetigo)也称为链球菌性脓疱疮或称结痂性脓疱疮,初起损害为小片红斑,很快发展成许多脓疱,脓疱易破,出现脓性分泌物,最后形成黄褐色的痂(图 6-2)。痂厚,黏着紧密,挤压后会流出脓液。局部淋巴结会产生疼痛和肿大,通常会伴有系统症状,如咽痛和发热。与大疱性脓疱疮相比,非大疱性脓疱疮起病急,并与年龄和季节无关。在特应性皮炎的患者中发病率较高。

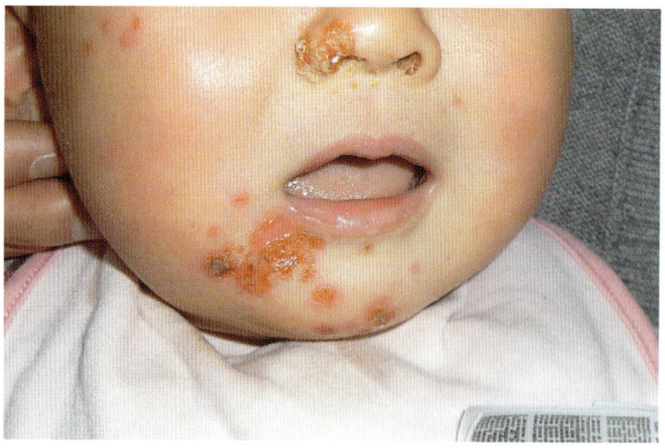

Fig. 6-2　Non-bullous impetigo

(图 6-2　非大疱性脓疱疮)

【Diagnosis and Differential Diagnosis】

A diagnosis of non-bullous impetigo can be established according to clinical features and culture results. It is difficult to distinguish non-bullous impetigo from Kaposi's varicelliform eruption, particularly in children with atopic dermatitis. The two conditions may occur simultaneously.

【诊断与鉴别诊断】

根据临床表现和细菌培养可以确诊。非大疱性脓疱疮与 Kaposi 水痘样疹很难区别,尤其是在患有特应性皮炎的儿童身上。这两种疾病可同时发生。

【Treatment】

Systemic antibiotics are absolutely the first line of treatment. Because some patients with non-bullous impetigo caused by *Streptococcus* may develop post-streptococcal glomerulonephritis, a urinalysis should be conducted during and 6 weeks after the infection. To prevent such complication, administration of oral antibiotics is usually continued 10 days after remission of the eruptions.

【治疗】

口服抗生素是一线的治疗手段。由于非大疱性脓疱疮可能会并发肾小球肾炎，所以链球菌所致的非大疱性脓疱疮的患者在患病期间及其后的6周都要进行尿液检查。为了防止发生肾炎，在皮损消退后还需继续口服10天抗生素。

Section Two　Staphylococcal Scalded Skin Syndrome

Staphylococcal scalded skin syndrome (SSSS) is also known as staphylococcal toxic epidermal necrolysis. It is caused by exfoliative toxins (ETs) released by *Staphylococcus aureus* in the epidermis. It occurs most frequently in infants and children under 6 years old. Fever and red rashes around the mouth or eyes appear first, followed by diffuse epidermal exfoliation with skin tenderness, erosion and blistering. Nikolsky's sign is positive for SSSS disease. Systemic management, supportive care, and the administration of antibiotics are the main treatments.

第二节　葡萄球菌性烫伤样皮肤综合征

葡萄球菌性烫伤样皮肤综合征(staphylococcal scalded skin syndrome, SSSS)，又名葡萄球菌性中毒性表皮坏死松解症，是由表皮的金黄色葡萄球菌产生的剥脱性毒素(exfoliative toxins, ETs)引起，最常发生于婴儿和6岁以下的儿童。以发热和口及眼周红斑起病，后广泛表皮痛性剥脱，露出糜烂面和发生大疱。尼氏征阳性。系统治疗、支持治疗和抗生素的应用是主要的治疗手段。

【Etiology and Pathogenesis】

SSSS is caused by ETs produced by *Staphylococcus aureus* in the epidermis. The infection occurs most commonly at sites such as nasopharynx, conjunctivae, external ears and umbilicus. ETs can also affect remote sites via blood circulation. This toxin is a serine protease that targets desmoglein-1 (a desmosome structural protein) leading to epidermolytic effects. As a result, a pemphigus foliaceus-like acantholysis and intraepidermal blisters on the upper epidermal layer occur.

【病因及发病机制】

SSSS由表皮的金黄色葡萄球菌产生的ETs引起。鼻咽、结膜、外耳和肚脐最易被感染。ETs能通过血循环而作用于远隔部位，ETs是一种丝氨酸蛋白酶，作用于桥粒芯糖蛋白-1(即桥粒的结构性蛋白)而产生表皮松解效应。在表皮浅层会出现落叶性天疱疮样的皮肤棘层松解和表皮上部表皮内大疱。

【Clinical Manifestations】

SSSS occurs most frequently in infants and children under the age of six; it is extremely rare in adults. It begins with erythema and blistering around the mouth, nostrils, and periocular area. Systemic symptoms such as a low grade fever (about 38 ℃ or higher), irritability, and anorexia are usually present. Typically, wrinkles and fissures around the mouth, eye discharge and crusting constitute the characteristic facial features of this disease. The erythema often begins on the flexural areas such as the neck, the axillary fossae, and groin; later the entire skin begins to exfoliate and erosions similar to burned skin are seen (Fig. 6-3). Skin at normal sites also exfoliates easily by friction (Nikolsky's sign is

【临床表现】

SSSS最常发生于婴儿和6岁以下的儿童，成年人很少发生。通常以口、鼻孔和眼周的红斑和大疱起病。伴有系统性症状，如发热至38 ℃或以上、易激惹和食欲不振。口周的皱褶和裂隙、眼分泌物和痂构成了独特的面部特征。红斑出现在颈部、腋窝和腹股沟等皱褶部位，同时整个身体的皮肤开始剥脱出现糜烂面，如烫伤样(图6-3)。正常部位的皮肤在摩擦下也易于剥脱(尼氏征阳性)，有剧烈的疼痛。通常不累及黏膜。头皮剥

positive). Sharp pain is present. Mucous membranes tend not to be affected and exfoliation on the scalp occurs in rare cases. SSSS begins to heal as exfoliation is accelerated by systemic administration of antibiotics. Usually, the entire course of SSSS is 1-2 weeks.

脱罕见。SSSS 患者在使用抗生素后剥脱加速并开始愈合,整个病程为 1～2 周。

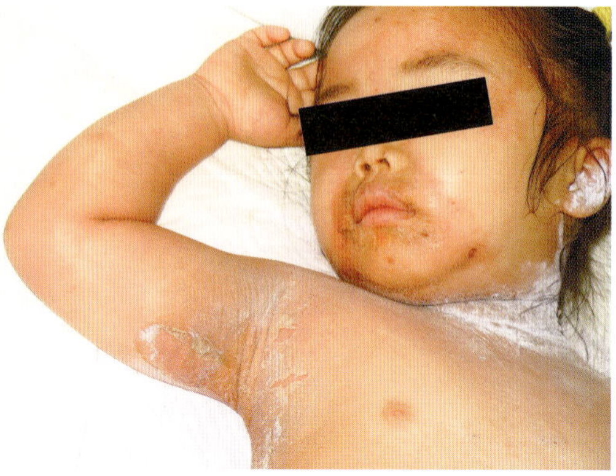

Fig. 6-3 Staphylococcal scalded skin syndrome(图 6-3 葡萄球菌性烫伤样皮肤综合征)

【Histopathology】

Acantholysis, epidermal clefts, and infiltration of polymorphous nuclear cells are observed beneath the horny cell layer and within the granular cell layer.

【组织病理】

在角质层下和颗粒细胞层中会出现棘层松解或裂隙和多形核细胞渗入。

【Diagnosis and Differential Diagnosis】

SSSS can be diagnosed by the characteristic facial features, burn-like widespread epidermal exfoliation, marked Nikolsky ' s sign, and the sparing of the oral mucosa. Most cases of toxic epidermal necrolysis(TEN)are induced by drugs. Histopathologically, the necrolysis is present in all epidermal layers and even in mucous membranes in TEN cases. Infants are rarely affected by TEN. In cases of generalized bullous impetigo, the characteristic facial features of SSSS are absent.

【诊断与鉴别诊断】

SSSS 可通过独特的面部特征、烫伤样的广泛的表皮剥脱、尼氏征强阳性及正常的口腔黏膜来诊断。大多数中毒性表皮坏死松解症是由药物导致的。从组织病理角度看,中毒性表皮坏死松解症是表皮全层的坏死,重者侵及黏膜。婴儿极少发生中毒性表皮坏死松解症。泛发性大疱性脓疱疮没有 SSSS 中独特的面部特征。

【Treatment】

Patients with SSSS should be hospitalized and treated with supportive care including rehydration with intravenous fluid and antibiotics that are effective against *Staphylococcus aureus*. The affected skin needs to be sterilized and treated with topical ointments that contain antibiotics and petrolatum. SSSS tends to have a good prognosis with proper treatment; however, the condition may deteriorate when sepsis or pneumonia occurs as a complication in infants and in immunocompromised adults.

【治疗】

应住院治疗。在治疗本病时要注意支持治疗,维持水、电解质平衡,并静脉给予对金黄色葡萄球菌有效的抗生素。在感染部位要保持无菌并局部应用包含抗生素和凡士林的药膏。SSSS 预后良好。然而,合并有败血症或肺炎的婴儿和免疫缺陷的成人 SSSS 会很严重。

Section Three Folliculitis

Folliculitis is a localized bacterial infection occurring within a single hair follicle. It manifests typically as small pustules

第三节 毛囊炎

毛囊炎(folliculitis)是单个毛囊发生的局限性细菌感染。毛囊炎是毛囊口部

surrounded by mild erythema at the orifice of the hair follicle. Folliculitis that occurs on the face during puberty is called acne vulgaris. It may progress to furuncle or carbuncle, where the inflammation extends deeply and involves more than one hair follicle. Skin cleansing and topical or oral antibiotic therapy are usually curative.

小的脓疱，周围有红晕。在青春期面部的毛囊炎称为寻常性痤疮。毛囊炎进一步发展，可形成疖(furuncle)或痈，这种情况通常炎症更深，同时累及多个毛囊单位。皮肤清洁及局部或口服抗生素都有一定的治疗效果。

【Etiology and Pathogenesis】

Folliculitis is infection in the hair follicle ordinarily initiated by *Staphylococcus aureus* or *Staphylococcus epidermidis*. It is often secondary to a minor trauma, obstruction of a hair follicle, scratching around a hair follicle, or topical application of glucocorticoids that allow significant bacterial multiplication.

【病因及发病机制】

毛囊炎是金黄色葡萄球菌或表皮葡萄球菌所致的毛囊感染。微小外伤、毛囊堵塞、搔抓毛囊周围或局部应用糖皮质激素可造成上述细菌的感染，进而导致毛囊产生炎症。

【Clinical Manifestations】

Pustules occur at hair follicle openings and are surrounded by an erythematous halo (Fig. 6-4). The crust is formed within several days, followed in most cases by healing without scarring. When multiple eruptions occur at the openings of the follicles (superficial folliculitis) on the face, especially during puberty, the condition is known as acne vulgaris. Under some circumstances, folliculitis may proceed to an intense inflammatory phase, furuncles (deep-seated folliculitis) (Fig. 6-5) or carbuncles (multiple lesions with more than one hair follicle involved). Deep-seated folliculitis particularly in the beard areas is also known as sycosis vulgaris.

【临床表现】

毛囊周围有红晕，毛囊口有脓疱(图6-4)。几天后形成痂，绝大多数情况下愈后不留瘢痕。青春期发生于面部多发的毛囊口的炎症(浅表性毛囊炎)称为寻常性痤疮。深在性毛囊炎伴随有严重感染症状时，在某些情况下可进展为疖(深在性毛囊炎)(图6-5)或痈(多个毛囊受累形成多发性皮损)。局限于胡须区的深在毛囊炎称为寻常性须疮。

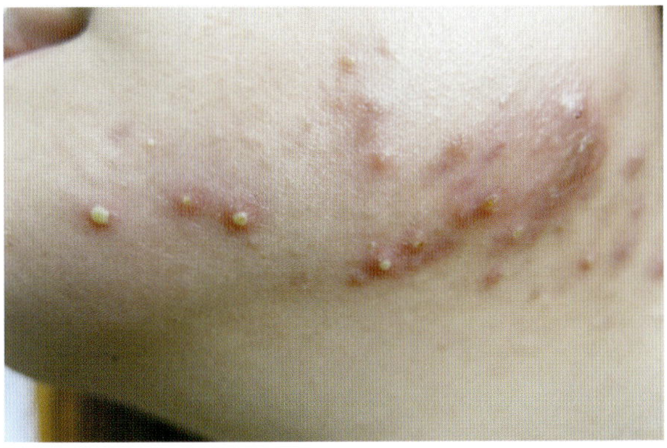

Fig. 6-4　Folliculitis(图 6-4　毛囊炎)

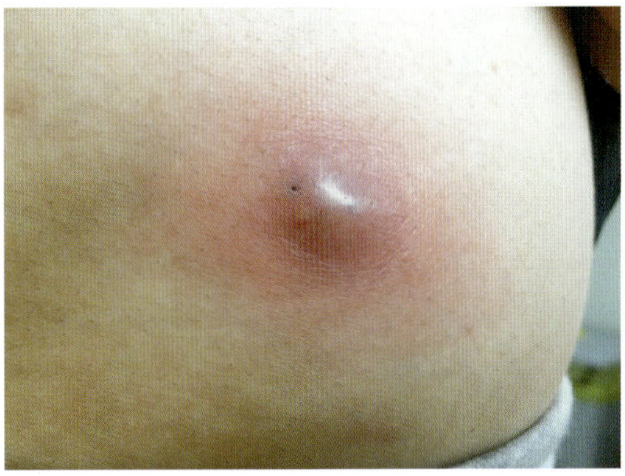

Fig. 6-5　Furuncle(图 6-5　疖)

【Diagnosis and Differential Diagnosis】

The diagnosis of folliculitis is based on clinical appearance. Bacterial culture can confirm the etiology. Folliculitis should be differentiated from furuncle and furunculosis.

【诊断与鉴别诊断】

根据皮损可以诊断。细菌培养可以确定病因。需与疖和疖病鉴别。

【Treatment】

In the mild form (few eruptions), treatment is not needed since folliculitis can heal spontaneously. Topical or oral antibiotics are only used in cases involving multiple follicles or deeper forms

【治疗】

当症状较轻、皮损较少时，毛囊炎可自愈，因此无需治疗。当皮损较多或发生深部毛囊炎时，可应用局部或口服抗

of folliculitis.

Section Four Erysipelas

Erysipelas is most often caused by group-A β-hemolytic streptococcal bacteria-*Streptococcus pyogenes*. The disease evolves rapidly with sudden fever. The face is most frequently affected. The lesions are edematous erythema with sharp margins and advancing borders. Severe painful and burning sensations are often present. Since most cultures for *Streptococcus pyogenes* are negative, antistreptolysin O (ASO) and antistreptokinase (ASK) measures are recommended in such circumstances. Penicillin is the first-line treatment for classical erysipelas. Patients with mild erysipelas can be treated orally with amoxicillin for 10-14 days. A randomized study indicated 5 or 10 days oral levofloxacin treatment can shorten the duration of treatment.

【Etiology and Pathogenesis】

Erysipelas is an acute purulent inflammatory disease that primarily affects the dermis. Although it is almost always caused by group-A β-hemolytic streptococcus (*Streptococcus pyogenes*), other groups, including group-B *Streptococcus pyogenes* (in newborns), *Staphylococcus aureus* and even *Pneumococcus* spp. , have also been documented in erysipelas. The pathogenesis of recurrent erysipelas is thought to be associated with local lymphatic blockage, localized skin barrier damage or inadequate treatment of erysipelas in the past, but the details remain unclear.

【Clinical Manifestations】

The lesions are sharply demarcated edematous erythema frequently found on the face and legs (Fig. 6-6). The disease may be accompanied by sudden chills and fever. The erythematous surface is tense and shiny due to swelling, and intense pain is often present as well. The eruptions spread rapidly and mark the border between infected and uninfected skin. Occasionally, bullae occur on the edematous erythema (erysipelas bullosa). A person with erysipelas on one side of the face is apt to be affected on the other side of the face within a short time. Systemic symptoms such as fever, nausea, and vomiting are commonly present. For most patients, the eruptions and fever disappear in about one week; however, certain individuals have a tendency to develop recurrent erysipelas on previously affected sites (commonly known as recurrent erysipelas).

【Laboratory Findings】

The elevated ASO and ASK may indicate an active streptococcal

生素治疗。

第四节 丹 毒

丹毒(erysipelas)通常由 A 组 β-溶血性链球菌(化脓性链球菌)感染所致。丹毒会引起突然的发热。脸部常受累。皮损表现为边界清楚的水肿性红斑并迅速蔓延。存在强烈的疼痛和皮肤灼热感。由于化脓性链球菌不易从细菌培养中得到,所以抗链球菌溶血素 O 试验(ASO)和抗链激酶(ASK)检测很有价值。青霉素类抗生素是传统丹毒的一线治疗手段,对不严重的门诊患者,10～14 天口服阿莫西林也是首选药物。一项随机研究表明 5 天或 10 天的左氧氟沙星口服治疗可使治疗时间缩短。

【病因及发病机制】

丹毒是主要累及真皮的急性化脓性感染性疾病。通常是 A 组 β-溶血性链球菌(化脓性链球菌)感染所致。其他组的化脓性链球菌(新生儿是 B 组)、金黄色葡萄球菌和肺炎球菌可引起类似于丹毒的症状。复发性丹毒的发病机制考虑与局部淋巴管堵塞、局部皮肤屏障破坏或不恰当的治疗有关,具体机制不清。

【临床表现】

皮疹为境界清楚的水肿性红斑,常常发生于面部和腿部(图 6-6),伴有突然发生的寒战和发热。由于肿胀,红斑表面紧张发亮。同时伴有剧烈的疼痛。皮疹迅速向外蔓延。受累与非受累皮肤间界线明显。在水肿性红斑的基础上可发生大疱(大疱性丹毒)。丹毒发生于面部时,一侧面部首先受累,很快另一侧也受到影响。可出现全身性症状,如发热、恶心和呕吐。大部分患者的皮疹和发热大约 1 周后会消失。然而,对于个别患者来说,皮疹可反复出现在原发部位,这种类型称为复发性丹毒。

【实验室检查】

抗链球菌溶血素 O(ASO)和抗链激

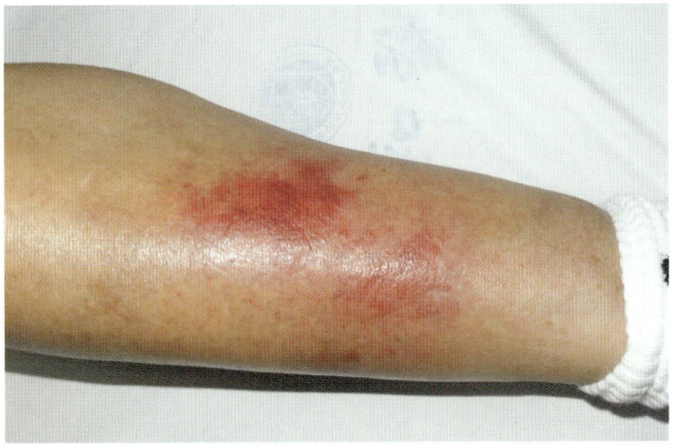

Fig. 6-6　Erysipelas(图 6-6　丹毒)

infection in patients, and an elevated erythrocyte sedimentation rate (ESR), leukocytosis (left shift of the nuclei in leukocytes), and a positive test of C reactive protein (CRP) may be observed. The positive rate for the detection of streptococcus from an affected skin sample or aspirated tissue fluid is low; however, it can be confirmed by PCR detection, and the latter technique is being used more frequently today for streptococcal bacteria detection.

酶(ASK)水平的提高提示患者链球菌的感染。可有血沉(ESR)加快,白细胞增多(白细胞核左移)和C反应蛋白(CRP)阳性。受累皮肤组织碎片或气道组织抽提液中的链球菌检出率低,但现在可用PCR进行证实,PCR可用于链球菌的检测。

【Diagnosis and Differential Diagnosis】

In general, the diagnosis of erysipelas is not difficult according to its tendentious site and the clinical features of the lesions. In fact, erysipelas is a superficial cellulitis of the skin, however, cellulitis usually mentioned is more deeply seated than erysipelas, and its erythematous edges are less clearly defined. Necrotizing fasciitis can be distinguished from erysipelas by the rapidly progressing necrotic lesions and intense systemic symptoms. Insect bites, thrombophlebitis, Sweet syndrome, herpes zoster, and carcinoma erysipelatodes also need to be differentiated from erysipelas.

【诊断与鉴别诊断】

根据其发病部位和临床特点一般不难诊断。丹毒实际上是一种皮肤浅表的蜂窝织炎,但常说的蜂窝织炎较丹毒的位置更深,同时红斑境界不像丹毒那样清楚。坏死性筋膜炎有迅速进展的坏死斑和显著的系统症状。同时,丹毒还需要与虫咬、血栓性静脉炎、Sweet综合征、带状疱疹和肿瘤性丹毒区别。

【Treatment】

Antibiotics such as penicillins and oral cephalosporins are adequate agents of choice. Treatment should continue 10 days after remission to avoid recurrence and to prevent complications from nephritis.

【治疗】

可用青霉素类抗生素和头孢菌素口服治疗。治疗需持续到症状减轻后10天,以预防疾病复发和肾炎并发症。

Section Five　Tuberculosis Cutis

第五节　皮肤结核

Tuberculosis (TB) cutis or cutaneous tuberculosis is essentially an invasion of the skin by *Mycobacterium tuberculosis*, or very rarely *M. avium-intracellulare* complex and *M. bovis*. Clinically, cutaneous TB can be further categorized into two groups: the more commonly seen "true" cutaneous tuberculosis, which is defined as the skin TB lesions resulting directly from mycobacteria inoculation on the skin; and the so-called "tuberculid" variety, which arises when the skin reacts to an endogenous source

皮肤结核(tuberculosis cutis or cutaneous tuberculosis)主要致病菌是结核分枝杆菌,偶尔也可由鸟分枝杆菌-细胞内复合群或牛型分枝杆菌侵入皮肤引起。临床上,皮肤结核可分为2大类,其中由外源性分枝杆菌直接感染皮肤,在原发感染部位产生皮损者称为真性皮肤结核,是皮肤结核中最常见的类型。结

of *M. tuberculosis*.

Cutaneous tuberculosis can be further classified into subtypes according to the clinical features, virulence of the mycobacteria, and the immune response of the patient. Most cases of cutaneous tuberculosis are secondary infections in patients who have a history of extracutaneous tuberculosis.

1. Tuberculosis cutis or cutaneous tuberculosis

1) Lupus vulgaris

This type was the most common among cutaneous tuberculosis in the past, but is rarely seen today. It is characterized by reddish-brown papules appearing on the face and neck, coalescing into elevated, sharply defined infiltrative plaques. The skin lesions result from a direct spread of extracutaneous tuberculosis either hematogenously or through lymphatics. It progresses slowly and can leads to squamous cell carcinoma occasionally.

【Etiology and Pathogenesis】

M. tuberculosis is thought to disseminate hematogenously or through lymphatics based on a fact that extracutaneous organs such as lung or lymph nodes are commonly involved earlier. In lupus vulgaris, tubercles on the skin resulting from hematogenous dissemination of the primary infection are considered to be the first sign of tuberculosis relapse.

【Clinical Manifestations】

A single or several reddish-brown papules first appear unilaterally on the face, neck or arm, coalescing into erythematous plaques. The surface of the plaques exfoliates with scarring in the centers. Papules tend to reappear on the scarring areas, and will gradually enlarge and coalesce, leading to the formation of large, firm, elevated plaques in the middle with small reddish-brown or brown nodules on the edges (Fig. 6-7). When pressed by a glass slide, the nodules are yellowish-brown resembling 'apple jelly'. Lupus vulgaris progresses extremely slow and can persist untreated for years. In addition to the lesions described above, ulceration and atrophy can occur, or even develop into squamous cell carcinoma. Lupus vulgaris can be present in flat macular, ulcerative, or proliferative hypertrophic forms.

【Histopathology】

Tubercles in the dermis consisting of epithelioid cells, Langhans giant cells may be seen accompanied by caseous necrosis.

【Diagnosis and Differential Diagnosis】

Lupus vulgaris is diagnosed by the clinical features, histopathology,

核疹则是皮肤对内源性结核分枝杆菌的过敏反应。

皮肤结核依据临床特征、细菌的毒力和患者的免疫反应进一步分为几种亚型。大多数皮肤结核的患者曾经有皮肤外结核病史，因此这些患者的皮肤结核是二次感染。

一、皮肤结核病

(一) 寻常狼疮

寻常狼疮(lupus vulgaris)曾经是皮肤结核的最常见类型，但现在少见，表现为面或颈部褐红色丘疹融合成隆起的境界清楚的浸润性斑块。该型是皮肤外结核经由血源性或淋巴性播散而来的结核分枝杆菌所致。进展缓慢，极少数情况下会进展为鳞状细胞癌。

【病因及发病机制】

可能与皮肤外器官的结核病灶通过血源性或淋巴性播散有关，这些病灶包括肺和淋巴结。在寻常狼疮中，结核复燃的首发症状是通过血源播散而在皮肤上形成结节。

【临床表现】

单个或多个褐红色的丘疹首先出现于面、颈部或手臂的单侧，融合成红色斑块。斑块表面剥脱，中央部形成瘢痕。丘疹再次出现于瘢痕部位，渐进反复扩大和融合。这一过程导致中央出现大而硬的隆起性斑块，其周围则为小的褐红色或褐色的结节(图 6-7)。用玻片压时，丘疹呈黄棕色，与苹果酱相似。寻常狼疮进展尤其缓慢，如不治疗，可多年不愈。除上述皮损外，寻常狼疮还可有溃疡和皮肤萎缩，有时可形成鳞状细胞癌。寻常狼疮根据临床特点可分为扁平斑片型、溃疡型和增生肥大型。

【组织病理】

真皮内可见由上皮样细胞和郎罕巨细胞组成的结节，并伴有干酪样坏死。

【诊断与鉴别诊断】

根据临床特征、组织病理和皮肤结

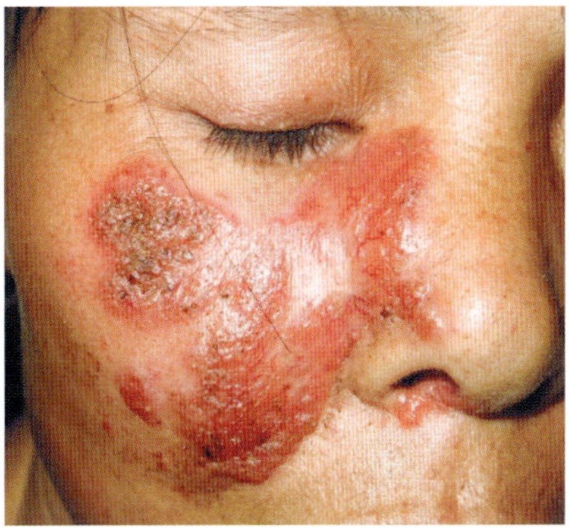

Fig. 6-7　Lupus vulgaris(图 6-7　寻常狼疮)

and a positive tuberculin skin test. Confirmation of *M. tuberculosis* can be carried out by PCR or culture.

Lupus vulgaris should be differentiated from chronic discoid lupus erythematosus, cutaneous sarcoidosis, tertiary syphilis, and sporotrichosis. Biopsy, skin tests, and cultures are usually helpful for differentiating this group of diseases.

【Treatment】

Lupus vulgaris responds well to antituberculous drugs. The prognosis in general is good, but often with scarring.

2) Scrofuloderma

This is the most common type of cutaneous TB, frequently involving the neck and trunk. The lesions begin with painless subcutaneous nodules that eventually form fistula and pus from the cold abscesses. The latter two appearances are very characteristic for this type of cutaneous TB. The causative agent-*M. tuberculosis*-is disseminated from an underlying extracutaneous TB locus to the skin. Cordlike scars are formed in most cases.

【Clinical Manifestations】

Scrofuloderma is descended from an existing active TB in extracutaneous locations such as the lungs, lymph nodes, bones, muscles or tendons. A painless light pink subcutaneous nodule called a cold abscess appears first and becomes softer, gradually forming a fistula from which pus is discharged. Later, ulceration and characteristic cordlike scarring develops at a previous scrofuloderma site. Slight localized fever and pain may be observed over entire course of the disease.

【Laboratory Findings】

Large quantities of *M. tuberculosis* can be found in the pus or biopsy specimens. The presence of mycobacteria can be confirmed

核菌素试验强阳性，寻常狼疮不难诊断，可通过 PCR 检查或细菌培养来鉴定结核分枝杆菌。

寻常狼疮需与慢性盘状红斑狼疮、皮肤结节病、三期梅毒和孢子丝菌病鉴别。皮肤活检、皮肤试验及细菌培养有助于确立诊断。

【治疗】

寻常狼疮对抗结核药物敏感。虽然寻常狼疮预后良好，但会留下明显的瘢痕。

（二）瘰疬性皮肤结核

瘰疬性皮肤结核(scrofuloderma)是皮肤结核最常见的类型，颈部和躯干最常累及。其通常以无痛性皮下结节起病，以瘘管形成和寒性脓肿脓液流出为特征，由结核分枝杆菌引起，是由皮肤外结核病灶播散到皮肤引起。多会形成束状瘢痕。

【临床表现】

瘰疬性皮肤结核是由肺部、淋巴结、骨骼、肌肉或肌腱处活动性结核进展直接传播至皮肤引起。皮肤上首先出现寒性脓肿，表现为无痛性微红的皮下结节。进而软化并在皮肤上形成瘘管，脓液从中流出。在原先瘰疬部位出现溃疡和特征性的束状瘢痕。整个病程中都有轻微的局限性发热和疼痛。

【实验室检查】

脓液和皮损组织中可见大量的结核分枝杆菌。PCR 检查和细菌培养可鉴定

by PCR or culture.

分枝杆菌。

【Treatment】

The treatments for scrofuloderma are the same as lupus vulgaris.

【治疗】

瘰疬性皮肤结核与寻常狼疮的治疗方法相同。

3) Warty lupus (Tuberculosis verrucosa cutis)

(三) 疣状狼疮(疣状皮肤结核)

【Etiology and Pathogenesis】

Warty lupus or tuberculosis verrucosa cutis, despite the name, is a variant of cutaneous tuberculosis. The indurated, warty skin lesions arise by inoculation of tubercle bacilli in an individual previously infected with *M. tuberculosis* who typically manifests a moderate or high degree of immunity to TB.

【病因及发病机制】

疣状狼疮(warty lupus)或疣状皮肤结核(tuberculosis verrucosa cutis)是皮肤结核的一种亚型,常发生于对结核分枝杆菌有中等到高度免疫力者,一般发生在原有感染的患者身上,在结核分枝杆菌种植部位产生硬结样的疣状损害。

【Clinical Manifestations】

Warty lupus occurs most frequently at the ends of extremities, dorsal surfaces of joints, and buttocks secondary to external stimulation or injury. Several small, asymptomatic, indurated wart-like papules with a slight inflammatory edge coalesce and enlarge to form erythematous verrucous plaques at the periphery. The lesions enlarge centrifugally and tend to heal in the center (Fig. 6-8). Warty lupus is an infection of the superficial layers, so ulceration is rare.

【临床表现】

疣状狼疮最常发生于四肢末端、关节的背侧面和臀部,继发于外部刺激或外伤。临床表现为几个小的无症状的硬结样疣状丘疹,外周为轻微的融合的炎性外沿,增大形成带有疣状外沿的红斑块。皮损向外沿扩展,中心趋向于愈合(图 6-8)。疣状狼疮是皮肤浅层的感染,不会发生溃疡。

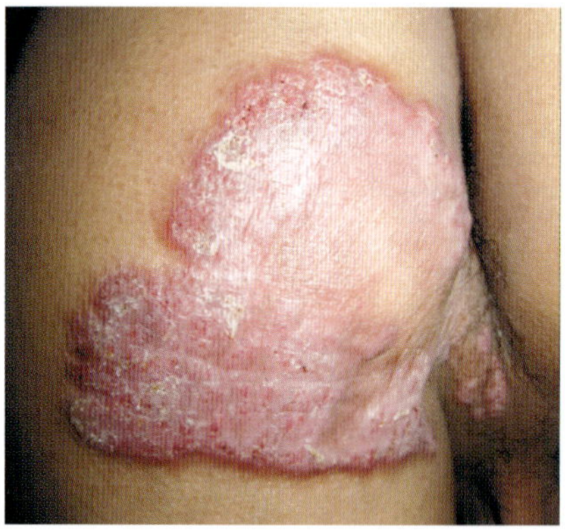

Fig. 6-8　Warty lupus/Tuberculosis verrucosa cutis(图 6-8　疣状狼疮/疣状皮肤结核)

【Histopathology】

Histopathologically, the epidermis shows hyperkeratosis and parakeratosis with marked acanthosis and papillomatosis. An inflammatory infiltration mainly composed of neutrophils accompanied by lymphocytes can also be found in the dermis. Abscesses occur occasionally, and tuberculoid structure with caseous necrosis may be observed.

【组织病理】

组织病理显示表皮角化过度伴角化不全,棘层明显肥厚,乳头瘤样增生,真皮内有以中性粒细胞为主、伴有真皮淋巴细胞的炎症细胞浸润,有时形成脓肿,偶见结核样结构伴干酪样坏死。

【Diagnosis and Differential Diagnosis】

Identification of *M. tuberculosis* can be made by PCR or by culture. A positive tuberculin skin test and typical pathological

【诊断与鉴别诊断】

可通过 PCR 检查或细菌培养来鉴定结核分枝杆菌。结合皮肤结核菌素试验

findings are helpful for diagnosis. Lupus vulgaris, chromomycosis, viral warts, and tinea cruris should be differentiated from warty lupus.

【Treatment】

Warty lupus responds well to antituberculous drugs.

2. Tuberculids

Tuberculids are the consequence of immune responses to an underlying tuberculosis focus. The immunogens are thought to be carried hematogenously by disseminated *M. tuberculosis* or tubercle bacilli that originate in a primary TB infection. Individuals with strong cell-mediated immunity to tuberculosis are easily affected.

1) Papulonecrotic tuberculid

This condition is a vasculitis caused by an allergic reaction to *M. tuberculosis*. It occurs mostly in young people, affecting most frequently the extensor surfaces of extremities, particularly on the elbows and knees. Multiple, dark red papules in 1 cm diameter or less appear first and later become pustules with ulceration. Scarring remains after healing. Because new papules appear continuously, even though the progress is slow, the clinical manifestation commonly presents as a mixture of new eruptions and old ones. Antituberculous drugs are effective.

2) Lichen scrofulosorum

Lichen scrofulosorum most frequently follows an initial infection of *M. tuberculosis* or BCG vaccination. Scattered or aggregated red follicular papules one to several millimeters in diameter appear on the trunk or extremities. Histopathologically, epithelioid cells and giant Langhans cells in granulomas are easily found in the dermis but without caseous necrosis. The evidence for *M. tuberculosis* is negative no matter what assays are used. Therefore, lichen scrofulosorum has been assigned to the class of tuberculids, as an allergic reaction against mycobacterial components. Antituberculous drugs and minocycline are also effective for this type of tuberculid. Most cases heal after several months' treatment.

Section Six　Leprosy

Leprosy, formerly known as Hansen's disease, is a chronic infection caused by *Mycobacterium leprae*. The infection mainly involves the skin and peripheral nerves. According to individuals' cellular immunity to *M. leprae*, leprosy is classified into tuberculoid leprosy (TT), lepromatous leprosy (LL), borderline leprosy, and indeterminate leprosy (IL). In TT, skin involvement takes the form

强阳性和皮肤病理检查所见不难诊断。疣状狼疮需与寻常狼疮、着色真菌病、病毒疣和股癣鉴别。

【治疗】

疣状狼疮对抗结核药反应良好。

二、结核疹

结核疹(tuberculids)是皮肤对体内结核病灶的免疫反应。这种免疫反应的免疫原来源于血源播散的人型结核分枝杆菌或结核分枝杆菌的初次感染。结核疹常常发生于有强烈的细胞介导的抗结核免疫反应的患者身上。

(一) 丘疹坏死性结核疹

丘疹坏死性结核疹(papulonecrotic tuberculid)是机体对人型结核分枝杆菌的过敏反应性血管炎。本病多见于青年人,好发于四肢伸面,尤其好发于肘部和膝关节。皮损表现为众多的暗红色丘疹,起先直径为 1 cm 或小于 1 cm,后形成脓疱和溃疡,愈后遗留瘢痕。丘疹连续出现,并且进展缓慢,新皮损与陈旧皮损共存。抗结核药有效。

(二) 瘰疬性苔藓性皮肤结核

瘰疬性苔藓性皮肤结核(lichen scrofulosorum)常于感染人型结核分枝杆菌或接种卡介苗之后发生。皮损表现为在躯干或四肢上分散或聚合分布的毛囊性丘疹,红色,直径为一毫米到数毫米。病理上真皮内有上皮样细胞和郎罕巨细胞,可形成肉芽肿,但无干酪样坏死,也找不到结核分枝杆菌。因此,瘰疬性苔藓性皮肤结核应是结核疹,是对分枝杆菌复合物的过敏反应。抗结核药和米诺环素对瘰疬性苔藓性皮肤结核有效。多数患者可在数月内痊愈。

第六节　麻　　风

麻风(leprosy)曾称为海森氏病(Hansen's disease),是麻风分枝杆菌造成的慢性感染性疾病。皮肤和外周神经最常受到侵犯。根据对麻风分枝杆菌的细菌免疫力强弱可将麻风分为四型:结核样型麻风(TT),瘤型麻风(LL),界线

of erythemas or a small number of papules accompanied by slightly reduced sensory perception. However, in LL, *M. leprae* spreads and proliferates in the entire body to form lepromas. A multidrug approach including dapsone is recommended for leprosy.

型麻风和未定型麻风(IL)。结核样型麻风临床表现为红斑、丘疹和感知觉的轻微减退。在瘤型麻风中，麻风分枝杆菌在全身中增殖并形成麻风结节。包括氨苯砜在内的多种药物疗法是主要的治疗手段。

【Etiology, Pathogenesis and Epidemiology】

Leprosy is an infection caused by *Mycobacterium leprae*. The mechanism of infection is not fully understood. As the pathogenicity of *M. leprae* is extremely low, the innate immunity in a normal person should eliminate the infection. In addition, the incubation period of leprosy is 3-5 years; therefore, the disease is extremely rare, but also very difficult to trace in a population. Leprosy occurs worldwide, but half of the patient population comes from Asia and Africa, accounting for 12 million cases.

【病因、发病机制及流行病学】

麻风是麻风分枝杆菌感染所造成的疾病。感染机制未完全阐明。由于麻风分枝杆菌的致病力极弱，所以机体的天然免疫通常可将感染菌清除。麻风病的潜伏期通常为3～5年。基于以上原因，麻风病例很少。全世界都有麻风患者，大约1200万患者分布在亚洲和非洲，占全世界麻风患者数目的一半。

【Clinical Manifestations and Classification】

Leprosy is divided into the subtypes listed below (Ridley-Jopling classification) according to the strength of the host's cellular immunity against *M. leprae*. Each subtype of leprosy varies in severity of the skin lesions and in peripheral nerve symptoms.

(1) Tuberculoid leprosy (TT): this type is the mildest form of leprosy. It occurs in hosts with strong cellular immunity. Sharply demarcated, localized, erythematous patches or papules appear singly or multiply. Color of papules may fade gradually accompanied by alopecia, reduced sensation, and disability of perspiration.

(2) Lepromatous leprosy (LL): *M. leprae* proliferates systemically in hosts who have impaired cellular immunity. A leproma (a mass of histiocytes containing large quantities of *M. leprae*) forms in the peripheral nerves, eyes, and lymph nodes. Multiple nodules appear on the skin. As the infection progresses, visual impairment, neuralgia, and deformity of face and extremities occur (leonine facies)(Fig. 6-9).

(3) Borderline leprosy (tuberculoid borderline (BT), lepromatous borderline (BL), borderline leprosy (BB)): the clinical condition is intermediate in severity between those of TT and LL. The number of patients with borderline leprosy has been increasing in recent years. The clinical manifestation is a mixture of the clinical features of TT and LL.

(4) Indeterminate leprosy (IL): this type of leprosy is easily

【临床表现和分类】

根据机体对麻风分枝杆菌细胞免疫的强弱可将麻风分为以下几类(Ridley-Jopling分类法)。皮损的严重程度和外周神经症状依不同的亚型而异。

(1) 结核样型麻风(TT)　此种类型是最轻微的一类麻风，宿主的细胞免疫力很强，皮损为边界清楚的局限的片状红斑，或者是单个或成片出现的丘疹，病程中，丘疹会褪色，伴有毳毛脱落、感觉减退和汗闭。

(2) 瘤型麻风(LL)　此型麻风是麻风分枝杆菌在细胞免疫缺陷的患者全身增殖引起的。在机体的外周神经、眼睛和淋巴结中会形成麻风结节，它由包含有大量麻风分枝杆菌的众多组织细胞组成。在皮肤上会出现多发的麻风结节。随着感染进程，患者会出现视力受损、神经痛和面部及四肢的变形(狮面)(图6-9)。

(3) 界线型麻风(界线类偏结核样型(BT)、界线类偏瘤型(BL)和中间界线型(BB))　此型临床情况介于结核样型麻风和瘤型麻风之间，近年来，界线型麻风的患病人数日益增多，此型麻风会出现结核样型麻风和瘤型麻风的多种复杂的临床特征。

(4) 未定型麻风(IL)　此种麻风容

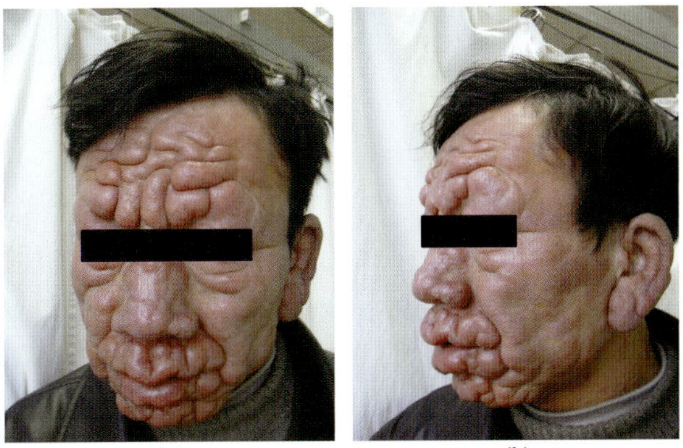

(a)　(b)

Fig. 6-9　Lepromatous leprosy(图 6-9　瘤型麻风)

misdiagnosed. Two or three flat, poorly demarcated, light pink patches with unclear border appear on the skin. Peripheral nerve symptoms are mild or absent. Histopathologically, this type of leprosy lacks the characteristic findings of leprosy, and evidence for bacilli are rare or absent. The WHO classification published in 1995 subdivided leprosy into multibacillary (MB) and paucibacillary (PB) subtypes according to either the bacterial populations found through skin smear examination or the numbers of skin lesions or of the nerves involved.

Lepra reaction: includes type Ⅰ and type Ⅱ reactions.

(1) (Jopling's) type Ⅰ reaction: it is believed to be caused by delayed-type hypersensitivity and occurs in BL, LL, BB, or BT, but particularly in BL. The patient's condition may transform to TT when the patient's cellular immunity increases, which is termed a reversal or upgrading reaction. Conversely, when the patient's cellular immunity attenuates the patient's condition will transform to LL, which is termed a degrading reaction. The former is more commonly seen while the latter is quite rare. Reversal reactions occur most commonly within 6 months to 1 year after initiation of chemotherapy and manifest as an abrupt exacerbation of the original skin lesions, which are tumid with a more clear border to the lesions, with new tumid lesions occurring on previously normal skin, occasionally accompanied by an abrupt onset of neuritis. Annular, concentric lesions or eczematous changes may also be found at this stage.

(2) (Jopling's) type Ⅱ reaction: is also known as erythema nodosum leprosum (ENL). Up to 75% of ENL cases occur in LL. ENL can also be seen in BL. It usually occurs in patients treated with chemotherapy after 1 or several years. Clinically, ENL presents as multiple tender bright red dermal or subcutaneous nodules like erythema nodosum on normal-appearing skin on the face, trunk, and extremities, accompanied by fever, anorexia,

易漏诊，皮损为 2～3 个扁平的淡粉色斑片，边界不清，外周神经症状轻微或无，皮肤活组织检查未发现麻风的典型损害。麻风分枝杆菌很少或无。WHO 在 1995 年颁布的分类法中，采用皮肤涂片查菌分类法和皮损或神经损害计数分类法将麻风分为多杆菌型(MB)和少杆菌型(PB)。

麻风反应(lepra reaction)：包括Ⅰ型和Ⅱ型麻风反应。

(1) Ⅰ型麻风反应　认为是由迟发性超敏反应引起，可见于 BL、LL、BB 或 BT，特别是 BL。患者细胞免疫增强时表现为病情向 TT 转变即逆向或升级反应，反之，患者细胞免疫降低时则表现为病情向 LL 转变，称为降级反应，大多数为前者，而后者罕见。逆向反应多见于开始化疗后 6 个月到 1 年内，表现为原有皮损突然加重、肿胀、边界更清楚、在正常皮肤上发生肿胀性损害、伴有或不伴有突发性神经炎等。可出现环形、同心圆状皮损或湿疹样改变。

(2) Ⅱ型麻风反应　又称麻风结节性红斑。75%的患者发生于 LL，也见于 BL 患者。常发生于化疗 1 年或数年后。表现为面部、躯干和四肢在正常皮肤上发生类似结节性红斑的多个疼痛性鲜红色真皮内或皮下结节，伴有发热、厌食、倦怠、关节痛、关节炎、神经炎、睾丸炎、

malaise, arthralgias, arthritis, neuritis, orchitis, or epididymitis. Targetoid, vesicular, pustular, ulcerative, or necrotic lesions may also be found. Neutrophilic leukocytosis can be detected. Dramatic response to treatment with thalidomide is found in more than 90% of patients, which is also of diagnostic value.

附睾炎等。可出现靶形、水疱、脓疱、溃疡或坏死性损害。患者外周血白细胞升高。90%的患者对沙利度胺反应良好，具有诊断价值。

【Laboratory Findings】

M. leprae is detected from the tissue fluid and/or pathological tissue of the lesions by acid-fast stain. The lepromin test may be used for classification of leprosy: it is strongly positive in TT and weakly positive in BB, BL and LL. However, the diagnostic value of the lepromin test is limited because the test gives false positivity under normal conditions. When direct detection of *M. leprae* is difficult, as in TT, PCR is indicated.

Serological anti-PGL-1 assay from a peripheral blood has some diagnostic value. The elevated immunoglobulin and false positive (BFP) serological reaction to syphilis may be observed in some cases.

【实验室检查】

通过对组织液和/或皮损病理组织的抗酸染色可找到麻风分枝杆菌。麻风菌素试验可用来对麻风进行分类：在结核样型麻风(TT)时示强阳性，在中间界线型(BB)、界线类偏瘤型麻风(BL)和瘤型麻风(LL)中示弱阳性。然而，麻风菌素试验的诊断价值有限是因为在正常状况下其可为假阳性。当直接寻找麻风分枝杆菌有困难时，可用其他方法，如在结核样型麻风(TT)中可用 PCR 检查找麻风分枝杆菌。

外周血中血清抗-PGL-1 有诊断价值。另外，有些患者可出现免疫球蛋白升高和梅毒血清学假阳性。

【Histopathology】

In tuberculoid leprosy (TT), no grenz zone can be observed. There are epithelioid granulomas, many Langhans giant cells, and lymphocytes in dermis. Acid-fast stain is negative. In the nodular lesions of lepromatous leprosy (LL), the epidermis is attenuated and there is a grenz zone between the overlying epidermis and nodular granulomatous infiltration composed mainly of macrophages and foamy cells with few lymphocytes. Numerous bacilli of *M. leprae* can be detected with acid-fast or Fite stain in macrophages or foamy cells.

【组织病理】

在结核样型麻风(TT)，无表皮下“无浸润带”，真皮内可见上皮样细胞肉芽肿，有较多淋巴细胞和郎罕巨细胞，抗酸染色阴性。在瘤型麻风(LL)结节性损害中，表皮变薄，表皮下有“无浸润带”，真皮内有主要由巨噬细胞和泡沫细胞组成的结节状肉芽肿性浸润，淋巴细胞较少。抗酸或 Fite 染色可见巨噬细胞或泡沫细胞内有较多的麻风分枝杆菌。

【Diagnosis and Differential Diagnosis】

Leprosy is diagnosed by skin lesions that are accompanied by reduced sensation, thickening of peripheral nerves, neurological disorders, laboratory findings, and histopathology.

Leprosy should be differentiated from tuberculosis, syphilis, cutaneous mycosis, and various diseases that are accompanied by peripheral nerve impairment including diabetes, syringomyelia, and mycosis fungoides.

【诊断与鉴别诊断】

麻风可通过皮损及与皮损伴随的感觉减退、外周神经肥厚、神经障碍、实验室检查及组织病理来诊断。

麻风需与结核病，梅毒，皮肤真菌病，伴有外周神经损害的疾病如糖尿病、脊髓空洞症和蕈样肉芽肿鉴别。

【Treatment】

Multidrug therapy consisting of dapsone, rifampicin and clofazimine is recommended by WHO. The therapy should be continued for 6 months in paucibacillary subtype cases and 2 years

【治疗】

WHO 推荐用氨苯砜、利福平和氨苯吩嗪多种药物联合治疗麻风。对少菌型患者，治疗需持续 6 个月，而多菌型患者

in multibacillary subtype cases until completely cured. In recent years, new quinolone antibiotics have also been used. NSAIDs are administered when the lepra reaction causes sharp pain.

的治疗需持续 2 年才算治疗充分。近年来，新喹诺酮类抗生素也用于治疗麻风。当麻风反应导致剧烈疼痛时可用非甾体类抗炎药治疗。

Section Seven　Dermatoses Caused by Atypical Mycobacteria

第七节　非典型分枝杆菌所致的皮肤病

Atypical mycobacteria, also known as Non-tuberculous mycobacteria (NTM) or environmental mycobacteria, are mycobacteria species other than those of the *Mycobacterium tuberculosis* complex or *Mycobacterium leprae*. NTM are ubiquitous acid-fast organisms which can produce a wide range of diseases including skin and soft tissue infections. Nowadays, more than 170 species of NTM have been identified, most of which have been incriminated in skin and soft tissue infections. Initially, NTM have been classified into Runyon groups based on colony morphology, growth rate, and pigmentation. As technology moves forward, this classification system is now made using rapid molecular diagnostic systems. Nonetheless, growth rates continue to provide practical means for identification species of NTM. On this basis, NTM can be categorized into rapidly growing mycobacteria (RGM) and slowly growing mycobacteria (SGM). Although RGM is weaker in pathogenicity than SGM, they both may cause disseminated diseases in immunocompromised hosts.

非典型分枝杆菌（atypical mycobacteria）是除结核分枝杆菌或麻风分支杆菌之外的分枝杆菌，又称为非结核分枝杆菌（non-tuberculous mycobacteria, NTM）、环境分枝杆菌。NTM 在环境中广泛存在，抗酸染色阳性，可以造成多种疾病，包括皮肤和软组织的感染。目前报道的非典型分枝杆菌已达 170 余种，它们大多都能引起皮肤和软组织的感染。最早，Runyon 根据集落的形态、生长速度以及是否产生色素，对非典型分枝杆菌进行分类。随着技术的发展，Runyon 分类法运用减少，临床采用快速的分子诊断系统对 NTM 进行分类。然而 NTM 仍可以根据其生长速度分为快生长菌（rapidly growing mycobacteria, RGM）和慢生长菌（slowly growing mycobacteria, SGM）。虽然 RGM 的致病性比 SGM 弱，但是仍然能够在免疫缺陷人群中引起播散性感染。

Most NTM species are easily isolated from the environment including water (both natural and municipal systems), soil, plants, and animals. Tap water is considered to be the major reservoir for NTM pathogens in humans, which has heightened concerns for public health.

大部分非典型分枝杆菌在环境中广泛存在，包括水源（自然和家庭内水源）、土壤、植物和动物。自来水被认为是人类感染非典型分枝杆菌的主要致病源，而这个问题已经引起了对公共卫生问题的关注。

Skin and Soft Tissue Infections

皮肤软组织感染

The increasing reports of NTM infections of skin and soft tissue in recent years have attracted significant attention in the medical community. Although the increase was first thought to reflect the increased population of immunosuppressed individuals, numerous reports have been documented in healthy individuals.

近年来，由于非典型分枝杆菌造成的皮肤、软组织感染病例数增多，引起了医学界的广泛关注。非典型分枝杆菌的感染并不代表免疫抑制人群的增加，因为大量的患者来自正常的群体。

However, most skin and soft tissue infections caused by NTM are nonspecific, and clinical presentations may present with abscesses, papules, plaques, nodules, sporotrichoid nodules, ulcers, draining sinus tracts, cellulitis, panniculitis, and folliculitis, etc. The manifestations of cutaneous NTM infection are polymorphous,

然而，大部分非典型分枝杆菌造成的皮肤、软组织感染的临床表现并没有特异性，可表现为脓肿、丘疹、斑块、结节、孢子丝菌样结节、溃疡、窦道、蜂窝织炎、脂膜炎、毛囊炎等。临床表现的多样

which make the diagnosis difficult; thus, a high index of suspicion in the appropriate clinical setting is necessary to make a prompt diagnosis. NTM infections should be considered in all patients with 'therapy resistant' cutaneous infections. Usually, cutaneous NTM infections develop after traumatic injury, surgery, or cosmetic procedures. It has been reported that cutaneous NTM infections can occur secondarily as a result of a disseminated mycobacterial disease, especially among immunosuppressed patients.

性导致诊断的困难，而根据临床指南来诊断疑似病例能够提高诊断的效率。临床所有治疗效果不佳的皮肤、软组织感染都需要考虑非典型分枝杆菌的感染。通常，皮肤非典型分枝杆菌感染患者有创伤史、手术史或美容操作史。也有文献报道，其可以继发于播散性分枝杆菌的二次感染，特别是在免疫缺陷患者中。

1. Swimming pool granuloma

一、游泳池肉芽肿

【Etiology and Pathogenesis】

The primary risk factor of *M. marinum* infections is exposure to aquatic environments or marine animals. Hence, these infections are commonly known as "swimming pool granuloma", also named as "fish-tank granuloma" or "aquarium granuloma". *M. marinum* is a slow-growing mycobacterium whose incubation period is 16 days. Typically, infections are seen in immunocompetent patients who have jobs or hobbies with exposure to fresh or salt water. Up to 45% of cases with confirmed *M. marinum* infection have a fish-related activity history. The main pattern of inoculation is trauma followed by exposure to water/fish environments. Most preceding lesions are superficial abrasions or negligible wounds. The duration from the onset of the symptoms until an actual visit to a clinic varies from 15 days to 3 years. Patients usually do not seek medical help until their symptoms get worse.

【病因及发病机制】

海鱼分枝杆菌感染的高危因素是接触水环境或海产品，其引起的皮肤感染最常见的是"游泳池肉芽肿"，又称为"鱼缸肉芽肿"或"水肉芽肿"。海鱼分枝杆菌是一种慢生长菌，接种后需要 16 天的生长期。患者通常为因职业或兴趣有淡水/海水接触史的免疫力正常者。45%的确诊病例曾有鱼的接触史。创面接触水域/鱼类环境而接种细菌。大多数患者起病时仅为浅表擦伤或轻微创口。患者从发病到病情严重而就医的过程一般是 15 天到 3 年。

【Clinical Manifestations】

Initially, a solitary, erythematous papule or nodule is found at the site of inoculation, often on an extremity. This can progress to a verrucous violaceous plaque and/or ulcer which producing a serosanguineous discharge (Fig. 6-10). Proximal extension of the infection may occur through lymphatic spread and 20% of patients present with a sporotrichoid distribution. Up to 29% of cases reported *M. marinum* invades deeper tissues, such as tendon

【临床表现】

起初，接种部位可见孤立的红色丘疹或结节，常常位于单个肢体。之后可以发展为疣状的紫色斑块和/或有血样分泌物渗出的溃疡(图 6-10)。感染可以沿淋巴管向近端扩散，20%患者呈孢子丝菌病样表现。在 29%的病例中，疾病还可侵袭深层组织，如腱鞘、囊腔、骨和

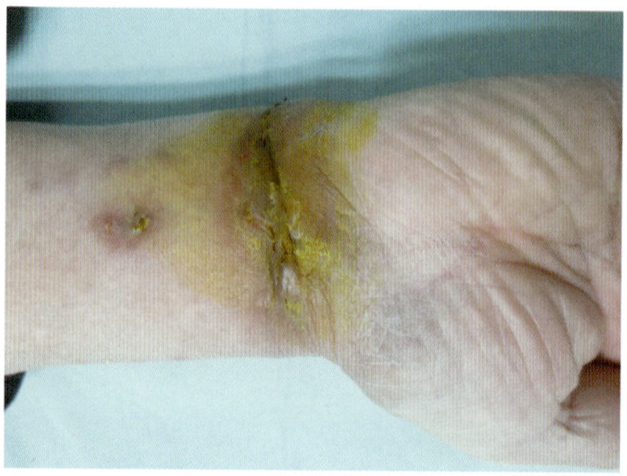

Fig. 6-10 Atypical mycobacterial infection(图 6-10 非典型分枝杆菌感染)

sheaths, bursae, bones, and joints. Deeper soft tissue invasion can be seen in all patients regardless of their immunologic state. Because the organism grows poorly at 37 ℃, systemic dissemination is rare and has been reported to occur only in immunocompromised patients.

关节组织。深层组织感染可见于免疫力正常或者抑制的患者。由于海鱼分枝杆菌在 37 ℃环境中生长受限，故此，系统性感染罕见，报道仅见于免疫抑制患者。

【Diagnosis and Differential Diagnosis】

The disease can be diagnosed by history of exposure after trauma, histopathologic manifestation, the results of acid-fast stain and cultures. On histopathologic sections, lesions caused by *M. marinum* show prominent epidermal changes, such as acanthosis, pseudoepitheliomatous hyperplasia, and exocytosis. Common histopathologic patterns include granulomatous inflammatory infiltrate with tuberculoid granuloma formation, sarcoidosis-like granulomas, or rheumatoid-like nodules. AFB may be seen in small quantities but may be neglected by regular microscopy. Only a part of the acid-fast staining on drainage material or tissue is positive. Usually, *M. marinum* colonies are seen after 10-28 days of incubation, but cultures should be observed for at least 6 weeks. The disease should be differentiated from tuberculosis cutis verrucosa, pyoderma, leishmaniasis, and sporotrichosis.

【诊断与鉴别诊断】

根据暴露病史、外伤史、组织病理、抗酸染色、培养结果可以诊断。海鱼分枝杆菌感染可致显著的表皮改变，如棘层肥厚、假上皮样增生和细胞外溢。典型的病理损害为类似结核性肉芽肿的肉芽肿性炎性浸润、肉样瘤样肉芽肿或风湿样肉芽肿。抗酸染色可能小部分阳性，但是常规病理检查往往没有发现。只有部分病例有分泌物或者组织抗酸染色阳性。组织培养一般需 10～28 天，培养基需要观察 6 周。临床需要和疣状皮肤结核、脓皮病、利什曼病和孢子丝菌病鉴别。

【Treatment】

Antimicrobials are the mainstays of successful treatment for *M. marinum*. In superficial cutaneous infections, clarithromycin, doxycycline, minocycline, and trimethoprim-sulfamethoxazole as monotherapy are effective. Multidrug therapy is recommended for more significant infections, especially when deeper structures are involved. In contrast to other NTMs, routine antimicrobial susceptibility testing of isolates of *M. marinum* is not required unless treatment fails. In cases of severe infections including the sporotrichoid distribution pattern, the most effective drugs seem to be a combination of rifampicin and ethambutol. Spontaneous remission has been reported with untreated infections in immunocompetent hosts. Surgical treatment is not usually recommended and is usually reserved for deeper infections of subcutaneous tissue such as tendon and/or bone.

【治疗】

抗感染治疗对海鱼分枝杆菌有效。对浅部皮肤感染，克拉霉素、多西环素、米诺环素和磺胺甲噁唑-甲氧苄啶单药治疗有效。联合治疗仅用于较严重感染患者，如深层组织受累。不同于其他非典型分枝杆菌感染，海鱼分枝杆菌感染，除治疗失败外不需要做药敏试验。在严重病例中，如孢子丝菌病样皮损患者，最有效的治疗方案是利福平联合乙胺丁醇。有免疫力正常的患者自愈的报道。手术治疗不推荐，常常会出现皮下组织的深层感染，如肌腱和骨。

2. Cutaneous *M. Kansasii* infection

二、堪萨斯分枝杆菌皮肤感染

【Etiology and Pathogenesis】

M. Kansasii typically causes pulmonary disease which resembles pulmonary tuberculosis. Unlike other NTM, it has not been found in soil or natural water supplies. Rather, it has been recovered consistently from dust and tap water in endemic areas. The immunocompromised state and contaminated water are the risk

【病因及发病机制】

堪萨斯分枝杆菌通常引起肺部疾病，表现与肺结核相似。该菌不易从环境中获取，存在于灰尘和水中，在高发区部分水源中可以分离。免疫抑制剂应用和污染水源暴露史是易感因素。很可能

factors of the disease. Primary cutaneous lesions may occur after a local trauma. The infection can also be caused via respiratory way.

通过呼吸或局部接种感染。

【Clinical Manifestations】

Disseminated disease can occur in immunosuppressed patients, but it typically remains as a localized indolent lesion confined to the skin in the immunocompetent persons. Cutaneous lesions may have a sporotrichoid distribution, and present as non-healing ulcers, nodules, and cellulitis.

【临床表现】

免疫缺陷患者的感染可能播散，而免疫正常患者的感染常常局限于皮肤，呈孢子丝菌病样分布，表现为经久不愈的溃疡、结节和蜂窝织炎。

【Diagnosis and Differential Diagnosis】

The diagnosis can be made with clinical manifestations and culture results. The immunocompromised state may be helpful in the diagnosis. Blood culture is valuable for disseminated infection. The disease should be differentiated from tuberculosis cutis verrucosa, syphiloma, chromomycosis, swimming pool granuloma, sporotrichosis, and bacterial cellulitis, etc.

【诊断与鉴别诊断】

根据临床表现和细菌培养能够确诊。免疫抑制状态病史对诊断有帮助。血培养对诊断播散性感染有价值。皮损需要与疣状皮肤结核、梅毒树胶肿、着色真菌病、游泳池肉芽肿、孢子丝菌病、细菌性蜂窝织炎等疾病鉴别。

【Treatment】

The traditional antituberculous agents as well as erythromycin, minocycline, and doxycycline have been effective in the treatment. Because of resistance, antibiotic selection should always be based on specific sensitivities.

【治疗】

许多药物，如抗结核药物和红霉素、米诺环素和多西环素治疗均有效，但是需要做药敏试验来选择治疗药物。

Min ZHENG(郑敏), Jiong ZHOU(周炯), Sui-qing CAI (蔡绥勍)

Chapter Seven Dermatoses Caused by Fungi

Section One Tinea Capitis

Tinea capitis is a superficial fungal infection of the scalp and hair caused by dermatophytes.

【Etiology】

The infections can be transmitted from humans to humans (either directly or indirectly) or from infected animals to humans. The most common causative fungi today in China for tinea capitis are *Microsporum canis* (*M. canis*), *Trichophyton violaceum* (*T. violaceum*), *Trichophyton mentagrophytes* (*T. mentagrophytes*), and *Trichophyton tonsurans* (*T. tonsurans*). Recently, *T. tonsurans replaced M. canis as the most common cause of tinea capitis in the United States* and Europe. However, in the years 1950 through 1970, *Trichophyton schoenleinii* (*T. schoenleinii*) and *Microsporum ferrugineum* (*M. ferrugineum*) species were common throughout China but are rarely seen today except in Xinjiang Province.

【Clinical Manifestations】

Tinea capitis is commonly classified into four types: tinea favosa, tinea alba, black-dot tinea and kerion.

(1) Tinea favosa: tinea favosa was very common in China in the 1950s and 1960s but is rarely seen today except in Xinjiang Province, where occasional outbreaks are still seen. It appears mostly in young children, and rarely in infants and adults. *T. schoenleinii* is the predominant pathogen. The initial lesion is erythema around the hair roots which then develops into a follicular pustule. After the pustule ruptures, a disc-like yellowish crust is left. Further, the lesions expand and coalesce into a cup-shaped crust called scutulae with a distinctive odor of cat urine. The scutula always adhere to the scalp in the center and the margins curve up. When the crust is torn off a bright-red moist erosion or a superficial ulcer will be left. The scutula is usually pierced by hair and the hair usually becomes bent and dry, and is easily broken. Atrophic scarring will result, destroying the follicles and leading to permanent alopecia if untreated (Fig. 7-1).

(2) Tinea alba: *M. canis* and *T. mentagrophytes* are the most common causative agents of tinea alba and *M. ferrugineum* is rarely seen today. Usually tinea alba occurs in childhood and undergoes spontaneous remission in adolescence. The lesions begin with multiple localized whitish scaly patches on the scalp. As the lesions progress, satellite scaly patches will occur around the initial ones.

第七章 真菌感染性皮肤病

第一节 头 癣

头癣(tinea capitis)是皮肤癣菌感染头皮和毛发引起的浅部真菌病。

【病因】

头癣由直接接触或间接接触患者或带病动物引起。我国目前常见致病菌为犬小孢子菌、紫色毛癣菌、须癣毛癣菌、断发毛癣菌等,而在欧美发达国家,近年来的主要致病菌为断发毛癣菌。二十世纪五六十年代我国常见的致病菌许兰氏毛癣菌、铁锈色小孢子菌等目前已极为罕见,仅见于我国新疆地区。

【临床表现】

头癣可分为黄癣、白癣、黑癣和脓癣4种类型。

(1) 黄癣(tinea favosa) 二十世纪五六十年代黄癣在我国很常见,目前我国罕见,仅偶见于新疆地区,偶有暴发发生。该病多在儿童期发病,偶见于幼儿和成人。主要病原菌为许兰氏毛癣菌。皮损初起为发根处皮肤发生红斑,继而出现毛囊性脓疱,脓疱破裂后形成碟形蜜黄色痂,随着病情发展,黄痂扩大融合形成杯状,边缘翘起,中心黏着,中央有头发穿过,嗅之有鼠臭味,称为黄癣痂(scutulae)。除去黄痂,露出鲜红湿润糜烂面或浅溃疡。患处头发干枯、弯曲、易折断。如不及时治疗,局部毛囊破坏,头发脱落,形成萎缩性瘢痕,导致永久性秃发(图7-1)。

(2) 白癣(tinea alba) 主要由犬小孢子菌和须癣毛癣菌引起。铁锈色小孢子菌引起者已非常罕见。多为儿童期患病,青春期后可自愈。初起为头皮出现数个白色鳞屑性局限斑片,很快向四周扩大,周围可出现卫星样小鳞屑性斑片。

The affected hairs will uniformly break 2-5 mm away from the scalp and the remnant hairs will become loose and easily pulled out. A white fungal sheath around the hair root is the feature of tinea alba (Fig. 7-2).

局部头发在离头皮 2～5 mm 处均匀一致折断，留下发桩。发桩松动易拔出，根部可见白套样菌鞘，具有特征性(图 7-2)。

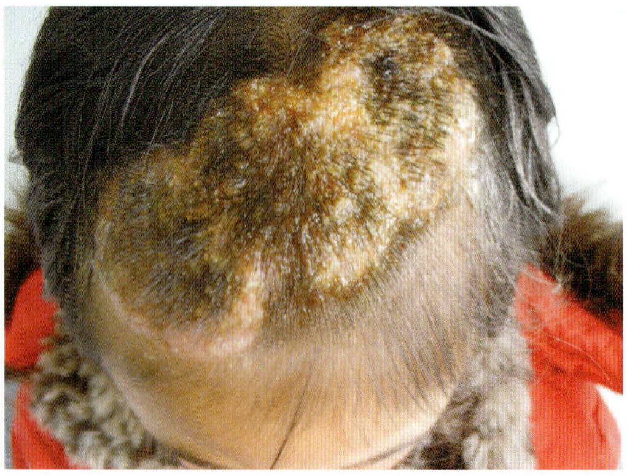

Fig. 7-1　Tinea favosa(图 7-1　黄癣)

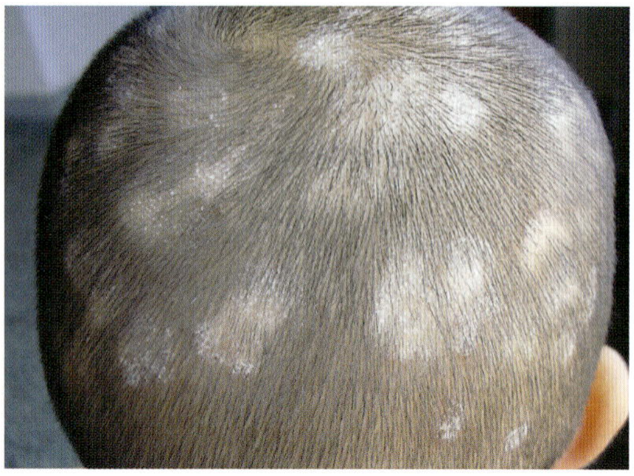

Fig. 7-2　Tinea alba(图 7-2　白癣)

(3) Black-dot tinea: the most common causative fungi are *T. violaceum* and *T. tonsurans*. Black-dot tinea can occur in children and adults. The initial rashes are pinhead-sized scaly, itching patches scattered over the entire scalp. The affected hairs will break off at the surface of the scalp and leave black dots. The hair follicles can be destroyed to leave atrophic scars and spotted alopecia in chronic cases (Fig. 7-3).

(4) Kerion: kerion is usually caused by *M. canis*, *T. mentagrophytes*, *T. rubrum* and *T. verrucosum*. The onset is acute. A soft, elevated, carbuncle-like swelling with fluctuation quickly develops. Some serous fluid or translucent pus will ooze when squeezed. The affected hairs become loose and broken, easily pulled out. Usually kerion lasts only a short time, but scarring and permanent alopecia may be seen afterwards(Fig. 7-4).

(3) 黑癣(black-dot tinea)　主要由紫色毛癣菌和断发毛癣菌引起。儿童和成人均可发病。初起皮损为头皮针尖大小鳞屑性斑片，稍痒，常散在分布。局部病发紧贴头皮折断，留下黑色小点。部分病程较长患者，可因毛囊破坏而形成瘢痕及点状秃发(图 7-3)。

(4) 脓癣(kerion)　脓癣多由犬小孢子菌、须癣毛癣菌、红色毛癣菌和疣状毛癣菌等引起。急性起病，患处出现红肿的痈状隆起，质地软，有波动感，用力挤压可有少许浆液或半透明脓液。皮损内毛发松动折断，易拔出。病程一般较短，愈后留有萎缩性瘢痕而形成永久性秃发(图 7-4)。

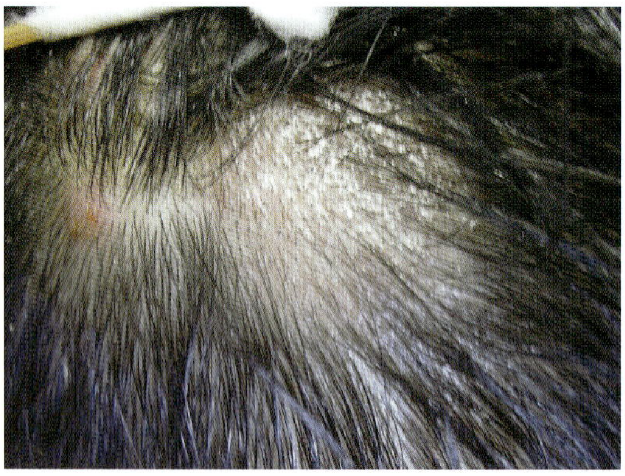

Fig. 7-3　Black-dot tinea(图 7-3　黑癣)

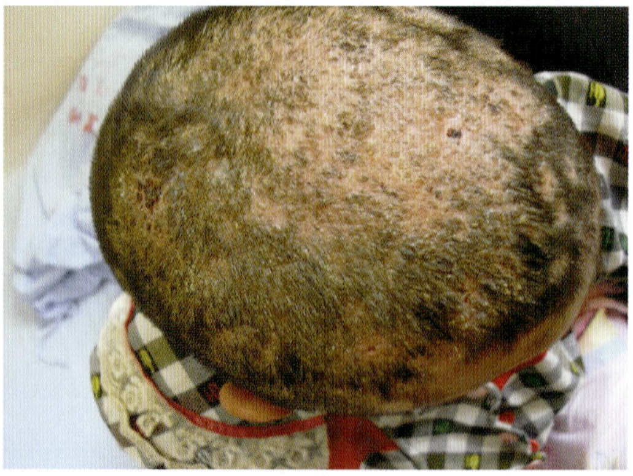

Fig. 7-4　Kerion(图 7-4　脓癣)

【Laboratory Findings】

(1) Direct microscopic examination: broken hair, scales and

【实验室检查】

(1) 真菌直接镜检　取断发、鳞屑或

scutulae are appropriate specimens for direct microscopic examination. Fungal hyphae and spores can be found by a 10% KOH examination. Because KOH examination may yield false-negative results in up to 15% of cases, patients suspected clinically of having an infection should be treated. Tinea capitis can be classified into three subtypes according to the invasion sites (all appearing on or near damaged hair) seen under microscopy.

黄癣痂经 10% KOH 直接镜检可发现菌丝和孢子。由于 KOH 镜检有 15% 的假阴性率，临床表现高度怀疑头癣感染的患者，即使 KOH 直接镜检阴性，也应进行治疗。在镜下，根据病发的不同感染部位（均位于或邻近病发），头癣可分为以下 3 种类型。

①Ectothrix type: the hair is surrounded by an orderly arranged sheath of tiny spores. Hyphae are occasionally found in the hair shaft. *M. canis* and *T. mentagrophytes* are the most frequent fungi for ectothrix type, as seen in tinea alba.

① 发外型：孢子位于发外，排列整齐，成团或成链状，偶尔发内可见菌丝，常见于犬小孢子菌和须癣毛癣菌引起的白癣。

② Endothrix type: abundant spores are found inside the hair shaft that either fill the hair shaft, or else the spores are arranged in lines along the hair shaft with discrete or clumped distribution. The affected hairs appear thicker, but are still casily broken. This type is commonly seen in black-dot tinea, normally caused by *T. violaceum* and *T. tonsurans*.

②发内型：孢子充满发内或在发内呈链状排列，稀疏或密集分布，病发直径增大，脆弱易断，常见于紫色毛癣菌和断发毛癣菌引起的黑癣。

③ Favus-like type: segmented hyphae of various diameters exist in the hair shaft along the axis of the hair shaft. Vacuola may sometimes appear inside the hair shaft. The hornlike hyphae may also be found in scutula. This type is seen in tinea favosa caused by *T. schoenleinii*.

③黄癣型：发内有粗细不一的分节菌丝，与毛发长轴平行，发内可有或无空泡，此外，取黄癣痂进行真菌检查可发现鹿角状菌丝，见于许兰氏毛癣菌引起的黄癣。

(2) Fungal culture: broken hair, scales and scutulae should be collected for culture. The colonies of fungi and their features under microscopy vary with species.

(2) 真菌培养　取断发、鳞屑或黄癣痂进行真菌培养，可见菌落生长。菌落形态和镜下特征依病原菌不同而不同。

(3) Wood's light: under Wood's light, the affected hair of tinea favosa will yield a dim green fluorescence, while the infected hair of tinea alba will be bright green. Black-dot tinea is always fluorescent-negative.

(3) 伍氏灯检查　黄癣病发暗绿色的荧光，白癣病发亮绿色的荧光，黑癣病无荧光。

【Diagnosis and Differential Diagnosis】

Diagnosis depends on the clinical features, fungal detection and Wood's light examination. Tinea capitis must be differentiated clinically from impetigo, seborrheic dermatitis, psoriasis, alopecia areata, and pityriasis amiantacea. The fungal examination will usually be the key point for the differentiation. Kerion should be differentiated from bacterial abscess. The latter has remarkable red swelling with pain and the affected hair can be loose but is not broken; also, bacterial culture is positive but fungal culture is negative.

【诊断与鉴别诊断】

根据临床特点、真菌检测、伍氏灯检查结果，一般可准确诊断。临床上，头癣有时应与下列疾病相鉴别：脓疱疮、脂溢性皮炎、银屑病、斑秃、石棉样糠疹等。鉴别主要依靠真菌检查。脓癣尚需与细菌性脓肿相鉴别。后者红、肿、热、痛明显，皮损内毛发松动但不折断，细菌培养阳性而真菌检查及培养均阴性。

【Treatment】

(1) Oral drugs: griseofulvin remains the first line treatment for tinea capitis. The dose ranges from 10 to 20 mg/(kg · d). Terbinafine and itraconazole are excellent alternatives. The doses of

【治疗】

(1) 口服药物　①灰黄霉素：首选药物，10～20 mg/(kg · d)，连续 2～4 周。②特比萘芬：体重＜20 kg，62.5 mg/d；

terbinafine are 62.5 mg/d for body weights below 20 kg;125 mg/d for body weights ranging from 20 to 40 kg and 250 mg/d for body weights above 40 kg, respectively. The dose of itraconazole is 3-5 mg/(kg・d)for children and 200 mg/d for adults. All treatments continue for 4-6 weeks.

体重为20～40 kg,125 mg/d;体重>40 kg,250 mg/d,连续2～4周。③伊曲康唑:儿童3～5 mg/(kg・d),成人200 mg/d,连续4～6周。

(2) Topical agents: topical antifungal agents such as miconazole cream, terbinafine cream are recommended. 5% sulfur ointment could also be used.

(2) 外用药物　外用抗真菌药物如咪康唑霜、特比萘芬霜等,5%硫黄软膏亦可使用。

(3) Hair shaving and washing: it is necessary to clean the hair daily with soap and shave infected hair regularly. Topical treatments are not adequate for kerion or tinea favosa, which usually require oral treatments.

(3) 洗头和剃发　每日用温水、肥皂洗头,定期剃除病发。对脓癣或黄癣,单纯外用药物还不够,常需口服治疗。

(4) Sterilization: sterilization is often used to prevent reinfection. Contaminated towels, hats, bedding, and combs should be boiled regularly to remove any causative fungi.

(4) 消毒　消毒是预防再感染的重要措施。患者使用的毛巾、帽子、枕套、床单、梳子等定期煮沸消毒。

(5) Other treatments: severe kerion may be treated with oral glucocorticoids for a short period to reduce inflammatory reactions and the possibility of scarring. If any secondary bacterial infection occurs, local or systemic administration of antibiotics should be helpful.

(5) 其他治疗　脓癣患者病情严重时可短期口服糖皮质激素,以减轻炎症反应和减少瘢痕形成。如继发细菌感染,可局部或系统使用抗生素。

Section Two　Tinea Corporis and Tinea Cruris

第二节　体癣和股癣

Tinea corporis is a superficial dermatophyte infection on the glabrous skin except palms, soles, and the groin. Tinea cruris is a superficial dermatophytic infection of the groin and adjacent area including perineum, buttocks and perianal area.

体癣是指发生于平滑皮肤部位的浅部真菌感染。股癣是特指发生在腹股沟、会阴部及臀间部位的浅表真菌感染。

【Etiology】

【病因】

The most common causative fungi for this condition are *T. rubrum*, *T. mentagrophytes* and *E. floccosum*. However, other dermatophytes such as *M. canis*, *M. gypseum*, *T. violaceum* and *T. tonsurans* can also be the cause of these infections occasionally.

体股癣的主要致病菌为红色毛癣菌、须癣毛癣菌和絮状表皮癣菌。犬小孢子菌、石膏样小孢子菌、紫色毛癣菌、断发毛癣菌等偶可引起感染。

【Clinical Manifestations】

【临床表现】

(1) Tinea corporis: tinea corporis includes all superficial dermatophyte infections of the glossy skin other than those involving the scalp, palms, soles, and the groin. The primary lesions are papules, vesicles or papulovesicles. As the primary rashes spread peripherally, one or more circular, sharply circumscribed, slightly erythematous, dry, scaly patches are likely to occur. These lesions often coalesce into large patches, in which the central part of the lesions resolves and leaves hyperpigmentation and scaling, while the border, composed of vesicles and papules, is more inflamed and actively expands (Fig. 7-5).

(1) 体癣(tinea corporis)　指发生于除头部、手足、腹股沟外的人体其他部位光滑皮肤的浅表皮肤癣菌感染,原发损害为丘疹、水疱或丘疱疹,以后皮损逐渐向四周扩展,形成环形或多环形、境界清楚的、淡红色、干燥、有鳞屑的斑片,可互相融合成大斑片。皮损中央消退,遗留色素沉着及脱屑,但由水疱和丘疹组成的边缘仍然活跃,并不断向四周蔓延(图7-5)。

(2) Tinea cruris: tinea cruris occurs most frequently on the

(2) 股癣(tinea cruris)　常发生于

upper and inner surfaces of the thighs and may extend downward to the perineum and backward around the anus and buttocks. It begins as papules, papulovesicles and small erythematous scaly patches that spread peripherally to form well-circumscribed circular or semicircular plaques. The center can self-resolve to leave hyperpigmentation and scaling, while the border may still have papules, vesicles or scales (Fig. 7-6).

大腿内上部，可延及会阴、肛周及臀部。开始为丘疹、丘疱疹及小片鳞屑性红斑，逐渐向四周蔓延扩大呈环形或半环形，边界清楚，由丘疹、水疱及结痂组成，中央部位可自愈，遗留色素沉着和脱屑(图7-6)。

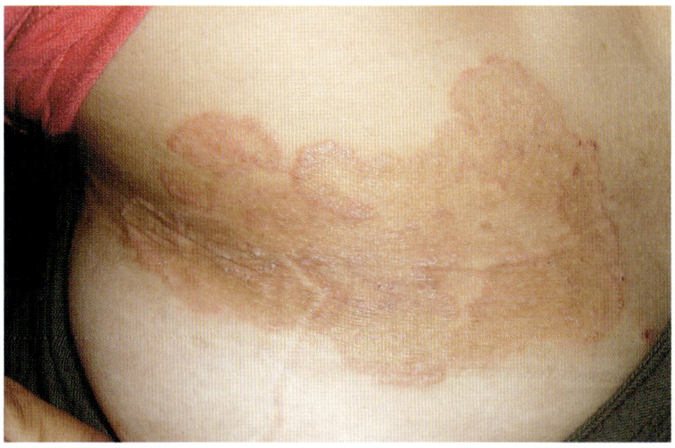

Fig. 7-5　Tinea corporis(图 7-5　体癣)

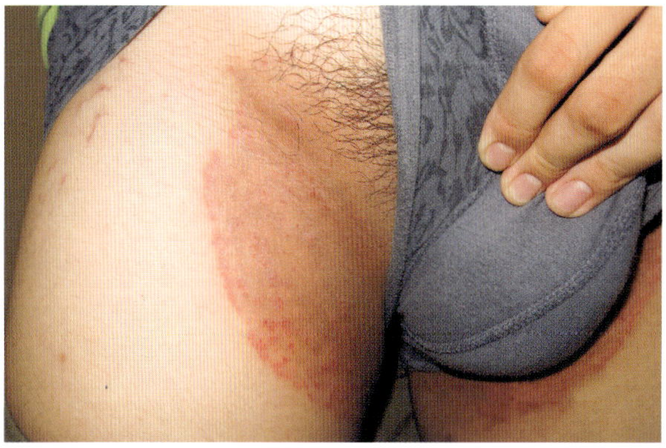

Fig. 7-6　Tinea cruris(图 7-6　股癣)

【Laboratory Findings】

(1) Direct microscopy: scrapings from the peripheries of lesions can be treated with 10% KOH for direct microscopic examination, and hyphae and spores should then be visible.

(2) Fungal culture: scrapings from the peripheries of lesions are inoculated on fungal culture media and fungal colonies will appear in 1-2 weeks. Different species possess different characteristics for colony morphology as well as distinct microscopic features.

【实验室检查】

(1) 真菌直接镜检　用 10% 的 KOH 处理皮损边缘皮屑，真菌直接镜检可找到菌丝和孢子。

(2) 真菌培养　皮损边缘皮屑真菌培养 1～2 周可见菌落生长。菌落和镜下特征视病原菌不同而各异。

【Diagnosis and Differential Diagnosis】

The diagnosis of tinea corporis and tinea cruris depends on the clinical manifestations and fungal detection by both direct examination and culture. Atypical conditions should be differentiated from eczema, lichen simplex chronicus, intertrigo and erythrasma.

【诊断及鉴别诊断】

根据临床表现和皮屑真菌镜检及培养结果可确诊。不典型的皮损尚需与湿疹、慢性单纯性苔藓、间擦疹、红癣等相鉴别。

【Treatment】

Topical treatment is sufficient for most cases. Topical administration of azoles such as miconazole, ketoconazole, clotrimazole and bifonazole, or allylamines (terbinafine and butenafine) are effective. Cases involving extensive skin areas or not reacting well to topical agents can be treated by combining topical with oral agents. In these cases, itraconazole 200 mg daily or terbinafine 250 mg daily are a good choice and the treatment should continue for 1-2 weeks. For tinea cruris, less irritating topical agents can be selected and the affected area should always be kept

【治疗】

多数病例外用药物即可。唑类抗真菌药物(如咪康唑、酮康唑、克霉唑、联苯苄唑等)或丙烯胺类抗真菌药物(如特比萘芬和布替萘芬等)外用均可取得良好效果。皮损泛发或单用外用药物效果欠佳病例可联合使用口服药物治疗。可选用伊曲康唑每日 200 mg 或特比萘芬每日 250 mg，连续服用 1～2 周。股癣患者应注意选用刺激性小的外用药物，同时

clean and dry as possible.

注意保持局部清洁干燥。

Section Three Tinea Manus and Tinea Pedis

第三节 手癣和足癣

Tinea manus and tinea pedis are superficial fungal infections caused by dermatophytes and involve fingers, finger webs, and palms for the former and toes, toe webs and soles for the latter.

手癣(tinea manus)和足癣(tinea pedis)是指皮肤癣菌侵犯指趾、指(趾)间、掌跖部所引起的浅部真菌感染。

【Etiology】

T. rubrum, *T. mentagrophytes*, *E. floccosum*, *T. megninii* together are responsible for the vast majority of cases of tinea manus and pedis. Tinea pedis tends to be spread by close contact with fungal contaminants. It has been noted that tinea pedis is an important infectious source for tinea manus. Epidermal swelling due to long-term immersion of the hands in water (perhaps for occupational reasons), hand abrasions due to frequent scrubbing, and erosion of the outer lipid layer caused by prolonged contact with detergents and organic solvents all increase the risks for tinea manus development.

【病因】

手足癣的病原菌主要为红色毛癣菌、须癣毛癣菌、絮状表皮癣菌、玫瑰色毛癣菌等。足癣发病与密切接触传染源有关;足癣是手癣的重要传染源,双手长期浸水引起表皮肿胀(可能由于职业因素)和经常摩擦受伤、长期接触洗涤剂及有机溶剂引起的外层脂质层的侵蚀等是手癣发病的重要诱因。

【Clinical Manifestations】

(1) Hyperkeratotic type: the diffuse hyperkeratotic erythema is perhaps the most remarkable lesion. The affected skin becomes coarse, scaly, dry and the sweat glands will cease to function. Rhagade occurs easily in winter and may lead to restrictions of movement in the extremities due to pain (Fig. 7-7).

(2) Scaly and papular type: the characteristic lesion is erythema and papules with clear boundary. At the edge of the erythema and papules, foliated scales adhere annularly or semi-annularly. Intense itching is the major symptom (Fig. 7-8).

【临床表现】

(1) 角化过度型 皮肤弥漫性角化过度性红斑,皮肤粗糙无汗,干燥脱屑。寒冷季节常发生皮肤皲裂,导致疼痛,影响活动(图 7-7)。

(2) 丘疹鳞屑型 境界较清楚的红斑、丘疹,边缘呈弧形或半环状,附着小片状脱屑,有明显痒感(图 7-8)。

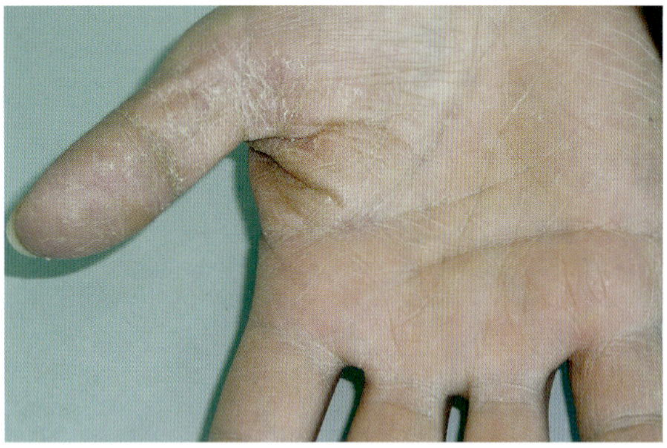

Fig. 7-7 Tinea manus and pedis-hyperkeratotic type
(图 7-7 手足癣-角化过度型)

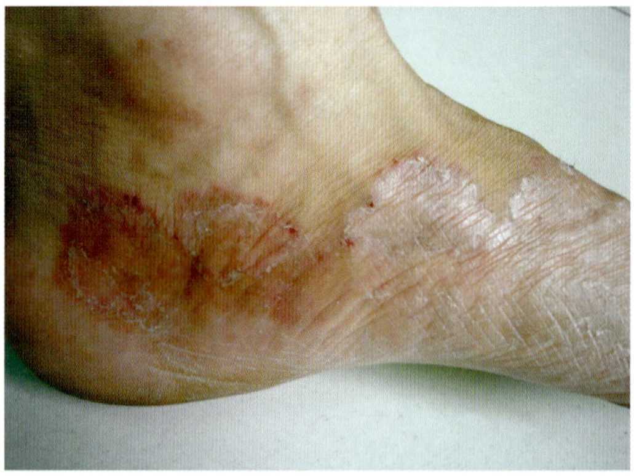

Fig. 7-8 Tinea manus and pedis-scaly and papular type
(图 7-8 手足癣-丘疹鳞屑型)

(3) Vesicular type: the initial lesions are deep-seated vesicles. The vesicles are in a sporadic or clustered arrangement and break only with difficulty. No obvious red halos are seen around the lesions. The vesicles will be absorbed in a few days, leaving scales,

(3) 水疱型 皮损初起为群集或散发小水疱,位置较深,疱壁不易穿破,周围无明显红晕,数天后水疱吸收出现脱屑。损害向四周不断扩大蔓延,水疱可

or else will coalesce to form bullae as the lesions spread. Again, intense itching is the predominant symptom for this type (Fig. 7-9).

融合为大疱,伴明显瘙痒(图 7-9)。

(4) Interdigital erosive type: whitish macerations appear in the interdigital area as the initial lesion. Erosions with red base and little exudation may be left after removing the surface (Fig. 7-10). The lesions usually give off a distinctive odor. The patients always have an unbearable itching.

(4) 趾/指间糜烂型 趾/指间浸渍发白,表皮剥脱后露出基底潮红的糜烂面,有少量渗液(图 7-10),有异臭。患者常自觉瘙痒难忍。

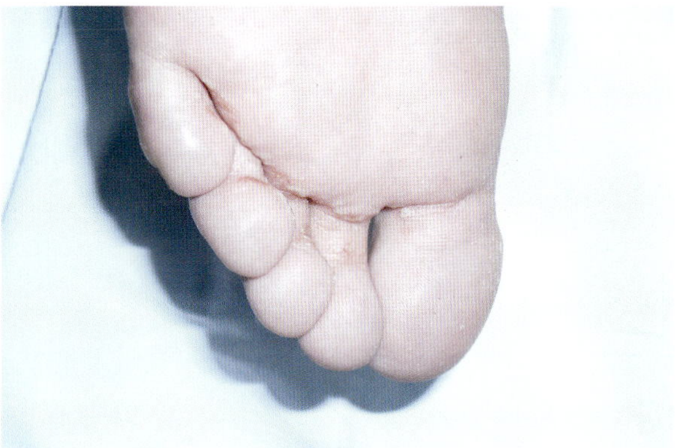

Fig. 7-9 Tinea manus and pedis-vesicular type
(图 7-9 手足癣-水疱型)

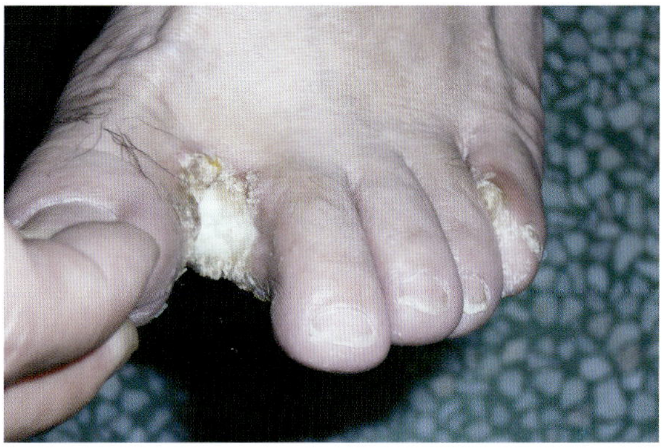

Fig. 7-10 Tinea manus and pedis-interdigital erosive type
(图 7-10 手足癣-趾/指间糜烂型)

【Laboratory Findings】

(1) Direct microscopic fungal examination: scrapings are taken from lesions and treated with a 10%-20% solution of potassium hydroxide (KOH) prior to fungal examination under the microscope. Hyphae and spores can be found in the scrapings.

(2) Fungal culture: scrapings taken from the lesions are inoculated on the fungal medium, and will grow into colonies after 1-2 weeks. The fungal colonies and the microscopic appearance of them will vary for different fungal species.

【实验室检查】

(1) 真菌直接镜检 刮取病变部位鳞屑,经 10%~20% KOH 液制片后直接镜检可发现菌丝和孢子。

(2) 真菌培养 取鳞屑真菌培养,1~2 周后可见菌落生长,菌落形态和镜下特征依病原菌不同而不同。

【Diagnosis and Differential Diagnosis】

The clinical manifestation, demonstration of the fungus by microscopic examination, and fungal culture together will establish the diagnosis. However, tinea manus and pedis should be differentiated from eczema, lichen simplex chronicus, chronic contact dermatitis, palmoplantar pustulosis, palmoplantar keratoderma and secondary syphilides. Fungal examination and culture are the key methods for differentiation.

【诊断及鉴别诊断】

根据临床表现、直接真菌镜检和培养,一般可准确诊断。临床上,手足癣有时应与下列疾病相鉴别:湿疹、慢性单纯性苔藓、慢性接触性皮炎、掌跖脓疱病、掌跖角皮症、二期梅毒疹等。真菌检查及培养是鉴别的关键。

【Treatment】

(1) Topical therapy: the precise formulations of antifungal agents should be selected according to the lesions. Moist compresses should be applied if a large amount of exudation exists. Methyl violet paste may be used after the exudation is controlled by previous treatments, or if maceration and erosion exist. If the

【治疗】

(1) 局部治疗 根据病变类型和皮损表现选择不同剂型的抗真菌药物。如渗液明显,应先进行湿敷;渗液减轻及有糜烂浸渍者可用龙胆紫糊剂;无明显糜烂、渗液皮损可选择各种抗真菌的霜剂

lesions appear to be without erosions or exudation, antifungal creams or gels may be applied instead. Keratolytics such as Whitfield's ointment or some retinoid ointment may also be used to promote healing for the hyperkeratotic type.

或凝胶等;角化过度型可加用韦氏膏、维A酸类等角质剥脱剂以提高疗效。

(2) Systemic therapy: oral agents may be used in cases with widespread infection, and in chronic or persistent cases. The most effective agents are terbinafine 250 mg/d and itraconazole 200 mg/d. Sometimes fluconazole 150 mg per week can also be used. The treatment should be continued for 2-4 weeks.

(2)系统治疗 适用于泛发或慢性迁延性病例。可给予特比萘芬 250 mg/d、伊曲康唑 200 mg/d 或每周给予氟康唑 150 mg,口服,疗程 2~4 周。

Section Four Onychomycosis

第四节 甲真菌病

Onychomycosis is a fungal infection of the nails and the subungual tissues.

由各种真菌引起的甲板或甲下组织感染称为甲真菌病(onychomycosis)。

【Etiology】

【病因】

The most common etiologic fungi of onychomycosis are *T. rubrum*, *T. mentagrophytes* and *E. floccosum*. However, other dermatophytes species such as *T. violaceum*, *T. tonsurans* and *T. schoenleinii* may also cause occasional nail infections. In addition, some non-dermatophytic molds such as *Candida* spp., *Scopulariopsis brevicaulis*, *Fusarium* spp., *Cephalosporium* spp., *Aspergillus* spp. and *Scytalidium* spp. have been associated with onychomycosis.

甲真菌病的主要致病菌为红色毛癣菌、须癣毛癣菌和絮状表皮癣菌。紫色毛癣菌、断发毛癣菌、许兰氏毛癣菌等也可致病。此外,念珠菌、短帚霉、镰刀菌、头孢霉、曲霉、柱顶孢霉等部分非皮肤癣菌亦可致病。

【Clinical Manifestations】

【临床表现】

Onychomycosis can be classified into four classic types based on the invasive paths of the pathogenic fungi and the clinical features.

根据致病菌入侵部位及甲板受累表现分为 4 种类型。

(1) Distal and lateral subungual onychomycosis (DLSO): this is the most common pattern of onychomycosis. The invasion begins at the distal edge of the nail plate and the lateral nail fold. From there the infection gradually spreads toward the nail bed and leads to subungual hyperkeratosis. The nail plate may be lifted up and becomes obviously thickened, brittle and opaque. The color of the nail plate may become brown, yellowish, green or gray. The distal edge of the nail plate may also crack with remarkable subungual hyperkeratosis (Fig. 7-11).

(1)远端侧缘甲下型 最常见的临床类型。初起感染部位为甲板远端和侧缘皮肤角质层,逐渐蔓延至甲床,引起甲下角质增生。甲分离,甲板增厚变脆、浑浊不透明,可变为棕色、黄色、绿色、灰白色等,甲板远端残缺,游离缘下角质堆积明显(图 7-11)。

(2) Superficial white onychomycosis (SWO): superficial white onychomycosis is characterized by well-circumscribed, irregular powdery white patches on the dorsal surface of the nail plate. In severe cases, the entire surface of the nail plate may be affected and the nail plate becomes brittle and easily broken(Fig. 7-12).

(2)白色浅表型 甲板表面有边缘清楚、形态不规则的粉末状白色斑片,严重者可累及全甲,甲脆、易破损(图7-12)。

(3) Proximal subungual onychomycosis (PSO): the infection starts from the posterior nail fold and produces a white patch. The patch may extend to the entire nail plate, but in this case the

(3)近端甲下型 感染初起于近端甲沟,病原菌入侵后在甲根部形成白斑,随着甲板生长,白斑可扩展至整个甲板,

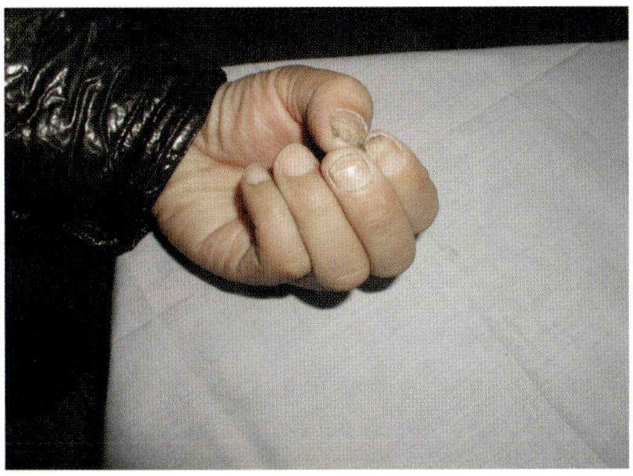

Fig. 7-11　Onychomycosis-DLSO
(图 7-11　甲真菌病-远端侧缘甲下型)

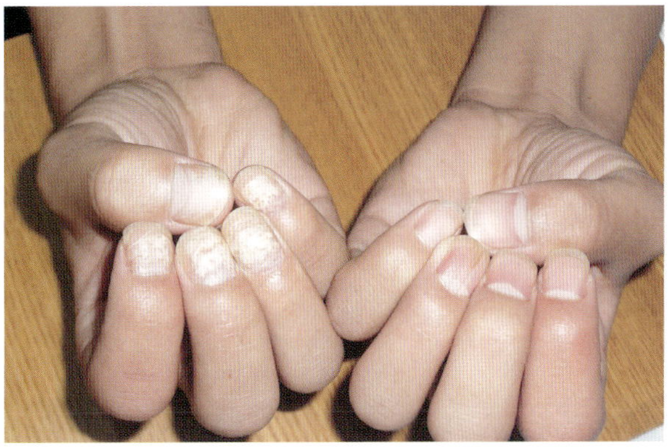

Fig. 7-12　Onychomycosis-SWO
(图 7-12　甲真菌病-白色浅表型)

subungual hyperkeratosis is not severe(Fig. 7-13). Infections due to *Candida* spp. or *Scytalidium* spp. should be taken into account if paronychia is also present.

(4) Total dystrophic onychomycosis (TDO): total dystrophic onychomycosis may result from any clinical forms of onychomycosis if left untreated. The fungus invades the entire nail plate and the entire nail becomes thick and brittle and the nail will then appear yellowish-brown with irregular surface. In severe cases, the nail may even break off and leave a hyperkeratotic nail bed(Fig. 7-14).

甲下角质堆积不明显(图 7-13)。如伴有甲沟炎,应考虑白念珠菌、柱顶孢霉感染的可能。

(4) 全甲营养不良型　上述三型如不及时治疗,都可能发展为全甲营养不良型。真菌侵入全甲,全甲增厚变脆,呈黄褐色,高低不平。严重者全甲消失,甲床裸露,角质增厚(图 7-14)。

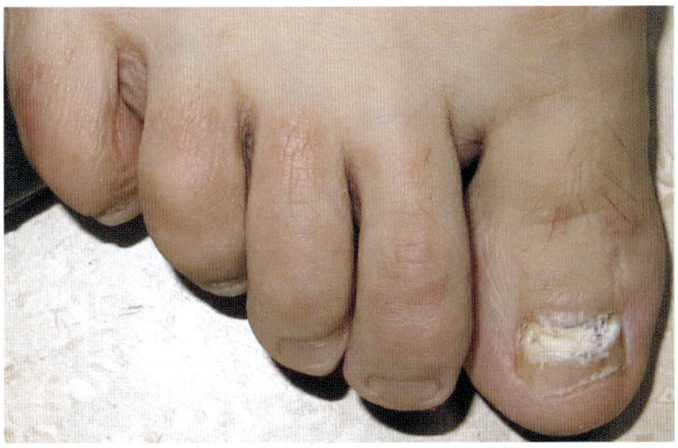

Fig. 7-13　Onychomycosis-PSO
(图 7-13　甲真菌病-近端甲下型)

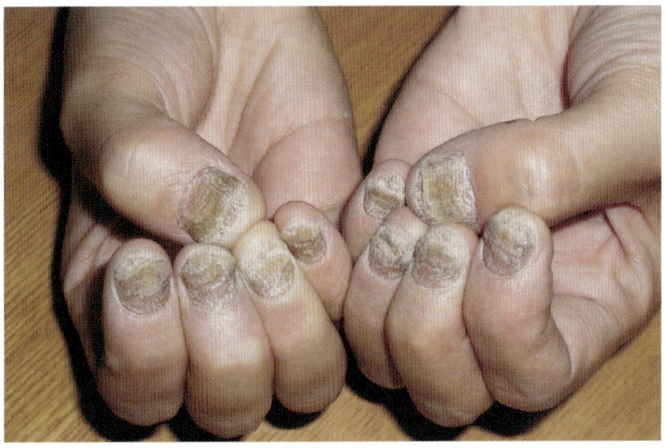

Fig. 7-14　Onychomycosis-TDO
(图 7-14　甲真菌病-全甲营养不良型)

【Laboratory Findings】

(1) Direct microscopic examination: nail clippings or scrapings near the nail bed should be suitable for direct microscopic examination. The specimens are treated with 10%-20% KOH before the examination. Hyphae and spores can be found under microscopy.

(2) Fungal culture: nail clippings or scrapings are inoculated onto the culture media and a fungal colony should be allowed to grow. The morphology of the colony and the microscopic appearance depend on the particular fungal species.

【实验室检查】

(1) 真菌直接镜检　取病变区和正常区交界部位、靠近甲床的甲屑,经 10%～20% KOH 液制片后直接镜检可发现菌丝和孢子。

(2) 真菌培养　取甲屑真菌培养,可见菌落生长。菌落形态和镜下特征依病原菌不同而不同。

(3) Histopathological examination: hyphae and spores can be found in the section of the affected nail and nail bed stained by PAS.

(3) 组织病理检查　病甲和受累甲床组织PAS染色可以找到菌丝和孢子。

【Diagnosis and Differential Diagnosis】

The clinical manifestations and positive fungal evidence from direct microscopic examination and fungal culture together give the principal support to a definite diagnosis. Numerous diseases such as psoriasis, pachyonychia congenita, leukonychia, eczema, acrodermatitis continua and lichen planus, can produce nail changes similar to onychomycosis. But symmetric involvement and negative demonstration of fungus by microscopic examination, by culture or by histopathological examination can be used to distinguish these diseases from onychomycosis.

【诊断与鉴别诊断】

临床表现及真菌检查阳性可以确诊。甲真菌病需与许多甲病相鉴别。银屑病、先天性厚甲症、白甲症、湿疹、连续性肢端皮炎、扁平苔藓等均可引起甲真菌病样的甲损害,但常累及多个指(趾)甲,对称分布,真菌检查阴性,甲病理检查无菌丝和孢子。

【Treatment】

(1) Oral agents: ① Itraconazole, 200 mg twice daily (usually taken with or after meals) for 1 week/monthly for 3-4 months, appears effective for any kind of onychomycosis caused by all fungi species. ② Terbinafine, 250 mg once daily for 6 to 12 weeks, is more effective for onychomycosis caused by dermatophytes. ③ Fluconazole, 150 mg once per week for 12 to 18 weeks or 150 mg two times a week for more than 4 months, is mainly prescribed in cases of onychomycosis caused by *Candida* spp. Oral agents in combination with topical ones will generally augment the therapeutic effect.

(2) Topical agents: topical agents can be applied in cases of SWO without involvement of the nail root and/or nail bed and for DLSO when the affected area less than 2/3 of the entire nail. The most effective agents are nail lacquers containing amorofine (5%) or ciclopirox (8%). However, topical therapies in general are much less effective than systemic antifungals and more than a year is needed to observe obvious effects.

【治疗】

(1) 口服药物　①伊曲康唑,200 mg,每日两次,饭时或饭后即服,连服7天,停21天为一个疗程,连续3～4个疗程以上,适用于各种真菌引起的甲真菌病;②特比萘芬,250 mg,每日一次,连续服用6～12周,主要用于治疗皮肤癣菌引起的甲真菌病;③氟康唑,150 mg,每周一次,连续服用12～18周,或150 mg,每周两次,连续4月以上,主要用于治疗念珠菌引起的甲真菌病。联合外用药物治疗可提高疗效。

(2) 外用药物　主要适用于治疗未累及甲根或甲床的白色浅表型及累及范围不超过甲板2/3的远端侧缘甲下型甲真菌病。目前比较有效的治疗药物有5%阿莫罗芬涂甲剂和8%环吡酮胺涂甲剂等。值得注意的是,外用药物治疗甲真菌病需要长期用药(一年以上),很少能根治,远不如口服药有效。

Section Five　Pityriasis Versicolor

Pityriasis versicolor, also known as tinea versicolor, is a superficial, chronic fungal infection of the *stratum corneum* of the epidermis caused by *Malassezia*.

第五节　花斑糠疹

花斑糠疹(pityriasis versicolor)又称为花斑癣,是由马拉色菌所引起的一种皮肤角质层的浅表的慢性真菌感染。

【Etiology and Pathogenesis】

Pityriasis versicolor is caused by *Malassezia*, which are opportunistic organisms found in the *stratum corneum* of normal skin in a yeast form. *Malassezia* can convert from the yeast-like phase into the hyphae phase under certain conditions, and then can

【病因及发病机制】

病原菌为马拉色菌。马拉色菌属条件致病菌,其酵母相存在于正常皮肤角质层。在某些诱因作用下,马拉色菌由酵母相转变为菌丝相,则具有感染力,侵

become the cause of a skin infection. The common predisposing factors for infection include high temperature, excessive sweating, systemic or topical use of glucocorticoids, topical use of greasy agents, malnutrition, extracellular accumulation of glycogen, chronic infections, pregnancy, and family susceptibility.

犯周围组织产生皮损。最常见诱因是高温和多汗，其次为全身或局部使用糖皮质激素、皮肤使用油脂类制剂、营养不良、细胞外糖原沉积、慢性感染、妊娠及家族易感性等。

【Clinical Manifestations】

Typical lesions appear to be guttate or nummular patches with fine scales. The patches are yellowish or brownish in dark skin and hypopigmented in pale skin. Sites of predilection are the chest, back, upper arms and the neck (Fig. 7-15). The disease may even occur on the face, abdomen, scalp, palms, soles and intertriginous areas, particularly in young adults. In some instances, follicular papules with mild inflammation are marked features of the eruptions. It can be found on the chest, back and abdomen.

【临床表现】

典型皮损为点滴至钱币大小斑片，上覆糠秕状鳞屑。深色皮肤上皮损色较深，呈黄色、棕色，白皮肤上皮损色淡发白。皮损最常见于胸、背、上臂、颈部（图7-15），也可见于面部、腹部、头皮、掌跖和间擦部位，尤其是青年人。有时皮损呈毛囊性丘疹，炎症反应轻微，好发于胸、背及腹部。

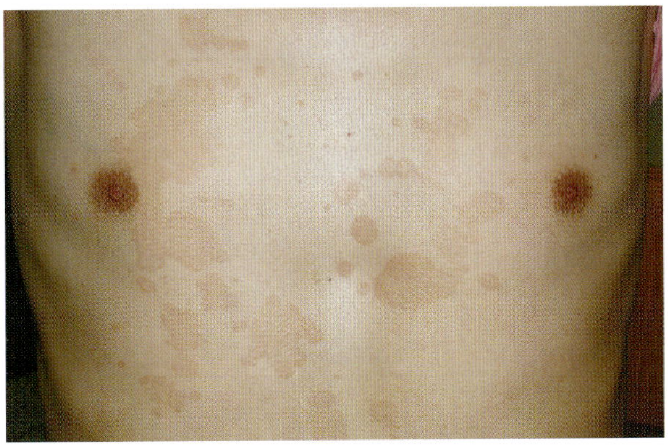

Fig. 7-15　Pityriasis versicolor（图 7-15　花斑糠疹）

【Diagnosis and Differential Diagnosis】

Diagnosis is based on the typical clinical manifestations and the microscopic examination. Microscopically, short, thick fungal hyphae and a large number of various sized, round or oval thick-walled spores 3-8 μm in diameter can be seen. Identification by culture is impractical with low positive rate and is not normally required to establish a diagnosis. Lesions that are imperceptible or doubtful may be examined under Wood's light in a dark room. The lesions associated with this disease will give a yellowish or brownish fluorescence.

【诊断及鉴别诊断】

根据典型的临床表现、皮损真菌镜检找到短粗菌丝和直径 3～8 μm 的圆形、卵圆形厚壁孢子即可诊断。培养阳性率低，通常不用于临床诊断。皮损不明显或可疑者可在暗室内行伍氏灯检查，皮损呈黄色或棕色荧光有助于诊断。

Pityriasis versicolor must be differentiated from vitiligo, pityriasis rosea, pityriasis alba, etc. Eruptions of vitiligo appear as well-demarcated depigmented patches, surrounded by hyperpigmentation, rarely with scales or itching. Moreover, microscopic examination for fungi is negative in vitiligo. Pityriasis rosea occurs on the trunk and limbs, and appears as numerous round or oval-shaped scaly macules with a rosy color. The long axis of the lesions on the trunk will lie parallel to the skin lines. This is a self-limiting disease without

本病应与白癜风、玫瑰糠疹、单纯糠疹等相鉴别。白癜风为边界清楚的色素脱失斑，边缘色素加深，一般无脱屑，无痒感，真菌镜检阴性；玫瑰糠疹好发于躯干及四肢近端，为圆形或椭圆形玫瑰红色斑疹，表面覆以糠秕状鳞屑，皮损长轴与皮纹走向一致。本病有自限性，不复发。单纯糠疹多发于儿童或青年人面

recurrence. Pityriasis alba usually occurs in children or adolescents, and the location is usually on the face. Microscopic examination is helpful here, in which neither hyphae nor spores can be found in this case.

部。真菌镜检均为阴性有助于诊断。

【Treatment】

Daily applications of any of the following topical agents have been used successfully: a 10%-20% aqueous solution of sodium hyposulfite followed by 4% dilute hydrochloric acid, imidazole, selenium sulfide shampoos or lotions, zinc pyrithione shampoos, sulfur preparations, salicylic acid preparations, propylene glycol lotions, benzoyl peroxide, etc. Systemic treatment is necessary if eruptions appear with a diffuse distribution or if topical drugs are not effective. Ketoconazole 200 mg daily for 10 days is effective. Oral itraconazole are also evolving treatment options, e. g. , 200 mg of itraconazole for 5-7 days, or else fluconazole 400 mg stat. The use of terbinafine has been shown to be ineffective via the oral route but useful as a topical preparation.

【治疗】

局部治疗通常有效，常用药物包括10%～20%硫代硫酸钠溶液涂搽数分钟后涂以4%稀盐酸溶液、咪唑类、硫化硒、吡硫锌、硫黄制剂、水杨酸制剂、丙烯甘油和过氧化苯甲酰等。对于皮疹泛发、久治不愈的患者可口服抗真菌药物，酮康唑每日200 mg，顿服，连续10天；伊曲康唑每日200 mg，顿服，连续5～7天；氟康唑400 mg，顿服；特比萘芬口服无效，外用有效。

Section Six *Malassezia* Folliculitis

Malassezia folliculitis is an inflammatory disease of the follicles caused by accelerated growth of *Malassezia*, which is considered to be normal skin flora. The common triggers of the disease include hyperhidrosis, seborrhea, and the systemic or topical use of glucocorticoids or antibiotics.

第六节 马拉色菌毛囊炎

马拉色菌毛囊炎(*Malassezia* folliculitis)是由马拉色菌在毛囊内大量繁殖引起的毛囊炎症。马拉色菌被认为是一种正常皮肤菌群。该病的常见诱因有多汗、皮脂溢出、局部或系统使用糖皮质激素及抗生素等。

【Etiology and Pathogenesis】

Malassezia, mainly *M. furfur*, *M. globosa*, and *M. sympodialisis*, are part of normal skin flora. Some predisposing factors such as hyperhidrosis, seborrhea, and the systemic or topical use of glucocorticoids or antibiotics promote the growth of *Malassezia* in the follicles. The metabolites produced by *Malassezia* then provoke the scaling that obstructs the follicular ducts and therefore leads to the rupture of the follicles. The follicular rupture elicits the inflammatory reaction that resembles very severe acne.

【病因及发病机制】

本病的病原菌马拉色菌(主要是糠秕马拉色菌、球形马拉色菌和合轴马拉色菌)是人体皮肤的正常菌群。在促发因素如多汗、皮脂溢出、局部或系统使用糖皮质激素或抗生素等的影响下，马拉色菌在毛囊内大量繁殖，其代谢产物刺激毛囊产生大量脱屑阻塞毛囊导管，导致毛囊扩张破裂引起炎症反应，出现类似严重痤疮的损害。

【Clinical Manifestations】

This disease is particularly prevalent in adolescents and young adulthood. It has a predilection for areas rich in sebaceous glands such as the upper back and chest. Occasionally, it may also involve the shoulders, face, neck, legs and scalp. The lesions appear as dome-shaped follicular red papules (Fig. 7-16) or more rarely as pustules. Mild pruritus may also be present. It sometimes appears in conjunction with acne, pityriasis versicolor or seborrheic

【临床表现】

多见于中青年，好发于皮脂腺丰富的部位，如上背、胸部，偶见于肩部、面部、颈部、小腿、头皮等。皮损表现为圆顶状红色毛囊性丘疹(图7-16)，间有脓疱。患者常有不同程度的瘙痒，本病常并发痤疮、花斑糠疹、脂溢性皮炎等病。

dermatitis.

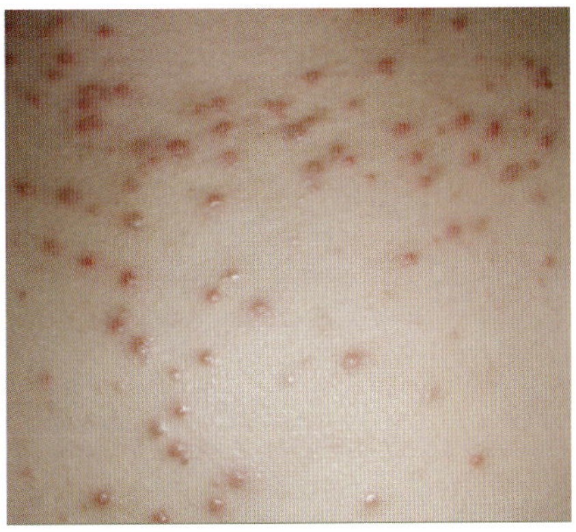

Fig. 7-16 ***Malassezia*** **folliculitis(图 7-16　马拉色菌毛囊炎)**

【Diagnosis and Differential Diagnosis】

Diagnosis of *malassezia* folliculitis depends on specific features of the eruptions and on microscopic examination. Microscopically, there are clusters of round or oval thick-walled spores and crescent-shaped hyphae.

The disease should be differentiated from acne vulgaris, papular forms of cutaneous candidiasis, bacterial folliculitis and eosinophilic pustular folliculitis. Acne vulgaris usually occurs on the face, chest and back, accompanied by black or white comedones. Papular forms of cutaneous candidiasis may have very similar lesions to *malassezia* folliculitis. However, in the former the papules are usually covered by ring-shaped scales and microscopic examination reveals pseudohyphae and spores. Patients with bacterial folliculitis will experience a shorter and more acute course with significant soreness. Pustules usually occur on the top of the red follicular papules of bacterial folliculitis in a very short time. The etiology of eosinophilic pustular folliculitis is still unknown, although it occurs mostly in men whose peripheral blood eosinophils are significantly increased. Histopathology shows large amount of eosinophils in the follicles.

【诊断及鉴别诊断】

根据临床表现，真菌镜检见成堆的圆形或卵圆形厚壁孢子或新月状菌丝可诊断。

本病应与寻常型痤疮、丘疹型皮肤念珠菌病、细菌性毛囊炎、嗜酸性脓疱性毛囊炎等鉴别。寻常型痤疮好发于颜面部、前胸及后背，伴有黑头及白头粉刺。丘疹型皮肤念珠菌病皮损与马拉色菌毛囊炎相似，但丘疹顶端常伴有圈状脱屑，真菌镜检可见假菌丝和芽孢。细菌性毛囊炎起病急、病程短，红色的毛囊性丘疹顶端迅速形成脓疱，有明显痛感。嗜酸性脓疱性毛囊炎病因不明，男性多见，外周血嗜酸粒细胞可显著升高，组织病理显示毛囊内有大量的嗜酸性粒细胞。

【Treatment】

Treatment of *malassezia* folliculitis is the same as for pityriasis versicolor.

【治疗】

马拉色菌毛囊炎的治疗同花斑糠疹。

Section Seven　Candidiasis

Candidiasis is the acute or chronic fungal infection of skin, mucosal membranes and/or internal organs caused by *Candida* spp.

第七节　念珠菌病

念珠菌病(candidiasis)是由念珠菌属引起的皮肤黏膜及内脏器官的急性或慢性感染。

【Etiology and Pathogenesis】

Candidiasis is an infection caused by the *Candida* spp. The common causative species in this genus include *C. albicans*, *C.*

【病因及发病机制】

念珠菌病是由多种念珠菌属感染引起的，常见病原菌为念珠菌属的白念珠

tropicalis, *C. krusei*, *C. stellatoidea*, *C. glabrata*, *C. guilliermondii*, *C. parapsilosis*, *C. paratropicalis*. These are opportunistic organisms and infections are usually only found in individuals who have locally or generally impaired immune response. *Candida albicans* remains the most common causative pathogen, but the frequency of non-*albicans* *Candida* infections has gradually increased in recent years.

菌、热带念珠菌、克柔念珠菌、星形念珠菌、光滑念珠菌、季也蒙念珠菌、近平滑念珠菌、伪热带念珠菌等，均为条件致病菌，常在局部或全身免疫力降低时发病。白念珠菌引起的感染最常见，近年来非白念珠菌感染的发病率有上升趋势。

【Clinical Manifestations】

(1) Mucous membrane candidiasis:

① Thrush: thrush most commonly occurs in the newborn. Adult patients with diabetes or AIDS, or undergoing long-term glucocorticoids and/or broad-spectrum antibiotic therapy, or those taking cytotoxic therapy or radiotherapy are also predisposed to thrush. Grayish white membranous plaques (pseudomembranes) are found on the surface of the mucous membrane of the tongue, soft palate or buccal mucosa. The base of these plaques is moist, reddish, and erosive (Fig. 7-17). Mucous ulceration may develop in severe cases, and is often painful.

② Vulvovaginal candidiasis: the lesion presents as congestion and swelling of the vaginal mucosa. Grayish white membranous plaques (pseudomembranes) may be found on the surface of the vaginal mucosa. The vaginal discharge is often thick and tenacious and the color becomes yellowish or cheese-like. Sometimes small membranous pieces can be found in the vaginal discharge (Fig. 7-18). Lesions can spread posteriorly to the perineum and around the anus, which will undergo remarkable swelling with intensive itching.

【临床表现】

(1) 黏膜念珠菌病

①鹅口疮(thrush)：常见于新生儿。成人鹅口疮常见于糖尿病患者、艾滋病患者、长期使用糖皮质激素和/或广谱抗生素患者，或接受化疗或放疗的肿瘤患者。损害为黏着于舌、软腭或颊黏膜上的灰白色假膜，基底为湿润的鲜红色糜烂面(图7-17)。严重病例可出现黏膜溃疡，患者自觉疼痛。

②外阴阴道念珠菌病(vulvovaginal candidiasis)：损害表现为阴道壁充血、水肿，阴道黏膜上可见灰白色假膜。阴道分泌物浓稠，呈黄色或乳酪样，有时混有豆腐渣样白色小块(图7-18)。皮损可扩展至肛周和整个会阴部，表现为外阴部明显红肿和剧烈瘙痒。

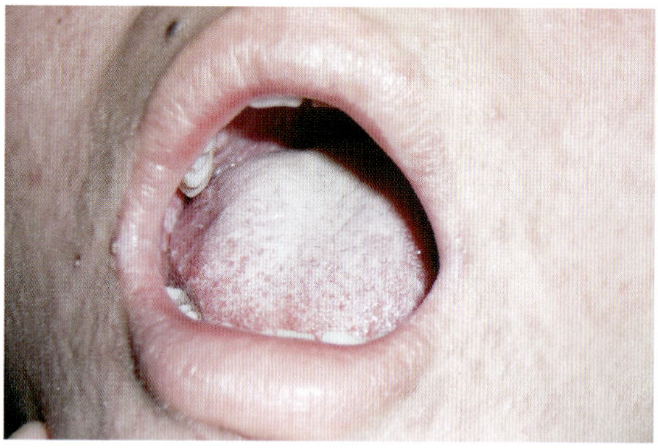

Fig. 7-17 Thrush
(图7-17 鹅口疮)

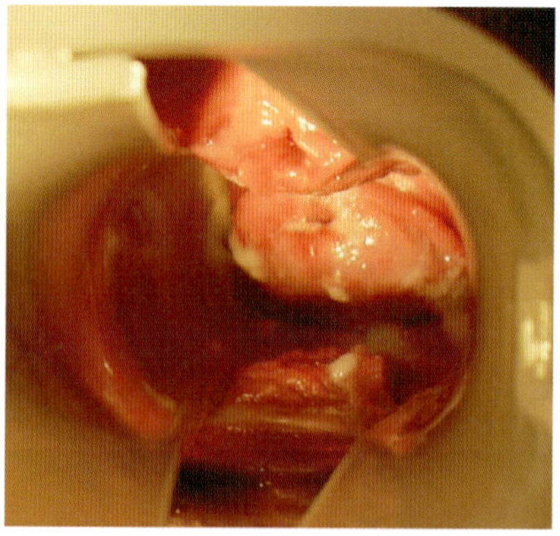

Fig. 7-18 Vulvovaginal candidiasis
(图7-18 外阴阴道念珠菌病)

③Candidal balanoposthitis: in this condition the lesions always occur on the glans, coronary sulcus, and the inner side of the prepuce, which are characterized by mild erythema with a dry smooth surface, or by superficial erosion and thin-walled pustules. Thrush-like grayish white pseudomembranes on the glans and

③念珠菌性包皮龟头炎(candidal balanoposthitis)：损害好发于龟头、冠状沟及包皮内叶，为轻度潮红斑片，表面干燥光滑，或为表浅糜烂及薄壁脓疱。严重病例龟头和冠状沟可出现鹅口疮样白

coronary sulcus can be found in some severe cases (Fig. 7-19).

(2) Cutaneous candidiasis:

① Candidal intertrigo: candidal intertrigo always arises in intertriginous areas, such as the armpits, groin, under the breasts, and in the umbilicus. The disease begins with erythema, papules or vesicles and gradually extends and coalesces to form a well-circumscribed erythema with vesicles on the surface. The vesicles may rupture to leave scaling or erosion with minimal exudation. Papules, vesicles or pustules may be scattered peripherally, but with a tendency to cluster (Fig. 7-20). Itching is a predominant complaint.

色假膜(图 7-19)。

(2) 皮肤念珠菌病

① 念珠菌性间擦疹(candidal intertrigo):损害常累及间擦部位，如腋窝、腹股沟、乳房下、脐部等。皮损开始为红斑、丘疹或小水疱，以后融合成边缘清楚的较大片状红斑，表面有水疱。水疱破裂后可出现脱屑或形成糜烂面，有少许渗液。皮损外周可见散在分布的丘疹、水疱或脓疱，但倾向于聚集(图7-20)。患者自觉瘙痒。

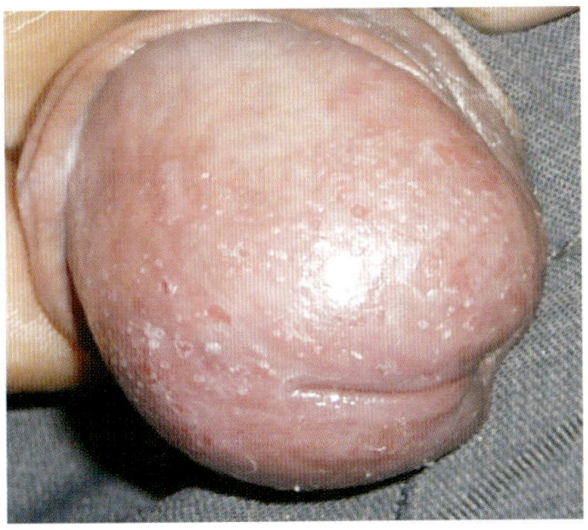

Fig. 7-19　Candidal balanoposthitis
(图 7-19　念珠菌性包皮龟头炎)

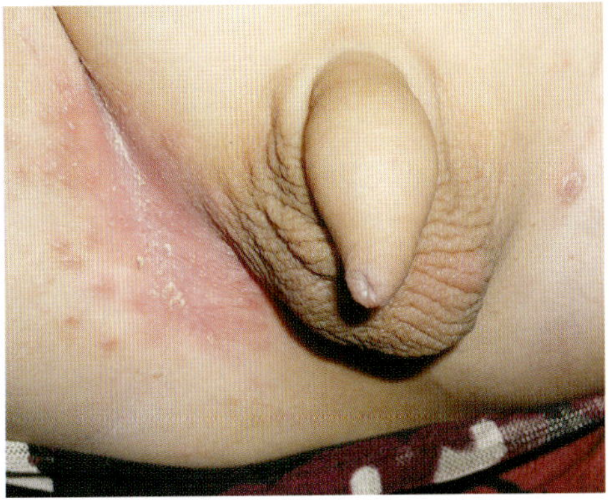

Fig. 7-20　Candidal intertrigo
(图 7-20　念珠菌性间擦疹)

② Erosio interdigitalis: this form of candidiasis is seen as macerated white skin on an erythematous base on the webs of the fingers and toes. If the macerated skin peels off, erosion surrounded by a collar of white epidermis is visible underneath (Fig. 7-21). This disease is often accompanied by candidal paronychia and onychomycosis.

② 念珠菌性指(趾)间糜烂(erosio interdigitalis):损害为指(趾)间红斑，表皮浸渍发白，脱落后形成糜烂，周边可见领圈样残留发白表皮(图 7-21)，常伴念珠菌性甲沟炎和甲念珠菌病。

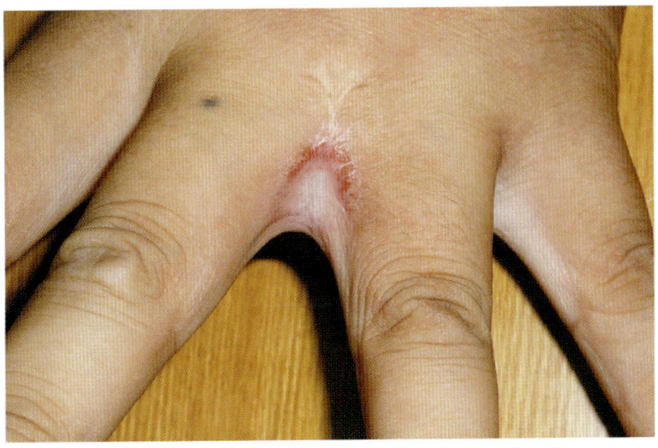

Fig. 7-21　Erosio interdigitalis (图 7-21　念珠菌性指(趾)间糜烂)

③ Candidal paronychia: it is usually a chronic condition that leads to the swelling of the paronychial tissue with occasional discharge of thin pus or exudation. The patients may feel mild pain.

③ 念珠菌性甲沟炎(candidal paronychia):病程呈慢性，表现为甲沟红肿，但很少化脓，有时有少量渗液，自觉稍痛。

④Pseudo diaper rash: the disease usually starts in the perianal region and is characterized by large irregular well circumscribed erythema with scattered papules, vesicles, macerated epidermis and scaling on the surface. Maculopapules, vesicles or papulovesicles may be scattered along the edges of the lesions. The disease may spread over the entire diaper area.

④念珠菌性尿布疹(pseudo diaper rash):皮损初起于肛周,为大片不规则、境界清楚的红斑,上面可见丘疹、水疱和浸渍的表皮及脱屑。皮损周围可有散在分布的斑丘疹、水疱和丘疱疹。皮损可蔓延至整个尿布区。

⑤Chronic mucocutaneous candidiasis: the patients often have inherited endocrinopathy or some defects in immunity. Onset is usually before the age of 3. The disease starts with thrush and perleche, followed by scaly erythematous hyperkeratotic lesions on the scalp, face and end of extremities. The hair becomes sparse. The hyperkeratotic, hornlike, or verrucous lesions on the forehead and nose are characteristic of the disease.

⑤慢性皮肤黏膜念珠菌病(chronic mucocutaneous candidiasis):患者多伴有遗传性内分泌异常或免疫功能低下。常在3岁以内开始发病,一般先出现鹅口疮和口角糜烂,以后头皮、面部、四肢末端出现红斑鳞屑性皮疹,伴角质增生。头发稀疏,前额、鼻部可出现疣赘样增殖性皮损,具有特征性。

⑥Candidal granuloma: this disease is characterized by papules with yellowish brown heavy crusts that adhere to the surface. The papules may sometimes protrude as cutaneous horns. The site of predilection is the face. The scalp, nails, trunk, lower extremities and the throat can occasionally be affected. Patients often have defects in immunity and lymphocytopenia.

⑥念珠菌性肉芽肿(candidal granuloma):特征性的皮损为丘疹,其上黏着厚的棕黄色痂,有时可突出如皮角状,常见于面部。头皮、指甲、躯干、下肢及咽部偶可出现。患者常伴免疫缺陷及淋巴细胞减少。

(3) Systemic candidiasis: systemic candidiasis always affects immunocompromised patients. Patients who are at high risk include those with malignancies especially leukemia or lymphoma, patients with AIDS, debilitated and malnourished patients, patients with transplants receiving immunosuppressive drugs for prolonged periods, patients being treated with glucocorticoids for long periods, or patients with indwelling intravenous catheters. The initial sign of systemic candidiasis may vary depending on the involvement of internal organs. The clinical findings include fever of unknown origin, pulmonary infiltration, gastrointestinal bleeding, endocarditis, renal failure, meningitis, osteomyelitis, endophthalmitis, peritonitis, and disseminated maculopapular exanthema. The cutaneous findings are erythema and maculopapules that become papular, pustular, and hemorrhagic, and may progress to necrotic ulcerating lesions.

(3) 系统性念珠菌病(systemic candidiasis)　好发于免疫功能低下者,这些高危者包括肿瘤(尤其是白血病和淋巴瘤)患者、艾滋病患者、虚弱和营养不良患者、需要长期使用免疫抑制剂的器官移植患者、长期接受糖皮质激素治疗的患者及静脉内导管插管患者。最初表现视累及器官不同而不同,可出现不明原因的发热、肺部浸润、胃肠道出血、心内膜炎、肾功能衰竭、脑膜炎、骨髓炎、眼内炎、腹膜炎或皮肤播散性斑丘疹等。皮肤表现初起为红斑及斑丘疹,随后发展为丘疹性、脓疱性、出血性皮损,如出现局部坏死,则可出现溃疡性损害。

(4) Candidid: candidid may develop after a candidal infection and the clinical manifestation is identical to dermatophytid, which is characterized by pinhead-sized clusters of sterile vesicular lesions mainly on the webs of the fingers or toes, or on the trunk. The eruptions should subside with anti-allergic treatments, or after the original candidal infection has resolved with treatment.

(4) 念珠菌疹(candidid)　可发生于念珠菌感染后,其临床表现与癣菌疹相同,常为成群的无菌性针头大小的水疱性损害,位于指趾间或躯干,给予抗过敏治疗或经治疗念珠菌初始感染部位恢复后皮疹可消退。

【Laboratory Findings】

【实验室检查】

(1) Direct microscopic examination: specimens should be collected according to the affected locations (e. g. , scales, mucous

(1) 直接镜检　根据感染部位不同采集不同标本,如鳞屑、黏膜刮取物、白

scrapings, vaginal discharges, sputum, urine, stools, blood, cerebrospinal fluid, or tissue biopsy). Direct microscopic examination should find pseudohyphae and round or oval spores.

(2) Fungal culture: the specimen should be inoculated on fungal culture media to find yeast-like colonies growing after 24-48 hours. The fungi species can be identified by biochemistry tests.

(3) Histopathological examination: pseudohyphae, hyphae and spores can be found in the affected tissue.

(4) Serological test: G-test can be used to measure the level of 1,3-β-glucan, which is a major structural component of yeast cell walls. The release of this molecule from yeast cells into serum provides evidence of the systemic fungal infection. The test differentiates fungal from bacterial infections but it is not specific for candidiasis.

带、痰、尿、粪、血、脑脊液、活检组织等。直接镜检见假菌丝、圆形或卵圆形芽孢。

(2) 真菌培养　将标本接种于真菌培养基上培养 24～48 h,可见酵母样菌落生长。通过生化试验可鉴定菌种。

(3) 组织病理检查　组织病理检查可找到假菌丝、真菌丝和芽孢。

(4) 血清学检查　G 试验通过检测血清中 1,3-β-葡聚糖(酵母细胞壁的主要结构成分,该分子从酵母细胞壁释放入血清中可提供系统性真菌感染的证据)水平判断是否存在系统性真菌感染,可帮助鉴别真菌与细菌感染,但对念珠菌感染无特异性。

【Diagnosis and Differential Diagnosis】

A definitive diagnosis is reached when the growth of of *Candida* spp. is found on fungal culture. Thrush should be differentiated from oral leukoplakia, lichen planus and tertiary syphilis. Vaginal candidiasis should be differentiated from trichomoniasis, which is a sexually transmitted vaginal infection caused by the protozoa *Trichomonas vaginalis*. Systemic candidiasis should be differentiated from other systemic fungal infections, tuberculosis, neoplasms and chronic bacterial infections.

【诊断与鉴别诊断】

所有患者的确诊必须有真菌镜检和/或培养阳性结果。鹅口疮需与黏膜白斑、扁平苔癣、三期梅毒等相鉴别。阴道念珠菌病应与阴道滴虫病相鉴别,后者是一种由阴道毛滴虫原虫引起的性传播性阴道内感染。系统性念珠菌病应与其他系统性真菌病、结核、肿瘤以及其他慢性细菌感染相鉴别。

【Treatment】

(1) Topical therapy: topical therapy is suitable for some cutaneous and mucous candidiasis. Nystatin ointment, nystatin glycerine, ketoconazole cream, miconazole cream or bifonazole cream can be selected. The formulation of topical antifungal agents should be appropriately selected according to the infected area and the rash type. Nystatin or miconazole vaginal suppositories can be used for the treatment of vaginal candidiasis.

(2) Systemic therapy: fluconazole, itraconazole and amphotericin B can be selected for systemic treatment. The doses and courses should be decided for each infection accordingly. New antifungal agents such as caspofungin, micafungin, voriconazole, or amphotericin B liposome are also available for the patients that are resistant to fluconazole and/or itraconazole or those that have intolerance to amphotericin B. Gastrointestinal candidiasis can be treated by oral administration of nystatin. Immunocompromised patients are better treated with the combination of immunomodulators and antifungal agents.

【治疗】

(1) 局部治疗　适用于部分皮肤和黏膜念珠菌感染,可选用制霉菌素软膏、制霉菌素甘油、酮康唑或咪康唑霜、联苯苄唑乳膏等,应根据不同部位和皮损类型选用合适剂型的外用抗真菌药物。阴道念珠菌病可选用制霉菌素栓剂或咪康唑栓剂等。

(2) 系统治疗　可选用氟康唑、伊曲康唑及两性霉素 B 等治疗,根据不同病变选择不同剂量和疗程。对于氟康唑和/或伊曲康唑治疗无效或不能耐受两性霉素 B 治疗的病例,可选用新型抗真菌药物卡泊芬净或米卡芬净、伏立康唑及两性霉素 B 脂质体进行治疗。消化道念珠菌病可口服制霉菌素治疗。具有免疫缺陷者可联合使用免疫调节剂和抗真菌剂治疗。

Section Eight　Sporotrichosis

Sporotrichosis is a chronic infection of skin, subcutaneous tissue and adjacent lymphatic vessels caused by saprophytic dimorphic fungus *Sporothrix schenckii*.

【Etiology and Pathogenesis】

Sporotrichosis is caused by *Sporothrix schenckii*, a saprophyte that lives in soil or on plants or on the trunks of trees. The infection can occur when *Sporothrix* contaminated soil or grass comes in contact with a pre-existing wound in the skin, or directly after contact with *Sporothrix*-contaminated thorns. The infection can involve the mouth, throat and even intestinal mucosa after contaminated vegetables or fruits are swallowed. Pulmonary infection is usually due to inhalation of the spores.

【Clinical Manifestations】

(1) Mucocutaneous sporotrichosis:

① Lymphangitic type: the initial lesion commonly occurs on exposed areas such as the hands, forearms, legs and ankles. The lesions are usually unilaterally distributed. The earliest manifestation may be a small painless hard nodule that does not adhere to the overlying skin. The nodules gradually grow larger and become adherent to the overlying skin which become violaceous in color. Necrosis in the center of the nodules followed by ulceration (called sporotrichotic chancre) could develop with a small amount of pus and elevated margins. The nodules may develop along the draining lymphatics and can look as if they are arranged in a line. These nodules can also ulcerate. The lymphatic ducts among the nodules may become hard and thick, and may resemble ropes (Fig. 7-22).

② Fixed type: fixed cutaneous sporotrichosis is characterized by a solitary lesion without spreading along the lymphatics. The lesions may appear as papules, nodules, scaly patches or as acneiform, granulomatous, verrucous or infiltrative plaques (Fig. 7-23).

③ Mucous type: the primary infection is caused by swallowing contaminated fruits or vegetables. Sometimes secondary mucous sporotrichosis will occur along with disseminated sporotrichosis. The most common infected areas are the mouth, throat and nasal mucosa. The infections begin with erythema and painful ulcerations and can develop with minimal pus. It may heal with scarring. Regional draining lymph nodes can become enlarged.

第八节　孢子丝菌病

孢子丝菌病(sporotrichosis)是由腐生的双相真菌申克孢子丝菌引起的皮肤、皮下组织及附近淋巴管的慢性感染性疾病。

【病因及发病机制】

病原菌为申克孢子丝菌，是土壤、植物、木材的腐生菌。外伤后接触申克孢子丝菌污染的土壤、花草，或被申克孢子丝菌污染的荆棘、木刺等刺伤，病原菌直接进入皮肤而引起感染。吞食带菌的蔬菜、水果可引起口腔、咽喉和肠黏膜感染。肺部感染多由吸入病原菌孢子引起。

【临床表现】

(1) 皮肤黏膜型孢子丝菌病

①淋巴管型：初起损害位于暴露部位，如手、前臂、小腿、踝等，多为单侧。开始为无痛质硬结节，不与皮肤粘连。随后结节逐渐扩大并与皮肤粘连，变为紫红色，中央坏死，形成溃疡，表面有稀薄脓液，可结痂，边缘隆起，称为孢子丝菌性下疳。同时，沿引流淋巴管走向先后出现新的结节，成串排列。新出现的结节也可出现坏死溃疡。皮损间的淋巴管可增粗、变硬呈索状(图 7-22)。

②固定型：皮损常单发，固定于初发部位，不沿淋巴管继续播散。皮损表现为丘疹、结节、鳞屑性斑片，或呈痤疮样、肉芽肿性、疣状、浸润性斑块(图 7-23)。

③黏膜型：可为原发性，由吞食污染的蔬菜、水果而引起。也可继发于播散性孢子丝菌病。病变多累及口腔、咽部和鼻黏膜。初起为红斑，以后逐渐形成溃疡，有少量脓性分泌物，常伴疼痛，愈后遗留瘢痕。局部引流淋巴结可肿大。

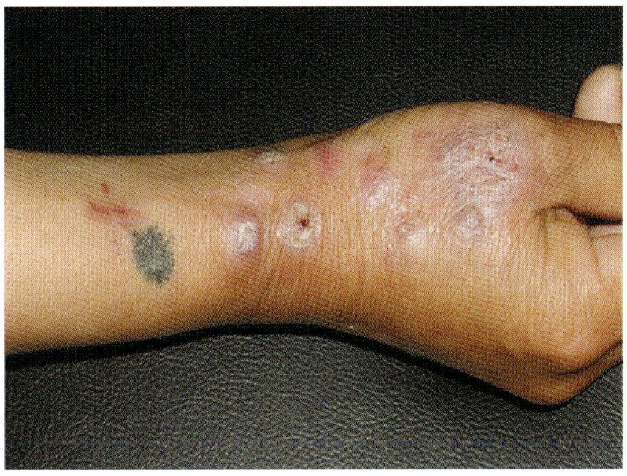

Fig. 7-22　Sporotrichosis-lymphangitic type

(图 7-22　孢子丝菌病-淋巴管型)

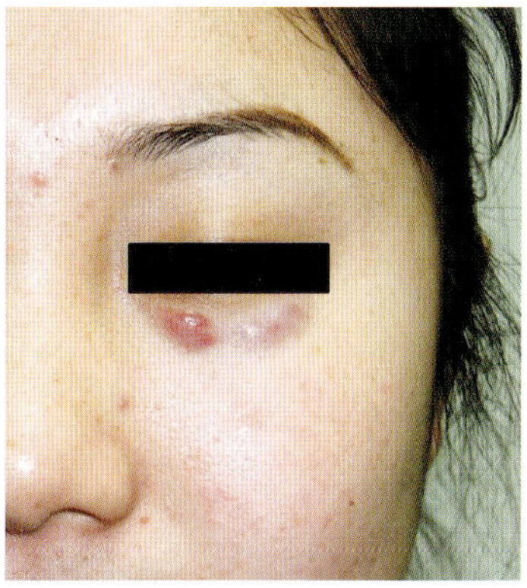

Fig. 7-23　Sporotrichosis-fixed type

(图 7-23　孢子丝菌病-固定型)

(2) Miscellaneous types:

① Extracutaneous type: extracutenous sporotrichosis is rarely seen. Pulmonary sporotrichosis is characterized by thin-walled cavities in the lung and lymphadenopathy of the hila, trachea and bronchi, which resembles pulmonary tuberculosis. Ocular sporotrichosis is usually a primary infection and always involves the conjunctiva and dacryocyst. Local lymph node enlargement is minimal here. Infections involving bone, periosteum and synovium can lead to arthritis mutilans and cause pain, swelling, deformity and limitation of movements in the joints. Sporotrichotic meningitis in which a markedly elevated protein levels and increased cell count would be found in the cerebrospinal fluid is rare, and fungal culture may find *S. schenckii* in this case.

(2) 其他类型

①皮肤外型:少见。肺部孢子丝菌病临床表现似肺结核,可形成薄壁空洞,肺门、气管及支气管淋巴结常肿大。眼孢子丝菌病主要累及结膜、泪囊等,多为原发性感染,局部淋巴结常无明显肿大。骨、骨膜及滑膜孢子丝菌病常引起残毁性关节炎,表现为关节肿痛变形及运动受限。孢子丝菌性脑膜炎极少见,当其发生时,脑脊液中蛋白和细胞明显增多,培养可找到申克孢子丝菌。

② Disseminated type: disseminated sporotrichosis always occurs in immunocompromised patients, diabetics, patients on long-term glucocorticoids and/or broad-spectrum antibiotic therapies, or those on cytotoxic therapy or radiotherapy. The clinical manifestations show disseminated subcutaneous nodules and internal involvement could also occur due to hematogenous dissemination, such as the kidneys, testicles, breasts, liver, spleen, thyroid, myocardium, etc. The constitutional symptoms include high fever and weight loss.

②播散型:多发生于免疫功能低下患者,糖尿病患者,长期使用糖皮质激素、广谱抗生素或进行化疗或放疗的患者。表现为全身播散性皮下结节,也可通过血行播散至肾、睾丸、乳腺、肝、脾、甲状腺、心肌等,引起相应症状。患者常有高热、体重减轻等全身症状。

【Laboratory Findings】

(1) Fungal culture: the samples for culture may be taken from pus, sputum or lesion scrapings. The inoculations should be cultured at 37 ℃ and at room temperature respectively. The characteristics of colonies at different temperatures and the morphology under microscopy will be important in identifying the species.

【实验室检查】

(1) 真菌培养　取脓液、痰、皮损刮取物等分别在室温和 37 ℃进行培养,可见菌落生长。根据不同温度培养下的菌落形态和镜下特征可以鉴定。

(2) Histopathological examination: the histopathological changes resemble an infectious granuloma. Asteroid bodies and cigar-shaped, round or oval spores may be found.

(2) 组织病理检查　表现为感染性肉芽肿性病变,可出现星状体。皮损中可见呈圆形、卵圆形或雪茄样的孢子。

【Diagnosis and Differential Diagnosis】

Diagnosis should be made according to the typical manifestations, positive fungal culture and spores found in the histopathological examination. Sporotrichosis should be differentiated from primary coccidioidomycosis, swimming pool granuloma, tuberculosis, syphilis, mycetoma, and pyoderma. Fungal culture and histopathological examination are helpful for differentiation.

【诊断与鉴别诊断】

根据典型临床表现、真菌培养阳性及组织病理检查发现孢子可明确诊断。需要与原发性皮肤球孢子菌病、游泳池肉芽肿、结核、梅毒、足菌肿、脓皮病等相鉴别。真菌培养和组织病理检查找到孢子可帮助鉴别。

【Treatment】

(1) Systemic therapy: 10% potassium iodide solution is the first line agent to treat mucocutaneous sporotrichosis. The usual dosage is 10 mL thrice daily. Itraconazole 100-200 mg daily or terbinafine 250 mg daily can be an effective alternative for patients allergic to or unresponsive to potassium iodide, or for those who have tuberculosis. The treatment should be continued for 3-6 months or at least 1 month after the lesions disappear. Potassium iodide is not effective for extracutaneous or disseminated sporotrichosis, which should be treated by amphotericin B in acute phase and followed by maintenance therapy with itraconazole.

(2) Miscellaneous therapies: local thermotherapy lasting for 30 minutes 2-4 times daily can be applied to isolated lesions. Surgery can be combined with medications in extracutaneous sporotrichosis.

【治疗】

(1) 系统治疗　皮肤黏膜型孢子丝菌病首选碘化钾治疗。一般采用10%碘化钾液,每次10 mL,每天3次。对碘化钾过敏、无效或有肺结核的患者,可采用伊曲康唑治疗,每日100～200 mg,连服3～6个月。也可采用特比萘芬250 mg/d,连续3～6个月。治疗应持续至皮损全部消退后至少1个月。皮肤外型和播散型孢子丝菌病碘化钾治疗无效,急性期可采用两性霉素B治疗,当病情改善后以伊曲康唑维持治疗。

(2) 其他治疗　局部温热治疗,适用于皮损数目少者,每日2～4次,每次30 min。皮肤外型孢子丝菌病在使用口服药物同时,必要时可行手术清创。

Section Nine　Chromoblastomycosis

Chromoblastomycosis is a fungal infection of skin and subcutaneous tissue caused by dematiaceous fungi.

第九节　着色芽生菌病

着色芽生菌病(chromoblastomycosis)是由暗色孢科真菌引起的皮肤和皮下组织局限性的感染。

【Etiology and Pathogenesis】

Chromoblastomycosis is caused by dematiaceous fungi. The most common causative agents are *Cladosporium carrionii*, *Fonsecaea compacta*, *Fonsecaea pedrosoi*, *Phialophora verrucosa*, *Rhinocladiella cerophilum*. The causative agents enter the skin and mucosa through wounds and lead to infections. Direct transmission from person to person never occurs.

【病因及发病机制】

着色芽生菌病主要由5种暗色孢科真菌引起,分别为卡氏枝孢霉、紧密着色真菌、裴氏着色真菌、疣状瓶霉和喙枝孢霉。致病菌通过伤口进入皮肤或黏膜而感染,人与人之间不直接传染。

【Clinical Manifestations】

Chromoblastomycosis usually affects the legs, feet or forearms. It begins as a small papule or nodule without obvious itching, and then it slowly spreads by the growth of satellite lesions, and which in turn finally coalesce to form tumorous or plaque-like lesions with verrucous hyperplasia. The color becomes dark brown. Ulceration usually occurs as well and is always covered by dark brown crusts. Some pus may ooze out by squeezing. The

【临床表现】

病变好发于小腿、足和前臂,初起为丘疹或小结节,无明显痒感。以后皮损缓慢扩大,周围出现卫星病灶并融合成肿瘤样或斑块状,表面疣状增生,呈污褐色,常有溃疡并结褐色痂,压之有少量脓液。皮损表面常有黑点,边缘清楚,周围皮肤呈暗红色或紫色浸润。陈旧性损害

lesion has a clear boundary and the skin around it appears dark red or purple due to inflammatory infiltration. Some black dots may appear on the surface. Healing with atrophy or hyperplastic scarring will take place at the center while the infection continues to spread peripherally at the edges. Some lesions can spread along the draining lymphantics and may ultimately lead to elephantiasis as seen in sporotrichosis or other deformity as the course is persistent and chronic(Fig. 7-24).

中央可自愈，遗留萎缩或肥厚性瘢痕，边缘可向四周扩展。损害可沿淋巴管播散，如孢子丝菌病样，病程慢性迁延，可引起象皮肿和畸形(图 7-24)。

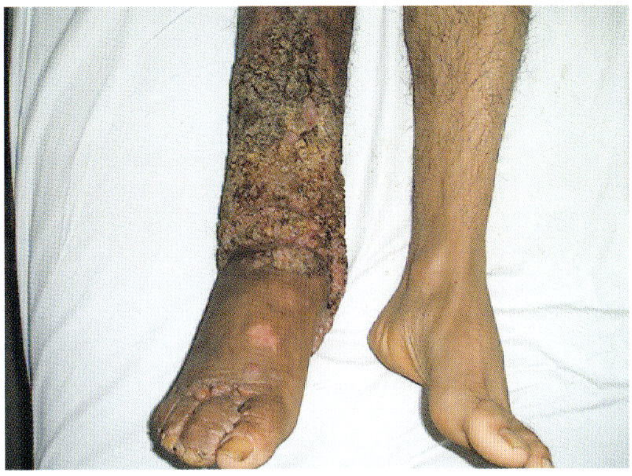

Fig. 7-24　Chromoblastomycosis(图 7-24　着色芽生菌病)

【Laboratory Findings】

(1) Direct microscopic examination: brown hyphae and/or brown septate, spherical spores with thick dark walls can be found by direct microscopic examination of samples of pus and scrapings.

(2) Fungal culture: cultures of pus and scrapings should show black, slowly growing colonies. The colonies and microscopic morphology will vary with different species.

(3) Histopathological examination: the histopathological changes are characterized by a granulomatous reaction. In chromoblastomycosis, the fungi appear single or in clusters of spherical brown septate spores (called sclerotic bodies) with thick cell walls. This is the characteristic tissue morphology of chromoblastomycosis. This morphologic feature differentiates chromoblastomycosis from phaeomycosis.

【实验室检查】

(1) 真菌直接镜检　取脓液、皮损组织刮取物行真菌直接镜检可发现棕色菌丝和/或棕色圆形厚壁分隔孢子。

(2) 真菌培养　取脓液、皮损刮取物进行真菌培养可见生长缓慢的黑色菌落。菌落形态和镜下特征依病原菌不同而不同。

(3) 组织病理检查　呈肉芽肿性改变。着色芽生菌病组织中可见单个或成堆棕色圆形厚壁分隔孢子，称为硬核体，这是着色芽生菌病的特征性改变，并以此与暗色丝孢霉病相鉴别。

【Diagnosis and Differential Diagnosis】

The diagnosis should be made depending on the typical clinical manifestations, direct microscopic finding of brown spores and hyphae, histopathological finding of brown hyphae and sclerotic bodies, and fungal culture with growth of dematiaceous fungi.

Chromoblastomycosis should be differentiated from cutaneous tuberculosis, syphilis, sporotrichosis and blastomycosis. The histopathological and direct microscopic fungal examinations with fungal culture could be of help for differentiation.

【诊断及鉴别诊断】

根据临床表现，真菌直接镜检发现棕色菌丝和孢子，病理检查发现棕色菌丝和硬核体，真菌培养有暗色孢科真菌生长，可明确诊断。

应与皮肤结核、梅毒、孢子丝菌病、芽生菌病等相鉴别。组织病理、真菌镜检和培养可帮助鉴别。

【Treatment】

(1) Systemic therapy: itraconazole 200-600 mg daily is often effective and the treatment should last at least for 6 months. Alternatively, amphotericin B 0.5-1.0 mg/kg daily combined with 5-flucytosin 100-200 mg/kg daily may also be effective and the treatment should be continued for more than 1 month. Potassium iodide can be used as an adjunctive therapy.

(2) Adjunctive therapy: local thermotherapy could be effective for some cases.

(3) Surgery: surgical excision for solitary or small lesions is the best treatment. For more numerous lesions, surgical excision and grafting of the affected areas can be applied, together with oral agents.

【治疗】

(1) 系统治疗　伊曲康唑 200～600 mg/d,疗程至少 6 个月;两性霉素 B 0.5～1.0 mg/(kg・d)与 5-氟胞嘧啶 100～200 mg/(kg・d)联合使用至少 1 个月。碘化钾亦可作为辅助治疗使用。

(2) 辅助治疗　局部热疗对部分病例有效。

(3) 手术治疗　孤立或小的皮损可采用手术彻底切除。对于病变广泛的病例,也可通过手术切除后植皮,并结合口服药物治疗。

Hui CHEN(陈辉), Xing-ping CHEN(陈兴平)

Chapter Eight　Dermatoses Caused by Arthropods and Aquatic Organisms

第八章　节肢动物和水生生物性皮肤病

Section One　Scabies

第一节　疥　　疮

Scabies is a contagious dermatosis caused by *Sarcoptes scabiei* infestation, and is characterized by papules or papulovesicles, burrows, and nodules on the thin and tender sites of the skin accompanied with intense pruritus.

疥疮（scabies）是疥螨寄生人体皮肤引起的接触传染性皮肤病，以皮肤薄嫩部位的丘疹或丘疱疹、隧道和结节，伴剧烈瘙痒为特征。

【Etiology and Pathogenesis】

【病因及发病机制】

The causative *Sarcoptes scabiei* (*S. scabiei*), also known as *Sarcoptes mite*, is categorized into two types: human and animal *S. scabiei*. The former more commonly infests human beings and usually spreads by close skin-to-skin contact with the infested individuals, or by indirect contact with contaminated clothing, beddings, or towels. Scabies is highly contagious and may be endemic in households or in schools.

疥螨又称疥虫，分人型疥螨和动物疥螨。人的疥疮主要由人型疥螨引起，通过密切接触疥疮患者而直接传染，或接触疥螨污染的衣服、被子、毛巾等间接传染。疥疮传染性强，容易在家庭或学校宿舍内相互传染。

The male *S. scabiei* dies soon after mating, whereas the fertilized female mite burrows into the *stratum corneum* to form a tunnel, where she eventually dies after laying 40-50 eggs. Usually, it takes 3-5 days for eggs to hatch into larvae, and another 3-4 days for larvae to become nymphs. The latter finally develops into an adult mite after two cycles of ecdyses (skin-shedding). The cumulative time from a deposited egg to a mature adult mite is around 15 days, but adult mites survive for no more than 2-3 days after leaving the host.

疥螨的雄虫在与雌虫交配后死亡，受精的雌虫钻入皮肤角质层内形成隧道并在隧道内产卵，产卵 40～50 个后死亡。虫卵经 3～5 天发育成幼虫，幼虫经 3～4 天发育成若虫，若虫经两次蜕皮后发育为成虫，从虫卵发育为成虫约需 15 天。但疥螨离开人体后只能存活 2～3 天。

【Clinical Manifestations】

【临床表现】

S. scabiei most commonly affects the thin and delicate sites of the skin such as interdigital webs, the lower abdomen, buttocks, genitalia, underneath the female breasts, antecubital fossae, and axillae, etc. The scalp and face of adults are seldom affected, but the entire body of children may be involved.

疥螨常侵犯皮肤薄嫩部位，如指缝、下腹部、臀部、外生殖器、女性乳房下、肘窝、腋窝等部位。成年人头面部不易受累，而婴幼儿任何部位均可受累。

The characteristic skin lesions of scabies include papules or papulovesicles, burrows, and nodules. Papules or papulovesicles of rice-grain size with a red halo are common on interdigital webs, the lower abdomen, and under female breasts (Fig. 8-1, Fig. 8-2). Burrows are slightly-elevated and grayish-colored straight lines of 2-10 mm in length appearing commonly seen on the finger webs, often with a papule or papulovesicle at its end where the female mite can usually be found. Typical scabietic nodules are brown or red with a diameter of 3-5 mm, often located on the penis and scrotum (Fig. 8-3, Fig. 8-4). Patients with scabies usually have intense pruritus accompanied by heavy scratching particularly at

特征性皮损包括丘疹或丘疱疹、隧道及结节。丘疹或丘疱疹常见于指缝、下腹部、女性乳房下等，米粒大小，周围有红晕（图 8-1，图 8-2）。隧道常见于指缝，呈灰白色线状微隆起损害，长为 2～10 mm，末端常有丘疹或丘疱疹，含有雌疥螨。结节常见于阴茎和阴囊，褐色或红色，直径 3～5 mm，称疥疮结节（图 8-3，图 8-4）。常伴剧烈瘙痒，夜间尤甚。由于搔抓可出现抓痕、血痂、湿疹样变等继发皮损或继发细菌感染。

night, resulting in secondary excoriation, crusting, eczematous lesions, or even bacterial infections.

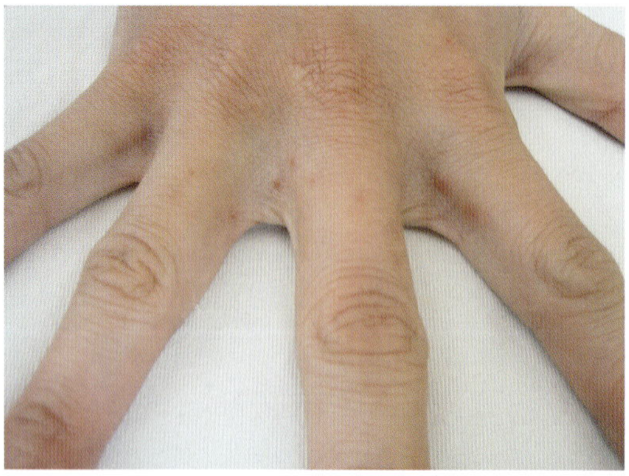

Fig. 8-1　Scabies-papules or papulovesicles on finger webs
(图 8-1　疥疮-指间丘疹或丘疱疹)

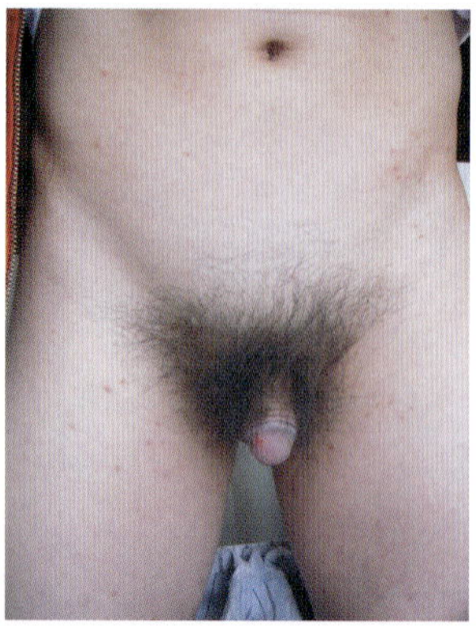

Fig. 8-2　Scabies-papules or papulovesicles in lower abdomen
(图 8-2　疥疮-下腹部丘疹或丘疱疹)

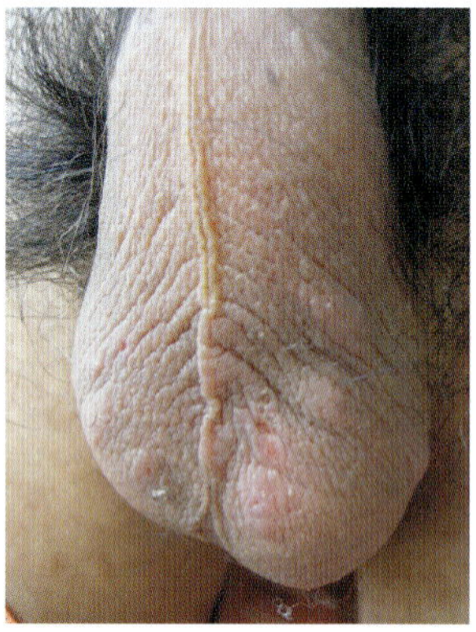

Fig. 8-3　Scabies-nodules on scrotum
(图 8-3　疥疮-阴囊结节)

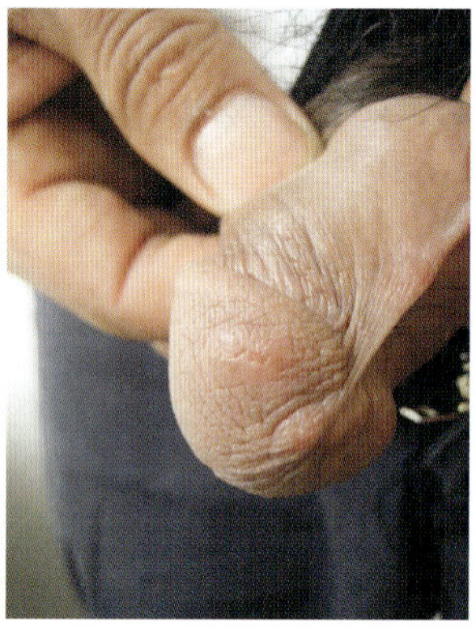

Fig. 8-4　Scabies-nodules on glans
(图 8-4　疥疮-龟头结节)

Crusted scabies (also known as Norwegian scabies) is an unusual type and occurs predominantly in patients with conscious disturbance or malnutrition, and in immunocompromised individuals, who typically present with a large amount of scales, crusts, verrucous hypertrophic plaques, or even erythroderma in severe cases. The crusts contain thousands to millions of *S. scabiei*, and are therefore heavily contagious.

结痂性疥疮(挪威疥)是疥疮的少见类型,主要见于意识障碍、营养不良和免疫抑制患者,表现为全身大量鳞屑、结痂,甚至呈疣状增生斑块,重者呈红皮病改变。痂内含大量疥螨,传染性极强。

【Diagnosis and Differential Diagnosis】

【诊断与鉴别诊断】

Diagnosis of scabies relies on contact history, typical skin lesions, intense pruritus especially at night, and positive findings of *S. scabiei* or its eggs in papulovesicles or tunnels under microscope. It should be differentiated from pediculosis, prurigo, papular urticaria, etc.

根据接触史、典型皮损、夜间剧痒,刮取指缝隧道或丘疱疹的组织液置显微镜下检查发现疥螨或其虫卵即可确诊。需与虱病、痒疹、丘疹性荨麻疹等鉴别。

【Prevention and Treatment】

【预防和治疗】

Close skin-to-skin contact with the infested individuals should be avoided. The patients' clothing and bed linens are recommended to be sterilized with boiling water. Intimate contacts-especially

应避免与患者皮肤接触。患者的衣服和被褥应煮沸消毒。密切接触者(包括家人)应同时接受检查和治疗。

family members-should be inspected simultaneously and treated if infested.

The major therapeutic regimen for scabies is topical scabicides. One of the following scabicides is of choice: 10% sulfur ointment (5% for infants and children) once daily for 5 days, 1% gamma benxene hexachloride (γ-666, lindane) cream twice daily for 2-3 days, or 25% benzyl benzoate emulsion once or twice daily for 2-3 days.

疥疮治疗以外用灭疥药物为主。可选用10%硫软膏(婴幼儿用5%)1次/天,连用5天;1%γ-六氯化苯(γ-666,林旦)乳膏,2次/天,连用2～3天;25%苯甲酸苄酯乳剂,1～2次/天,连用2～3天。

Topical scabicides must be kept over the whole body surface (except the head and face of adults) during the entire procedure of treatment, and should be washed off 24 hours after the last application. A repeated treatment with the same scabicides in a two-week interval is necessary for patients who suffer a recurrent attack. Because γ-666 has neurotoxic properties, the total dosage of 1% γ-666 cream must be no more than 30 g, and children under the age of two, pregnant or breast-feeding women are contraindicated for use of 1% γ-666 cream.

外用药应从颈部以下(儿童应包括头面部)搽遍全身,治疗期间应始终保持皮肤上有药,最后1次用药24 h后将药物洗去。若有复发,可在间隔2周后重复治疗。因γ-666有神经毒性,1% γ-666乳膏总量不超过30 g,2岁以下儿童、孕妇、哺乳期妇女禁用。

For scabietic nodules, topical use or intranodular injection of glucocorticoids, and cryotherapy with liquid nitrogen are effective approaches.

疥疮结节可外用糖皮质激素霜或皮损内注射糖皮质激素治疗,也可采用液氮冷冻治疗。

Oral antihistamines are helpful for alleviating intense pruritus. Antibiotics may be used in cases of secondary bacterial infections. A single dose (200 mg/kg) of ivermectin was reported to be effective for crusted scabies, endemic scabies, scabies resistant to regular therapy, and recurrent scabies.

瘙痒严重者可口服抗组胺药。继发细菌感染时可使用抗生素。伊维菌素200 mg/kg单剂口服对结痂性疥疮、流行性疥疮、常规治疗抵抗的疥疮和反复感染的疥疮有效。

Section Two Paederus Dermatitis

第二节 隐翅虫皮炎

Paederus dermatitis is an acute irritant dermatitis caused by contact with the toxic body fluids of the Paederus beetle.

隐翅虫皮炎(paederus dermatitis)是接触隐翅虫体内毒性体液引起的急性刺激性皮炎。

【Etiology and Pathogenesis】

【病因及发病机制】

The causative agent for paederus dermatitis is *Paederus beetle*, which belongs to paederus genus *Insecta* class and *Coleoptae* order. The adult *Paederus beetle* is 7-10 mm long and 0.5 mm wide, and has a black head, an orange chest, a pair of transparent wings, and two spines on its tail. *Paederus beetles* always lives in moist places like meadows, or under stones. *Paederus beetles* are phototropic; tending to hide in the daytime and fly towards any lights at night. When *Paederus beetles* land on human skin or are accidentally crushed in one's bed, the highly acidic (pH=1-2) toxins from its genital organ flow out to cause an irritant dermatitis in a few hours or within 1-2 days.

隐翅虫属昆虫纲,鞘翅目,其中的毒隐翅虫属引起隐翅虫皮炎。虫体长7～10 mm,宽0.5 mm,头呈黑色,胸呈橘黄色,有1对透明膜翅,附2个尾刺。隐翅虫栖居于草木间或石头下潮湿之处,昼伏夜出,有向光性,夜间常围绕日光灯飞行。若停留于人体皮肤上被打碎或在床上被压碎后,虫体生殖器内一种强酸性(pH=1～2)毒液流出,接触皮肤后可于数小时到1～2天引起皮炎。

【Clinical Manifestations】

Paederus dermatitis is common in summer and autumn, especially in rainy seasons. It occurs predominantly on exposed parts of the body such as the face, neck, and extremities. The typical skin lesion is a patchy or linear edematous erythema with grouped papules, vesicles, or pustules on its top surface (Fig. 8-5), often accompanied with adjacent lymphadenopathy. If eyelids or scrotum are affected, extremely severe swelling may occur. Localized symptoms including burning sensation, pruritus, and pain are common, but systemic symptoms such as fever or dizziness may appear in severe cases. The disease may last for one week, and temporary hyperpigmentation may be left after resolution of the inflammatory skin lesions.

【临床表现】

隐翅虫皮炎好发于夏秋季节,尤以雨季多见。皮损多见于面部、颈部、四肢等暴露部位。典型皮损为线状、斑片状水肿性红斑,其上有密集丘疹、小水疱或脓疱(图 8-5),附近淋巴结常肿大。损害若发生于眼睑或阴囊则肿胀明显。自觉灼热、瘙痒或疼痛,重者出现发热、头晕等全身症状。病程约 1 周。愈后留有暂时性色素沉着。

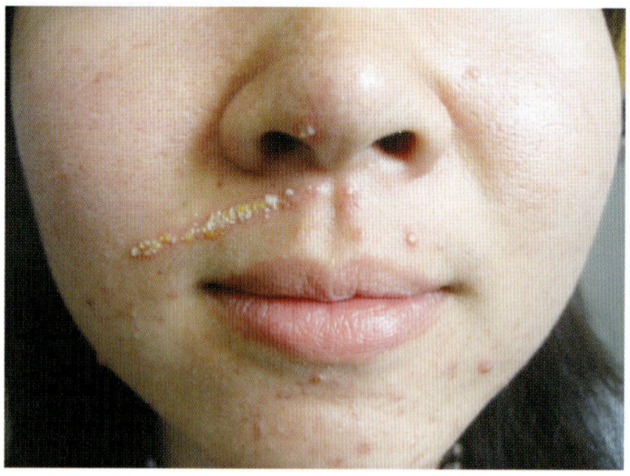

Fig. 8-5　Paederus dermatitis(图 8-5　隐翅虫皮炎)

【Diagnosis and Differential Diagnosis】

Diagnosis of paederus dermatitis is not difficult, given the seasonal incidence, contact history, patchy or linear edematous erythema on exposed parts, as well as the symptoms of pain or itching. It should be differentiated from impetigo or eczema.

【诊断与鉴别诊断】

根据发病季节、隐翅虫接触史、身体暴露部位线状或斑片状水肿性红斑、自觉瘙痒灼痛等特点,诊断不难。需与脓疱疮和湿疹鉴别。

【Prevention and Treatment】

The key approach to prevent from paederus dermatitis is to avoid contact with *Paederus beetle*. Keeping window screens closed at night and sleeping under mosquito nets are practical measures for prevention. If a *Paederus beetle* lands on the skin or bed, try to remove it away by gently prodding rather than crushing it.

In case of contact with the toxic body fluid of the *Paederus beetle*, rinsing the affected skin as early as possible with soap and water is recommended. Topical use of calamine lotion is effective for eliminating skin lesions. With regard to severe swelling, solutions of 1 : 8000 potassium permanganate, 0. 1% rivanol, normal saline, 3% boric acid, or 5% sodium bicarbonate may be chosen for wet dressing. Oral antihistamines are of choice for pruritus relief. Short-term use of glucocorticoids is necessary for

【预防和治疗】

预防的关键在于避免接触隐翅虫,夜间应关好纱窗,睡眠时放下蚊帐。如遇虫体落在皮肤上或床上,轻轻弹去即可,不要打碎或压碎虫体。

如不慎接触到隐翅虫体内毒液,尽早用弱碱性溶液如肥皂水清洗皮肤。外用炉甘石洗剂可使皮损迅速消退,肿胀明显者可选用 1 : 8000 高锰酸钾、0. 1% 依沙丫啶、生理盐水、3% 硼酸、5% 碳酸氢钠等溶液湿敷。口服抗组胺药可减轻瘙痒,重者可短期使用糖皮质激素。继发细菌感染时可使用抗生素。

severe cases. Antibiotics should be used in cases of secondary bacterial infections.

Section Three Pediculosis

Pediculosis is a contagious dermatosis caused by repeated biting and blood sucking of the head louse, body louse, or pubic louse.

【Etiology and Pathogenesis】

The causative louse is an arthropod, which can cling to human skin, hair, or clothes with its claws and lives on blood drawn from its host.

Pediculosis is transmitted by direct skin-to-skin contact or by indirect contact with louse-contaminated clothes or beddings. When the louse pierces human skin and begins sucking blood, it deposits its saliva, digestive juices, or fecal materials into the skin, resulting in pruritus and skin inflammation. In addition, as a disease carrier, the body louse is capable of transmitting diseases such as epidemic typhus, louse-borne relapsing fever, or trench fever, etc.

【Clinical Manifcstations】

(1) Pediculosis capitis: pediculosis capitis (also known as head lice) most frequently affects children. Erythematous macules and papules are usually found at the biting sites on scalp accompanied with intense pruritus. Epidermal exfoliations, bloody crusts, and even serous exudations may develop due to repeated scratching, which sometimes let the hairs glue together and produce a bad smell. Impetigo, furuncle, or adjacent lymphadenopathy may also be present if accompanied by secondary bacterial infections. Head lice are always found on the scalp and hairs. However, the nits which grasp the hair shafts tightly are more commonly seen. At the same time, the affected hairs are always dry and lusterless.

(2) Pediculosis corporis: body lice and their nits reside in the collars, seams, and crotches of clothing. Skin lesions including erythemas, papules, wheals, and scratch marks are often found on the dorsum of the body. Lichenification, hyperpigmentation, or secondary bacterial infections (e. g. , impetigo, furuncle) may follow intense scratching.

(3) Pediculosis pubis: pubic lice often inhabit the pubic hairs but may also affect hairs in the perianal area, the lower abdomen, and the axillae, eyelashes, or eyebrows as well. Pubic lice are generally transmitted by sexual activity. The noticeable skin lesions include papules, petechiae, scratch marks, and bloody crusts usually accompanied by intense pruritus. Secretions or blood-fed pubic lice are often found in or on patient's underwear. Folliculitis or furuncle

第三节 虱 病

虱病(pediculosis)是头虱、体虱、阴虱等寄生人体皮肤反复叮咬、吸血所致的传染性皮肤病。

【病因及发病机制】

虱为节肢动物，利用其足爪抓附于皮肤、毛发或衣物上，并通过吮吸宿主的血液而生存。

虱病通过人与人之间直接接触传染，或接触被虱污染的衣物而间接传染。当虱用口器刺入皮肤吸血时，其唾液、排泄物等注入皮肤可引起瘙痒和皮肤炎症。体虱还可传播斑疹伤寒、回归热、战壕热等疾病。

【临床表现】

(1) 头虱病(pediculosis capitis) 主要累及儿童。头虱叮咬处皮肤可见红斑、丘疹，伴剧烈瘙痒。反复搔抓后可出现表皮剥蚀、血痂，甚至浆液渗出，使头发粘连，散发出臭味。若继发细菌感染可发生脓疱疮或疖及颈部淋巴结肿大。头皮和头发上常可见虱体，但更常见到发干上黏附虱卵。受累头发干燥、无光泽。

(2) 体虱病(pediculosis corporis) 体虱及其卵主要寄生于内衣衣领、衣缝、裤裆等处。体虱叮咬主要见于背部，叮咬处可见红斑、丘疹、风团、抓痕，剧烈搔抓后可出现苔藓样变、色素沉着，继发细菌感染则出现脓疱疮、疖等。

(3) 阴虱病(pediculosis pubis) 阴虱主要寄生于耻骨部阴毛，也可见于肛周、下腹部、腋下、睫毛、眉弓等处。多由性接触传播。皮损为丘疹、瘀点、抓痕、血痂，伴剧痒。内裤上可粘有虱的排泄物和血渍。剧烈搔抓可继发毛囊炎或疖。皮肤和阴毛上可见阴虱及虱卵紧附

may follow intensive scratching. The pubic lice and/or their nits are often found to attach tightly to pubic skin and hairs (Fig. 8-6), but the nits sometimes cling to the lower parts of hair shaft so tightly that they are difficult to be located.

(图 8-6),有时虱卵抱于毛干下段而不易被发现。

【Diagnosis and Differential Diagnosis】

The diagnosis of pediculosis can be made without much difficulty, given a contact history, characteristic skin lesions, localized pruritus, and observation of the lice (Fig. 8-7) or their nits. The condition should be differentiated from scabies or eczema.

【诊断与鉴别诊断】

根据虱病接触史、皮疹特点和局限性瘙痒诊断不难,若发现虱体(图 8-7)或虱卵即可确诊。需与疥疮和湿疹鉴别。

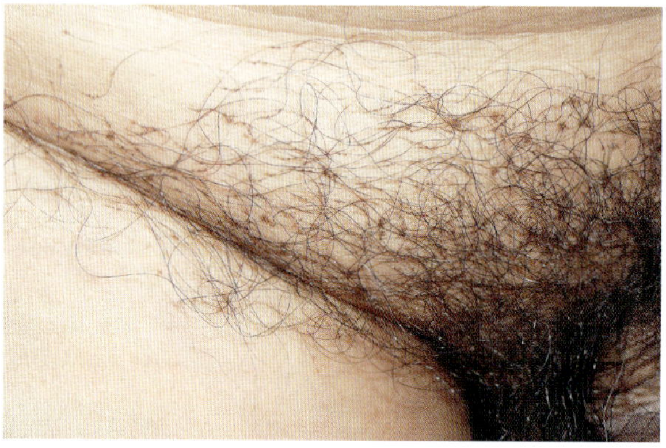

Fig. 8-6 Pediculosis pubis(图 8-6 阴虱)

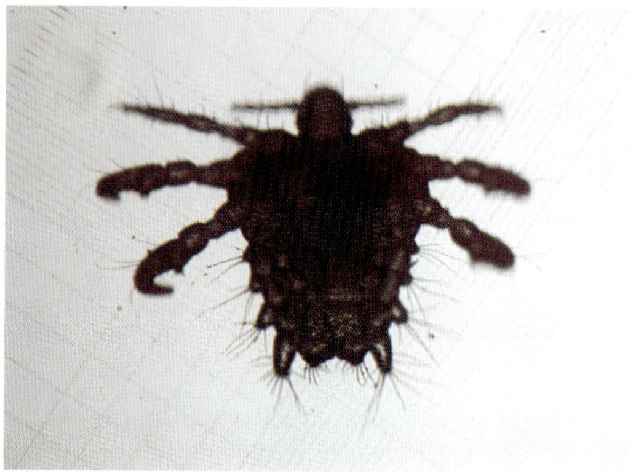

Fig. 8-7 Pediculosis-pubic lice(图 8-7 阴虱-阴虱体)

【Prevention and Treatment】

The first recommendation for treatment of pediculosis capitis is hair shaving. For patients who are unwilling to shave, a double-edged fine-tooth comb is recommended to comb away the lice and their nits followed by topical use of 50% tincture of radix stemona, 25% benzyl benzoate emulsion, or 1% gamma benxene hexachloride (γ-666) cream twice daily for a total of 2 days. The scalp should be cleaned with plenty of hot water and soap on the third day. Alternatively, a 1 : 1 mixture of coal tar and plant oil may be applied to the scalp, and the affected hairs are then rubbed with the hands and wrapped in a towel every night for a total of 3 days. The mixture should finally be washed off with warm water and soap on the fourth day.

For treatment of pediculosis corporis, the patients' clothing and bedding should be disinfected with boiling water or by sun exposure after cleansing. Patients with pediculosis pubis should have their pubic hair shaved off and burnt completely. Then, 10% sulfur ointment, or 1% γ-666 cream emulsion should be used topically to kill the lice and nits. Oral antihistamines are helpful for alleviating pruritus.

All clothing and fomites from patients, such as caps, scarfs, pillowcases, underwear, quilts, or the used combs, must be disinfected with boiling water after the patients have healed.

【预防和治疗】

治疗头虱病时最好先剃头,不愿剃头者可用密篦子将虱体及卵篦尽后,选用 50% 百部酊、25% 苯甲酸苄酯乳剂、1% γ-666 乳膏等外搽,2 次/天,共 2 天,第 3 天用大量热水肥皂洗头。亦可用煤焦油与植物油等量混合后,搽在头皮和头发上用手揉搓均匀,再以毛巾包扎,1 次/晚,连用 3 天,第 4 天用温水肥皂洗头。

治疗体虱病时应将患者用过的衣被等煮沸消毒,不能煮沸的可在烈日下暴晒后洗净再用。治疗阴虱病时应先剃去阴毛,包在纸中焚烧。局部外搽 10% 硫软膏、1% γ-666 乳膏等以杀死虱体和虱卵。口服抗组胺药物可减轻瘙痒症状。

虱病患者治愈后,其用过的物品如帽、头巾、枕套、内衣、浴巾、被褥,以及梳子、篦子等均应用热水烫洗,以消灭虱体和卵。

Section Four　Bee and Wasp Sting

Bee sting refers to the localized and systemic reactions to the injected venom through the stinger of a toxic gland of the honeybee, wasp, or mutillid.

【Etiology and Pathogenesis】

Bees and wasps are *hymenoptera* insects and include many kinds. The causative insects for bee and wasp stings include the honeybee, wasp, scollid, mutillid sphecidae, etc., among which the honeybee sting is the most common. Bees and wasps have stingers on their tails linked to their toxic glands. The stingers penetrate into the skin and inject the venom from their toxic glands into the skin when attacking humans, resulting in localized or systemic reactions. Male honeybees never sting, female honeybees sometimes sting humans, but only in self-defense, whereas the worker honeybees often sting human skin. Worker honeybees have tubular stingers with an inverse clasp on its head top, which are often fractured in penetrating the human skin and often remains in the skin after they leave. Wasps are often social and like to live in nests in forest trees, caves, or under eaves. When humans are near their nests, thousands of wasps may rush out and sting the exposed skin.

The components of venom from the toxic gland differ with the type of bee or wasp. Honeybee venom has two kinds: acid venom from a big secretary gland containing hydrochloric acid, formic acid, etc.; and alkaline venom from a small secretary gland mainly containing neurotoxins. Wasp venom also contains inflammatory mediators, such as histamine, serotonin, bradykinin, or antigenic substance, which have stronger toxicities than those from honeybees and may cause severe systemic allergic reactions.

【Clinical Manifestations】

The initial reactions to bee sting are pruritus, burning sensation, or pain at the sting sites. Erythematous macules, swelling, wheals, even vesicles, bullae, or necrosis may quickly develop at or around the sting sites, always with a petechial punctum on the central top surface of the skin lesions where the remains of the stinger may often be found. If a patient is stung simultaneously by a large number of bees, systemic reactions such as nausea, vomiting, dizziness, headache, or fever are likely to develop. In such severe cases, anaphylactic shock or even death may also occur in minutes if untreated promptly. Delayed serum sickness-like anaphylactic reactions characterized by fever, urticaria, and arthralgia may develop in 7-14 days after being stung.

第四节　蜂　蜇　伤

蜂蜇伤(bee sting)是蜜蜂、黄蜂、蚁蜂等蜇人时将其毒液注入皮肤引起的局部或全身反应。

【病因及发病机制】

蜂为膜翅目昆虫，种类繁多，常见的蜇人蜂有蜜蜂、黄蜂、蚁蜂、土蜂、细腰蜂等，以蜜蜂蜇人最常见。蜂的尾部有毒刺和毒腺相连，蜂蜇人时毒刺刺入皮肤，毒腺中的毒液通过毒刺注入皮肤而致病。蜜蜂的雄蜂不蜇人，雌蜂仅在自卫时蜇人，工蜂的毒刺呈管状，顶端还有倒钩，蜇人后离开时毒刺常折断在皮肤内。黄蜂常巢居在山林树丛、山洞和房檐下，喜群居，当人从其巢穴附近经过时，黄蜂常蜂拥而上蜇伤人暴露皮肤。

蜂的毒液成分随蜂的种类不同而有差异。蜜蜂的毒液有两种：大分泌腺分泌的酸性毒液，主要含盐酸、蚁酸等；小分泌腺分泌的碱性毒液，主要含神经毒。黄蜂的毒液还含有组胺、5-羟色胺、缓激肽等炎症介质和抗原性物质，毒性更强，可引起严重的全身过敏反应。

【临床表现】

人被蜂蜇伤时局部皮肤即感瘙痒或灼痛，迅速出现红肿、风团，重者出现水疱、大疱，甚至组织坏死，蜇伤处中央常有一瘀点，该处常可发现残留的毒刺。若同时多处被蜇伤，可出现恶心、呕吐、眩晕、头痛、发热等全身中毒症状。严重者在数分钟内即引起中毒性休克，救治不及可致死亡。蜂蜇伤后7～14天还可发生血清病样迟发型超敏反应，出现发热、荨麻疹、关节痛等表现。

【Diagnosis and Differential Diagnosis】

Diagnosis of bee stings is not difficult if the patient has a clear history of being stung, given swelling or wheals at or around the sting sites, and the accompanying symptoms. However, it may be confused with mite dermatitis or papular urticaria, especially when the patient cannot confirm a clear history of being stung.

【诊断与鉴别诊断】

根据蜂蜇伤史，蜇伤局部红肿、风团，局部和全身症状等，诊断不难。需与螨皮炎、丘疹性荨麻疹等鉴别，特别是蜇伤史不确定者。

【Treatment】

The broken stingers, if present, should first be pulled out from the affected skin. Topical use of a wet compress with 10% ammonia chloride, 5% sodium bicarbonate (for honeybee stings), or diluted acetic acid (for wasp stings), and even ice packs, can relieve the symptoms.

Oral antihistamines and analgesics may alleviate pruritus and relieve pain. 1% ipecac hydrochloric acid alkali solution (3 mL) or 2% procaine hydrochloride solution (2-4 mL) should be injected perilesionally if the stung area is heavily inflammed or intensely painful. Glucocorticoids should be administered as early as possible in severe cases. Anti-shock approaches must be administered immediately if patients have the symptoms of anaphylactic or toxic shock.

Beekeepers should wear protective masks and gloves before taking honey. Playing with or chasing the flying bees or wasps should be avoided to prevent from defensive stings by the agitated bees or wasps. Wasp nests on trees or under eaves should be removed or annihilated using protective measures.

【治疗】

首先应检查蜂蜇伤处有无折断的毒刺，如发现有，应立即拔除。局部外搽10%氨水或5%碳酸氢钠溶液(蜜蜂蜇伤)、稀醋酸(黄蜂蜇伤)，或以冰袋冷敷，可减轻局部症状。

口服抗组胺药和止痛药可减轻瘙痒和疼痛症状。如蜇伤处疼痛剧烈，可在损害近端或周围皮下注射 1%盐酸吐根碱溶液 3 mL 或 2%盐酸普鲁卡因溶液 2～4 mL。症状严重者，尽早使用糖皮质激素。有过敏性或中毒性休克症状者立即进行抗休克治疗。

养蜂者应在取蜂蜜前戴好防护面罩和手套。发现蜂飞时，切勿嬉戏或追赶，避免激怒蜂而被其蜇伤。发现树上或房檐下有黄蜂巢穴，应在防护措施保护下予以摘除，彻底消灭。

Section Five Microbasic Dermatitis

Microbasic dermatitis, also known as jellyfish dermatitis or medusa dermatitis, is an acute skin inflammation caused by contact with the nematocysts of jellyfish, sea anemones, or coral. Severe systemic reactions to nematocystic toxins may appear in severe cases. As the names indicate here, jellyfish dermatitis is only one type of microbasic dermatitis.

第五节 刺胞皮炎

刺胞皮炎(microbasic dermatitis)，旧称海蜇皮炎或水母皮炎，是由海蜇、海葵、珊瑚等含刺胞动物的刺胞刺蜇皮肤引起的急性炎症，重者有严重的全身反应。海蜇皮炎是刺胞皮炎中的一种。

【Etiology and Pathogenesis】

The nematocystic animals, formerly known as coelenterates, are divided into the medusa class, leech class, and coral class, most of which live in the sea. Jellyfish is a term for hundreds of kinds of medusa, which grow into their mature form from June to October every year. They look like umbrellas when floating in water. A jellyfish has 8 tentacles; each of them bears a large number of tight clusters of nematocysts on its surface. Once a jellyfish's tentacles contact with human skin, its nematocyst ejects and penetrates into human skin to release a large amount of toxic fluid. This toxic fluid

【病因及发病机制】

刺胞动物，旧称腔肠动物，分为水母纲、水蛭纲和珊瑚纲，绝大多数生活在海中。海蜇是数百种水母的通称，每年 6—10 月份成熟，呈伞形浮于水面。海蜇有 8 个触手，每一触手上都有密集的刺胞。当触及人皮肤时，刺胞弹开，将刺丝刺入皮肤并注入大量毒液。毒液内所含类蛋白、肽类、组胺、5-羟色胺、致痛剂等物质引起局部或全身反应。

consists of proteinoids, peptides, histamines, 5-hydroxy tryptamine, algogenic substances, etc., which cause local or systemic toxic reactions.

【Clinical Manifestations】

Microbasic dermatitis is most common in summer and autumn, and mainly occurs in fishermen, aquaculture workers, seawater swimmers and divers, or individuals who contact with broken pieces of nematocystic animals at the beach. The patient often has a history of being stung by nematocystic animals such as jellyfish while fishing, swimming or diving in the sea, or wading alongside the beach.

After being stung by a nematocystic animal, a sharp pain may occur immediately, and pruritus or a burning sensation may develop in several minutes. Erythema, papules, wheals, petechia, or ecchymosis appear quickly on the sting sites; some of the papules are soon converted into vesicles or bullae. Since the tentacles of the jellyfish are string-like, the skin lesions are likely present in forms of linear, striped, or even lash-like marks. If the patient is stung simultaneously by several tentacles, the skin lesions may have a "map-like" appearance. The patients often have intense pruritus. Usually, the skin lesions begin to regress in 2-3 days and resolve completely in 1-2 weeks.

When the patient is stung by extremely toxic nematocystic animals or by nematocystic animals at multiple body sites, severe systemic reactions including discomfort, nausea, vomiting, muscular pain, hypotension, or even anaphylactic shock may occur. These may quickly lead to death if left untreated.

【Diagnosis and Differential Diagnosis】

The seasonal onset, a history of being stung by nematocystic animals, and characteristic skin lesions with accompanying symptoms provide the necessary diagnostic clues in most cases.

【Prevention and Treatment】

In general, contact with nematocystic animals should be avoided. The nematocysts attached to the skin should be scraped away as quick as possible, and the affected area should be washed immediately with sea water.

A cold wet compress with saturated alum solution, 1% ammonia chloride, or 10% sodium bicarbonate should be applied onto the affected areas. Oral antihistamines and intravenous injection of 10% calcium gluconate solution are useful in alleviating symptoms. In severe cases with symptoms of anaphylactic shock such as low blood pressure, antishock medications must be administered immediately. Direct contact with nematocystic animals

【临床表现】

多见于夏秋季。渔民、养殖场工人、海水浴者和潜水者好发，海边淌水者可因接触刺胞动物碎片污染的海水而发病，患者常有下海捕捞或游泳时被海蜇等刺胞动物蜇伤史。

皮肤被刺伤时有锐痛感，数分钟后即有痒痛、麻痛，或烧灼感。蜇伤局部皮肤出现红斑、丘疹、风团、瘀点和瘀斑，有的丘疹很快变成水疱或大疱。因海蜇触手呈长条形，皮疹亦多呈条状或线状，甚至形如鞭打痕迹。若同时接触多个触手，则皮疹可呈特殊的地图形，常伴有剧痒。皮疹在2～3天开始消退，经1～2周痊愈。

如果多处被蜇，或被毒性较强的刺胞动物严重蜇伤，则可引起全身不适、恶心、呕吐、肌肉疼痛，甚至血压下降，发生中毒性或过敏性休克。如不及时抢救，可导致死亡。

【诊断与鉴别诊断】

根据发病季节、与刺胞动物接触史、特殊形态的皮疹及伴随症状，一般容易诊断。

【预防和治疗】

应尽量避免接触刺胞动物。接触刺胞动物后应尽快粘去皮肤表面的刺胞，并立即用海水冲洗。

蜇伤局部选用饱和明矾、1%氨水、10%碳酸氢钠等溶液冷湿敷。内服抗组胺药物、静脉推注10%葡萄糖酸钙溶液等可减轻症状。有血压下降等休克症状者，应立即进行抗休克治疗。下海捕捞或游泳时，切勿直接用手接触海蜇等刺胞动物。

while fishing or swimming should be avoided.

Section Six Papular Urticaria

Papular urticaria, also known as acute prurigo simplex, is an allergic dermatosis commonly affecting children. It is characterized by urticaria-like red edematous papules accompanied with intense pruritus.

【Etiology and Pathogenesis】

Papular urticaria is an allergic reaction of sensitive individuals to insect bites. The common causative insects include mosquitoes, fleas, mites, and bugs. However, gastrointestinal disturbances, food intolerance, and environmental changes may trigger this condition as well.

【Clinical Manifestations】

Papular urticaria is most commonly seen in spring and autumn, and mainly affects young children. The skin lesions of papular urticaria are often sparsely distributed on the exposed parts of the body, e. g. , the trunk and extremities. The typical skin lesions are spindle-shaped urticaria-like edematous papules of mungbean to soybean size, sometimes with a vesicle on its central top surface (Fig. 8-8), and always accompanied with intense pruritus. Erosion and crust formation may follow persistent scratching. With secondary bacterial infections, e. g. , folliculitis and impetigo, the patient may have fever and adjacent lymphadenopathy. The skin lesions tend to appear and recess in episodes, with each episode lasting for 3-7 days. After recession, hyperpigmentation or firm papules or nodules may be left.

第六节 丘疹性荨麻疹

丘疹性荨麻疹(papular urticaria),又称急性单纯性痒疹,是儿童常见的一种过敏性皮肤病,以红色风团样丘疹为特征,伴剧烈瘙痒。

【病因及发病机制】

丘疹性荨麻疹系敏感个体被蚊子、跳蚤、螨虫、臭虫等昆虫叮咬引起的过敏反应。此外,胃肠功能紊乱、食物不耐受、环境变化等也可诱发本病。

【临床表现】

多见于春秋季节,儿童好发。皮疹多散在分布于躯干、四肢等暴露部位,典型皮疹为绿豆至黄豆大小的纺锤形红色水肿性风团样丘疹,部分顶端有小水疱(图 8-8),瘙痒明显。搔抓后可出现糜烂、结痂。继发细菌感染时出现毛囊炎、脓疱疮等,伴发热和淋巴结肿大。皮疹常成批发生,每批皮疹持续 3～7 天,消退后留下色素沉着,或质硬丘疹、结节。

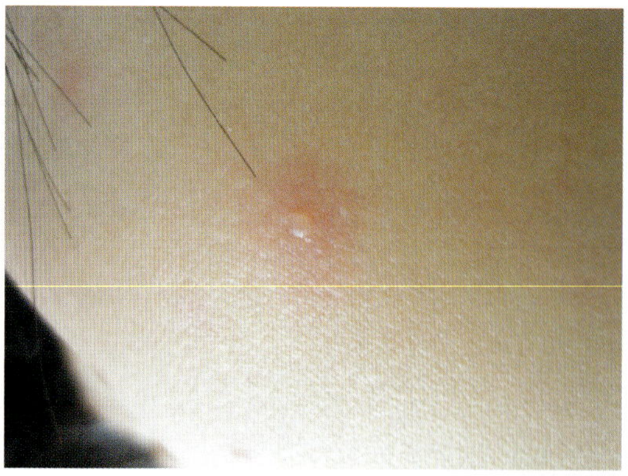

Fig. 8-8 Papular urticaria(图 8-8 丘疹性荨麻疹)

【Diagnosis and Differential Diagnosis】

The seasonal tendency, patient's age, characteristic skin lesions, and accompanied pruritus altogether strongly suggest a diagnosis of papular urticaria. However, this condition sometimes needs to be differentiated from urticaria, varicella, or prurigo.

【诊断与鉴别诊断】

根据好发季节和年龄、特征性皮疹和伴随瘙痒症状,容易诊断。需与荨麻疹、水痘、痒疹等相鉴别。

【Prevention and Treatment】

(1) Prevention: the living environment should be kept clean and hygienic, and contact with insect-infested pets should be avoided. Insecticides should be applied if necessary. Ingestion of potentially allergenic or spoiled food should also be avoided, and gastrointestinal disturbances or intestinal parasite infestations should be treated when they present.

(2) Systemic therapy: oral antihistamines are helpful for relieving intense pruritus. An intravenous injection of 10% calcium gluconate is necessary for patients with widespread skin lesions. Short-term and systemic use of glucocorticoids may be indicated for severe cases. Antibiotics should be used for patients with bacterial infections.

(3) Topical therapy: topical preparations such as 0.5% to 1% menthol-calamine lotion, 2% camphor cream, and glucocorticoid creams are effective for eliminating skin lesions. For erosive or exudated lesions, solutions of 3% boric acid or 0.02% furacilin should be used in moist compresses. Antibiotics (e. g., 2.5% mupirocin ointment, 2% fusidic acid cream) are necessary for secondary bacterial infections.

【预防和治疗】

(1) 预防　搞好环境和居室卫生，避免接触患病宠物，必要时喷洒杀虫剂。避免摄入鱼、虾等易致敏食物和变质食物，治疗肠道疾病和清除肠道寄生虫。

(2) 系统治疗　口服抗组胺药可减轻瘙痒症状，皮疹广泛者静脉注射 10% 葡萄糖酸钙溶液，严重者可短期使用糖皮质激素。伴有细菌感染者使用抗生素。

(3) 外用治疗　可外搽 0.5%～1% 薄荷炉甘石洗剂、2%樟脑霜、糖皮质激素霜等。伴糜烂渗出者以 3% 硼酸、0.02%呋喃西林等溶液湿敷。继发细菌感染时外搽 2.5%莫匹罗星软膏、2%夫西地酸乳膏等。

Guan-qing WANG(王官清), Zhen-ling LU(卢珍玲)

Chapter Nine　Dermatitis and Eczema

第九章　皮炎和湿疹

Section One　Contact Dermatitis

第一节　接触性皮炎

Contact dermatitis is an inflammatory reaction of the skin resulting from direct contact with certain external substances. It presents with erythemas, swelling, papules, vesicles, and even bullae.

接触性皮炎(contact dermatitis)是接触外源性物质后导致的皮肤炎症性反应，表现为红斑、肿胀、丘疹、水疱，甚至大疱。

【Etiology and Pathogenesis】

【病因及发病机制】

Contact dermatitis can be divided into two categories according to the etiology: irritant contact dermatitis (ICD) and allergic contact dermatitis (ACD).

接触性皮炎根据发生的原因，可以分为刺激性接触性皮炎和变态反应性接触性皮炎两种。

(1) ICD: accounts for the majority of contact dermatitis cases. The skin lesions are caused by the direct effect of an irritant on the skin, which presumably would affect anybody under similar circumstances.

(1) 刺激性接触性皮炎　占接触性皮炎的大多数，由接触物直接刺激引起。如果暴露充分，任何人接触后均可以发生。

(2) ACD: the causative substances are less irritating in general, and the condition only occurs in specific individuals who are allergic to these substances.

(2) 变态反应性接触性皮炎　此型皮炎的接触物质往往不具有强烈刺激性，仅仅是有过敏素质的人接触该物质方能发病。

【Clinical Manifestations】

【临床表现】

The dermatitis is generally confined to the site of exposure, but it may spread beyond the exposed area, and may even become generalized in severe cases. The clinical manifestations vary according to the specific chemical or agent, the concentration of the irritants, the manner of contact, and the individual's sensitivity. Acute contact dermatitis may present with erythema, edema, bullae, and even necrosis, with intense burning and stinging sensations (Fig. 9-1). However, in cases of chronic contact dermatitis, hyperkeratosis, lichenification, and fissures are more likely.

皮炎一般发生在和变应原接触的部位。但是，严重患者皮损可能会超出接触范围甚至泛发。临床表现根据接触物的性质、浓度、接触方式和个人反应性的不同而表现多样。急性接触性皮炎表现为红斑、水肿、大疱和坏死，伴烧灼和刺痛感(图 9-1)。若为慢性接触性皮炎，则主要表现为角化过度、苔藓化和皲裂形成。

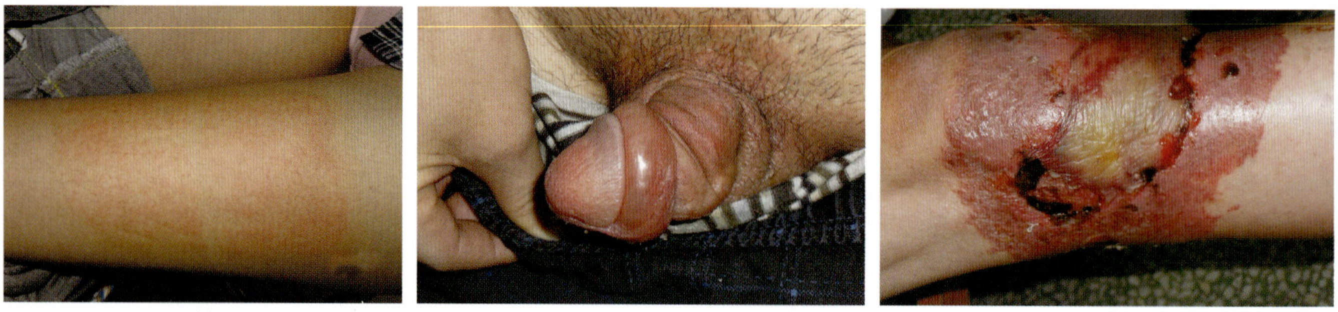

(a)　(b)　(c)

Fig. 9-1　Contact dermatitis(图 9-1　接触性皮炎)

【Diagnosis and Differential Diagnosis】

The diagnosis is based on clinical presentation and a history of exposure to the suspected irritant(s). Patch testing is performed to diagnose allergic contact dermatitis. Contact dermatitis should be differentiated from a number of dermatoses including atopic dermatitis, as well as dyshidrotic eczema, palmar psoriasis, tinea manus and pedis, and erythema multiforme, etc.

【诊断与鉴别诊断】

根据致敏物接触史和临床检查可确诊。斑贴试验可用来协助诊断变态反应性接触性皮炎。需与特应性皮炎、汗疱疹、手掌银屑病、手足癣和多形红斑等相鉴别。

【Treatment】

It is important to identify and avoid the substances that are the cause of the dermatitis. If contact is not completely avoidable, one should wash the skin thoroughly and immediately with cool water after contact to a known allergen or irritant. Treatment usually consists of medications that help with symptomatic improvement and healing of any rash. Glucocorticoids and antihistamines are the most commonly used medications for contact dermatitis. Topical drugs should be prescribed according to the type and location of the rash. In the acute stage, calamine lotion should be applied for redness and swelling, along with 3% boric acid solution for any exudative lesions. In the subacute stage, corticosteroid creams or zinc oxide oil is appropriate for less exudative eruptions, while corticosteroid cream is recommended for any rash without exudation. In the chronic stage, anti-inflammatory ointments are preferred for the lesions.

【治疗】

首要的是要确定和避免再接触致敏物。如果接触了已知的过敏原或者刺激物后，要立刻用冷水冲洗。药物治疗主要是缓解症状，加快皮损消退。糖皮质激素和抗组胺药是最常用的药物。外用药可以根据皮损的性质和部位选用不同的剂型。急性期红肿明显时选用炉甘石洗剂，渗出较多时选用 3% 硼酸溶液湿敷；亚急性期有少量渗出时选用糖皮质激素霜剂或氧化锌油，无渗出时选用糖皮质激素霜剂；慢性期宜选用具有抗炎作用的软膏。

【Specific Type of Contact Dermatitis】

(1) Cosmetic dermatitis: an inflammation of the skin occurring on areas that have been exposed to cosmetics. It manifests as erythema, papules, papulovesicles, even vesicles or bullae in severe cases, appearing in an area previously exposed to the cosmetic substance (often an area on the face), accompanied by a stinging or burning sensation. The lesions are usually well demarcated. When a medical history is taken, any use of cosmetics (e. g., type and duration) and details of daily activities should be included. The physician should also carefully examine the site, extent, morphology, and pattern of lesions, which in turn may help to determine the type of cosmetics that have been used. Definitive diagnosis necessitates the use of patch testing to determine the source of the allergy. Once the likely causative cosmetic agent has been determined, the patient should avoid subsequent contact with that substance and others that may carry the same allergen. Topical treatment with glucocorticoid ointments, lotions, or creams is helpful in most cases. Systemic treatment with antihistamines can be chosen, and glucocorticoids may be required for severe cases.

【特殊类型的接触性皮炎】

(1) 化妆品皮炎　由化妆品引起的皮肤炎症。表现为接触部位红斑，丘疹，丘疱疹，严重者可出现水疱、大疱，常边界清楚，大多发生于颜面部，自觉针刺感或烧灼感。诊断需仔细询问化妆品的使用种类和时间及日常活动等情况，仔细检查受累位置、程度、皮损形态和类型，常有助于分辨出使用的化妆品种类。斑贴试验可以协助诊断化妆品皮炎。治疗主要是立即停止使用致敏化妆品。局部治疗包括使用糖皮质激素软膏、洗剂或者霜剂。系统治疗可以用抗组胺药，必要时可以使用糖皮质激素。

(2) Photocontact dermatitis: a delayed-type hypersensitivity

(2) 光接触性皮炎　指皮肤黏膜接

mucocutaneous reaction in response to a photoantigen applied to the skin in subjects previously sensitized to the same substance at the time of UVA exposure. Lesions occur on areas exposed to the sun, and appear as erythema or hyperpigmentation, with eczematous, lichenoid, and lupus erythematosus-like reactions. The avoidance of sunlight or the use of sunscreen agents may be effective in preventing photocontact dermatitis.

触光敏性物质致敏后，再次接触该物质经日光照射而发生的迟发型变态反应性皮肤病。在光暴露部位发生，表现为红斑、色素沉着、湿疹样、苔癣样或红斑狼疮样皮损。患者应避光，外出可用遮光剂。

(3) Systemic contact dermatitis: an inflammatory skin disease that may occur in persons with contact allergy when they are exposed to a hapten orally, transcutaneously, intravenously, or by inhalation. Lesions are polymorphous appearing as erythema, papules, plaques, vesicles and involving at least two sites, one of which is remote. Systemic therapy should be pursued including oral antihistamine, vitamin C, and 10% calcium gluconate intravenously, and corticosteroid when necessary.

(3) 系统性接触性皮炎　在已具有接触致敏的个体，当半抗原通过口服、透皮、静脉注射或吸入进入机体到达皮肤而发生的一种炎症性皮肤病。表现为红斑、丘疹、斑块、水疱等多形皮疹，两个以上部位发生，且其中一个为远隔部位。治疗应加强系统抗过敏治疗(内服抗组胺药物、维生素C，静脉注射10%葡萄糖酸钙溶液等，必要时系统使用糖皮质激素)。

Section Two　Eczema

第二节　湿　疹

Eczema is the term for a group of inflammatory skin disorders characterized by polymorphous and recurrent eruptions with severe itching.

湿疹(eczema)是指一组皮损多形、瘙痒剧烈、易复发的炎性皮肤病。

【Etiology and Pathogenesis】

The exact cause of eczema is unknown, but it is thought to be an interaction of exogenous and endogenous factors. Exogenous factors such as infections, environment, and climate conditions may affect the development of eczema. Some food may aggravate eczema in some individuals. Endogenous factors, including chronic digestive problems, gastrointestinal dysfunction, insomnia, fatigue, and even emotional changes, can induce and aggravate the eczema. Eczema is an overactive response of the immune system to unknown triggers which are heritable or come from the environment. Eczema is typically classified as a delayed-type hypersensitivity reaction (Type Ⅳ).

【病因及发病机制】

湿疹的确切病因还不是很清楚，涉及各种内外因素的相互作用。外因(如感染、环境、气候条件)可以诱发湿疹。某些食物也可以加重湿疹。内因(如慢性消化系统疾病、胃肠道功能紊乱、失眠、劳累和情绪变化)也可以诱发或加重湿疹。湿疹是免疫系统对未知的刺激因素的一种过度反应，涉及遗传和环境，属于Ⅳ型迟发型超敏反应。

【Clinical Manifestations】

This disease can be divided into three categories according to eruption and the clinical progress: acute, subacute, and chronic eczema.

【临床表现】

根据病程和皮损特点可以分为三种类型：急性、亚急性和慢性湿疹。

Acute eczema: abrupt onset, may appear on any part of the body. The skin lesions appear symmetrically and are polymorphic. At first, an erythema appears on the affected area, which later develops into papules, vesicles, erosions, exudation, crusts, etc. The skin rash is often spread over a large area without distinct borders

急性湿疹：起病突然，可以累及任何部位，皮损对称多形，开始时为红斑，然后演变成丘疹、水疱、糜烂、渗出、结痂等。皮损常常融合成片，边界不清(图9-2)。有剧烈瘙痒感。如果得到正确的

(Fig. 9-2). Itching is common and severe. The condition usually improves after 2-3 weeks of proper treatment but tends to recur. After repeated recurrences it tends to become chronic.

治疗，常在 2～3 周内好转，但其容易复发，反复发作者可转为慢性。

Subacute eczema: acute eczema, when not properly treated, is likely to evolve into subacute eczema. The main eruption types of subacute eczema are papules, scales, and crusts, and occasionally vesicles and mild erosions (Fig. 9-3). Patients usually complain of severe pruritus.

亚急性湿疹：急性湿疹如果没有得到恰当的治疗可以转为亚急性湿疹。亚急性湿疹的主要皮损是丘疹、鳞屑和结痂，有少许的水疱和轻度糜烂（图 9-3）。仍然有剧烈瘙痒。

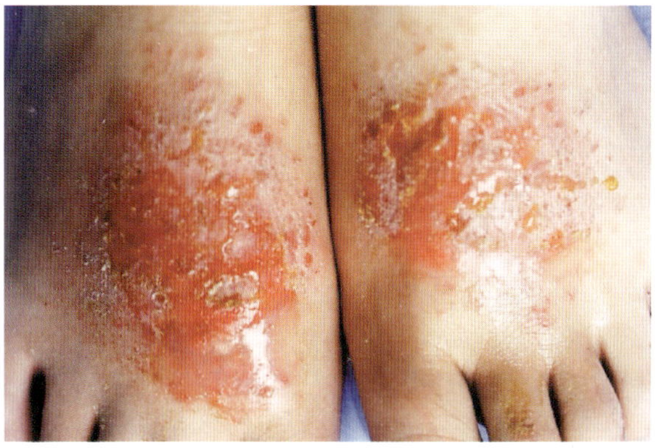

Fig. 9-2　Acute eczema(图 9-2　急性湿疹)

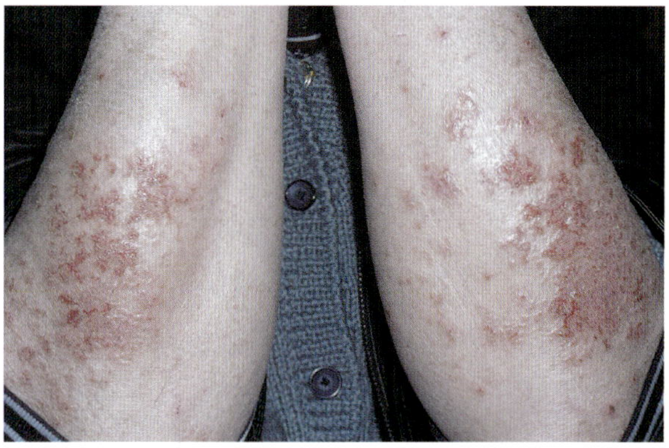

Fig. 9-3　Subacute eczema(图 9-3　亚急性湿疹)

Chronic eczema: chronic eczema usually evolves from acute or subacute eczema, although some cases are chronic from the beginning. The skin of the affected part becomes thick, coarse and hard, often dark red or brown with scales. The borders are more pronounced than in acute cases. Erosions, exudation, or crusts with a limited amount of papules or vesicles can occasionally be found in the surrounding area (Fig. 9-4). Separated episodes of severe itching are common. For a chronic case, eczema may last for months or years in either severe or mild forms from time to time, frequently relapsing into the acute or chronic forms.

慢性湿疹：虽然慢性湿疹可以一开始就表现为慢性，但大多数来源于急性和亚急性湿疹。受累部位的皮肤增厚、粗糙、变硬，呈暗红色或者棕色，常附有鳞屑。边界比急性湿疹清楚。有些皮损偶尔边缘有一些糜烂、渗出、结痂和少量的丘疹或者水疱（图 9-4）。瘙痒呈阵发性。慢性湿疹可以持续数月到数年，临床表现可轻可重，可在急性和慢性之间反复。

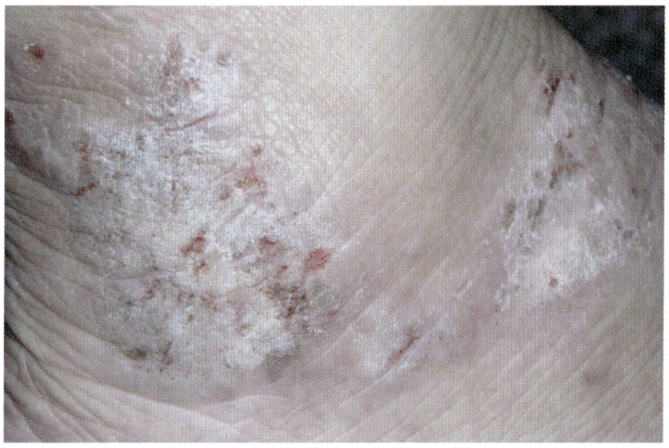

Fig. 9-4　Chronic eczema(图 9-4　慢性湿疹)

【Treatment】

The primary goal for the treatment of eczema is to reduce itching and inflammation, and prevent worsening of the condition.

【治疗】

湿疹的治疗目的是控制瘙痒，减轻炎症和避免恶化。

(1) General management: carefully investigate the patient's work environment, lifestyle, diet, hobbies, and emotional changes, and determine whether an underlying chronic disorder is involved, in order to identify possible triggers for eczema for that individual. Removal or avoidance of the triggers is then a necessary step for eczema control. Exogenous irritants such as hot water, severe scratching, and substances that cause individual sensitivity should also be managed. Among these irritants, foods such as fish, shrimp, strong tea, coffee, or wine should be avoided in allergic patients.

(1) 一般治疗　寻找该病发生的原因,仔细了解患者的工作环境、生活习惯、饮食、嗜好和思想情绪变化,并对全身情况进行全面体检,以明确有无慢性疾病,去除这些致病因素。避免各种外界刺激,如热水、过度搔抓以及其他患者对其敏感的物质。避免各种易致敏的食物,如鱼、虾、浓茶、咖啡、酒类等。

(2) Systemic therapy: antihistamines are effective in managing itching. If necessary, two kinds of antihistamines can be used together or alternately. Since itching often occurs at night, these medications are best administered then. Non-sedating antihistamines (the second generation of antihistamines) are preferred over sedating types. Oral or injected glucocorticoids act quickly to control an outbreak of eczema, but their long-term use is discouraged since the condition is not a life-threatening one and glucocorticoids carry unpleasant and potentially harmful side effects. Antibiotics should be prescribed if an infection occurs.

(2) 系统治疗　抗组胺药能有效地止痒。必要时可以两种抗组胺药联用或者交替使用。因为湿疹瘙痒常发生在晚上,可以在晚上服药。首选第二代抗组胺药物。本病并不危及生命,口服或者注射糖皮质激素虽能很快地控制湿疹的发作,但是因其有潜在的副作用,不能长期使用。如有感染,可以选用抗生素。

(3) Topical therapy: the principles for the treatment of eczema are similar to those of contact dermatitis. Drug selection depends on the exact type of eruption and drug availability. Moist compresses are needed in cases with edema and erythema or erosion and exudation. For subacute eruptions, occlusion with zinc oxide paste can be used. Topical glucocorticoids are always the first line of treatment for moderate and severe forms of eczema.

(3) 局部治疗　治疗原则和接触性皮炎相同,根据不同的皮损和药物剂型用药。如急性湿疹有明显红肿或者渗出糜烂者应该用溶液湿敷。亚急性者可以选用糊剂包敷。局部糖皮质激素制剂治疗对于中到重度的湿疹常是第一线的用药。

Section Three　Atopic Dermatitis

第三节　特应性皮炎

Atopic dermatitis is an itchy, chronically relapsing inflammatory skin condition in individuals with hyper-allergic tendencies.

特应性皮炎(atopic dermatitis, AD)是一种与遗传过敏素质有关的瘙痒性慢性复发性炎症性皮肤病。

【Etiology and Pathogenesis】

【病因及发病机制】

1. Etiology

一、病因

(1) Genetic factors: genetic factors play an important role in atopic dermatitis as other atopic conditions may present in the individual or family members. Through epidemiologic studies, it is noted that the child is at a higher risk for some atopic condition if either one of the parent shows the atopic trait. Recently, studies of genetic links to this spectrum of disease have identified a number of genes that are related to different atopic syndromes. For example, filaggrin mutation can induce atopic dermatitis because of damage to skin barrier function.

(1) 遗传因素　遗传背景在特应性皮炎的发病中起了重要的作用,患者或其家族成员常有先天性"特应性"体质。流行病学研究显示,父母具有特应性体质,则其子女通常具有更高发展成特应性体质的危险性。通过基因连锁研究已证实一些基因与各种"特应性"表现相关联。丝聚蛋白基因突变导致皮肤屏障功能破坏,可诱发本病。

(2) Allergens: various food-derived allergens or even aeroallergens

(2) 变应原　各种吸入或食入的变

can trigger an anaphylactic response when ingested or inhaled by susceptible patients.

(3) Environmental factors: many environmental factors can also influence the clinical course of atopic dermatitis. These include the specific season, psychological factors, sudden changes in temperature or weather, and even occupational factors.

2. Pathogenesis

(1) Allergic mechanisms: one of the assured characteristics of the atopic immune system is its capacity to generate IgE antibodies in response to allergens. The key to determine the course and outcome is the differentiation pathway followed by $CD4^+$ helper T lymphocyte activation. The immune response proceeds as follows: precursor Th0 cells can be differentiated into either Th1 or Th2 cells according to induction by external factors; atopic dendritic cells produce significant amounts of prostaglandin E2 (PGE2), which helps skew T-cell differentiation towards the Th2 phenotype. These Th2 cells 'modulate' or assist B lymphocytes to produce immunoglobulins (Igs), thereby inducing IgE synthesis. Recent advances in pathogenesis of AD emphasize the importance of proinflammatory cytokines such as IL-13.

(2) Non-allergic mechanisms: some non-allergic conditions are also important for atopic dermatitis development such as dysfunction of the blood vessels at the local area, dry skin due to increased transepidermal water loss and decreased water retention, weakness or failure to maintain skin moisture due to the increase or decrease of various lipids at the surface of the skin, or through abnormalities in sweat glands or sebaceous glands.

应原进入体内均可能引起患者皮肤的过敏反应。

(3) 环境因素 许多环境因素均可影响特应性皮炎的临床过程,包括季节、精神因素、温度变化、环境气候的急剧变化、职业等。

二、发病机制

(1) 变态反应性机制 特应性皮炎免疫状态的特征是能够产生针对变应原的 IgE 抗体,而影响此过程的关键在于 $CD4^+$ 辅助性 T 细胞 (Th)的分化路径。在外界因素作用下,Th0 细胞主要分化为 Th1 和 Th2 两种细胞。特应性免疫中的树枝状细胞(DC)可产生明显增多的前列腺素 E2(PGE2),它可以促使 Th0 细胞朝 Th2 表型分化。Th2 细胞能协助 B 细胞产生免疫球蛋白(包括 IgE)。最近研究进展强调前炎症细胞因子(包括白介素-13)在特应性皮炎发病机制中的重要性。

(2) 非变态反应性发病机制 包括血管机能的失调、皮肤经表皮水分丢失增加和水保留降低导致干性皮肤、各种脂质成分的降低或增加而使角质层的保湿作用减弱,以及皮脂腺与汗腺的功能失调。

【Clinical Manifestations】

Atopic dermatitis is an itchy, chronic, relapsing dermatitis that is slightly more common in males than in females. The age of onset is between 2 and 6 months in the majority of cases, but it may start at any age. It is known to occur even earlier than 2 months of age in some cases. Intense itching is a predominant symptom of atopic dermatitis. The features and distribution of the eruptions vary with age. There are three phases for this disease: the infantile phase, the childhood phase and the adolescent and adult phase.

Infantile phase: this phase is also known as infantile eczema. The age of onset is around 2 to 3 months. The lesions most frequently start on the face, particularly on the cheeks, forehead, or scalp, but may occur elsewhere on the body, such as the trunk and limbs. The lesions consist of intensely itchy erythema and discrete or confluent edematous plaques, which may become exudative and crusted as a result of rubbing (Fig. 9-5).

【临床表现】

特应性皮炎是一种瘙痒性、慢性、复发性皮炎,男性比女性稍为多见,可发生于任何年龄,但多数发病年龄始于出生后 2～6 个月,也有部分病例在出生后 2 个月内发病。剧痒为本病突出的主观症状。本病在不同的年龄阶段具有不同的特点,通常分为三个阶段:婴儿期、儿童期、青年成人期。

婴儿期:亦称为婴儿湿疹,通常在出生后第二或第三个月开始发生。皮损主要发生在面部,特别是两颊、额及头皮,也可发生于任何部位包括躯干、四肢。皮损主要为红斑和散在或融合的水肿性斑片,伴明显瘙痒,搔抓后可出现渗出及结痂(图 9-5)。

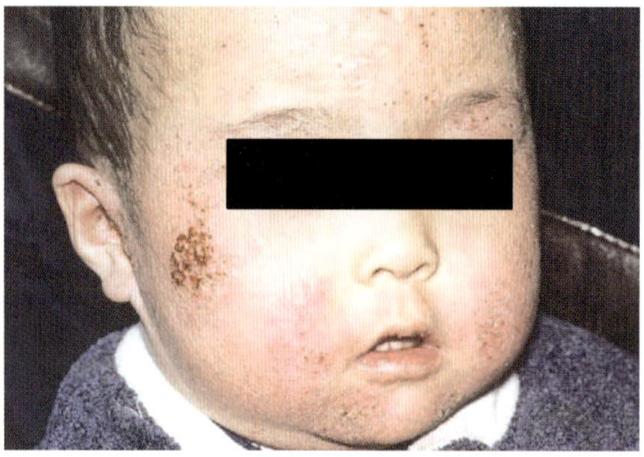

Fig. 9-5　Atopic dermatitis-infantile phase(图 9-5　特应性皮炎-婴儿期)

Childhood phase: lesions become less acute in general upon leaving the infantile stage. Therefore, affected areas are likely to be less exudative, be drier, and have more papules. The lesions often present typically as slightly scaly, infiltrative lichenified plaques. The predilection sites are the antecubital and popliteal fossae, the flexor areas of the wrists, eyelids, face, and the skin around the neck. The lesions tend to appear over non-exposed parts of the body as widely scattered, excoriated papules 2-4 mm in diameter (Fig. 9-6). Pruritus is constant. A chronic, fluctuating course is typical and will continue into adolescence and adulthood in some cases.

儿童期：在儿童期，很少有急性皮损发作，皮损渗出减少趋于干燥，并出现较多的丘疹。典型皮损为有少量鳞屑的浸润性苔藓化斑块，多见于肘前、腘窝、腕屈侧、眼睑、面部及颈部。非暴露部位常见 2～4 mm 孤立的抓破的丘疹散布(图 9-6)。儿童期亦有剧烈瘙痒。病程为慢性、波动性，部分可迁延不愈一直持续至青年成人期。

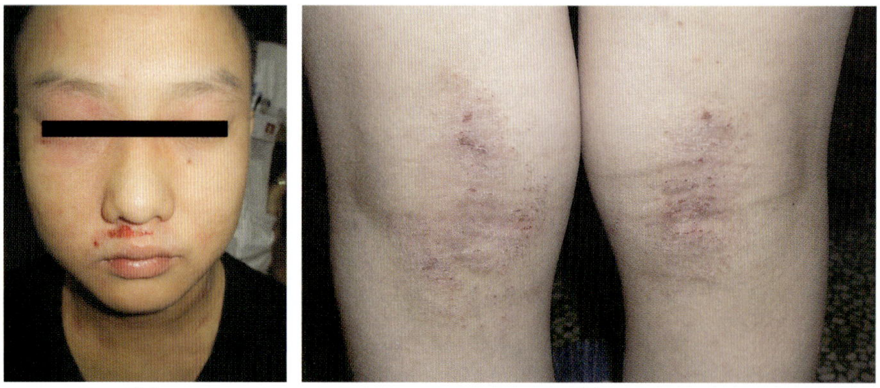

(a)　(b)

Fig. 9-6　Atopic dermatitis-childhood phase(图 9-6　特应性皮炎-儿童期)

Adolescent and adult phase: the clinical manifestation is quite similar to that in late childhood. Localized erythema, papules, and lichenified and infiltrated plaques with gray scales and hyperpigmentation can occur on the elbows, popliteal fossae, front and sides of the neck, face, and the dorsa of the hands. In general, the lesions are found most frequently on the flexor areas (Fig. 9-7).

青年成人期：皮损与儿童期晚期类似，多为局限性干燥红斑或丘疹，融合后皮肤浸润肥厚而呈苔藓样变，覆灰白色鳞屑，或有色素沉着，主要发生在肘、腘窝、颈前及侧部，亦可发生于面、手背等处，皮疹以屈侧为重(图 9-7)。

【Diagnosis and Differential Diagnosis】

【诊断与鉴别诊断】

The diagnosis of atopic dermatitis is usually based on history and clinical findings. Williams' diagnostic criteria are often adopted, in which a severe and current itching symptom or a history of itching recalled by parents in combination with three or more

本病根据病史和临床表现做出诊断。常采用 Williams 的特应性皮炎诊断标准。Williams 的特应性皮炎诊断标准为皮肤瘙痒史(或由其父母提供孩子有

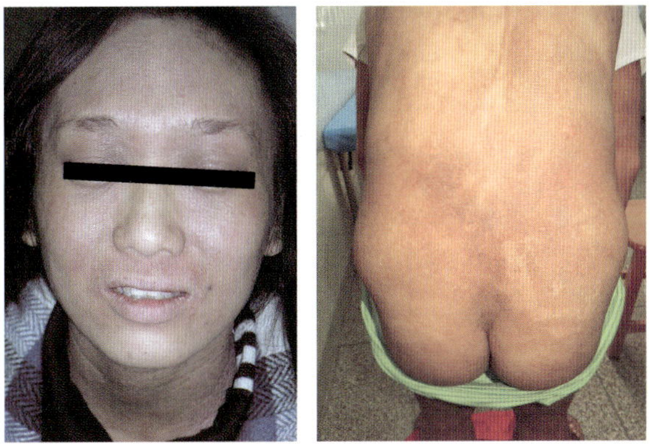

(a)　　(b)

Fig. 9-7　Atopic dermatitis-adolescent and adult phase(图 9-7　特应性皮炎-青年成人期)

items described below is of value for diagnosis: ①a history of skin crease involvement (including cheeks in children under 10 years); ②a history of other atopic diseases such as asthma or hay fever in the same patient or a history of any atopic disease in a first-degree relative in children under 4 years; ③a history of generally dry skin; ④visible flexural dermatitis (or dermatitis of cheeks/forehead and outer aspects of limbs in children under 4 years); ⑤an onset earlier than 2 years old (only applies for children over 4 years old).

Dermatoses resembling atopic dermatitis may be seborrheic dermatitis (especially in infants), irritant and allergic contact dermatitis, nummular eczema, scabies, psoriasis, etc. The infantile phase of atopic dermatitis may need to be differentiated from immunodeficiency syndrome.

【Treatment】

(1) General management: in order to alleviate the clinical symptoms, trigger factors should be avoided. Supportive measures include keeping the patient away from environmental irritants (for example, by wearing soft cotton clothes); avoiding scratching or scraping of the affected areas; avoidance of excessive cleaning; prompt use of moisturizers after bathing; maintaining optimal temperature and humidity indoors; prevention of irritation due to sweating; and avoiding allergens such as house dust, wool, artificial fibers, and fungi. It should be recommended to adjust the diet to limit exposure to possible food allergens.

(2) Systemic therapy: oral agents are sometimes necessary in order to alleviate itching and anaphylaxis. In such cases antihistamines (mainly H1-receptor antagonists) are most commonly used. Different types of antihistamines may be alternatively applied for patients who require long-term therapy, but the use of systemic glucocorticoids should be avoided. Antibiotics can be used for short periods if infections occur.

(3) Topical therapy: the principles of topical therapy are

搔抓史)，加上如下 3 条或 3 条以上条件：①屈侧皮肤受累史(10 岁以下儿童包括颊部)；②个人史中有其他过敏性疾病如哮喘或花粉症，或 4 岁以下儿童的一级亲属中有过敏性疾病病史；③全身皮肤干燥史；④屈侧有湿疹(或 4 岁以下儿童面颊、前额部以及四肢伸侧的湿疹)；⑤2 岁前发病(适用于大于 4 岁者)。

需要鉴别的疾病有脂溢性皮炎(特别是在婴儿期)、刺激性及变应性接触性皮炎、钱币状湿疹、疥疮、银屑病等。婴儿期还需与免疫缺陷综合征相鉴别。

【治疗】

(1) 一般治疗　原则主要是减少本病的激发因素，使症状减轻或缓解。尽量避免各种外界刺激，如穿宽松、纯棉衣服；不要用力搔抓和摩擦；避免过度的皮肤清洗，洗浴后用润肤露；温度及湿度适宜；减少汗液分泌的刺激；尽量减少环境中的变应原，如屋尘、毛、人造纤维、真菌等；注意饮食及消化功能。

(2) 系统治疗　主要为脱敏及止痒。可给予口服抗组胺制剂，主要是 H1 受体拮抗剂，需长期治疗者，可定期更换抗组胺制剂的种类。避免系统应用糖皮质激素。有感染时，可短期应用抗生素。

(3) 局部治疗　原则与湿疹相同。

similar to those for eczema management. In general, oil-or petrolatum-based ointments are preferred for the chronic lesions that are characteristic of atopic dermatitis-particularly when lichenification is prominent-while creams are optimal for treating acute and subacute lesions without exudation. When lesions are exudative, moist compresses are needed first, and cream or ointments will be suitable for the lesions once exudation has been improved or stopped. Regardless of the formulations described above, moisturizers should be included in all treatments. Recently, topical immunomodulatory agents such as 0.03%-0.1% tacrolimus and 1% pimecrolimus ointments have shown some effectiveness against this disease.

慢性皮损特别是苔藓化明显者选用油脂类软膏,急性及亚急性非渗出皮损选用乳膏,渗出明显皮损要先湿敷,待渗出减少或停止后再选用乳膏或软膏。常用保湿剂。近年来,局部免疫调节剂也常被推荐使用,如 0.03%～0.1%他克莫司软膏和 1%吡美莫司软膏。

(4) Immunosupressive drugs: MTX, cyclosporin, mycophenolate mofetil, and azathioprine are also beginning to be prescribed for some severe cases. However, caution is warranted due to the possible side reactions of these drugs.

(4) 免疫抑制剂 对严重病例,可采用甲氨蝶呤、环孢素、霉酚酸酯、硫唑嘌呤等治疗,但应充分权衡利弊。

Section Four Perioral Dermatitis

第四节 口周皮炎

Perioral dermatitis is a chronic papulopustular and eczematous dermatitis affecting the perioral area, chin, nose, nasolabial groove, and even periorbital regions.

口周皮炎(perioral dermatitis)是发生在唇周、颏、鼻、鼻唇沟甚至眼周等处的慢性丘脓疱和湿疹样皮肤病。

【Etiology and Pathogenesis】

The etiology of perioral dermatitis is unknown; however, the overuse of topical glucocorticoids for minor skin problems on the face often precedes manifestation of this disease.

【病因及发病机制】

病因不明。本病发生前常有面部使用糖皮质激素不当的病史。

【Clinical Manifestations】

This disease occurs mostly in young women from 23 to 35 years of age, although a distinct papular variant may occur in children. Typically, small red or pink papules and papulovesicles develop on the skin surrounding the mouth. A clear zone of several millimeters between the vermilion border and the affected skin is commonly seen, which gives a 'ring' appearance around the mouth (Fig. 9-8). Occasionally, the skin around the eyes may also be involved. Mild itching or burning sensation may occur. Perioral dermatitis can persist for months or years.

【临床表现】

本病主要发生在 23～35 岁的年轻女性,也有一部分丘疹型在儿童中出现。典型皮损为口周小的红色或粉红色的丘疹和丘疱疹。在唇红与受累皮肤之间有一数毫米未受累带,看起来像在口周形成"环"(图 9-8)。有时候,眼周皮肤也受累。有轻微痒或烧灼感。可反复发作数月或者数年。

【Diagnosis】

The diagnosis of perioral dermatitis can be made based on the special location and morphological features of the lesions.

【诊断】

根据发病部位和皮损的形态特点可做出诊断。

【Treatment】

An oral antibiotic such as minocycline or tetracycline is often needed for perioral dermatitis. Treatment may need to be continued for several months to prevent recurrence. For milder cases or for pregnant women topical antibiotic creams may also be used. A

【治疗】

治疗口周皮炎常需要口服抗生素(如米诺环素或四环素)。为防止复发,治疗需要持续数月。轻微病例或孕妇可以局部使用抗生素软膏。严重者可短期

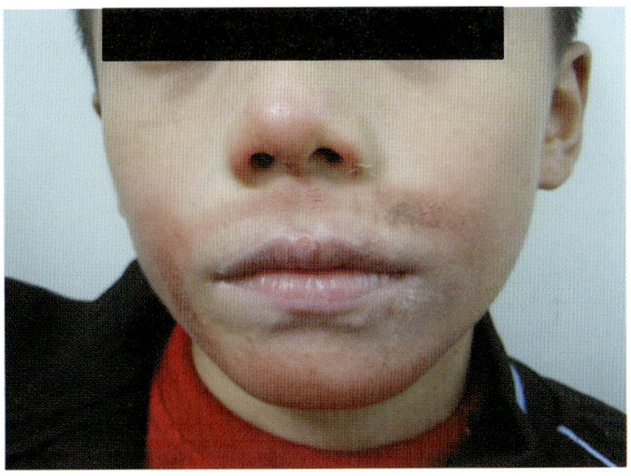

Fig. 9-8　Perioral dermatitis(图 9-8　口周皮炎)

glucocorticoid cream should only be used as a temporary measure in severe cases. Topical tacrolimus or pimecrolimus may also be effective.

应用糖皮质激素霜。他克莫司或吡美莫司局部使用也有效。

Yong-chu HUANG(黄永初),Xing-ping CHEN(陈兴平)

Chapter Ten Urticaria

Urticaria is defined as a localized edema caused by increased vasopermeability of the skin and mucosa.

【Etiology and Pathogenesis】

1) Etiology

The etiology of urticaria is quite complicated. A number of factors listed below have been associated with urticaria development; however, these only account for roughly a quarter of all cases. For the remainder (and especially for most chronic cases), the causes are still not clear.

(1) Medications: almost any medication is capable of causing urticaria. Penicillin is one common example.

(2) Food and additives: the most common causes of urticaria are proteins from animal sources such as fish, shrimp, crab, meat, and eggs; however plant-derived proteins such as nuts and food additives (including food colorings, spices, preservatives, yeast, salicylic acid, and citric acid) also can be triggers for this disease.

(3) Infections: infection caused by viruses, bacteria or parasites.

(4) Insect stings: wasps, hornets or bees.

(5) Physical irritants: include mechanical stimuli, cold, heat, and sunlight.

(6) Emotional and/or endocrine changes: mental stress, emotional instability, menstrual cycles or pregnancy.

(7) Systemic diseases: 7%-9% of systemic lupus erythematosus is accompanied by urticaria. In addition, lymphoma, carcinoma, hyperthyroidism, rheumatic fever, rheumatoid arthritis, and diabetes are all able to cause urticaria.

(8) Heritable factors: heritable urticaria includes hereditary familial urticaria syndrome, familial cold urticaria, familial localized heat urticaria, and erythropoietic porphyria.

2) Pathogenesis

The key mediator of urticaria is histamine, which is released from mast cells in the skin. Along with histamine, other mediators such as leukotrienes, cytokines, and chemokines are also released from these mast cells during degranulation. These mediator chemicals have a variety of effects on tissues: they increase vascular

第十章 荨　麻　疹

荨麻疹(urticaria)是一种由于皮肤、黏膜血管渗透性增加而出现的局限性水肿反应。

【病因及发病机制】

(一) 病因

荨麻疹病因很复杂，约 1/4 的病例与下述因素有关，而 3/4 患者找不到原因，尤其是慢性荨麻疹。

(1) 药物　许多药物能引起本病，尤其是青霉素。

(2) 食物及食物添加剂　动物蛋白，如鱼、虾、蟹、肉类、蛋类；植物性食物，如坚果等；食物中加入的色素、调味品、防腐剂、酵母、水杨酸、柠檬酸等。

(3) 感染　细菌、病毒和寄生虫感染均可引起荨麻疹。

(4) 昆虫叮咬　黄蜂、蜜蜂等昆虫叮咬。

(5) 物理因素　如机械刺激、冷、热、日光等。

(6) 精神因素和/或内分泌改变　精神紧张、感情冲动、月经、妊娠。

(7) 内科疾病　系统性红斑狼疮有 7%～9%的患者有荨麻疹。另外，淋巴瘤、癌肿、甲状腺功能亢进、风湿病和类风湿关节炎、糖尿病等均可以引起荨麻疹。

(8) 遗传因素　包括遗传性家族性荨麻疹综合征、家族性冷荨麻疹、家族性局限性热性荨麻疹、红细胞生成性原卟啉病。

(二) 发病机制

由肥大细胞释放的组胺是荨麻疹发病机制中的关键炎性介质。肥大细胞脱颗粒后释放组胺和其他产物，如白三烯、细胞因子和趋化因子。这些产物引起血管通透性改变，内皮细胞黏附分子上调，

permeability, up-regulate endothelial cell adhesion molecules, provoke leukocyte movement and adhesion, and also enhance chemotaxis and transendothelial migration of leukocytes along the endothelial layer of blood vessels. As a result, a weal-and-flare reaction occurs.

白细胞滚动、吸附、趋化和跨内皮细胞迁移。由此,引起风团的发生。

Triggers that can stimulate mast cell degranulation can be divided into two groups: immunological triggers and non-immunological triggers. With immunological triggers, type Ⅰ hypersensitivity reaction plays an extremely important role in urticaria development, while type Ⅱ and type Ⅲ hypersensitivity reactions often only play a minor role. The non-immunological triggers for urticaria can stimulate mast cells directly. Two good examples of this type of triggers are bacterial toxins and crayfish (when eaten).

刺激肥大细胞脱颗粒的反应可以分为两种:免疫性和非免疫性。与免疫有关的荨麻疹主要是由Ⅰ型变态反应所致,偶尔也涉及Ⅱ型和Ⅲ型变态反应。非免疫性的,如细菌毒素、喇蛄等物质则可以直接刺激肥大细胞脱颗粒。

【Clinical Manifestations】

The skin rashes of urticaria are red, raised wheals that often disappear spontaneously after a short period. Rashes lasting longer than 24 hours are rare. The lesions resolve without scarring; however, the condition is quite apt to recur, even several times (Fig. 10-1). In some cases, urticaria presents only as an angioedema. Severe itching is a common complaint from patients, but some other systemic symptoms such as nausea, vomiting, hypotension, and increased heart rate can also occur in severe cases.

【临床表现】

皮疹为突然发生的红色、隆起的风团,常在短时间内自行消退,很少超过24 h,消退后不留痕迹,但是可以在一定时期内反复发生(图10-1)。少数表现为血管性水肿。患者感瘙痒剧烈。严重病例会出现恶心、呕吐、血压下降和心率加快等表现。

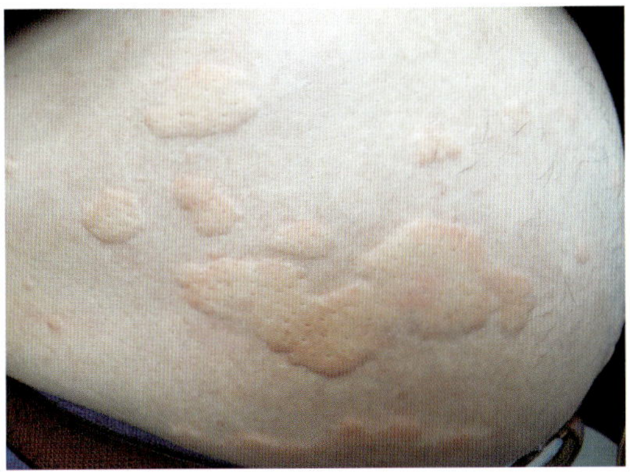

Fig. 10-1 Urticaria(图 10-1 荨麻疹)

Urticaria can be divided according to onset and clinical manifestation into the following groups (Tab. 10-1).

根据发病模式,结合临床表现,荨麻疹可做如下分类(表10-1)。

Tab. 10-1 Classification and definition of urticaria(表 10-1 荨麻疹的分类及定义)

Classification(类别)	Type(类型)	Definition(定义)
spontaneous (自发性)	acute spontaneous urticaria(急性自发性荨麻疹)	spontaneous hives and/or angioedema<6 weeks (自发性风团和/或血管性水肿发作<6周)
	chronic spontaneous urticaria (慢性自发性荨麻疹)	spontaneous hives and/or angioedema≥6 weeks(自发性风团和/或血管性水肿发作≥6周)

续表

Classification(类别)	Type(类型)	Definition(定义)
inducible(诱导性)		
1. physical (1. 物理性)	factitious urticaria (dermographism)(人工荨麻疹(皮肤划痕症))	hives within 1-5 min after pressure(Fig. 10-2)(机械性切力后 1～5 min 内局部形成条状风团,图 10-2)
	cold urticaria(冷性荨麻疹)	hives resulting from contact with cold, wind, liquid, air (遇到冷的物体、风、液体、空气等在接触部位形成风团)
	delayed pressure urticaria (延迟压力性荨麻疹)	hives occurring 30 min to 24 h after pressure is applied to the skin, often persisting for several days (垂直受压后 30 min 至 24 h 局部形成红斑样深在性水肿,可持续数天)
	heat contact urticaria (热接触性荨麻疹)	hives after the skin has been exposed to heat (皮肤受热后形成风团)
	solar urticaria (日光性荨麻疹)	hives within minutes of exposure to ultraviolet or visible light (暴露于紫外线或可见光后形成风团)
	vibratory urticaria or angioedema (振动性荨麻疹或血管性水肿)	redness and swelling several minutes after skin vibration (皮肤被振动刺激后数分钟出现局部发红和肿胀)
2. non-physical (2. 非物理性)	cholinergic urticaria (胆碱能性荨麻疹)	small (2-3 mm) wheals surrounded by an erythematous halo that follows sweating events and elevation in body temperature due to factors such as physical exercise, spicy foods, and emotional strain (皮肤受热刺激比如运动、进食辛辣食物、情绪激动时诱发的直径 2～3 mm 风团,周边有红晕)
	aquagenic urticaria (水源性荨麻疹)	hives resulting from contact with water (接触水后诱发风团)
	contact urticaria (接触性荨麻疹)	hives that occur on the skin after direct contact with an offending substance (皮肤接触一定物质后诱发风团)
	exercise-induced urticaria (运动诱导性荨麻疹)	hives or angioedema induced by exercise accompanied by other anaphylatic symptoms often occur within several minutes to 4 hours of ingesting a specific type of food(运动诱发的风团、血管性水肿,可伴有其他的过敏症状,常在进食某些特异性食物数分钟至 4 小时内发生)

Cited from: Chinese guideline for diagnosis and treatment of urticaria, 2014(摘自:中国荨麻疹诊疗指南,2014 版)

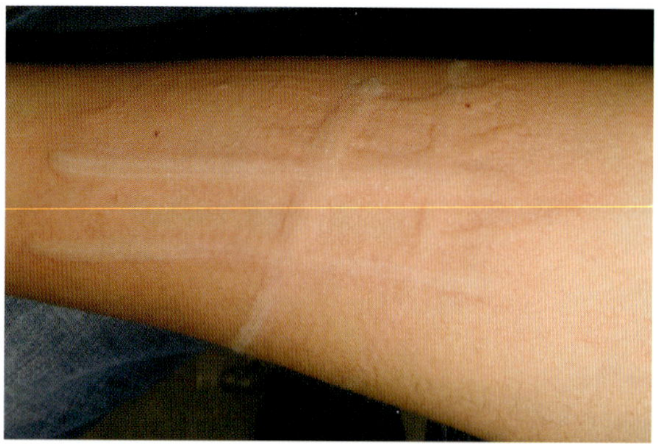

Fig. 10-2　Dermographism(图 10-2　皮肤划痕症)

【Laboratory Findings】

The significance of laboratory tests for urticaria diagnosis is still controversial. Laboratory testing for acute urticaria is not indicated unless some other particular medical conditions are

【实验室检查】

进行实验室检查还存在很大的争议。对急性荨麻疹一般不用实验室检查,除非有线索提示特别的病因。如持

suspected. Evaluation of the complement system, including total complement (CH50), C3, and C4 should be considered for patients with prominent angioedema and for patients with urticarial lesions lasting more than 24 hours. Blood cell count and differentiation should be tested when infection is suspected.

续性血管性水肿和超过 24 h 的荨麻疹，可以检查补体系统，包括总补体(CH50)、C3、C4。怀疑有感染时，可以直接做血细胞计数和分类。

Physical challenge tests can be performed when dermographism is suspected. Selected food exclusion tests can be performed when food allergy is suspected. Light and hot water tests are helpful to diagnose solar urticaria and heat contact urticaria respectively. Inducing high body temperature through exercise or hot water baths may be used to identify cholinergic urticaria.

如果怀疑皮肤划痕症，可以行机械刺激试验。怀疑食物过敏时，可行食物排除试验。光、热水试验可分别用于诊断日光性荨麻疹和热接触性荨麻疹。运动和热水可以诱发胆碱能性荨麻疹。

【Diagnosis】

Diagnosis is rather simple based on history and physical examination but the analysis of the root cause or causes is often difficult.

【诊断】

根据病史和体检，本病诊断容易，但是确定病因常较困难。

【Treatment】

The principles of therapy for urticaria are to avoid the causes and control the symptoms.

(1) Antihistamines: H1 receptor blockers are the first line of therapy for urticaria. They are effective in relieving the pruritus and rash of acute urticaria in most cases. Non-sedating or mildly sedating antihistamines are preferred for urticaria. A 2-to 4-fold increase in the routine dosage is suggested for chronic urticaria if the effect is not satisfactory.

(2) Vitamins: vitamins K and B12 may be useful in some cases of chronic urticaria.

(3) Antibiotics: effective in cases caused by infections.

(4) Epinephrine: the efficacy of epinephrine in acute urticaria is controversial. If angioedema is present with urticaria, 0.3-0.5 mg of epinephrine should be administered intramuscularly.

(5) Glucocorticoids: this group of drugs can stabilize mast cell membranes and inhibit further histamine release. It can also reduce the inflammatory effects of histamine and other mediators; therefore, it is suitable for severe acute or serum sickness urticaria.

(6) Miscellaneous drugs/combinations not included above: several medications are available to reduce permeability of the blood vessels, for example calcium and vitamins C and P in combination with antihistamines.

【治疗】

荨麻疹的治疗原则是去除病因和控制症状。

(1) 抗组胺药　H1 受体拮抗剂是治疗荨麻疹的一线用药。在大多数急性荨麻疹病例，这类药物能有效地缓解瘙痒和皮疹。首选第二代非镇静或低镇静抗组胺药物。慢性荨麻疹疗效不佳时，第二代抗组胺药物可增加到常规剂量的 2～4 倍。

(2) 维生素　维生素 K 和维生素 B12 对某些慢性荨麻疹患者可能有效。

(3) 抗生素　对由感染引起的病例有效。

(4) 肾上腺素　治疗急性荨麻疹尚有争议。如果同时伴有血管性水肿，可以立即肌内注射 0.3～0.5 mg 的肾上腺素。

(5) 糖皮质激素　能稳定肥大细胞膜，抑制进一步的组胺释放。还能减少组胺和其他介质的炎症作用。适用于严重的急性或血清病型荨麻疹。

(6) 其他药物　降低血管通透性的药物，如钙剂、维生素 C 和维生素 P 可与抗组胺剂联合使用。

Yong-chu HUANG(黄永初), Xing-ping CHEN(陈兴平)

Chapter Eleven　Adverse Cutaneous Reactions to Drugs

Adverse cutaneous reactions to drugs, also known as drug eruptions, are one of the most common types of adverse drug reactions (ADRs), and the unwanted or unintended cutaneous or mucocutaneous inflammatory reactions induced by agents via either systemically (typically by ingestion, inhalation, injection, or via suppository), or direct topical application to the surface of the skin. The drugs capable of causing drug eruptions are quite diverse and the clinical appearances vary with the drugs that have been used and the individual's condition when the drugs are administered. Therefore, the severity of this disease ranges from mild to life-threatening, with multiple organ and system involvement in severe cases.

【Etiology】

No single mechanism can fully explain all drug eruptions, but some of the factors that predispose to such conditions are listed below.

(1) Individual factors: theoretically, drug eruptions can develop in any individual. In reality, responses to a particular drug vary widely among the human population. Additionally, the responses to medicines in the case of a single individual can change over time. Factors which may contribute to the development of an adverse drug reaction include genetic factors (idiosyncrasy), certain enzyme deficiencies, underlying immune status, etc.

(2) Drug factors: although any drug may cause drug eruptions, it is true that certain drugs have a known tendency to cause certain types of drug reactions, or are at greater risk to induce drug eruptions than other drugs in the same group. For example, amoxicillin and ampicillin are among the usual suspects for adverse drug reactions, being far more prone to cause drug eruptions than cephalosporins. Drugs that commonly cause drug eruptions include ① antibiotics: semisynthetic penicillins, sulphonamides, cephalosporins, tetracyclines, chloromycetins, etc.; ② antipyretics and analgesics: aspirin, acetaminophen, etc.; ③ sedative hypnotics and antiepileptics: phenylbutazone, phenytoin, carbamazepine, etc.; ④ heterologous serum products and vaccines: antitetanic serum, antivenin, rabies vaccine, etc.; ⑤ some biological products; ⑥ herbal medicines.

(3) Other factors: infections, especially viral infections, play an important role in the onset, progression, exacerbation, and refractoriness of drug eruptions. Human herpes virus 6 (HHV-6)

第十一章　药物的皮肤不良反应

药物的皮肤不良反应也称为药疹(drug eruptions),是药物不良反应(ADRs)中最常见的表现之一,是药物通过口服、吸入、注射、栓剂或外用药吸收等各种途径进入人体后引起的非预期的皮肤或皮肤黏膜的炎症反应。引起皮肤不良反应的药物种类繁多,其临床表现依使用的药物及个体的不同而多种多样,病情轻重不等,严重者可累及多个系统,甚至危及生命。

【病因】

药疹的发生机制较为复杂,下面这些因素均可导致药疹的产生。

(1) 个体因素　理论上讲,任何个体都有可能发生药疹,但是,对某种特定的药物而言,人群中不同个体对药物反应的敏感性差异很大,即使是同一个体在不同时期对药物的敏感性也可不同,其原因包括遗传因素(过敏体质)、某些酶的缺陷、机体免疫状态的影响等。

(2) 药物因素　绝大部分药物都可能导致药疹,但某些类型的药物更倾向于引起某些类型的药疹,或在同一类型的药物中较其他的药物更易引起药疹,如阿莫西林、氨苄西林比头孢菌素类更易引起药疹。临床上易引起药疹的药物有:①抗生素,包括半合成青霉素、磺胺类、头孢霉素类、四环素类、氯霉素类等;②解热镇痛药,如阿司匹林、对乙酰氨基酚等;③镇静催眠药及抗癫痫药,如苯巴比妥、苯妥英钠、卡马西平等;④异种血清制剂及疫苗,如破伤风抗毒素、蛇毒免疫血清、狂犬病疫苗等;⑤生物制剂;⑥中草药。

(3) 其他因素　根据已有文献,感染尤其是病毒感染在药疹的发生、发展、加重以及难以治愈中起重要作用,人类疱

has been linked to drug eruption with eosinophilia and systemic symptoms (DRESS). It has also been noted that HIV patients have an abnormally high risk for drug eruptions.

疹病毒 6(HHV-6)与伴嗜酸性粒细胞增多和系统症状的药疹(DRESS)综合征的发病密切相关。HIV 感染者的高药疹发生已被重视。

【Pathogenesis】

【发病机制】

The pathogenesis of adverse drug reactions is quite complicated, but can be simply divided into hypersensitivity and non-hypersensitivity mechanisms, the former being more common.

药物不良反应的发病机制复杂，可分为超敏反应机制和非超敏反应机制，其中以超敏反应机制占多数。

(1) Hypersensitivity mechanism: the majority of adverse drug reactions are mediated by an immune mechanism. In this group, the immune-mediated drug hypersensitivity to a particular drug depends not only on the drug's molecular properties, but also on the host's metabolic behavior in light of the drug, such as uptake and excretion, genetic background, and medical condition when receiving the drug. In general, drugs with high molecular weights such as serum, vaccine or biological products, are complete antigens that can stimulate an immune response by themselves; however, most drugs used in clinical settings have low molecular weights and act as haptens (partial antigens), which cannot elicit an immune response unless they are attached to a large carrier (such as a protein) to form complete antigens. The substances causing immune-mediated hypersensitivity are not limited to the medication itself, but may also include the drug's various metabolites, excipients (inert ingredients) or even impurities mixed in with the drugs.

(1) 超敏反应机制　多数药物不良反应通过免疫机制介导。一种药物激发超敏反应的能力由多种因素所决定，包括药物的分子特性、药物代谢的个体差异(包括吸收和排泄)、免疫遗传背景及接受药物时个体的状况等。大分子药物(如血清、疫苗及生物制品)本身即为完全抗原，能激发免疫反应，而多数小分子药物属半抗原，本身不能激发免疫反应，需在机体内与蛋白等载体结合为完全抗原后，才能激发超敏反应。引起超敏反应的物质既可以是药物的原形，也可为其降解产物、赋形剂甚至杂质。

Different types of hypersensitivity have been associated with adverse drug reactions. In particular, they have been classified according to symptoms as: type Ⅰ response, which mimics an urticarial reaction; type Ⅱ, which presents as a purpuric reaction; type Ⅲ, which is vasculitis-like and type Ⅳ, similar to exfoliative dermatitis, morbilliform exanthema or eczematous reaction. Some drug eruptions are also due to allergic hypersensitivity modes such as photosensitivity and drug-induced lupus erythematosus syndrome, although the mechanisms are as yet undetermined.

各型超敏反应均可发生于药物不良反应，如Ⅰ型(荨麻疹型反应)、Ⅱ型(紫癜型反应)、Ⅲ型(血管炎型反应)、Ⅳ型(剥脱性皮炎、麻疹型或湿疹型反应)，此外还有一些药物不良反应由未知类型超敏反应介导，如光敏性反应、药物性红斑狼疮综合征等。

The common characteristics of drug eruptions with the hypersensitivity mechanism are listed below.

与超敏反应机制有关的药物的皮肤不良反应具有如下共同的特点。

① There is an incubation period of 4-20 days for a first time user, or within several minutes to 24 hours in cases of a previously exposed and sensitized individual.

①有一定的潜伏期，首次用药一般需 4～20 天出现临床表现，已致敏者再次用药，可在数分钟至 24 h 内发病。

② For any given drug, the eruptions occur only in an idiosyncratic minority of individuals.

②只发生于少数有过敏体质的服药者。

③ The severity of the condition does not correlate with the pharmacodynamic effects, toxicological effects, nor even with the dosage prescribed. Severe drug eruptions can take place in a high

③皮损及病情轻重与药物的药理及毒理作用、剂量无相关性，高敏状态下，即使极小剂量药物也可致严重的药疹。

sensitized individual even at very low doses.

④ The clinical manifestation of drug eruptions vary among individuals for the same drug, and even vary over time for a given patient.

④临床表现复杂，皮损形态各种各样，同一种药物在不同的个体，或一种药物致敏同一患者不同时期可发生不同类型药疹。

⑤Cross-sensitivity and polyvalent sensitivity may sometimes occur during peak stages of hypersensitivity. The former refers to sensitivity to one drug that predisposes an individual to sensitivity to one or more other drugs that are chemically related; the latter refers to circumstances where the individual is sensitive to one or more other drugs that are not chemically related to the "index" or promoter drug.

⑤在高敏状态下可发生交叉过敏及多价过敏现象，前者是指机体被某种药物致敏后，若再用与该种药物化学结构相似或存在共同化学基团的药物也可发生过敏反应；后者是指个体处于高敏状态时，同时对多种化学结构无相似之处的药物发生过敏。

⑥In general, the course of drug eruption is self-limiting and the use of anti-allergic drugs and glucocorticoids is usually effective.

⑥病程有一定的自限性，抗过敏和糖皮质激素治疗常有效。

(2) Non-hypersensitivity mechanism: the common features of drug eruptions with non-hypersensitivity mechanism are listed below.

(2) 非超敏反应机制　这类药疹的共同特点如下。

①Non-immunologic activation of immunological effect pathways: in other words, this type of reaction is activated by a direct response between the drug and certain immunological components rather than by an antigen-antibody reaction. For example, aspirin may cause urticaria by histamine released directly from the mast cells; in a similar way, radiographic contrast agents may induce a skin rash through some complement activation; for another example, skin lesions can be induced by NSAIDs (nonsteroidal anti-inflammatory drugs) that increase the leukotriene level in the skin by inhibiting cyclooxygenase activity.

①免疫效应途径的非免疫活化：这类反应是通过药物与免疫效应成分的直接作用而不需要抗原抗体反应引起。某些药物(如阿司匹林)可直接诱导肥大细胞脱颗粒释放组胺而引起荨麻疹；造影剂则通过激活补体效应途径引起过敏；部分药物(如非甾体类抗炎药)可通过抑制环氧化酶使白三烯水平升高而引起皮损。

②Overdoses and accumulation of drugs: overdoses are common among old people and in patients with renal dysfunction. However, drug eruptions may occur even with a therapeutic dosage in some patients due to some abnormality in regards to drug uptake, metabolism or excretion. Accumulation resulting from delayed excretion and/or long-term use of some drugs therefore may give rise to drug eruptions, as exampled by acneiform lesions induced by potassium iodide after application for a long period.

②过量反应和蓄积作用：过量反应多见于老年人和肾功能不良者，因对药物吸收、代谢、排泄速度存在个体差异，故常规剂量也可出现过量反应；蓄积作用主要见于某些药物排泄缓慢或用药时间过久，如碘化钾长期使用引起的痤疮样皮损。

③Deficiencies or functional inhibition of the enzymes for drug metabolism: the patient with genetic or others defects is unable to produce or maintain the enzymes that are required for drug metabolism; consequently, this will interfere with the normal drug metabolic pathway and rate and increase the likelihood for inducing drug eruptions. For instance, phenytoin hypersensitivity syndrome occurs in individuals with epoxide hydrolase defects.

③药物代谢酶的缺陷或功能抑制：由于遗传因素或其他原因使参与药物代谢的酶缺陷或功能抑制，影响药物的正常代谢途径和速度而诱发药疹，如苯妥英钠超敏反应综合征通常发生在环氧化物水解酶缺陷的个体。

【Clinical Manifestations】

【临床表现】

The clinical presentation of drug eruptions is complicated,

药疹的临床表现复杂，可以以任何

since it may virtually mimic almost any cutaneous disease. The following list is the common types of drug eruptions in clinical practice and intended to reflect the extraordinary diversity of adverse drug reactions which a physician may have to face on some occasions.

皮肤病的形式出现。下面介绍一些常见的临床类型，可见医师所要面临的多样性及复杂性。

(1) Fixed drug reactions or fixed drug eruptions: fixed drug reactions are very common. The category is so named because the lesions appear repeatedly at the same location of the body whenever the patient is exposed to a particular drug. The exact mechanism of fixed drug eruptions remains unknown. Common causative agents are sulfonamides, antipyretics, analgesics, barbiturates and tetracyclines, etc. Lesions may occur on any particular part of the body; however, there appears to be a preference for the mucocutaneous junctions around the lips and genitalia. A typical lesion is a solitary, round or oval, well defined, violaceous, edematous erythema, 1-4 cm in diameter. Vesicles or bullae may occur in severe cases. The involved mucosa may present with erosions and exudations (Fig. 11-1). Patients usually feel a mild pruritus, but this can be painful if a secondary infection takes place. The erythema may resolve in about one week after the medication is withdrawn, leaving a permanent postinflammatory hyperpigmentation, which is characteristic for this disease. As more episodes recur, the number of lesions may increase and the affected area may extend somewhat beyond the initial rash.

(1) 固定型药物反应(fixed drug reactions)或固定型药疹(fixed drug eruptions) 很常见，因每次用药后皮疹在同一部位重复出现，所以命名为固定型药疹。发病机制不清楚。常由磺胺类、解热镇痛类、巴比妥类和四环素类等引起。皮疹可出现在身体的任何部位，好发于口唇和生殖器皮肤和黏膜交界处。典型皮损为圆形或类圆形界限清楚的水肿性暗紫红色斑，直径为 1～4 cm，常为 1 个，严重者红斑上可出现水疱或大疱，黏膜处易糜烂渗出(图 11-1)。自觉轻度瘙痒，如继发感染可自觉疼痛。停药 1 周左右红斑可消退，遗留持久的炎症后色素沉着，具有特征性。随着复发次数的增加，皮损数目也可增多，面积可扩大。

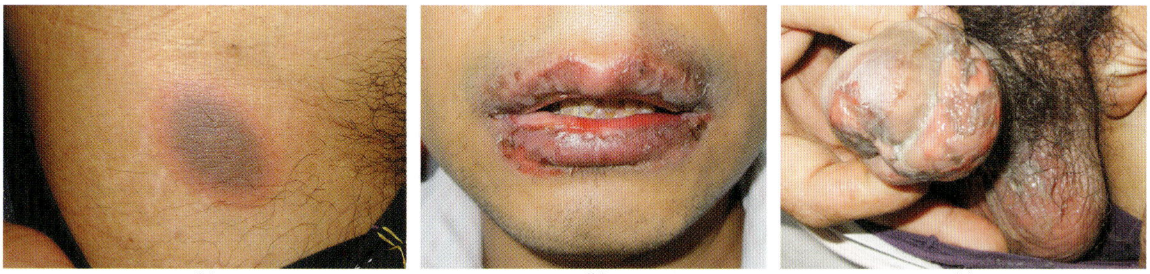

(a)　(b)　(c)

Fig. 11-1　Fixed drug reactions(图 11-1　固定型药物反应)

(2) Urticarial reactions: urticarial reactions are a relatively common type of drug eruption. Medications that cause this type of drug reaction are either acting on a hypersensitivity basis or on a non-hypersensitivity mechanism. The former is often triggered by serum products, penicillins and beta-lactam antibiotics, etc. The latter is commonly induced by aspirin and nonsteroidal anti-inflammatory drugs.

(2) 荨麻疹型反应　较常见，药物可通过超敏反应及非超敏反应机制引起荨麻疹型反应，前者多由血清制品、青霉素及 β-内酰胺类抗生素等引起，后者以阿司匹林和非甾体类抗炎药为最常见的诱发因素。

The clinical appearance of this type of drug eruption resembles that of acute urticaria (Fig. 11-2); however pruritic wheals or angioedema may flush readily and persist longer than those in acute urticaria. Urticaria is often the only symptom, but it may

临床表现与急性荨麻疹相似，表现为瘙痒性风团或血管性水肿(图 11-2)，但潮红更为明显，持续时间较长。荨麻疹可以作为唯一的症状出现，同时可伴

occasionally be accompanied by a serum sickness-like reaction, presenting as fever, arthralgia, lymphadenopathy and even proteinuria, and in severe cases allergic shock may occur. Chronic urticaria may result from an excessively slow excretion of the causative drug or from chronic exposure to some allergic antigen.

有血清病样症状，如发热、关节疼痛、淋巴结肿大甚至蛋白尿等，严重可并发过敏性休克。若致敏药物排泄缓慢或因不断接触过敏原，则可表现为慢性荨麻疹。

(3) Exanthematous reactions, morbilliform or scarlatiniform reactions, maculopapular reactions: this is the most common form of adverse cutaneous drug reaction. These are usually induced by penicillins (especially semisynthetic penicillins), sulfonamides, antipyretics, analgesics, barbiturates and other drugs. It is characterized by erythematous macules, usually mixed with extensive small papules (Fig. 11-3). The lesions tend to occur within the first week of the initiation of therapy but may appear later, or may even appear 10 days after the medication has been terminated. The onset is sudden, and usually accompanied by systemic symptoms such as fever, chills, etc.

(3) 发疹型反应(exanthematous reactions)、麻疹样或猩红热样型反应(morbilliform or scarlatiniform reactions)、斑丘疹型反应(maculopapular reactions)

最常见的皮肤药物不良反应，常因青霉素(尤其是半合成青霉素)、磺胺类、解热镇痛类、巴比妥类及其他药物引起。其特征是红斑，常伴有泛发性小丘疹(图11-3)。皮损多在首次用药1周内出现，也可在1周后出现，甚至在停药后10天内发生。发病突然，可伴发热、寒战等全身症状。

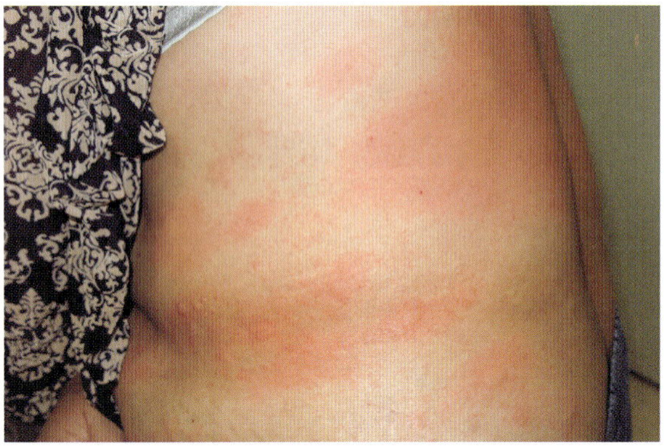

Fig. 11-2　Urticarial reactions(图 11-2　荨麻疹型反应)

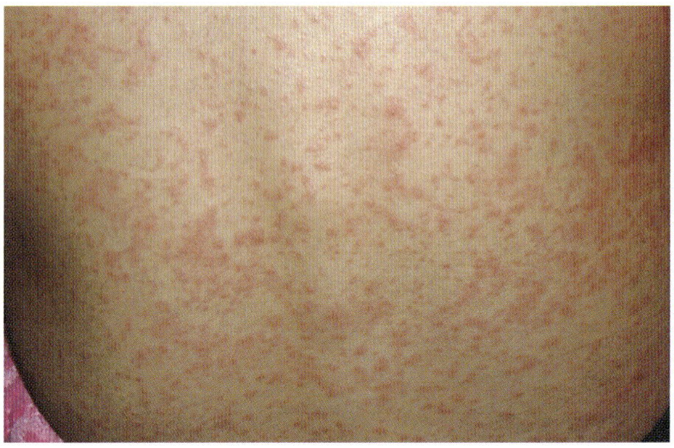

Fig. 11-3　Exanthematous reactions(图 11-3　发疹型反应)

The lesions of morbilliform reactions are similar to those of measles, which are pin-head or milium-sized red papules that are often distributed symmetrically. They tend to spread over the entire body, most commonly on the trunk. Small petechiae may occur in severe cases. Pruritus is usually prominent, which also distinguishes a drug eruption from a viral exanthem.

麻疹样型反应类似麻疹，皮损为针头或粟粒大小红色丘疹，双侧对称分布，可全身泛发，以躯干为多，严重者可伴发小出血点，瘙痒明显，可与病毒疹相鉴别。

The lesions of scarlatiniform reactions are diffuse, vivid red erythema, or rice grain to bean-sized red macules or maculopapules in a concentrated symmetric distribution. Usually, the lesions erupt first on the face and neck, spread to the trunk and limbs, and then extend rapidly over the entire body within 1-4 days with the predilection areas being the groin, axilla and the flexor surfaces on the extremities. The lesions are apt to coalesce and resemble scarlatina, but with apparent itching. The course is 1-2 weeks. The resolution of lesions is often followed by branny desquamation. In some patients the condition may evolve to severe drug eruptions if

猩红热样型反应呈弥漫性鲜红色斑或米粒至豆大红色斑疹或斑丘疹，密集对称分布，常从面颈部开始向躯干四肢蔓延，1～4天内遍布全身，尤以腹股沟、腋窝部或四肢屈侧更为明显，皮损可融合扩大，酷似猩红热的皮损，但瘙痒明显。病程1～2周，皮损消退后可伴糠状脱屑。若不及时治疗，部分患者可向重型药疹发展。

proper treatment is not begun immediately.

(4) Eczematous drug reactions: the patient usually has a history of contact dermatitis, where the skin has been exposed and sensitized to some topically administrated penicillin, streptomycin, or sulfonamide. A generalized eczematous eruption that resembles the appearance of allergic contact dermatitis may then develop upon systemic administration of the same or a cross-reacting drug. The lesions appear in various sizes and types, from erythematous macules, and small papules, to small papulovesicles or vesicles that usually coalesce and spread over the entire body, followed by erosions and exudations. The chronic lesions are similar to chronic eczema and show thickened, dry skin, accompanied by varying degrees of pruritus. The course is usually protracted, commonly over one month.

(4) 湿疹型药物反应　患者多因以前接触或外用青霉素、链霉素、磺胺等药物后使局部皮肤致敏引起接触性皮炎，再次使用相同或化学结构相似的药物后出现全身泛发性湿疹样改变。皮损表现为大小不等的红斑、小丘疹、小丘疱疹及水疱，常融合成片，泛发全身，可继发糜烂、渗出。慢性者皮肤肥厚、干燥，类似慢性湿疹，伴有不同程度瘙痒。病程较长，常在 1 个月以上。

(5) Purpuric drug reactions: drugs may induce anaphylactoid purpura. The common causative drugs are antibiotics, barbiturates, diuretics, etc. This condition is mediated by type Ⅱ hypersensitivity (thrombocytopenic purpura) or by type Ⅲ hypersensitivity (vasculitis). Purpuric lesions commonly occur on both lower limbs, with bilateral and symmetric distribution, and in severe cases it may involve the trunk and extremities. Mild cases present as red pinhead-to bean-sized petechiae and/or ecchymoses, either discrete or having a grouped distribution (Fig. 11-4). The lesions are slightly elevated, but do not blanch when pressed, and are sometimes accompanied by wheals or hemorrhagic bullae. In severe cases, the lesions are accompanied by arthralgia, abdominal pain, hematuria, blood in stool, etc.

(5) 紫癜型药物反应　药物可引起过敏性紫癜，常见引起此型反应的药物有抗生素、巴比妥类、利尿剂等，可通过Ⅱ型超敏反应(引起血小板减少性紫癜)或Ⅲ型超敏反应(引起血管炎)介导。皮损好发于双下肢，两侧对称，严重者可累及躯干和四肢。轻者表现为针头至豆大红色瘀点和瘀斑，散在或密集分布(图 11-4)，稍隆起，压之不褪色，可伴有风团或血疱。病情严重者可伴有关节肿痛、腹痛、血尿和便血等表现。

(6) Erythema multiforme drug reactions: the most common causative drugs are antipyretics, analgesics, sulfonamides, barbiturates, etc. Erythema multiforme can present as mild or severe. Patients with the mild form usually present with fever and influenza-like prodromal symptoms before the lesions appear; the lesions are symmetrically distributed and predispose to the distal portions of the extremities. The most characteristic feature is iris lesion, which is a well-defined edematous macule, ranging in size roughly from the size of a nail to the size of a coin, round or oval, with concentric rings of erythema and a purplish red or vesicular "bull's eye" center (Fig. 11-5). Pruritus is apparent for most patients but painful lesions may occur if the mucosal membrane of oral and genitalia becomes involved. In patients with the severe form of the disease, the condition begins with a more severe prodrome, and skin involvement is more generalized. The skin lesions may present as bullae, erosions and exudations with oral, ocular and genital mucosa more severely involved, all accompanied

(6) 多形红斑型药物反应　多形红斑型药物反应多由解热镇痛类、磺胺类及巴比妥类等药物引起。根据病情分为轻型和重型，轻型反应常在发热和流感样前驱症状后发生皮损，多对称分布，好发于四肢远端，典型皮损为指甲至钱币大小、圆形或椭圆形水肿性红斑，境界清楚，边缘潮红，中心暗紫红色，形如虹膜状，中央常出现水疱(图 11-5)，自觉瘙痒，累及口腔及外生殖器黏膜时可疼痛；重型反应，发病前有较重的前驱症状，皮损泛发全身，并可出现大疱、糜烂及渗出，尤以口、眼、外生殖器黏膜受累严重，出现剧烈疼痛，伴有高热、外周血白细胞升高、肝肾功能损害及继发感染等，病情凶险，可导致患者死亡。

by high fever, severe pain and leukocytosis, liver or renal dysfunction, secondary infection, etc. Without immediate treatment, these conditions can lead to death.

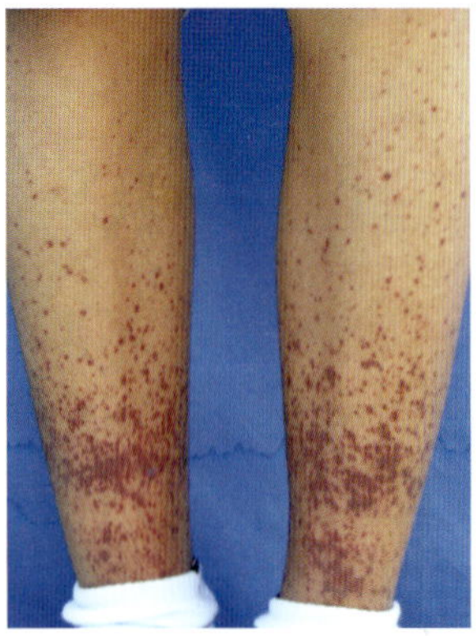

Fig. 11-4　Purpuric drug reactions

(图 11-4　紫癜型药物反应)

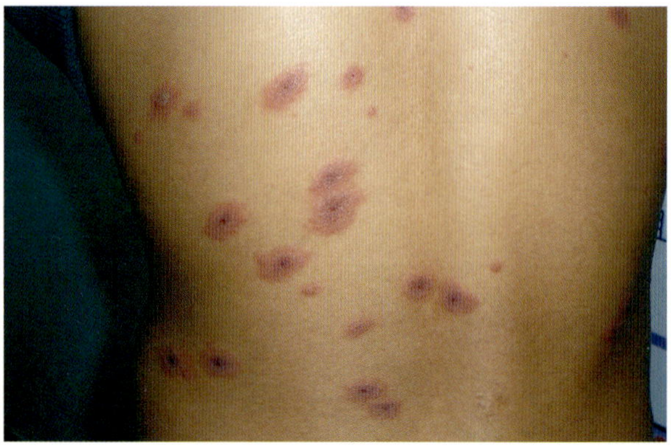

Fig. 11-5　Erythema multiforme drug reactions

(图 11-5　多形红斑型药物反应)

(7) Bullous drug reactions (Stevens-Johnson syndrome and toxic epidermal necrolysis): bullous or epidermal necrolysis drug reactions are the most severe adverse drug reactions. Bullous drug reactions may manifest as Stevens-Johnson syndrome (SJS) or toxic epidermal necrolysis (TEN), but the two conditions have very similar causative agents, mechanisms, and clinical and histopathological findings, with the single obvious exception of body surface area (BSA) involvement. SJS has less than 10 percent of body area involvement and TEN is more than 30 percent, with the range between the two being known as SJS/TEN overlap. The overall mortality rates are 5%-12% for SJS and over 30% for TEN.

The commonly causative drugs of bullous drug reactions are allopurinol, sulfonamides, antipyretics, analgesics, antibiotics, or barbiturates. The onset is acute, and lesions at first may resemble morbilliform or scarlatiniform drug reactions, but then evolve rapidly into purplish red or dark red patches overlaid with variously sized flaccid bullae. Epidermolysis on erythematous macules spread quickly over the entire body. Nikolsky's sign is positive. Erosions are easily formed even by gentle pressure, from which large amounts of exudation will seep to give a burn-like appearance. Haphalgesia is prominent. The mucosae of the oral cavity, eyes, respiratory and gastrointestinal tracts can all be involved (Fig. 11-6, Fig. 11-7). Severe constitutional symptoms, such as high fever, nausea, diarrhea, delirium, and even coma are likely. Significant internal organs impairment may accompany the disease. As a consequence of secondary infections, liver and renal failure,

(7) 大疱型药物反应(bullous drug reactions)(Stevens-Johnson 综合征(Stevens-Johnson syndrome, SJS)和中毒性表皮坏死松解症(toxic epidermal necrolysis, TEN)) 大疱型或表皮坏死松解型药物反应是最严重的药物不良反应，可表现 Stevens-Johnson 综合征(SJS)或中毒性表皮坏死松解症(TEN)，二者的药物因素、发病机制、临床表现和组织病理均相似，最重要的不同是前者累及的体表面积范围小于10%，而后者大于30%。累及体表面积在二者之间的是 SJS 与 TEN 的重叠型。SJS 的总死亡率为5%～12%，而 TEN 的大于30%。

大疱型药物反应常由别嘌呤醇、磺胺类、解热镇痛类、抗生素、巴比妥类等引起。起病急骤，部分患者发病开始可似麻疹样型或猩红热样型药物反应，迅速发展为紫红色或暗红色斑片并迅速波及全身，在红斑处出现大小不等的松弛性水疱和表皮松解，尼氏征(Nikolsky's sign)阳性，稍受外力即形成糜烂面，伴大量渗出，如烫伤样外观。皮肤触痛明显。口腔、眼、呼吸道、胃肠道黏膜均可受累(图 11-6，图 11-7)。全身中毒症状较重，可有高热、恶心、腹泻、谵妄、昏迷等全身症状。可伴有显著的内脏损害，如抢救不及时常因继发感染、肝功能衰竭、肾功能衰竭、电解质紊乱、内脏出血等而

electrolyte imbalance and visceral hemorrhage, patients may die if treatment is not begun immediately.

死亡。

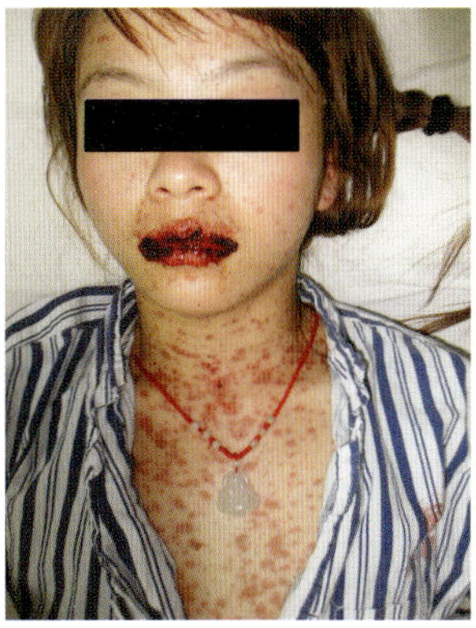

Fig. 11-6　Stevens-Johnson syndrome
(图 11-6　Stevens-Johnson 综合征)

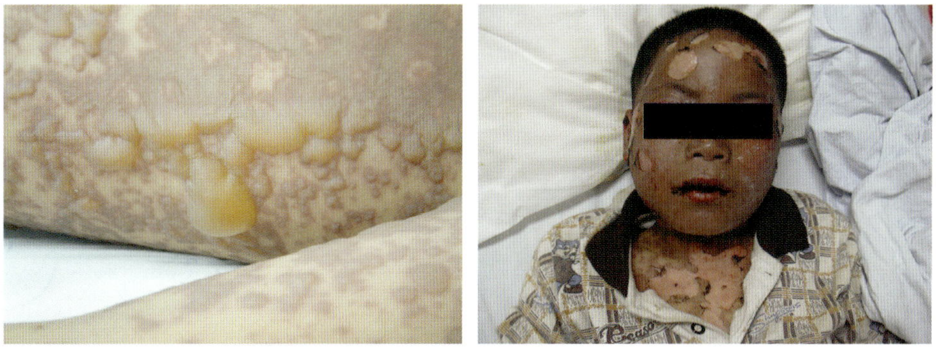

(a)　(b)

Fig. 11-7　Toxic epidermal necrolysis
(图 11-7　中毒性表皮坏死松解症)

(8) Exfoliative dermatitis drug reactions: this type of drug reaction is commonly caused by long term of using sulfonamides, barbiturates, antipyretics, analgesics, antiepileptics. For the first exposure to a suspected drug, the latent period for most patients is over 20 days. The patient will present with fever, malaise and other prodromal symptoms. The eruptions initially present as morbilliform or scarlatiniform lesions or large patches without prodromal symptoms. If the causative drugs are not discontinued or if they are not properly countered, the lesions tend to coalesce into generalized erythema and swelling over the entire body, with the face and hands being particularly affected. Vesicles, erosions and exudates with a putrid odor may develop later. Usually the erythematous swelling will begin to subside within 2-3 days, followed by a large number of scaly or foliate desquamations over the entire surface of the body (Fig. 11-8). Glove-or socks-like desquamations of the palms and soles may also be exhibited. Alopecia and/or shedding of finger-or toenails may also occur. The mucosae of the oral cavity and eyes can be involved, which will then present as oral erosions, dysphagia, conjunctival congestion, photophobia, etc. The patients often also present with constitutional symptoms, such as chills, fever, or vomiting with superficial lymphadenopathy. In severe cases, bronchopneumonia, drug hepatitis, renal failure, and granulocytopenia may occur. The course of the disease may become chronic. If the condition is not treated in time, the patient may die of general organ failure or secondary infections.

(8) 剥脱性皮炎型药物反应　剥脱性皮炎型药物反应常由磺胺类、巴比妥类、解热镇痛类、抗癫痫药等引起，多为长期用药后发生。首次发病潜伏期多在20天以上，发病前有发热、全身不适等前驱症状。皮损初始多呈麻疹样或猩红热样，可因继续用药或治疗不当所致，也可一开始即为泛发性大片损害而无前驱症状。皮损逐渐加重并融合成全身弥漫性红斑、肿胀，尤以面部及手部为重，可伴发水疱、糜烂和渗出，渗液有臭味，经2～3天后皮肤红肿开始消退，全身出现大量鳞片状或落叶状脱屑(图 11-8)，掌跖部则呈手套或袜套状剥脱，头发、指(趾)甲也可脱落。可累及口腔黏膜和眼结膜，出现口腔糜烂、吞咽困难、眼结膜充血和畏光等，常伴有寒战、发热、呕吐等全身症状，表浅淋巴结常肿大，严重者可伴有支气管肺炎、药物性肝炎、肾功能衰竭、粒细胞缺乏等。病程较长，如不及时治疗，严重者常因全身衰竭或继发感染而死亡。

(9) Acneiform drug reactions: acneiform drug reactions commonly develop after long-term uses of iodides, bromides, glucocorticoids and contraceptives. The lesions are similar to acneiform lesions, presenting mainly as follicular papules and

(9) 痤疮样型药物反应　痤疮样型药物反应多因长期应用碘剂、溴剂、糖皮质激素和避孕药等药物引起。皮损为毛囊性丘疹、丘疱疹等痤疮样皮损，多发生

papulovesicles on the face, chest and back (Fig. 11-9). This type of drug eruptions progresses slowly and usually without systemic symptoms.

于面部及胸背部(图 11-9),病程进展缓慢,一般无全身症状。

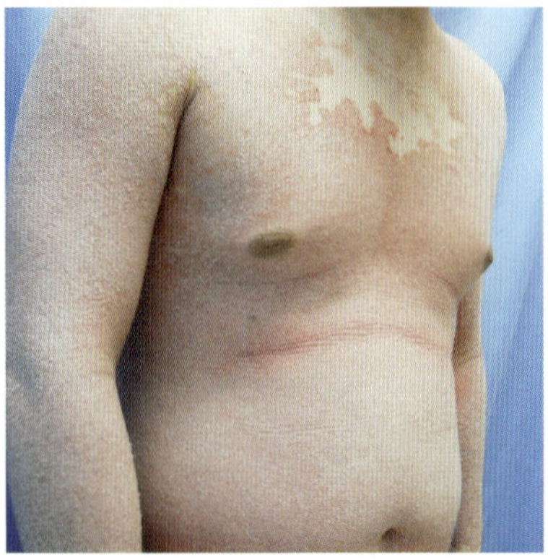

Fig. 11-8　Exfoliative dermatitis drug reactions
(图 11-8　剥脱性皮炎型药物反应)

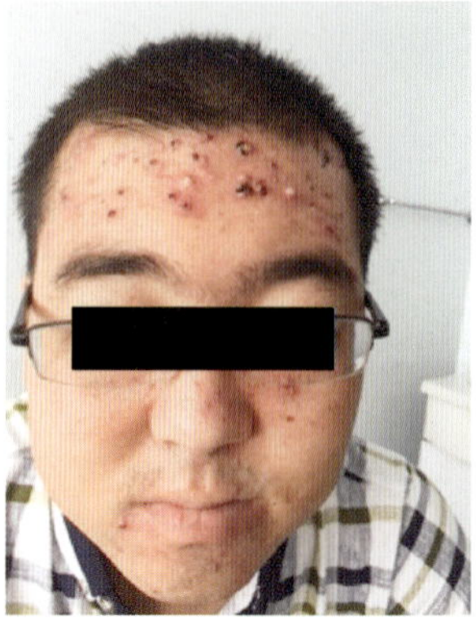

Fig. 11-9　Acneiform drug reactions
(图 11-9　痤疮样型药物反应)

(10) Photosensitive drug reactions: photosensitive drug reactions commonly develop only when ingestion of the offending drug (such as chlorpromazine, sulfonamides, tetracyclines, griseofulvin, psoralen, quinolones, thiazides, or contraceptives, etc.) is followed by exposure to sunlight or ultraviolet radiation. Clinically, the majority of cases fall into two types of presentations. The first type is phototoxic drug reactions, which begin with a burning sensation on the sunlight exposed area 7-8 hours after exposure and resemble sunburn. The condition can occur in anybody and severity is correlated with drug dose and amount of ultraviolet radiation received. The reaction resolves quickly once the causative drug is terminated, and so it does not require prior exposure or any immune response. The second common type of reaction is photoallergic drug reactions, which occur only in a relatively small number of patients. The immune system is involved. By contrast with the phototoxic type of drug reaction, there is a period of latency and the lesions are eczematous, lichenoid and pruritic occurring on both exposed and unexposed areas. It has a more protracted course.

(10) 光敏型药物反应　光敏型药物反应多因使用氯丙嗪、磺胺类、四环素类、灰黄霉素、补骨脂、喹诺酮类、酚噻嗪类及避孕药等,经日光或紫外线照射而引发,可分为两类。①光毒反应性药物反应,多于曝光后 7～8 h 发病,仅于曝光部位出现与晒斑相似的皮损,有烧灼感,任何人均可发病,反应与药物剂量和照射剂量相关,停药后很快消退;不需要既往接触史也不需要免疫系统的参加。②光变态反应性药物反应,仅少数人发病,有免疫系统的参与,有一定的潜伏期,于曝光部位和非曝光部位出现皮损,表现为湿疹样或苔藓样,瘙痒,病程较长。

(11) Drug hypersensitivity syndrome: drug hypersensitivity syndrome (DHS) is sometimes also called drug eruption with eosinophilia and systemic symptoms (DRESS) syndrome. Patients with DHS or DRESS share the characteristic features of fever, rash, and internal organ involvement. Other valuable diagnostic features are: ①rash develops more than 3 weeks after the inciting medication is first administered, often occurs with the first exposure to the medication; ②symptoms last longer (>2 weeks) after discontinuation of the causative drug; ③ fever (>38 ℃); ④multiple organ involvement; ⑤ eosinophilia (>1500 absolute

(11) 药物超敏反应综合征　药物超敏反应综合征(drug hypersensitivity syndrome, DHS)又称为伴嗜酸性粒细胞增多和系统症状的药疹(drug eruption with eosinophilia and systemic symptoms, DRESS)综合征,DHS 或 DRESS 具有发热、皮疹和内脏受累的共同特点,其特异性诊断要点包括:①用药后皮损发生时间晚(3 周以上),且常见于初次用药的患者;②停止致敏药物后症状持续时间长

eosinophilia); ⑥ lymphocyte activation including lymphocytosis, atypical lymphocytosis and lymphadenopathy; ⑦ often companied by reactivation of HHV-6, HHV-7, EBV, and CMV.

(2 周以上);③发热(超过 38 ℃);④多器官受累;⑤嗜酸性粒细胞增多症(超过 1.5×10^9/L 的绝对计数的嗜酸粒细胞增多);⑥淋巴细胞活化(淋巴细胞增多,异型淋巴细胞,淋巴结肿大);⑦经常有疱疹病毒 HHV-6、HHV-7、EBV 和 CMV 的再激活。

Seven major medications/classes of medication are implicated in DRESS as follows: ①anticonvulsants: phenobarbital, lamotrigine and phenytoin; ② long-acting sulfonamides: sulfamethoxazole, sulfadiazine, and sulfasalazine, but not related medications such as —sulfonylureas, thiazine diuretics, furosemide, and acetazolamide; ③allopurinol; ④nevirapine; ⑤abacavir; ⑥dapsone; ⑦minocycline. Vancomycin has also recently been recognized as a cause.

绝大多数的 DRESS 主要由以下七种药物引起:①抗癫痫药(苯巴比妥、拉莫三嗪与苯妥英钠);②长效磺胺药(磺胺甲噁唑、磺胺嘧啶、柳氮磺吡啶,但不包括磺脲、噻嗪类利尿剂、呋塞米与乙酰唑胺);③别嘌醇;④奈韦拉平;⑤阿巴卡韦;⑥氨苯砜;⑦米诺环素。万古霉素进近来也被认为是一种诱发药物。

The onset is sudden and clinical manifestations include fever, rash, lymphadenopathy, and internal organ involvement. Abnormal blood tests may also be seen. The initial lesions resemble morbilliform lesions, which appear on the face, upper trunk and upper extremities and later become exfoliative dermatitis-like lesions (Fig. 11-10). Facial swelling is characteristic for this syndrome. Vesicle formation results from upper dermal edema and sterile pustules or purpura may occur on occasion. The mortality rate of this syndrome is close to 10% if diagnosis and/or treatment are delayed, usually by complications of liver or renal involvement.

该病发病突然,临床表现包括发热、皮损、淋巴结肿大、血液学异常及内脏受累。早期皮损为面部、躯干上部及上肢的麻疹样皮损,可演变为剥脱性皮炎样皮损(图 11-10)。面部水肿具有特征性,真皮浅层水肿可导致水疱形成,也可出现无菌性脓疱和紫癜。如未能及时发现和治疗,本病死亡率在 10%左右,死因多为肝或肾受累的并发症。

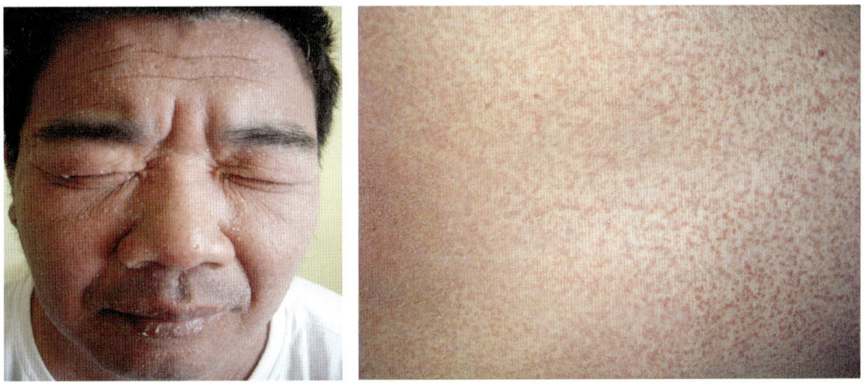

(a)　　(b)

Fig. 11-10　Drug hypersensitivity syndrome(图 11-10　药物超敏反应综合征)

(12) Other types: here we include acute generalized exanthematous pustulosis (AGEP), drug-induced pigmentation, drug-induced systemic lupus erythematosus, and lichenoid reactions, etc.

(12) 其他类型药物反应　其他类型药物反应包括急性泛发性发疹性脓疱病(acute generalized exanthematous pustulosis, AGEP)、药物诱导的皮肤色素沉着和系统性红斑狼疮及苔藓样反应等。

Clinically, severe cases of erythema multiforme drug eruptions, epidermal necrolysis drug reactions (SJS and TEN),

临床上将重症多形红斑型药物反应、表皮坏死松解型药物反应(SJS 及

exfoliative dermatitis drug eruptions and DHS or DRESS are all categorized as severe adverse cutaneous drug reactions.

TEN)、剥脱性皮炎型药物反应及药物超敏反应综合征称为重型药物皮肤不良反应。

【Diagnosis and Differential Diagnosis】

The diagnosis of drug eruptions relies on a positive history of drug administration, a latent period tied to the timeline of the treatment, the typical clinical features noted above, and consistent exclusion of any other skin conditions with similar lesions or exanthematous infections. Drug eruptions are often marked by vivid color and a prominent pruritus which quickly subsides once the offending drug is withdrawn. However, the determination of the exact causative drug may be difficult sometimes, especially when more than two kinds of drugs are being administered. Nevertheless, the diagnosis needs to be made after a comprehensive analysis of the patient's previous experience with the drugs, history of drug reactions, and correlation of current drug use to the onset of the lesions. Morbilliform or scarlatiniform drug reactions should be distinguished from measles and scarlet fever. Bullous epidermolytic drug reactions should be distinguished from staphylococcal scalded skin syndrome. In cases of genital fixed drug reactions, once the lesions start to rupture, a quick diagnosis should be made to distinguish the condition from genital herpes or chancre.

【诊断与鉴别诊断】

根据明确的服药史、潜伏期及各型药物反应的典型临床皮损进行诊断，同时需排除具有类似皮损的其他皮肤病及发疹性传染病。通常药物的皮肤副反应皮损颜色鲜艳，瘙痒更明显，且停用致敏药物后较快好转。但要准确判断致敏药物有时比较困难，特别是服用两种以上的药物时，应结合过去的服药史、药物反应史及此次用药与发病的关系等信息加以综合分析。麻疹样型或猩红热样型药物反应需与麻疹或猩红热进行鉴别，大疱性表皮松解型药物反应需与葡萄球菌性烫伤样皮肤综合征进行鉴别，生殖器部位的固定性药物反应出现破溃时，应与生殖器疱疹、硬下疳等进行鉴别。

【Treatment】

The principles for drug eruptions management that the physicians need to follow are as follows: to discontinue all suspected drugs immediately, to accelerate the excretion of the sensitizing drug if possible, to eliminate or repress the drug reactions, and to treat complications when they appear.

【治疗】

药疹的治疗首先是停用可疑过敏药物，加速药物的排泄，尽快消除药物反应，防止和及时治疗并发症。

(1) Mild drug reactions: the lesions may disappear spontaneously after the offending drugs are withdrawn. Antihistamines and vitamin C are often prescribed. If necessary, prednisone treatments may be started in moderate doses (30-60 mg/d) and gradually tapered off after the lesions have subsided. Calamine lotion and glucocorticoid cream may be used topically in patients who mainly present with erythema and papules. Cold moist compresses with a 3% boric acid solution may be effective in cases with erosions and exudation, and zinc oxide oil can be applied alternately with the compresses.

(1) 轻型药物反应　停用致敏药物后，皮损多自行消退。可给予抗组织胺药物和维生素 C 等，必要时给予中等剂量的泼尼松(30～60 mg/d)，皮损消退后可逐渐减量直至停药。皮损若以红斑、丘疹为主者可外用炉甘石洗剂或糖皮质激素霜，以糜烂渗出为主者可用 3% 硼酸溶液冷湿敷，湿敷间歇期可选用氧化锌油外用。

(2) Severe drug reactions

① Glucocorticoids: high dosages of glucocorticoids should be used as early as possible. For example, 300-400 mg of hydrocortisone or 10-20 mg of dexamethasone may be given intravenously once a day. The response should be observed over 3-5

(2) 重型药物反应

①糖皮质激素：及早足量应用糖皮质激素，一般可给氢化可的松 300～400 mg/d 静滴，或地塞米松 10～20 mg/d 静滴，糖皮质激素如足量，病情应在 3～5

days to determine if this dose is sufficient. If not, the glucocorticoid dose should be increased (e. g., adding 1/3 or 1/2 of the initial dose) to achieve better results. Alternatively, methylprednisolone can be given intravenously in a dose of 1 gram daily for 3 days. No matter what glucocorticoid is chosen, a tapering regimen should be followed as soon as the skin rash begins to lighten, no more new lesions appear, and the fever decreases.

天内控制，如未满意控制应加大剂量（增加原剂量的1/3～1/2）；病情严重者可选用甲泼尼龙，1 g/d 静脉注射，连续 3 天，以控制病情，待皮损颜色转淡、无新发皮损、体温下降后逐渐减量。

At present, the use of systemic glucocorticoids for the treatment of severe drug reactions is still controversial. The majority of published results show that systemic glucocorticoids do not alter the course of the illness but can increases the risk of infection, prolong the time of wound healing and promote the chance of gastrointestinal bleeding. Therefore, some have suggested that these patients should receive either intravenous immunoglobulin (IVIG) or cyclosporine therapy, especially for TEN. In such cases, patients should be treated with IVIG as early as possible. IVIG 1 g/kg daily for three days or 0.4 g/kg daily for 5 days or cyclosporine 3-5 mg/kg should be administered either orally or intravenously. The duration of cyclosporine therapy ranges from 8-24 days. A tapering schedule must be initiated once reepithelization occurs over the lesions.

目前，系统应用糖皮质激素治疗重症药疹仍然存在争议，大多数发表的文章认为系统应用糖皮质激素不能改变疾病的病程并可能增加感染的风险、延长愈合的时间和促使消化道出血。这些患者应该接受静脉应用免疫球蛋白（IVIG）或环孢素治疗，特别是 TEN，越早使用 IVIG 越好。静脉应用免疫球蛋白每日每公斤体重 1 g，连用 3 天或每日每公斤体重 0.4 g，连用 5 天，环孢素每日每公斤体重 3～5 mg 口服或静脉应用，不同的报道应用的时间不同，为 8～24 天，当表皮开始愈合时开始减量。

IVIG can inhibit Fas-Fas ligand mediated apoptosis and reduce the progression of the disease and the risk of death. Cyclosporine also has anti-apoptosis properties that may hasten the onset of reepithelization and therefore arrest further progression of the disease. However, IVIG treatment is not recommended for elderly patients or for patients with impaired renal function.

静脉应用免疫球蛋白能阻断 Fas 和 Fas 配体介导的凋亡，并能减轻疾病的进展和死亡的风险，环孢素具有抗凋亡的特性和减少表皮完全愈合的时间，有助于阻断疾病的进展。不推荐老年人和肾功能不全的患者使用 IVIG。

Infliximab and plasmapheresis are effective for SJS and TEN.

英利昔单抗及血液透析对 SJS 和 TEN 有肯定效果。

② Prevention and treatment of secondary infections: good nursing practice is absolutely essential in severe cases or patients with generalized lesions. Sterile and isolation measures should be emphasized at all times and care must be taken to limit the chance of infection. Attending physicians should also be cautioned on cross-sensitization and polyvalent sensitization when prescribing antibiotics for such patients. In general, the optimal selection of antibiotics is based on bacterial culture and drug sensitivity tests. However, a broad spectrum antibiotic that is not likely to be sensitized may be prescribed when it is needed before receiving the microbial sensitivity results. The possibility of an infection caused by drug-resistant bacteria or other causative agents such as fungi needs to be considered when the infection responds poorly to broad-spectrum antibiotics. Therapeutic schemes must often be adjusted according to therapeutic effectiveness for each patient.

②防治继发感染：对严重病例和皮损广泛者，良好的护理至关重要，应强调消毒隔离，医护人员在治疗和护理过程中要做到无菌操作，尽可能减少感染的机会；如有感染存在，选用抗生素时应注意避免使用易过敏药物（特别注意交叉过敏或多价过敏）。一般应根据细菌培养和药敏试验结果选用抗生素。在细菌学检查结果报告出来之前，应选用广谱、不易致敏的抗生素。如对广谱抗生素治疗效果不佳时应注意耐药菌的存在或其他感染（如真菌）的可能，并按具体的情况及时调整治疗方案。

③ Strengthening supportive therapy: hypoalbuminemia, fluid and electrolyte imbalances caused by high fever, difficulty in swallowing, and abundant exudations from extensive erosion surface or skin sloughing should all be treated immediately. Maintaining a normal blood volume is very important for effective treatment. If necessary, fresh blood, plasma, and/or serum protein should be given to the patient to maintain normal colloid osmotic pressures, which should decrease the exudation effectively. Corresponding care should be given to patients with internal organ involvement. Energy mixtures may be of benefit for some patients when given in appropriate amounts. Finally, it should be remembered that high dosages of glucocorticoids may themselves be responsible for side effects such as infection, alimentary canal stress ulcers, and hypertension.

③加强支持疗法：由于高热、进食困难、创面大量渗出或皮肤大片剥脱等常导致低蛋白血症和水、电解质紊乱，应及时加以纠正，同时注意维持血容量，必要时可输新鲜血液、血浆或血清蛋白以维持胶体渗透压，可有效减少渗出；对内脏受累者要及时做相应处理。应酌情给予能量合剂。应注意预防大剂量糖皮质激素引起的不良反应，如并发的各种感染、消化道应激溃疡和高血压等。

④ Strengthening care and topical therapy: the diet for severe patients should contain large amounts of protein and carbohydrates. The ward should be warm, airy, isolated and able to be sterilized at regular intervals. For patients with extensive lesions and severe exudation, drying the skin can be accomplished with moist compresses containing either a saline or 3% boric acid solution. This treatment with moist compresses can also be combined with exposure of the affected lesions to air or red and blue light alternately to promote healing. When eye membranes are involved, the eyes should be washed at regular intervals to decrease the likelihood of re-infection, and also to prevent the adhesion of the corneas, eyelids and conjunctiva. When the patient complains of difficulty in closing his or her eyes, oil gauze can be used to cover the eyes in order to avoid further corneal damage. Attention must also be drawn to other available methods of treatment such as oral rinses with sodium bicarbonate when oral membrane is involved, and bedsore prevention should also be employed as needed.

④加强护理和外用药治疗：应给予高蛋白、高碳水化合物饮食，病室温暖、通风、隔离、定期消毒。对皮损面积广、糜烂渗出重者，局部可用3%硼酸溶液或生理盐水湿敷，或以暴露干燥创面和湿敷相交替治疗，也可以采用红蓝光治疗。累及眼睛黏膜者应特别注意护理，定期冲洗以减少感染及防止角膜、眼睑球结膜粘连，闭眼困难者可用油纱布覆盖以防角膜长久暴露而损伤；口腔黏膜损害要注意口腔清洁，可用碳酸氢钠漱口。注意防止褥疮的发生。

Yu-xue GAO(高玉雪)

Chapter Twelve　Pruritic and Neurogenic Dermatoses

第十二章　瘙痒性和神经功能障碍性皮肤病

Section One　Psychogenic Pruritus

第一节　精神性瘙痒症

Pruritus can be an objective symptom for many skin diseases and sometimes for systemic diseases as well. On the other hand, psychogenic pruritus is defined as pruritus appearing in the absence of any skin pathology or any known underlying medical diseases. The clinical features of pruritus can be divided into localized and generalized pruritus.

瘙痒是许多皮肤病和系统性疾病具有的一种自觉症状。精神性瘙痒症(psychogenic pruritus)是一种只有皮肤瘙痒而缺乏皮肤病理或潜在的疾病的表现,一般分为局限性和全身性。

【Etiology and Pathogenesis】

【病因及发病机制】

The causes of pruritus vary among patients and the mechanisms are often quite complex. It is generally believed that the causes involve internal factors, external factors, or both. Psychogenic pruritus may even occur simultaneously with objective (i. e. ,non-psychogenic)pruritus due to either primary skin diseases or systemic illnesses such as diabetes mellitus, uremia, biliary cirrhosis,hyper-or hypothyroidism,hematological diseases,visceral tumors,and allergic diseases. Usually such underlying diseases will promote a generalized pruritus throughout the body. Other factors that may trigger such intensive pruritus include pregnancy, irregular menstruation, medicine, food, mental anxiety, or changes in weather (e. g. , temperature, humidity) or living environment or personal habits or clothing (including detergents).

病因复杂。一般认为致病因素包括内因、外因或两者兼有。精神性瘙痒症可以与器质性(非精神性)瘙痒症伴发,这可以是由某些皮肤病或某些系统性疾病,如糖尿病、尿毒症、胆汁性肝硬化、甲状腺功能亢进症或减退症、血液病、内脏肿瘤、变应性疾病引起。这些因素常引起全身性瘙痒症。其他如妊娠、月经不调、药物或食物、精神焦虑、气候改变(如温度,湿度)、环境、生活习惯或衣着(包括洗涤剂)等也可引起全身性瘙痒症。

On the other hand, besides those mentioned above, localized pruritus is usually related to localized factors such as haemorrhoids, anal fissures, pinworm infections, hyperhidrosis and scratching. Recently, studies have shown that pruritus-related receptors are enriched in both the dermal papilla layer and in the epidermal free nerve endings of unmyelinated C fibers. Pruritus is also associated with a variety of conducting mediators, and it is now believed that both central and peripheral factors have an impact on itchiness.

局限性瘙痒症的发生除以上因素外,常与痔疮、肛裂、蛲虫感染、多汗及搔抓等局部因素有关。近年来研究发现,介导瘙痒的多种受体位于真皮乳头及表皮的无髓C纤维游离神经末梢上。瘙痒也与多种传导介质相关,目前认为其中枢和外周都有致痒作用。

【Clinical Manifestations】

【临床表现】

(1) Pruritus universalis: itching can involve the whole body at the onset, or evolve from one specific site at the very beginning to the whole body. The pruritus tends to be paroxysmal, usually aggravated at night. The degree of pruritus varies with individuals and the course of disease in a giving individual. Excoriation, crusting, hyperpigmentation, lichenification, or secondary infections usually result from repeated rubbing and scratching (Fig. 12-1).

(1) 全身性瘙痒症　瘙痒可开始即为全身性,或局限于一处,继而扩展全身。常为阵发性,尤以夜间为重。瘙痒的程度不尽相同,长期过度搔抓,皮肤常继发抓痕、血痂、色素沉着、苔藓样变、继发感染等(图 12-1)。全身瘙痒症可表现为:①老年性瘙痒症(主要发生于老年患

Generalized pruritus may manifest as: ① pruritus senilis (usually induced by decreased function of the sebaceous glands, dry skin and excessive washing occurring mainly in elderly people); ② pruritus hiemalis(triggered by lower temperature or sudden climate change in winter); ③pruritus aestivalis (provoked by high temperature and over-sweating in summer); ④ aquagenic pruritus (itching occurs when the patient contact with water of any temperature).

者，与皮脂腺的功能下降、皮肤干燥及过度洗涤有关)；②冬季瘙痒症(发生于冬季，与低温、气候的突然改变有关)；③夏季瘙痒症(由于夏季高温及出汗过多诱发)；④水源性瘙痒症(在接触任何温度的水后发生瘙痒)。

(2) Pruritus localis: itching sensation is restricted to localized areas, such as the vulval area, anal region, scalp, legs, palmoplantar areas or the external auditory canal.

(2) 局限性瘙痒症　局限性瘙痒症多局限于身体某一部位，常见于外阴、肛门、头皮、小腿、掌跖、外耳道等。

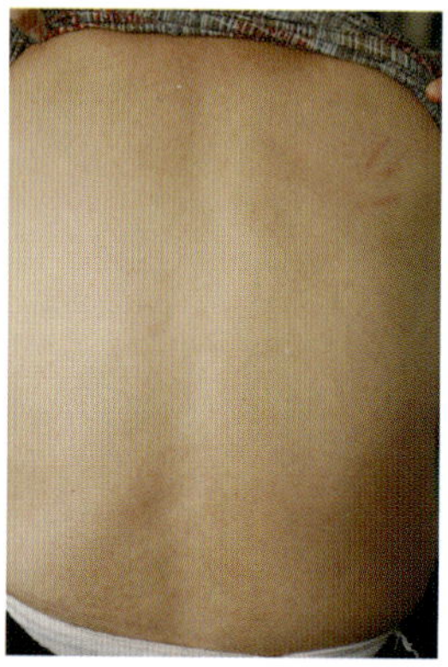

Fig. 12-1　Psychogenic pruritus(图 12-1　精神性瘙痒症)

【Diagnosis and Differential Diagnosis】

The diagnosis can be readily established according to the extent of pruritus or the presence of secondary signs without primary skin lesions. General physical examination and laboratory analysis is needed to search for the more fundamental causes. It is necessary to separate psychogenic pruritus from pruritus resulting from scabies and eczematoid dermatitis, papular urticaria, urticaria, and drug eruption. Psychogenic pruritus should also be distinguished from pruritus associated with underlying diseases.

【诊断与鉴别诊断】

根据全身性或局限性瘙痒仅有继发改变而无原发损害，易于诊断。为了寻找致病因素，常需做全面的体格检查和实验室检查。需与疥疮、湿疹样皮炎、丘疹性荨麻疹、荨麻疹、药疹相鉴别。同时需要鉴别精神性瘙痒症与由疾病引起的瘙痒症。

【Treatment】

Identify the causes of the pruritus carefully and give corresponding treatment. It is important to eliminate pruritus-inducing factors, such as alcohol, coffee, and spices; therefore some changes in lifestyle may be necessary. Application of antihistamines, moisturizers and UV (either UVA or UVB) irradiation may also be effective. For pruritus universalis, starch baths, bran baths, or mineral baths may be useful. When routine treatments for pruritus localis are ineffective, isotope or superficial X-ray treatment is recommended.

【治疗】

仔细查找病因并争取相应治疗，注意避免各种引起瘙痒的因素如酒、咖啡及刺激性食物，必要时应改变生活习惯。应用各种抗组胺类药物和外用润肤局封剂，或应用紫外线(UVA，UVB)照射均有效。全身性瘙痒症可行淀粉浴、糠浴或矿泉浴。局限性瘙痒症经多元治疗无效时，可考虑用同位素或浅层X线。

Section Two　Prurigo

Prurigo is a group of chronic or acute inflammatory dermatoses

第二节　痒　疹

痒疹(prurigo)为一组急性或慢性炎

characterized by intensive pruritic wheal-like papules or nodules.

【Etiology and Pathogenesis】

The etiology of prurigo is unknown. The disease is regarded to be in association with allergic reaction, maybe also with a number of postulated triggers, including neuropsychiatric diseases, inherited atopic background, insect bites, drug or food allergies, sunlight, infections, functional disorders of the gastrointestinal (GI) tract, and endocrine disorders.

【Clinical Manifestations】

(1) Acute prurigo:

①Simple acute prurigo: also known as papular urticaria, occurs most commonly in children or juveniles but may affect an entire household at once. It is common in the spring and autumn and often related to arthropod bites, such as ants, fleas, bedbugs and mites. This type of prurigo may also be caused by digestive disturbances or allergic reactions to certain substances. Secondary infections may follow after persistent rubbing and scratching. The symptoms last only for one to several weeks, but tend to recur if the underlying cause is not eliminated. The typical lesions are red, wheal-like papules, 1-2 cm in diameter. In some cases, papulovesicles, vesicles or bullae may be seen in the centre of each papular lesion. The lesions cluster easily but tend not to fuse. Patients generally have no systemic symptoms (see Chapter Eight).

②Prurigo adultorum: also known as temporary or transient prurigo, this is more common in adolescent and middle-aged women over the age of 30. Systemic symptoms may present prior to any skin lesions, including fatigue, headaches, insomnia and gastrointestinal disorders. The eruptions are usually on the trunk and the extensor surfaces of the extremities, especially the elbow and knee areas. However, the scalp, face, and hips can also be affected, presenting as millet-to soybean-sized, multiple firm papules, round or slightly flattened at the top, and of pink or normal skin color. The lesions are scattered or isolated, or may gather into clusters but do not fuse (Fig. 12-2). Itching is intense; wheal-like skin lesions and papulovesicles may appear after scratching, and with continued scratching these may eventually evolve into lichenification and pigmentation. The course of this type is in general chronic and persistent.

(2) Chronic prurigo:

①Prurigo infantilis: also known as Hebra's prurigo or early-onset prurigo, and mostly affects children under 3 years of age. The eruptions are most likely to appear on the extensor aspects of the

症性皮肤病，其特征为具有强烈瘙痒性风团样丘疹或结节等。

【病因及发病机制】

原因不明，多与变态反应有关，也可能与神经精神因素、遗传过敏体质有关，还可能与其他因素（如虫咬、药物或食物过敏、日光、病灶感染、胃肠道功能紊乱及内分泌障碍等）有关。

【临床表现】

(1) 急性痒疹

①急性单纯性痒疹（simple acute prurigo）：也称为丘疹性荨麻疹，多累及儿童及青少年，常见一个家庭中同时发病，春、秋季节多发，常与某些节肢动物，如蚁、蚤、蠓、臭虫及螨等的叮咬有关，也可能由消化障碍或对某些物质过敏而引起。自觉瘙痒，反复搔抓可继发感染，一般急性单纯性痒疹发疹一周至数周，病因未去除可反复发生。皮损为红色风团样丘疹，直径为 1～2 cm，损害中央常有丘疱疹、水疱或大疱，皮损易群集，少融合。患者一般无全身症状（参见第八章）。

②成人痒疹（prurigo adultorum）：又称暂时性或一过性痒疹。多见于中青年，以 30 岁以上女性多见。发病前常有疲乏、头痛、失眠及胃肠功能失调等全身症状。好发于躯干及四肢伸侧，肘、膝部明显，也可累及头皮、面部、臀部。基本皮损小米至黄豆大小，淡红或肤色，多发性坚实圆形或顶部略扁平的丘疹，散在分布，亦可聚集成簇，但不融合（图12-2）。瘙痒剧烈，搔抓后出现风团样皮损及丘疱疹，反复搔抓可出现苔藓样变和色素沉着。病情慢性迁延。

(2) 慢性痒疹

①小儿痒疹（prurigo infantilis）：又称 Hebra 痒疹（Hebra's prurigo）或早发性痒疹，多见于 3 岁以前的幼儿，好发于

extremities, presenting as soybean-sized wheal-like papules (Fig. 12-3), which then become firm, skin-colored papules, known as prurigo kuntchen, accompanied by intense itching. Lichenification, eczematoid lesions, and secondary infections may occur. After the eruptions subside, areas of hyperpigmentation are left at the lesion sites. The patient will also usually experience malnutrition, anemia, weight loss, gastrointestinal disorders, anxiety, etc. The course of this disease is chronic, and it can alleviate or self-heal when the patient reaches adolescence.

四肢伸侧,基本皮损为黄豆大小风团样丘疹(图 12-3),继而转变为肤色质硬小结节,即痒疹小结节(prurigo kuntchen)。瘙痒剧烈,易出现苔藓样改变、湿疹样变或继发感染。皮疹消退后留有色素沉着。患儿多伴营养不良、贫血、消瘦、胃肠功能紊乱、情绪急躁等,本病经过慢性,到青年期可缓解或自愈。

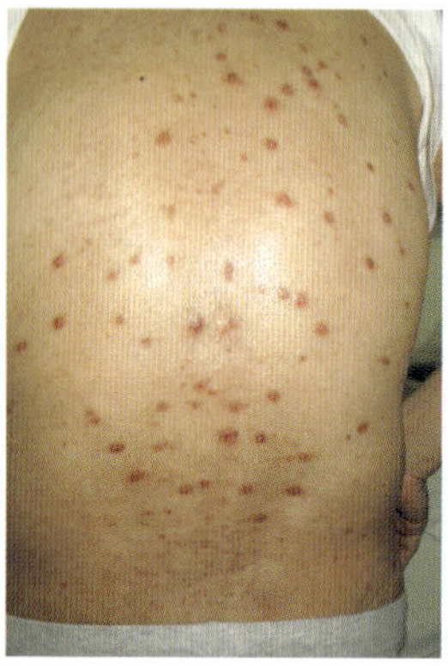

Fig. 12-2　Prurigo adultorum(图 12-2　成人痒疹)

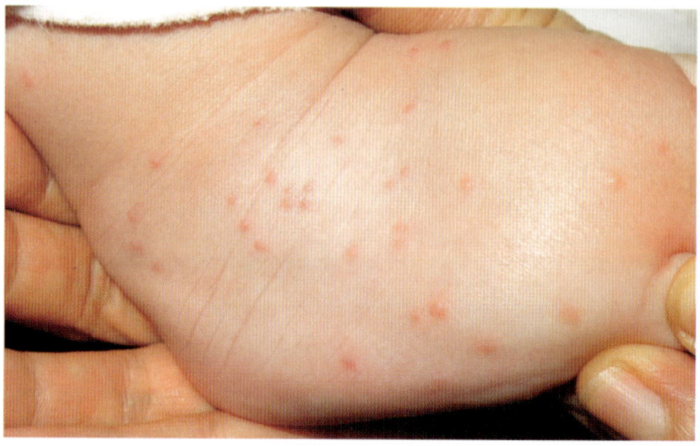

Fig. 12-3　Prurigo infantilis(图 12-3　小儿痒疹)

② Prurigo nodularis: often appearing on the extremities, especially on the extensor surfaces of the lower extremities. Prurigo nodularis occurs most commonly in adult women. An indefinite number of the nodules are arranged in strips and have a chronic and persistent course. At first the characteristic eruptions are hard, red, edematous papules that may evolve into yellow-colored, dome-shaped nodules with rough surfaces, randomly scattered, accompanied by intense itching. The secondary changes from picking and scratching are commonly seen in patients, and include hemorrhagic crust formation, excoriation and lichenification (Fig. 12-4).

②结节性痒疹(prurigo nodularis):好发于四肢,以小腿伸侧多见,多见于中青年及年长女性。皮损数目不定,结节有时呈条状排列,呈慢性经过,经久不愈。皮损初起为水肿性红色坚实丘疹,逐渐呈黄色或更大的半球状结节,表面粗糙,常散在分布。瘙痒剧烈,可因搔抓致结节顶部出现血痂、抓痕和苔藓样变(图 12-4)。

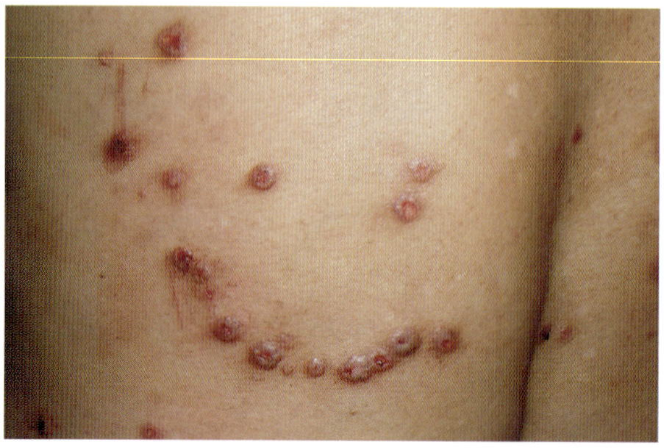

Fig. 12-4　Prurigo nodularis(图 12-4　结节性痒疹)

(3) Symptomatic prurigo: a special type of prurigo occurring in pregnant atopic women (see in patients with prurigo gestationis) or patients with tumors (such as lymphoma or leukemia). The etiology is unclear but it may relate to endocrine disorders. The skin lesions are wheal-or erythema multiforme-like papules, accompanied by intense itching. Secondary lesions may develop after scratching, and may present with excoriation, crust and hyperpigmentation, etc.

(3) 症状性痒疹(symptomatic prurigo)　这种特殊类型痒疹常发生于具有过敏体质的妊娠妇女(见于妊娠痒疹)或肿瘤(如淋巴瘤或白血病)患者。病因不明，可能与内分泌障碍有关。基本损害为风团样或多形红斑样丘疹，伴剧痒，搔抓后可出现表皮剥脱、血痂、色素沉着等变化。

【Histopathology】

The pathology change of prurigo is non-specific chronic inflammation, presenting as epidermal hyperkeratosis and parakeratosis, acanthosis, and intraepidermal edema. Mild intradermal edema and lymphocyte infiltration around the blood vessels can be seen in the dermis.

【组织病理学】

本病的病理变化为非特异性慢性炎症，表现为表皮角化过度及角化不全、棘细胞层肥厚、表皮内水肿、真皮内轻度水肿、血管周围有淋巴细胞浸润。

【Diagnosis and Differential Diagnosis】

According to the age of onset, predilection sites of the rash, wheal-like papules or papules, remaining firm papules after the initial rashes fade and intense itching, diagnosis can be easily made. However, it is necessary to determine the type of prurigo and to differentiate them from papular urticaria, dermatitis herpetiformis, scabies, lichen planus, primary cutaneous amyloidosis, verruca vulgaris, etc.

【诊断与鉴别诊断】

根据发病年龄、皮疹好发部位、只发风团样丘疹或丘疹、皮疹消退后遗留坚实的小丘疹、瘙痒剧烈，易于诊断。应确定痒疹的类型，并需与丘疹性荨麻疹、疱疹样皮炎、疥疮、扁平苔藓、原发性皮肤淀粉样变、寻常疣等病相鉴别。

【Treatment】

Avoidance of contributing factors is a crucial step in the management of this disease, for example preventing further insect bites, reducing local stimulation and treating the primary diseases.

(1) Topical therapy: the main purpose for the treatment of prurigo is to reduce the inflammation and relieve itching; therefore the application of topical glucocorticoids and keratolytics can be effective. For nodular lesions, intralesional injection of glucocorticoids may be more effective.

(2) Systemic therapy: antihistamines, procaine, vitamin C and calcium agents are all effective. A short term, low dosage regimen of glucocorticoids can be given when the treatment described above is not effective. UVA or PUVA may also be effective for intractable lesions.

(3) Physical therapy: starch baths or mineral baths can relieve the itching; prurigo nodularis can be treated with cryotherapy or laser, radioisotope or superficial X-ray therapy. UVA phototherapy or PUVA therapy are known to have some effect on recalcitrant lesions.

【治疗】

除去各种致病因素，治疗重在预防，如预防虫咬、避免局部刺激、治疗原发疾病等。

(1) 局部治疗　以消炎、止痒为主，也可以应用糖皮质激素和角质剥脱剂。结节性皮损采用糖皮质激素皮损内注射可能效果更好。

(2) 系统治疗　可应用抗组胺药、普鲁卡因、维生素 C、钙剂等。对上述方法疗效不佳的患者可短期系统使用小剂量糖皮质激素。顽固的病例可用 UVA 或 PUVA。

(3) 物理治疗　淀粉浴、矿泉浴可使瘙痒减轻，结节性痒疹可进行液氮冷冻、激光治疗、放射线同位素贴敷或浅 X 线放射治疗。UVA 光疗或 PUVA 治疗对顽固性皮损有一定疗效。

Section Three　Factitious Dermatitis

Factitious dermatitis is a self-inflicted skin disease caused by the intentional actions of the patients. This can occur on the skin, hair, nails or mucosa by mechanical means or chemical substances. These patients may intentionally hide their behavior when being interviewed by doctors.

【Etiology and Pathogenesis】

The condition is more commonly seen in females. Some studies have shown that factitious dermatitis is found more easily in health-care workers and their family members. Others consider this disease to be a behavioral dermatosis that reflects a mental illness.

【Clinical Manifestations】

Cutaneous lesions of factitious dermatitis vary with the irritant or irritants, which are most likely mechanical inducements rather than chemical substances. The skin lesions may sometimes resemble other dermatoses, but usually have a peculiar appearance with clear margins, mostly found asymmetrically in areas easily accessed by the hand. Erythema, vesicles, erosion and necrosis may appear locally, but lesions can show up as stab wounds with sharp angles and straight edges, or may be arranged eccentrically and irregularly, depending on the mechanical tools used, i. e., fingernails, knives, scissors and nails (Fig. 12-5). Chemical burns may exhibit a striped or guttate pattern. In any case the root cause of the damage is usually concealed by the patients.

第三节　人工皮炎

人工皮炎(factitious dermatitis)是指患者采用机械手段或化学物质,有意制造的自伤性皮肤损害,包括皮肤、毛发、指甲或黏膜。通常该类患者会有意识地隐蔽自己的行为。

【病因及发病机理】

女性多见,既往研究表明较多见于健康护理工作者和其家庭。也有人认为人工皮炎是精神性疾病的行为性皮肤病。

【临床表现】

人工皮炎的损害可因刺激物不同而相异,常见的刺激物多为机械性,少数为化学性的。皮损可类似其他皮肤病,但通常有明显的边界清楚的奇特外观,病变大多分布于手容易触及的部位,常不对称。患者以指甲或刀、剪、钉等利器机械性损伤皮肤,因此人为损害的形态常常是稀奇古怪的。局部可发生红斑、水疱、糜烂、坏死等,可呈刺伤外观,通常有尖角和直边,或呈离心性和不规则形状(图 12-5)。如因液体化学品灼伤,则可见到化学品在皮肤上流滴时造成的条状或点滴状的损害。患者常常隐瞒其损伤皮肤的行为。

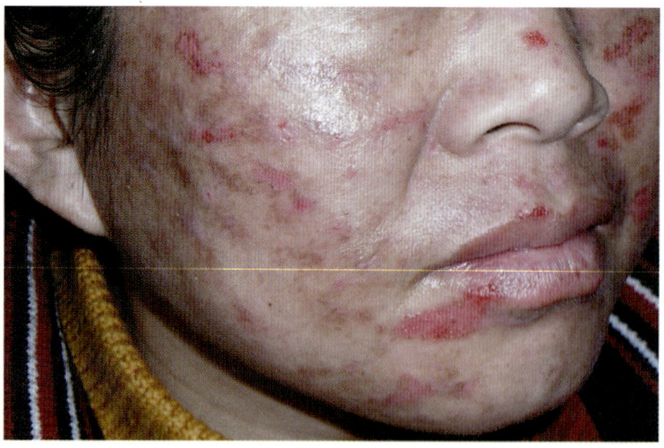

Fig. 12-5　Factitious dermatitis(图 12-5　人工皮炎)

【Diagnosis and Differential Diagnosis】

Since the patients tend to hide their self-inflicted skin behavior, it may be difficult to obtain a clear history to determine likely causative agents. Therefore one should seek the information from the family members of the patients for a diagnosis. When

【诊断与鉴别诊断】

常因患者隐瞒其自伤皮肤的行为,难得到明确的病史而造成诊断困难。如能从患者的家属那里取得真实的病史,将对诊断有重要意义。检查时如发现奇

peculiar skin lesions are found during examination on patients with hysterical personalities or behavior, which cannot be explained by accidental injury or by other causes, the primary diagnosis can be given.

特的皮肤损害，不能用意外损伤或其他原因解释，再加上患者有癔症性格或行为时，即可初步诊断。

【Treatment】

The primary target is nevertheless to first treat the dermatosis, and carefully analyze and record the patient's mental state. Proper treatment for psychosis should be given in time, and the prognosis of this disease is unpredictable.

【治疗】

首要治疗皮肤病、认真分析其精神状况，对精神性疾病应予及时治疗，本病预后难以估计。

Section Four　Lichen Simplex Chronicus

第四节　慢性单纯性苔藓

Lichen simplex chronicus is also known as neurodermatitis, which is a common chronic cutaneous neurological dysfunctional dermatosis. It is characterized by skin lichenification and paroxysmal intense itching.

慢性单纯性苔藓（lichen simplex chronicus）又称为神经性皮炎（neurodermatitis），是一种慢性常见的皮肤神经功能障碍性皮肤病。以皮肤的苔藓样变和阵发性剧痒为特征。

【Etiology and Pathogenesis】

The etiology of lichen simplex chronicus is still unclear, but central nervous system dysfunction is clearly related to the occurrence of the disease. The onset of this dermatosis is usually insidious, and develops gradually. Repeated mechanical friction or scratching of a localized area on a chronic basis will result in thickening of the skin. Psychiatric factors (fatigue, tension, anxiety, emotional agitation), endocrine dyscrasia, gastrointestinal dysfunction, nutrition or lack thereof, and topical irritation (woolen goods, chemicals, infections) have all been thought to be important in the development of or in the exacerbation of such conditions.

【病因及发病机制】

病因不明，中枢神经系统的功能失调与本病的发生有明显关系。起病常较隐伏，并逐渐进展，反复的机械性摩擦或搔抓某一局部会导致皮肤增厚，神经精神因素（疲劳、紧张、焦虑、情绪易激动）、内分泌失调、胃肠道功能障碍、饮食、局部刺激（毛织品、化学物品、感染病灶）都可能是主要的诱因或加重因素。

【Clinical Manifestations】

Lichen simplex chronicus is a chronic and recurrent skin disorder without exudate tendencies. The condition is divided into localized and disseminated types, according to the area (s) affected.

【临床表现】

本病呈慢性经过，易反复，无渗出倾向，根据病变范围分为局限型及播散型。

(1) Localized type:

Most commonly seen in young and middle-aged people. The disease has a predilection for the neck, extensor surfaces of the extremities, waist, eyelids, perineum, scrotum, pubic region, and external parts of the ear. At the beginning, the rash manifests as groups of flat papules, of millet to soybean size, round or polygonal in shape, and then these gradually infuse into lichenoid plaques with clear margins, red, brown or skin-colored, smooth or with very few scales on the surface (Fig. 12-6). It is characterized by intense itching, to the point of affecting sleep and work.

（1）局限型

多见于青壮年，皮疹好发于颈项、四肢伸侧、腰、眼睑、会阴、阴囊、阴阜、外耳等部。皮疹初为成群的粟粒至黄豆大小扁平丘疹，圆形或多角形，渐融合成边界清楚的苔藓样斑块，淡红、黄褐色或正常肤色，表面光滑或有少量鳞屑（图 12-6）。皮疹剧痒，影响睡眠和工作。

(2) Disseminated type:

This type has a predilection to occur in the adults and elders.

（2）播散型

①好发于成年人及老年人；②皮疹

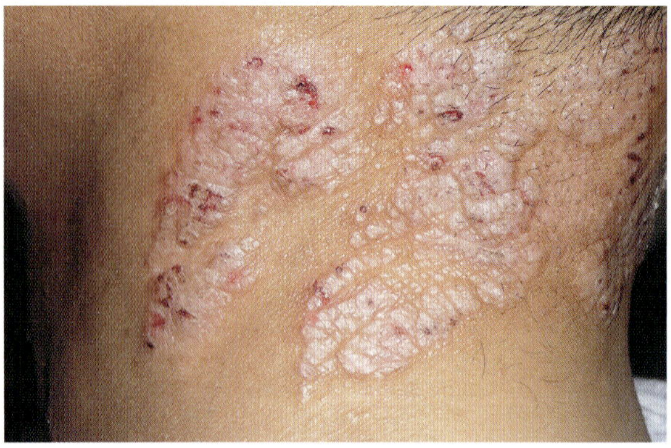

Fig. 12-6　Lichen simplex chronicus(图 12-6　慢性单纯性苔藓)

The lesions consist mainly of lichenifications, with pigmentation, accompanied by excoriation and blood crusts distributed all over the body. The patients usually experience intense itching.

散发全身;③皮损多呈苔藓样变,有色素沉着,伴有抓痕、血痂;④剧痒。

【Histopathology】

Hyperkeratosis, acanthosis, elongation of the rete ridges are displayed in the epidermis. In the dermis, capillary dilation, perivascular lymphocyte infiltration, fibroblast proliferation and fibrosis are present.

【组织病理】

表皮角化过度,棘层肥厚,表皮突延长,真皮毛细血管扩张,血管周围淋巴细胞浸润,成纤维细胞增生,呈纤维化。

【Diagnosis and Differential Diagnosis】

The diagnosis of lichen simplex chronicus is easy, based on the predilection sites, such as neck, lumbosacral, fossa cubitalia, classic lichenoid lesions, chronic course, no exudate tendency and intense paroxysmal itching. It should be differentiated from chronic eczema, atopic dermatitis, lichen planus, localized cutaneous amyloidosis, and pruritus.

【诊断与鉴别诊断】

根据皮疹好发于颈侧、腰骶部、肘窝等部位,皮损为典型的苔藓样变,病程呈慢性经过,无渗出倾向,阵发性剧痒的特点,易于诊断。需与慢性湿疹、特应性皮炎、扁平苔藓、局限性皮肤淀粉样变、瘙痒症等相鉴别。

【Treatment】

Make sure patients understand the etiology and course of the disease, remove the psychological stresses, stop cigarette smoking, alcohol consumption and spicy food, and avoid rubbing and other irritations such as over wash with hot water wherever possible. If underlying diseases such as athopia, gastrointestinal disorder, endocrine disorder and infections become involved, the patient should be treated accordingly. In severe cases, oral antihistamines, topical application or intralesional injection of glucocorticoid agents can be prescribed to control symptoms.

【治疗】

让患者了解本病的病因、病程,解除精神紧张,限制烟酒及辛辣食物,避免搔抓、摩擦、热水洗烫等方法止痒。如有精神衰弱、胃肠功能紊乱、内分泌紊乱、感染等,应给予相应治疗。严重者,可口服抗组胺类药、局部外用或皮损内注射糖皮质激素制剂。

Lie-hua DENG(邓列华)

Chapter Thirteen Erythematous, Papular and Squamous Dermatoses

第十三章 红斑、丘疹及鳞屑性皮肤病

Section One Erythema Multiforme

第一节 多形红斑

Erythema multiforme (EM) is an acute inflammatory dermatosis characterized by typical target-or iris-shaped lesions on the skin. Mucosa are often affected with a high recurrence rate.

多形红斑(erythema multiforme)是一种以靶形或虹膜状红斑为典型皮损的急性炎症性皮肤病,常伴发黏膜损害,易复发。

【Etiology】

The etiology of EM is complicated, but most cases can be traced to some infection, usually caused by herpes virus, especially in recurrent cases. While EM minor or herpes simplex-associated erythema multiforme (HAEM) is strongly associated with a preceding herpetic infection, Stevens-Johnson syndrome (SJS) and toxic epidermal necrolysis (TEN, see Chapter Eleven) are usually induced by medications. Mycoplasma pneumoniae is the second major cause of EM but may be the major cause of pediatric EM. Nevertheless, some overlaps exist in this spectrum of diseases. For example, herpes virus accounts for 6% to 10% of SJS cases, and mycoplasma is responsible for up to 25% of cases. Other causative factors include chronic infective diseases, foods, and physical factors such as cold, sunlight, and radiation. The characteristic lesions may also be found in other diseases such as rheumatic fever, connective tissue diseases, malignant tumors, etc.

【病因】

病因复杂,大多数多形红斑的病例与感染有关,疱疹病毒是最常见的原因,尤其是复发的病例。轻型多形红斑或单纯疱疹相关的多形红斑与疱疹病毒感染明显有关,而 Stevens-Johnson 综合征和中毒性表皮坏死松解症常表现为药物的不良反应(参见第十一章)。肺炎支原体是多形红斑的次要原因和儿童多形红斑的重要致病原因。然而,这一病谱有重叠,6%～10%的 Stevens-Johnson 综合征的病因是疱疹病毒,而 25%的是支原体。慢性感染病灶、食物及物理因素(如寒冷、日光、放射线等)均可引起本病,某些疾病(风湿热、结缔组织病、恶性肿瘤等)也可出现多形红斑样皮损。

【Pathogenesis】

The pathogenesis of EM remains unclear. However, recent studies suggest that cell-mediated immune reactions may play an important role in pathogenic process, as activated T lymphocytes are found in lesions of EM. The epidermis is infiltrated with $CD8^+$ T or suppressed T-cells, whereas the dermis displays a slight influx of $CD4^+$ helper T-cells. EM minor is closely associated with HLA-DQ3 while EM major is more often related to abnormalities in drug metabolism.

【发病机制】

多形红斑的发病机制还不清楚。近年研究则认为细胞介导的免疫反应在多形红斑的发病中起重要作用,多形红斑皮损中有激活的 T 细胞,其中 $CD8^+$ T 细胞或抑制性 T 细胞在表皮中占主导地位,而 $CD4^+$ 辅助 T 细胞则主要分布于真皮。此外还发现轻型多形红斑与 HLA-DQ3 密切相关,而重型多形红斑则与药物异常代谢相关。

【Clinical Manifestations】

EM occurs most often in children and young women during spring or fall. It is a self-limiting disease but will frequently recur. The onset is acute, and prodromal symptoms include chills, fever, headache, weakness of the limbs, arthralgia, and myalgia. The eruptions tend to be polymorphous composed of erythematous macules, maculopapules, papules, vesicles, bullae, purpura, and

【临床表现】

多累及儿童和青年女性。春秋季节易发病,病程自限性,但常复发。常起病急,前驱症状可有畏寒、发热、头痛、四肢乏力、关节及肌肉酸痛。皮损呈多形性,可有红斑、斑丘疹、丘疹、水疱、大疱、紫癜和风团等,这些皮损可同时出现。根

wheals that may all appear simultaneously. EM can be broadly classified into erythema-papule type EM, vesicle-bulla type EM, and EM major (Stevens-Johnson syndrome) by its variant clinical manifestations.

据皮损形态不同可将本病分为红斑-丘疹型、水疱-大疱型及重症型。

(1) Erythema-papule type EM: this is the most common type of EM, characterized by mild systemic symptoms and high recurrence rate. It begins with papules and sharply demarcated, vivid red, round or oval erythema varying in size from 0.5 to 1.0 cm, appearing predominantly on the face, neck, and extensor surfaces of the distal extremities. The rashes then extend gradually on its borders to form a typical "target-" or "iris-" like lesion. These lesions are usually dark red and wheal-like, with a duskier, purpuric center. In severe cases, vesicles may occur centrally (Fig. 13-1). The mucosa of the oral cavity or of the eyes can be involved in this type of EM. Most patients report mild pruritus, pain or burning. The lesions often resolve within 2-4 weeks, leaving transient hyperpigmentation.

(1) 红斑-丘疹型　此型常见，发病较轻，全身症状不重，但易复发。好发于面颈部、四肢远端伸侧皮肤，皮损主要为丘疹和红斑，初为 0.5～1.0 cm 大小圆形或椭圆形水肿性红斑，颜色鲜红，境界清楚，向周围逐渐扩大；典型皮损为暗红色斑或风团样皮损，中央为青紫色或为紫癜，严重时可出现水疱，形如靶形或虹膜样皮损(图 13-1)。口腔、眼等黏膜也可被累及。有瘙痒或轻度疼痛和灼热感。皮损 2～4 周消退，可留有暂时性色素沉着。

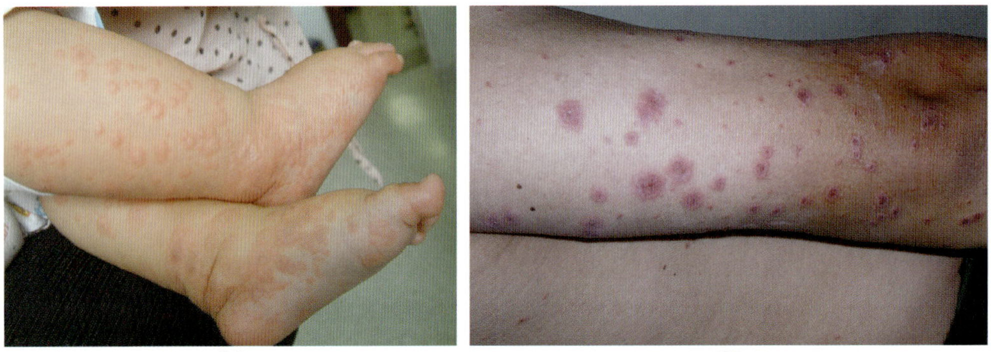

(a)　　(b)

Fig. 13-1　Erythema-papule type EM(图 13-1　红斑-丘疹型多形红斑)

(2) Vesicle-bulla type EM: the vesicle-bulla type EM often evolves from the erythema-papule type EM, accompanied by apparent systemic symptoms. Serous vesicles, bullae, and hemorrhagic bullae surrounded by dark red halos often appear on the skin of the distal extremities (Fig. 13-2), and may quickly spread centripetally to the entire body surface. Mucosa of the oral cavity, nose, eyes, and genitalia may be involved, with accompanying erosions and severe exudation.

(2) 水疱-大疱型　此型常由红斑-丘疹型发展而来，常伴全身症状。皮损为浆液性水疱、大疱或血疱，周围有暗红色晕(图 13-2)。除四肢远端外，可向心性扩散至全身，口、鼻、眼及外生殖器黏膜也可出现糜烂，渗出较严重。

(3) EM major: this is also known as Stevens-Johnson syndrome. In contrast to the two types of EM described above, EM major is characterized by a sudden onset, extensive skin lesions, and severe internal organ involvement. The lesions start with vivid or dark red iris-like edematous, erythematous macules or ecchymosis that enlarge and coalesce, quickly spreading over the entire body. Vesicles, bullae, or hemorrhagic lesions can develop over the surface of the erythematous macules or ecchymosis. Nikolsky's sign is

(3) 重症型　此型又称为 Stevens-Johnson 综合征，与上述两型不同，重症型多形红斑发展急骤，皮损广泛，有严重的内脏受累。皮损为水肿性鲜红色或暗红色虹膜样红斑或瘀斑，迅速扩大，相互融合，泛发全身，其上出现水疱、大疱或血疱，尼氏征阳性。累及口腔、眼睛、外阴、肛门等多部位黏膜(图 13-3)，口腔黏

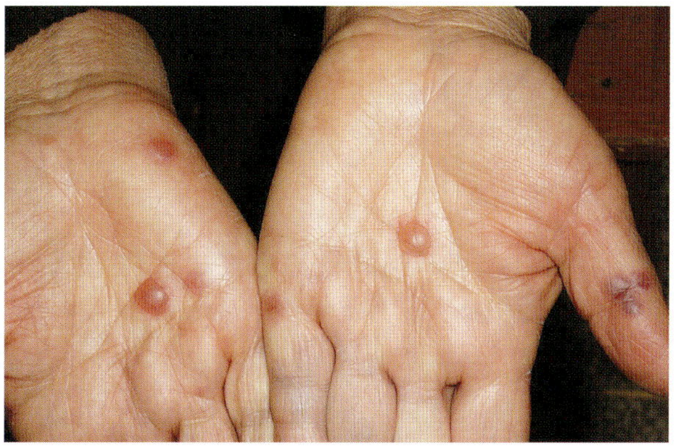

Fig. 13-2　Vesicle-bulla type EM(图 13-2　水疱-大疱型多形红斑)

positive. The mucous membranes are extensively affected throughout the body, including the oral cavity, eyes, genitalia, anus, etc. (Fig. 13-3). On the oral mucosa, erosive areas are typically covered by gray-white pseudomembranes. Visceral involvement includes pneumonia, gastrointestinal hemorrhage, necrotic pancreatitis, and liver damage. Septicemia may be caused by secondary infections. This serious condition may quickly lead to organ failure without proper treatment. The mortality rate of EM major is 5%-15% in severe cases when untreated.

膜可发生糜烂，表面可出现灰白色假膜，可导致肺炎、消化道出血等。可发生坏死性胰腺炎、肝功能损害，也可因继发感染引起败血症，若不及时抢救，短时期可进入衰竭状态，死亡率为5%～15%。

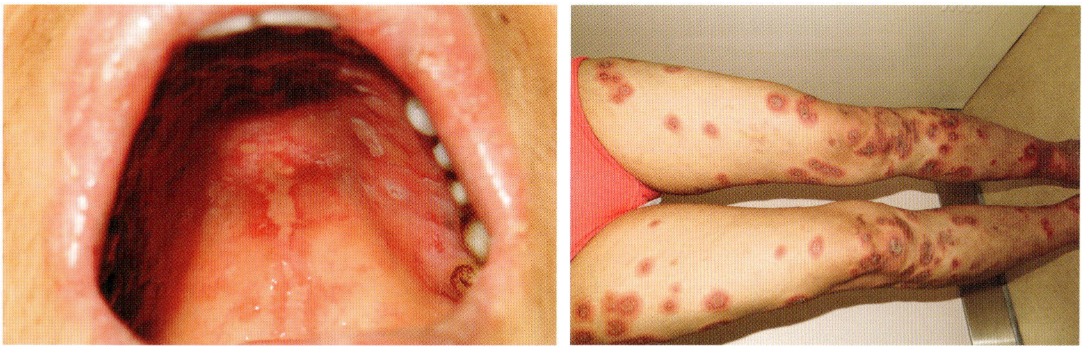

(a)　(b)

Fig. 13-3　EM major(图 13-3　重症型多形红斑)

【Histopathology】

The histopathologic features of EM vary with the specific clinical types. The main changes are keratinocyte necrosis, liquefaction degeneration of the basal cells; subepidermal vesiculation; edema, dilated vessels, extravasation of red blood cells, and infiltration of lymphocytes and a few eosinophils around the blood vessels in the upper dermis.

【组织病理】

各型的组织病理因临床类型不同而有所差异，基本改变为角质形成细胞坏死，基底细胞液化变性，表皮下水疱形成，真皮上部水肿、血管扩张、红细胞外渗、血管周围淋巴细胞及少数嗜酸粒细胞浸润。

【Diagnosis and Differential Diagnosis】

EM is usually diagnosed and classified by its clinical appearance and the patient's age. A skin biopsy may be needed occasionally to confirm the diagnosis. Among the conditions to be considered in a differential diagnosis for EM are chilblains, lupus

【诊断与鉴别诊断】

根据本病的发病年龄及典型临床表现，可对本病进行诊断和分型，必要时进行活检以助确诊。本病应与冻疮、红斑狼疮、大疱性类天疱疮、二期梅毒等进行

erythematosus, bullous pemphigoid, secondary syphilis, etc.

【Treatment】

Treatment of EM begins with determination and removal of the trigger factors (e. g., a suspected medication), although that is not always possible. Mild cases typically exhibit fewer symptoms and therefore often need no treatment at all beyond removal of the causative agent(s) since the lesions will heal spontaneously within weeks. However, patients with EM major need to be treated immediately since this may be life-threatening.

(1) Topical treatment: the principle of topical treatment includes the use of anti-inflammatory, astringent, and antipruritic agents along with prophylactic measures to prevent infection. Topical calamine lotion and glucocorticoid creams may be considered for lesions without erosions. 3% boric acid or normal saline moist compresses can be used for lesions with exudation and erosions. 0.5% neomycin cream and mupirocin ointment is effective in preventing bacterial infections in ulcerations. In severe cases, special care must be taken for mucous eruptions of the oral cavity and eyes to prevent eyelid adhesion and possible blindness.

(2) Systemic treatment: in mild cases, oral antihistamines may be sufficient. However, in severe cases, systemic glucocorticoids, given early and in adequate doses, will probably shorten the course of the disease. For example, oral prednisone 1-1.5 mg/(kg · d), or an equivalent amount of intravenous hydrocortisone, dexamethasone, or methylprednisolone may be used. Once the acute inflammation has been controlled, the dose of any of these glucocorticoids should be gradually reduced. At the same time, supportive measures such as maintaining electrolyte levels and fluid balance, and ensuring adequate caloric intake, particularly including protein and vitamins, are all helpful. Antibiotics should be given only in response to a specifically diagnosed bacterial infection. If the EM recurs frequently, antiherpetic medications (acyclovir, valacyclovir, or famciclovir) can be used for suppression. If patients with recurrent EM show no response to all the treatments above, azathioprine may need to be considered, or even thalidomide if the patient is not pregnant.

鉴别。

【治疗】

应积极寻找病因(尽管不容易),疑为药物引起者应停用一切可疑致敏药物。轻症患者多在数周内自愈,仅需对症处理;重症患者可危及生命,需积极治疗。

(1) 局部治疗　治疗原则为消炎、收敛、止痒及预防感染。无糜烂处可外用炉甘石洗剂或糖皮质激素霜,有渗出糜烂时可用3%硼酸溶液或生理盐水湿敷,局部破溃者可外用0.5%新霉素霜、莫匹罗星软膏等防止感染,加强口腔、眼部护理,防止眼睑粘连和失明。

(2) 系统治疗　轻症患者口服抗组织胺药。重症患者应尽早给予足量糖皮质激素以缩短病程,如泼尼松 1～1.5 mg/(kg · d)口服或等效剂量的氢化可的松、地塞米松、甲泼尼龙静滴,病情控制后逐渐减量,同时给予支持疗法,维持水、电解质平衡,保证热量、蛋白质和维生素的需要;合并感染时及时给予抗感染治疗。如果多形红斑复发频繁,可用抗疱疹病毒药物(阿昔洛韦、万昔洛韦或泛昔洛韦)抑制疗法,如果病情复发其他方法治疗无效时,可选用硫唑嘌呤或沙利度胺治疗(患者未妊娠)。

Section Two　Psoriasis

Psoriasis is a common, chronic, recurring, inflammatory disease of the skin, whose typical lesions are scaly plaques and papules. The disorder may affect people of any age, but it is most common in young adults, with both sexes affected equally. The morbidity rate of psoriasis in the world population is 0.1%-3.0%; in China specifically it is 0.123%. Psoriasis becomes worse or relapses

第二节　银　屑　病

银屑病(psoriasis)是一种常见的易复发的慢性炎症性皮肤病,典型皮损为鳞屑性斑块和丘疹,可发生于任何年龄,但多发生于青壮年,无明显性别差异,自然人群发病率为 0.1%～3%,我国为 0.123%。春冬季节易复发或加重,而夏

during winter and spring for most people and tends to improve in summer and autumn.

【Etiology and Pathogenesis】

The exact cause of psoriasis is not yet fully understood. Today, most hypotheses start from the assumption that the disease is an immune-mediated disorder, in which the hyperproliferation of keratinocytes is the consequence of interaction among multigenetic components and environmental factors.

(1) Genetic factors: studies on census, pedigree, genetics (e. g., twin studies), and HLA all strongly suggest a genetic predisposition to psoriasis. About 20% of psoriatic patients report a family history of the condition, and those patients usually report an onset earlier in life than those with no family history. The chance for an offspring to develop psoriasis is about 16% if one parent is affected by the disease and the likelihood goes up to 50% when both parents are affected. Histocompatibility antigen studies have shown that the class Ⅰ antigens A1, A13, A28, B13, B17, B37, and Cw6 (in which Cw6 shows the strongest association with this disease), and the class Ⅱ antigen DR7 are more likely to be expressed in psoriatic patients as compared to normal individuals. The genome-wide linkage analysis has identified seven loci since 1994 that have been associated with psoriasis. These are located at distinct chromosomal regions 1p, 1q, 3q, 4q, 6p, 17q, and 19p. Recent developments in genomic wide association studies in China indicate that genetic polymorphisms at the epidermal differentiation complex of chromosomes also contribute to psoriatic susceptibility.

(2) Environmental factors: epidemiological studies for the prevalence of psoriasis in monozygotic twins suggest a 70% chance of one twin developing psoriasis if the other has developed the condition, but only a 20% chance for dizygotic twins. These findings indicate that the hereditary factors are neither a necessary nor a sufficient trigger for psoriasis, and that environmental factors also play an important role in its occurrence. Several common environmental factors may influence the onset or the severity of psoriasis, including infection, emotional stress, trauma, surgical incision, pregnancy, cigarette smoking, and certain types of drugs.

Infections are considered a major promoting or exacerbating factor for psoriasis, particularly for the guttate variant. A history of acute streptococcal infection of the throat is common in guttate psoriasis, and furthermore the condition of the skin is always improved with antibiotic therapy.

(3) Immune factors: one distinct histopathological feature of psoriasis vulgaris is lymphocyte and monocyte infiltrates, especially T lymphocytes found in the dermis at psoriatic lesions under

秋季节多缓解。

【病因及发病机制】

银屑病的确切病因尚不清楚。目前认为，银屑病是遗传因素与环境因素等多种因素相互作用的多基因遗传病，通过免疫介导的共同通路最终引起角质形成细胞发生增殖。

（1）遗传因素　人口调查、家系、双胞胎及 HLA 研究均支持银屑病的遗传倾向。20%左右的银屑病患者有家族史，且有家族史者发病早于无家族史者。父母一方患有银屑病，其子女银屑病的发病率为 16%左右；而父母同患银屑病时，其子女银屑病的发病率为 50%。HLA 系统中Ⅰ类抗原 A1、A13、A28、B13、B17、B37 和 Cw6 和Ⅱ类抗原 DR7 在银屑病患者中表达的频率高于正常人，其中 Cw6 位点与银屑病相关最明显。自 1994 年以来，通过全基因组扫描已经确定的银屑病易感基因位点有位于 1p、1q、3q、4q、6p、17q、19p 等区域的 7 个位点。最新的中国基因组关联分析研究表明，表皮分化区域基因多态性也影响银屑病的易感性。

（2）环境因素　流行病学研究显示，双生子中同卵双生子共患银屑病占 70%，双卵双生子共患银屑病只有 20%，提示仅有遗传因素不足以引起发病，环境因素在诱发银屑病中起重要作用。最易促发或加重银屑病的因素是感染、精神紧张、外伤、手术、妊娠、吸烟和某些药物作用等。

感染一直被认为是诱发或加重银屑病的主要因素，例如，点滴型银屑病发病前常有咽部急性链球菌感染史，给予抗生素治疗后病情常可好转。

（3）免疫因素　寻常型银屑病皮损处淋巴细胞和单核细胞浸润明显，尤其 T 细胞真皮浸润是银屑病的重要病理特

microscopy. Perhaps these T lymphocytes participate in the occurrence and progress of the disease even though their precise role in the pathologic process is still unclear. It has been speculated that activated T lymphocytes move from the dermis into the epidermis and then release a variety of cytokines (IL-1, IL-6, IL-8, IFN-γ, TNF-α, IL-17, IL-23, etc.). These signaling molecules will induce keratinocyte proliferation and at the same time will cause more inflammation-producing cells to arrive at the site of the original proliferation, which in turn attracts even more T lymphocytes, inducing further inflammation, and then repeating the cycle. An accelerated proliferation of epidermal basal cells is another pathophysiological characteristic of psoriasis, presenting with cell mitotic cycle durations as short as 37.5 hours, and an epidermal turnover time of 3-4 days. Other histopathological changes include parakeratosis and the lack of a granular layer.

征，说明T细胞参与该病的发生与发展，虽然其在银屑病病理过程中的确切作用还不清楚。推测皮损中活化的T细胞从真皮移入表皮并释放出一系列细胞因子(IL-1、IL-6、IL-8，IFN-γ、TNF-α，IL-17，IL-23等)，这些信号分子刺激角质形成细胞增生，导致更多的炎症产生细胞到达增生部位，并因此吸引更多的T细胞，进一步加重炎症反应，如此循环。银屑病的病理生理的一个重要特点是表皮基底层角质形成细胞增殖加速，丝状分裂的周期缩短为37.5 h，表皮更替时间缩短为3～4天，组织病理出现角化不全，颗粒层消失。

【Clinical Manifestations】

Psoriasis may be categorized into psoriasis vulgaris, psoriasis arthropathica (psoriatic arthritis), pustular psoriasis, and erythrodermic psoriasis according to their respective clinical patterns. More than 99% of cases can be classified as psoriasis vulgaris, and the remaining three types listed above (except psoriatic arthritis) are frequently the result of the exacerbation of psoriasis vulgaris caused by triggers such as strongly irritating topical treatments, the sudden withdrawal of systemic glucocorticoids or immunosuppressants, infection, or even mental stress.

【临床表现】

根据银屑病的临床特征，可分为寻常型、关节病型(银屑病关节炎)、脓疱型及红皮病型，其中寻常型占99%以上，其他类型(银屑病关节炎除外)多由寻常型银屑病外用刺激性药物，突然停止系统使用糖皮质激素、免疫抑制剂以及感染，精神压力等诱发。

(1) Psoriasis vulgaris: this type of psoriasis begins with red papules or maculopapules that gradually becomes well-demarcated red plaques in a variety of morphologic patterns (guttate, nummular, geographic, ostraceous, etc.), covered with thick silvery scales (Fig. 13-4). Scraping off these lamellar scales is similar to scraping off wax drippings ("candle wax" phenomenon), which then exposes a shiny reddish translucent film on the surface of the lesion (film phenomenon). When the scales are removed completely, punctuate spots of bleeding appear within a few seconds (Auspitz's sign). The candle wax phenomenon, the reddish film, and the punctate bleeding are all important diagnostic clues for psoriasis. The degree of pruritus will vary from patient to patient.

(1) 寻常型银屑病(psoriasis vulgaris)

初期皮损为红色丘疹或斑丘疹，逐渐扩展成为境界清楚的红色斑块，有多种形态(如点滴状、钱币状，地图状、蛎壳状等)，上覆厚层银白色鳞屑(图13-4)，刮除成层鳞屑，犹如轻刮蜡滴(蜡滴现象)，刮去银白色鳞屑可见淡红色发光半透明薄膜(薄膜现象)，剥去薄膜可见点状出血(Auspitz征)。蜡滴现象、薄膜现象和点状出血对银屑病有诊断价值。自觉不同程度瘙痒。

The lesions may occur anywhere on the body surface, with a predilection for the extensor surfaces of the limbs, scalp, nails, and especially in the elbows, knees, and sacral region. The lesions are generally symmetrical in their distribution. Lesions on the scalp are usually covered with thicker scales than the lesions on exposed body sites, particularly along the margin of the hair. Hairs on the lesions usually have a bunched appearance (Fig. 13-5). The lesions

皮损可发生于全身各处，以四肢伸侧、头皮、甲，特别是肘部、膝部、骶尾部最为常见，常呈对称性。头皮皮损鳞屑一般比身体暴露部位厚，常超出发际，头发呈束状(图13-5)；乳房下、腋下和肛门、生殖器等皱褶部位皮损为无鳞屑的境界清楚红斑(反向性银屑病)。甲可受

in the intertriginous areas such as the inframammary region, axilla, anus, and genitalia show well demarcated erythema but a lack of scales (psoriasis inversa). The nails frequently show a pattern of multiple pits on the surface of the nail plate (thimble-like pitting) and onycholysis (separation of the nail from the nail bed), sometimes with subungual hyperkeratosis.

累,表现为"顶针状"凹陷,甲剥离,有时可见甲下角化过度。

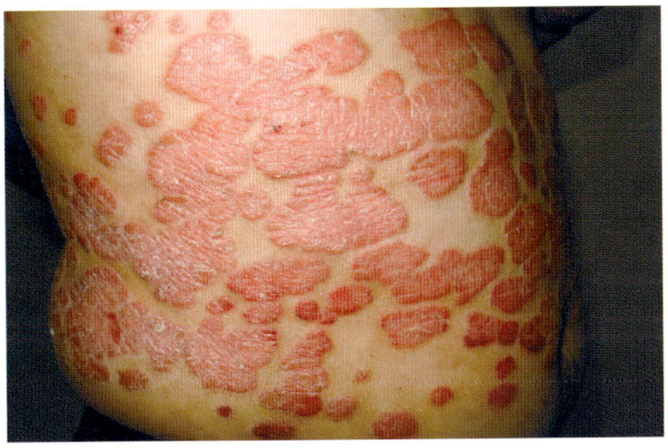

Fig. 13-4　Psoriasis vulgaris-plaque type
(图 13-4　寻常型银屑病-斑块状)

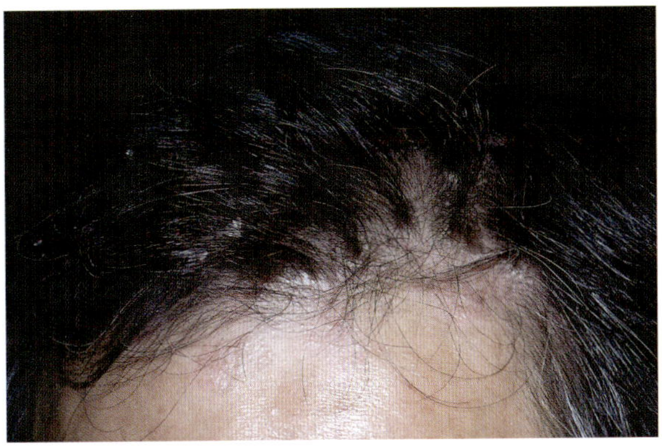

Fig. 13-5　Bunched hair in psoriasis vulgaris
(图 13-5　寻常型银屑病束状发)

The clinical course of psoriasis vulgaris can be divided into three phases: ①active stage, where new lesions appear continuously but old lesions remain unresolved. Here inflammatory infiltration is so prominent that redness is often seen around the lesions. A characteristic feature is an isomorphic response (Koebner's phenomenon), where new lesions appear on sites injured by needle injections, scratching, surgical incision, etc.; ② quiescent stage, where there are no signs of aggravation or remission for the old lesions, but no new lesions appear, and finally; ③resolution stage, in which the inflammation of the skin decreases, demonstrated by shrinking or flattening of the lesions and post-inflammatory hypo- or hyperpigmentation.

寻常型银屑病根据病情发展可分为三期:①进行期,新皮损不断出现,旧皮损无消退,皮损炎性浸润明显,周围皮肤可发红,针刺、搔抓、手术及其他损伤可导致受损部位出现典型的银屑病皮损,称为同形反应或 Koebner 现象;②静止期,原皮损稳定,无新皮损出现;③退行期,皮损缩小变平,炎症基本消退,遗留色素减退或色素沉着斑。

Acute guttate psoriasis (also known as eruptive psoriasis) most commonly affects the young. Usually this condition appears as an acute process and follows a streptococcal upper respiratory tract infection. The lesions often start appearing on the trunk and spread over the entire body within a few days. There are numerous small red papules covered by a few silvery scales (Fig. 13-6). Pruritus varies with the patient. This type of psoriasis usually can be resolved in a few weeks with an appropriate treatment, but a small subgroup of patients will develop chronic psoriasis.

急性点滴状银屑病(guttate psoriasis)又称为发疹性银屑病,常见于青年,发病前常有上呼吸道的链球菌感染病史。起病急骤,数天可泛发全身,躯干突然出现大量小的红色丘疹,覆以少许鳞屑(图 13-6),痒感程度不等。经适当治疗皮疹可在数周内消退,少数患者可转化为慢性病程。

(2) Psoriasis arthropathica: it is also known as psoriatic arthritis. 5%-8% of patients with psoriasis eventually develop psoriatic arthritis. Psoriatic arthritis typically runs a chronic course. Psoriasis lesions usually precede the onset of joint

(2) 关节病型银屑病(psoriasis arthropathica)　又称为银屑病关节炎,有 5%～8%的银屑病患者可出现关节炎症状。关节病型银屑病病程为慢性,关

symptoms. Psoriatic arthritis can affect any particular joint, but is more common in the large joints of the lower extremities, the distal joints of the fingers and toes, and even the back and sacroiliac joints. Marked nail damage often accompanies digital joint arthritis. The involved large joints may resemble a rheumatoid arthritis with joint malformation (Fig. 13-7). However, unlike rheumatoid arthritis, the rheumatoid factor in psoriatic arthritis is usually negative. Patients with spine and sacroiliac joint involvement show a strong correlation with HLA-B27 antigen.

节病变常在皮损后出现。任何关节均可受累，尤其是下肢的大关节和指、趾远端关节，甚至脊椎和骶髂关节。伴有明显甲损害者更易出现指、趾关节炎；大关节可出现关节畸形，类似类风湿关节炎(图13-7)，但与后者不同的是银屑病关节炎的类风湿因子常为阴性。脊椎及骶髂关节受累患者常与 HLA-B27 存在密切关联。

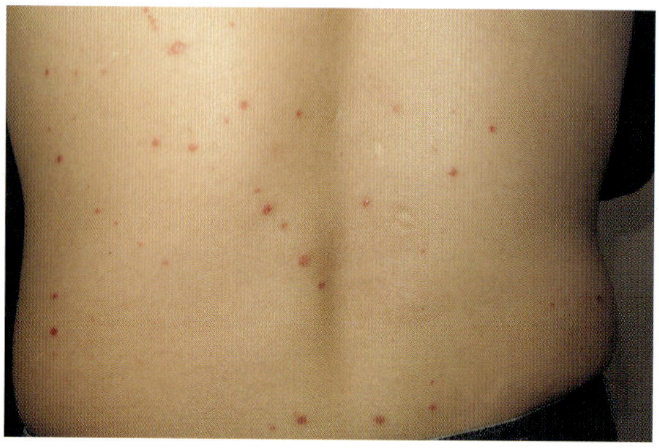

Fig. 13-6　Psoriasis vulgaris-guttate type
(图 13-6　寻常型银屑病-点滴状)

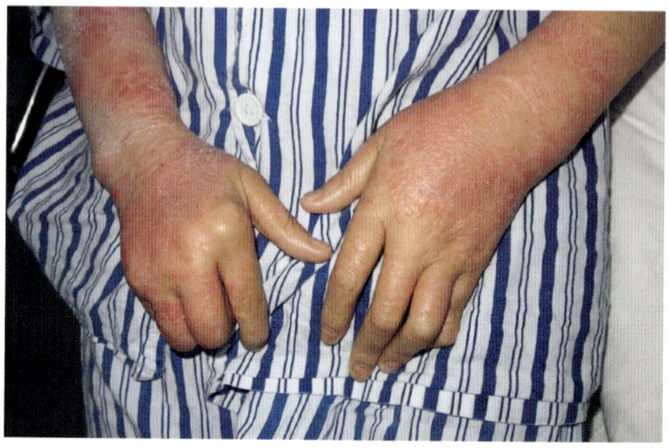

Fig. 13-7　Psoriasis arthropathica
(图 13-7　关节病型银屑病)

(3) Erythrodermic psoriasis: this type of psoriasis appears as inflammation and exfoliation of the skin over most of the body surface, in which the small normal-appearing areas look like islands. There is generalized redness and swelling of the skin covered with bran-like scales (Fig. 13-8) which may be accompanied by fever and lymphadenopathy. The course of this condition is more persistent and also is more likely to recur.

(3) 红皮病型银屑病(erythrodermic psoriasis)　红皮病型银屑病表现为全身大部分皮肤广泛的炎症和脱屑，皮肤呈弥漫性潮红、浸润肿胀并伴有大量糠状鳞屑，其间可有正常皮肤(皮岛)(图13-8)，可伴有发热、全身淋巴结肿大等全身症状。病程较长，易复发。

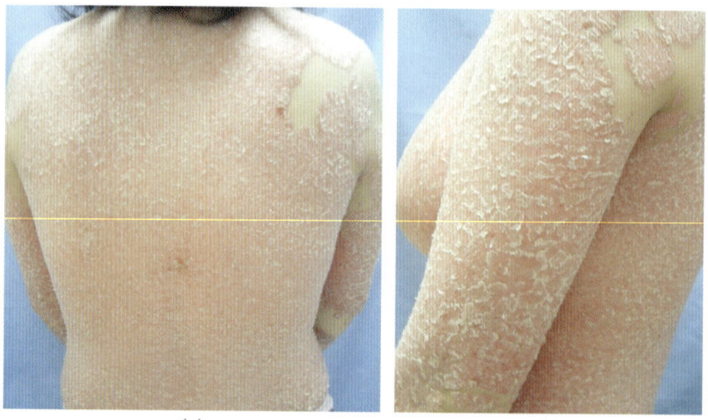

(a)　(b)

Fig. 13-8　Erythrodermic psoriasis(图 13-8　红皮病型银屑病)

(4) Pustular psoriasis: there are two forms of pustular psoriasis, generalized pustular psoriasis and localized pustular psoriasis.

① Generalized pustular psoriasis: here the pustules have a

(4) 脓疱型银屑病(pustular psoriasis)　脓疱型银屑病分为泛发性和局限性两型。

①泛发性脓疱型银屑病：常急性发

sudden onset and can spread quickly over the entire body. The yellow to yellow-white, pinhead to milium-sized, superficial, sterile, and small pustules occur in groups around old lesions of psoriasis vulgaris or in normal skin, and may coalesce, thereby forming large lakes of pus (Fig. 13-9). The skin around the pustules is often red, inflamed and can be painful. Attacks are often preceded by chills, high fever, and other constitutional signs. The patients may present fissured tongue, and thickened and turbid fingernails or toenails when the tongue and nails are involved. Usually the pustules dry up to form crusts within 1-2 weeks, but recurrent attacks can take place. The conditions can be progressive in some patients, presenting with severe symptoms and death from secondary infection and multiple organ failure.

病，皮损可迅速发展至全身，在寻常型银屑病皮损或正常皮肤上迅速出现黄色或黄白色的针尖至粟粒大小浅表性无菌性小脓疱，常密集分布融合成脓湖（图 13-9），脓疱周边的皮肤常发红，伴有炎症，可有疼痛感，常伴有寒战、高热等全身症状。患者可有沟状舌，指、趾甲受累时可出现肥厚浑浊。经过 1～2 周脓疱可干燥结痂，病情缓解，但可反复发作。患者可因继发感染、全身衰竭而死亡。

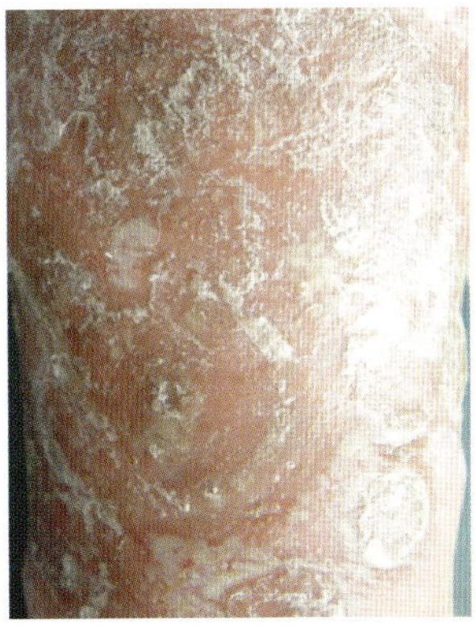

Fig. 13-9　Generalized pustular psoriasis(图 13-9　泛发性脓疱型银屑病)

② Localized pustular psoriasis: the sterile pustules are distributed symmetrically at the palms and soles only, especially in the thenar or hypothenar eminences or in the central portion of the palms and soles. For each episode, crops of small pustules develop on the erythematous areas and may rupture and crust or desquamate within 1-2 weeks, but new pustules will keep appearing under the scales. The process runs a chronic course with only a slight chance of significant remission. Nails are often involved in these patients, with punctate depressions, transverse grooves, longitudinal ridges, onycholysis, and subungual pus.

②局限性脓疱型银屑病：皮损局限于手掌及足跖，对称分布，好发于大、小鱼际及掌跖中部，皮损为成批发生在红斑基础上的无菌小脓疱。经 1～2 周脓疱破裂、结痂、脱屑，新脓疱又可在鳞屑下出现，病程慢性，经久不愈，仅少数显著消退。甲常受累，可出现点状凹陷、横沟、纵嵴、甲剥离及甲下积脓等。

【Histopathology】

The microscopic features of psoriasis reflect the increased cellular activity of the epidermis and the alterations of the dermis. Common changes in psoriasis vulgaris include hyperkeratosis and parakeratosis, with Munro microabscesses within the parakeratotic areas in the epidermal layer; thinning or absence of a granular layer; acanthosis with elongation of the epidermal rete ridges; clubbing of the dermal papillae; thinning of the prickle layer just above the clubbed dermal papillae; dilation of the capillaries in the

【组织病理】

银屑病的镜下特征表现为表皮细胞的活动性增加和真皮的改变。寻常型银屑病的常见表现为表皮角化过度伴角化不全，角化不全区可见 Munro 微脓肿，颗粒层变薄或消失，棘层增厚，表皮突向下延伸；真皮乳头呈杵状，其上部棘层变薄，真皮乳头内及真皮浅层毛细血管扩张充血，血管周围可见淋巴细胞为主的

papillae and superficial dermis; and dermal perivascular inflammatory cell infiltration consisting primarily of lymphocytes. Bearing similar histopathologic features to psoriasis vulgaris, erythrodermic psoriasis usually has more prominently dilated capillaries in the superficial dermis. Pustular psoriasis more likely presents Kogoj spongiform pustules, but parakeratosis and elongated rete ridges are less marked in that case.

炎症细胞浸润。红皮病型银屑病的病理变化为真皮浅层血管扩张充血更明显，其余变化与寻常型银屑病相似。脓疱型银屑病表现为Kogoj微脓肿，但角化不全及表皮突延伸不明显。

【Diagnosis and Differential Diagnosis】

The diagnosis of psoriasis and clinical classification is mainly based on the clinical appearance. Biopsy of skin lesions may be necessary to make a definitive diagnosis when only some suggestions of psoriasis are seen. It should be differentiated from the following diseases.

(1) Seborrheic dermatitis: psoriatic lesions on the scalp should be differentiated from seborrheic dermatitis. The latter usually has a less demarcated erythema with fine greasy yellow scales. The hair may be sparse, thin, or shedding, but never has a bunched appearance.

(2) Tinea capitis: should be differentiated from psoriasis with scalp lesions. The lesions of tinea capitis are commonly covered with grayish white flaky scales. Hairs are easily shed or broken off. Fungal examination is positive for tinea capitis, and the condition occurs less frequently in adults but more commonly in children.

(3) Secondary syphilids: in most cases, patients have a history of primary chancre. Typical lesions for secondary syphilis are brown in color and occur frequently on the palms and soles, but are accompanied by oral lesions, alopecia areata, condylomata lata, and lymphadenopathy.

(4) Pityriasis rosea: this should be differentiated particularly from guttate psoriasis. The lesions of pityriasis rosea are oval, rather than circular, and tend to align with skin lines. Scales are typically collarette in form. A large precursor patch (herald patch) often precedes the generalized rashes by a few days to a few weeks. Lesions usually occur on the upper trunk.

(5) Nummular eczema: for this condition the lesions are less well defined than the plaques of psoriasis. There may be exudation or crust, but no candle wax phenomenon; however, the pruritus is always quite intense. Lesions commonly appear on the trunk and the distal extremities but less commonly on the scalp and extensor surfaces of elbows and knees.

【诊断与鉴别诊断】

主要根据典型的临床表现进行诊断和分型，当诊断可疑时有必要进行皮损活检以明确诊断。需要与以下疾病进行鉴别。

(1) 脂溢性皮炎　头皮银屑病应与之鉴别，后者皮损为边缘不清的红斑，上覆细小、黄色、油腻的鳞屑。毛发可稀疏、变细、脱落，但无束状发。

(2) 头癣　头癣常需与头皮银屑病相鉴别。头癣的皮损上覆灰白色糠状鳞屑，有脱发和断发，易查到真菌。成人少见，多见于儿童。

(3) 二期梅毒疹　有硬下疳史，皮损呈褐色，典型皮损位于掌跖部位，可伴有口腔改变、斑秃、扁平湿疣及淋巴结肿大。

(4) 玫瑰糠疹　玫瑰糠疹特别需与点滴型银屑病相鉴别。前者皮损为椭圆形，而非圆形，沿皮纹走行。鳞屑呈衣领形，在发疹前几天到几周常先出现一母斑(先驱斑)。皮疹多于躯干上部出现。

(5) 盘状湿疹　皮疹境界不如银屑病那样清楚，可有渗出和结痂，无蜡滴现象，瘙痒剧烈。皮疹很少累及头皮、肘膝伸侧，易累及躯干及肢体远端。

【Treatment】

(1) Topical therapy: almost all of the topical glucocorticoid preparations (creams or ointments) are significantly effective in

【治疗】

(1) 局部治疗　局部应用糖皮质激素霜剂或软膏治疗银屑病有明显疗效，

suppressing the skin lesions. However, long-term use of high potency glucocorticoids, especially on large areas of the body, guarantees the development of side effects, which may include hypertension, osteoporosis, diabetes, peptic ulcers, and psychological changes. Regarding psoriasis treatment, more caution is needed because a "rebound" effect (pustular or erythrodermic psoriasis) can accompany the abrupt cessation of systemic use of glucocorticoids. Retinoic acid at concentrations of 0.025%-0.1% in cream or 0.05%-0.1% at Tazarotene gel has been proven to be considerably effective in plaque-type psoriasis. Alternatively, the vitamin D3 analogues, such as calcipotriene, are also effective, but should not be applied on the face and skin folds. The skin conditions may even better improved when treated with a combination formula of calcipotriene and betamethasone dipropionate than with either agent alone. Various keratoplastic preparations such as coal tar, anthralin, or salicylic acid ointment may be helpful in some cases.

应注意其不良反应，大面积长期应用强效或超强效激素可引起全身不良反应，如高血压、骨质疏松、糖尿病、消化性溃疡及精神症状。用激素治疗银屑病时须特别注意"反跳"效应，在突然停用糖皮质激素后甚至可诱发脓疱型或红皮病型银屑病；维A酸霜剂常用浓度为0.025%～0.1%，其中0.05%～0.1%的他扎罗汀凝胶治疗斑块型银屑病疗效较好；维生素D3衍生物如钙泊三醇也有较好的疗效，但不宜用于面部和皱褶部皮肤；钙泊三醇、倍他米松软膏联合外用比两种成分单独应用效果好。也可选用各种角质促成剂(如焦油制剂、蒽林软膏、水杨酸软膏等)。

(2) Systemic treatment: retinoids are suitable for the treatment of all types of psoriasis, such as etretinate administered orally in dosages of 0.75-1.0 mg/(kg·d). Immunosuppressants are prescribed mostly for erythrodermic psoriasis, pustular psoriasis, and psoriasis arthropathica. The medication frequently used in this group is methotrexate given orally in a dosage of 10-25 mg/week for an adult patient, but the weekly dosage may not exceed 50 mg. Other choices include cyclosporine and tacrolimus. Antibiotics should be given to patients with apparent infections or generalized pustular psoriasis. Oral or parenteral glucocorticoid treatment is indicated only for severe or life-threatening forms of the condition, such as erythrodermic psoriasis, acute psoriasis arthropathica, and generalized pustular psoriasis; it is usually not indicated for psoriasis vulgaris. The dose of glucocorticoids should be reduced when being combined with immunosuppressive agents or retinoids. To minimize side effects and to increase effectiveness, glucocorticoids should be used for a short time and the patient gradually weaned in order to avoid the rebound effect described above. Immunomodulators may be used in patients with compromised cellular immunity.

(2) 系统治疗　维A酸类药物适用于各型银屑病，如阿维A酯0.75～1.0 mg/(kg·d)口服；免疫抑制剂主要用于红皮病型、脓疱型、关节病型银屑病，常用药为甲氨蝶呤，成人剂量为每周10～25 mg口服，每周剂量不超过50 mg，也可用环孢素、他克莫司等；伴有明显感染或泛发性脓疱型银屑病患者应使用抗生素类药物；糖皮质激素主要用于严重的和危及生命的银屑病，如红皮病型银屑病、急性关节病型银屑病和泛发性脓疱型银屑病，一般不用于寻常型银屑病，与免疫抑制剂、维A酸类药物联用可减少用药剂量，为尽量减少副作用和提高疗效，应短期应用并逐渐减量以防止病情反跳；免疫调节剂可用于细胞免疫功能低下者。

(3) Biological agents: a number of biological agents have been used recently for the treatment of patients with severe psoriasis and psoriatic arthritis. The mechanism focuses mainly on two targets: T-cells, and cytokines such as TNF-α, IL-12/23 and IL-17. Two biological agents (alefacept and efalizumab) target T-cell function, but the use of the latter has been discontinued because of severe side effects. Other biological agents are infliximab, adalimumab, and

(3) 生物制剂　近年来生物制剂被引入治疗中重度银屑病和银屑病关节炎。主要针对两个靶点：T细胞和细胞因子，包括TNF-α、IL-12/23和IL-17。2种干扰T细胞功能的生物制剂(阿法西普和依法利珠单抗，依法利珠单抗因严重副作用而停用)，3种抑制TNF-α的单

golimumab (which are monoclonal antibodies inhibit TNF-α), etanercept (which inhibits soluble TNF-α receptors), and ustekinumab (which acts directly on IL-12 and IL-23 P40 subunits). Because these agents are expensive and also have potential for secondary infections such as tuberculosis, physicians should carefully consider the therapeutic indications and contraindications .

克隆抗体(英利昔单抗、阿达木单抗和戈利木单抗),1种抑制TNF-α的可溶性受体((依那西普),1种直接作用于IL-12和IL-23的p40亚基的单克隆抗体(优特克单抗,ustekinumab)。其价格昂贵且可能导致潜在的感染如结核病的发生,因此要严格掌握其适应证和禁忌证。

(4) Physical therapy: photochemotherapy (PUVA, psoralen plus UVA), UVB radiation (particularly narrowband UVB), excimer laser and bath therapy may all be used, together or separately.

(4) 物理治疗　光化学疗法(PUVA,即补骨脂联合UVA)、UVB光疗(尤其是窄波UVB)、准分子激光、浴疗等均可联合或单独应用。

(5) Traditional Chinese herbs: traditional Chinese herbs may be helpful when the condition of the patient warrants their use.

(5) 中医治疗　可根据病情给予中药治疗。

Section Three　Parapsoriasis

第三节　副银屑病

Parapsoriasis refers to a group of cutaneous diseases with unknown causes that are characterized by papules, erythema, and scales; by the absence of subjective symptoms; and by resistance to normal treatment. Since the clinical features always mimic psoriasis, they are grouped under the name of parapsoriasis.

副银屑病(parapsoriasis)是一组病因不明,以丘疹、红斑、鳞屑为特征的皮肤病,常无自觉症状,不易治愈。由于其临床特征与银屑病相似,故称为副银屑病。

【Etiology】

【病因】

The causative agents remain unclear for this group of diseases. No clear correlations with environmental factors or infection have been found to date, although there may be indications of a sensitized state arising from a focal inflammatory reaction. Nevertheless, adequate evidence is still lacking for this or any other theory.

本病病因不明,与环境因素和感染的关系也不明显,可能与病灶致敏有关,尚缺乏确切证据。

【Clinical Manifestations】

【临床表现】

This disease is sub-classified into four types based on the clinical features that present. They are parapsoriasis guttata, parapsoriasis en plaques, parapsoriasis lichenoides, and parapsoriasis varioliformis.

根据临床表现本病分为四型:点滴型、斑块型、苔藓样型及痘疮样型。

(1) Parapsoriasis guttata: this is the most common form of parapsoriasis, and is also known as pityriasis lichenoides chronicus. Usually the lesions affect both sides of the trunk, thighs and upper arms. The scalp, face, palms, soles, and mucous membranes are rarely affected. Typical lesions of parapsoriasis guttata are light red or brownish-red, pinpoint to milium sized macules or maculopapules, with fine flaky scales covering the surface of the lesions (Fig. 13-10). However, unlike psoriasis there is no punctate bleeding when scraping the scales (Auspitz's sign). The course of the disease tends to be chronic. However, the condition tends to resolve spontaneously in most cases after a certain time.

(1) 点滴型副银屑病(parapsoriasis guttata)　此型最为常见,又称为慢性苔藓样糠疹。好发于躯干两侧、大腿和上臂等,常不累及头、面、掌跖及黏膜。其典型皮疹为淡红色或红褐色针尖至粟粒大小的斑疹或斑丘疹,表面覆着细薄鳞屑(图13-10)。不同于银屑病,本病无点状出血(Auspitz征)。病程慢性,多数患者经一段时间后常可自愈。

(2) Parapsoriasis *en* plaques: this is a less common form of

(2) 斑块型副银屑病(parapsoriasis

parapsoriasis. The lesions more often affect the trunk and proximal extremities, while generally sparing the mucosa. This disease is characterized by well-defined; round, oval or irregular; and light red or brownish plaques covered by fine flaky scales (Fig. 13-11). Eruptions can be mildly itchy or asymptomatic but lichenoid atrophy or hypertrophy may occur after years or decades. Some patients with large plaque lesions may progress into mycosis fungoides (MF).

en plaques) 此型较为少见,常累及躯干及四肢近端,不侵犯黏膜。皮损表现为边界清楚的淡红色或褐色斑块,圆形、椭圆形或不规则形,上覆细薄鳞屑(图 13-11),可轻度瘙痒或无症状。病久历经数年或数十年后可出现苔藓样萎缩或增厚,少数大斑块型副银屑病可发展为蕈样霉菌病。

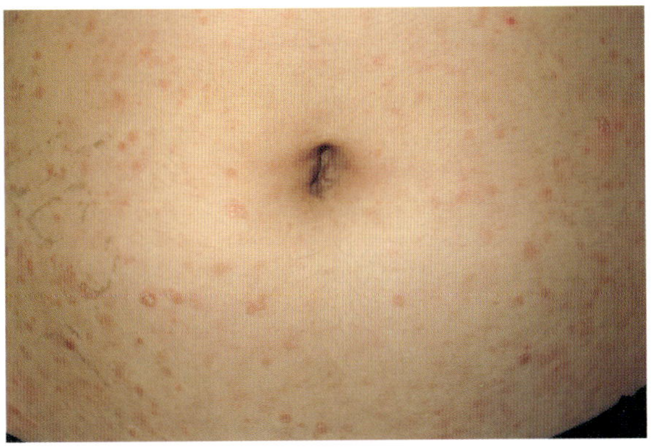

Fig. 13-10 Parapsoriasis guttata

(图 13-10 点滴型副银屑病)

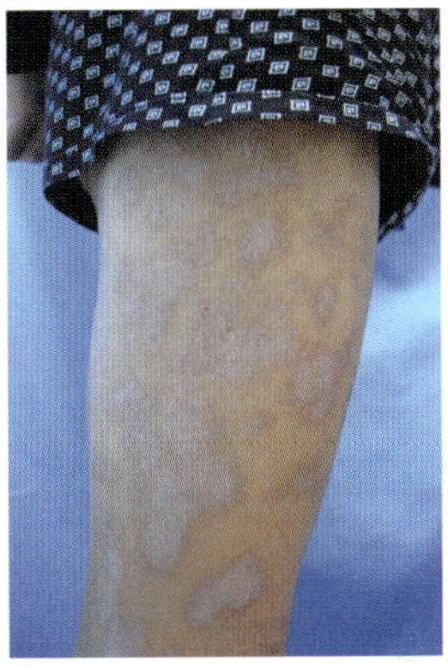

Fig. 13-11 Parapsoriasis en plaques

(图 13-11 斑块型副银屑病)

(3) Parapsoriasis lichenoides: the rash often appears from both sides of the neck, the trunk, and the breasts. The lesions are characterized by red or brownish-red, small, flat-topped, lichenoid scaly papules that tend to coalesce into reticular plaques. This form of parapsoriasis will eventually develop into mycosis fungoides for most cases. However, this disease was also mistakenly classified into the parapsoriasis en plaques group in some studies.

(3) 苔藓样型副银屑病(parapsoriasis lichenoides) 皮疹常累及颈部两侧、躯干、乳房等处。典型皮损为红色或红褐色扁平苔藓样鳞屑型小丘疹,聚集成网状斑块。此型多数可发展为蕈样霉菌病,有报道将其归为斑块型副银屑病中。

(4) Parapsoriasis varioliformis: this is also known as pityriasis lichenoides *et* varioliformis acuta (PLEVA). The rash often involves the trunk, the flexor surfaces of the upper extremities and the axillary regions. The lesions are characterized by yellowish or brownish-red, pinpoint to soybean-sized, round papules and papulovesicles. Vesicles can also be seen on occasions. The lesions tend to be hemorrhagic, with necrosis and crusting (Fig. 13-12). Once healing has begun, they leave superficial varioliform scars. The disease is self-limiting and chronic in most cases.

(4) 痘疮样型副银屑病(parapsoriasis varioliformis) 痘疮样型副银屑病又称为急性痘疮样苔藓状糠疹(pityriasis lichenoides *et* varioliformis acuta, PLEVA),常累及躯干、上肢屈侧及腋下。典型皮损为淡黄色或红褐色针尖至黄豆大小圆形丘疹、丘疱疹,偶有水疱,易出血、坏死及结痂(图 13-12),愈后可留有痘疮样表浅瘢痕。病程自限,多数为慢性。

【Diagnosis and Differential Diagnosis】

Parapsoriasis is difficult to diagnosis at both the clinical and histological levels, especially when it is necessary to make a definite differential diagnosis between parapsoriasis and an early stage of mycosis fungoides. With a chronic course and typical clinical features, parapsoriasis should be considered only when other erythrosquamous dermatoses have been excluded. The differential diagnosis includes MF, psoriasis, lichen planus, pityriasis rosea,

【诊断与鉴别诊断】

无论从临床和病理本病的诊断均较困难,尤其是必须与早期蕈样霉菌病进行鉴别诊断时更是如此。根据慢性病程及皮损特点,难以诊断为其他红斑鳞屑型皮肤病时应考虑本病。本病应与蕈样霉菌、银屑病、扁平苔藓、玫瑰糠疹、丘疹坏死性结核疹及淋巴瘤样丘疹病等疾病

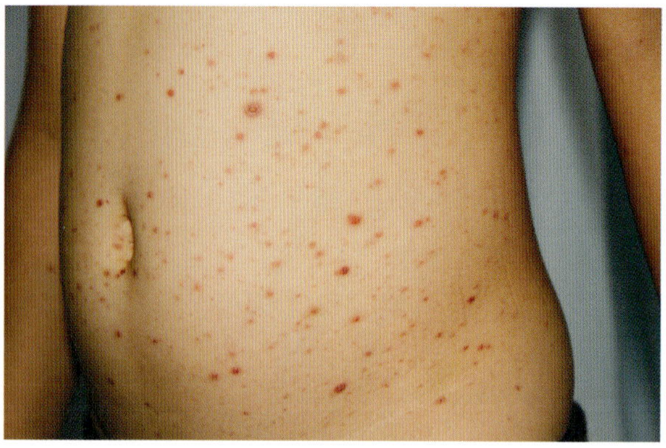

Fig. 13-12　Parapsoriasis varioliformis(图 13-12　痘疮样型副银屑病)

papulonecrotic tuberculid, and lymphomatoid papulosis, etc.

【Treatment】

There is no special long-term treatment for this disease, but it can be managed reasonably well by the following methods.

(1) Topical therapy: topical glucocorticoid creams or ointments or keratolytic agents (urea ointment, tretinoin creams, etc.) can be effective.

(2) Systemic therapy: antihistamines, vitamin complexes, and methotrexate may be sufficient to treat patients with small plaques; however, oral glucocorticoids may bring a more effective clinical response in severe cases of parapsoriasis varioliformis, especially when combined with immunomodulators. For pityriasis lichenoides, systemic antibiotics such as erythromycin can be effective.

(3) Physical therapy: phototherapy with either broad or narrow-band UVB or PUVA or herbal bath therapy can be effective in inducing remission.

鉴别。

【治疗】

目前本病尚无特效治疗方法。可采用以下方式综合治疗。

(1) 局部治疗　局部外用糖皮质激素霜剂或软膏或角质剥脱药(尿素软膏、维A酸霜等)有效。

(2) 系统治疗　抗组胺药、多种维生素、甲氨蝶呤等均可应用，特别是皮损为较小的斑块，病情严重的痘疮样副银屑病可口服糖皮质激素，亦可应用免疫调节药。对苔藓样糠疹系统使用抗生素(如红霉素)有效。

(3) 物理疗法　宽波或窄波UVB或PUVA及中药沐浴疗法均有效。

Section Four　Pityriasis Rosea

Pityriasis rosea is a common, mildly inflammatory cutaneous disorder. It typically presents as oval, rose-colored macules or maculopapules covered with fine scales. The course of pityriasis rosea is often self-limiting.

【Etiology】

The cause of pityriasis rosea is unclear. It is believed to be associated with a viral infection (HHV-7 and HHV-6), and cellular immune response may also be involved in the occurrence of this disease.

【Clinical Manifestations】

Pityriasis rosea most commonly affects people between the ages of 15 and 40, and is especially common in spring or autumn. Women are more frequently affected. The disease usually begins with a single, rose-colored, oval erythematous macule on the trunk,

第四节　玫瑰糠疹

玫瑰糠疹(pityriasis rosea)是一种常见的轻度炎症性皮肤病。其典型皮损为覆有糠状鳞屑的椭圆形玫瑰红色斑疹、斑丘疹，病程常为自限性。

【病因】

本病病因不明，现认为与病毒(人类疱疹病毒HHV-7及HHV-6)感染有关，细胞免疫反应可能参与了本病的发生。

【临床表现】

本病好发于15～40岁人群，春秋季多发，女性患者多见。大多数情况下，可在躯干、颈部或四肢的近心端先出现一孤立的玫瑰红色椭圆形红斑(前驱斑或

neck, or proximal extremities, known as a herald patch or mother patch. This precursor patch is typically 1-3 cm in diameter and covered with fine scales. After 1-2 weeks, numerous variable sized red patches begin to appear on the trunk, arms, legs or other parts of body. Similar to the herald patch, these rashes are usually in a symmetrical distribution, round or oval, 0. 2-1. 0 cm in diameter, covered by collarette scales at the borders. Typically, the long axes of the macules run along the lines of cleavage of the skin (Fig. 13-13)

母斑)，直径为 1～3 cm，上覆有糠状鳞屑。常在 1～2 周后，躯干、四肢及身体其他部位将逐渐出现大小不等的红色斑片，形同母斑，常对称分布，圆形或椭圆形，直径为 0. 2～1 cm，边缘覆衣领状鳞屑，长轴与皮纹平行(图 13-13)。

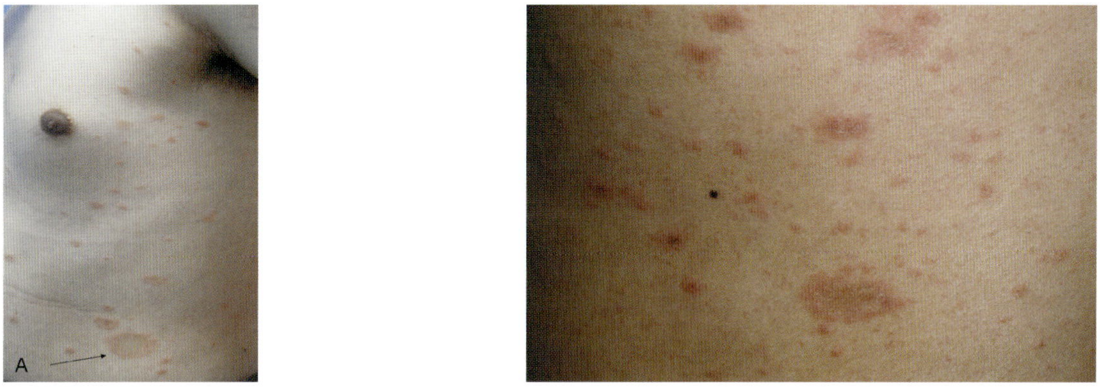

(a)　(b)

Fig. 13-13　Pityriasis rosea, herald patch is arrowed

(图 13-13　玫瑰糠疹，箭头所示为母斑)

The majority of patients with this disease will have mild or severe pruritus, and occasionally there may be other symptoms such as fatigue and aching. The disease is often self-limiting. The patches usually begin to fade spontaneously in 2-4 weeks and often clear in 6-8 weeks. In a minority of patients, the patches may last several months or years. Recurrence is uncommon once the skin heals.

多数患者可伴有或轻或重的瘙痒，偶有疲劳、疼痛等其他症状。本病常为自限性，斑疹常在 2～4 周开始自行消失，6～8 周痊愈，也有少数患者数月至数年仍不痊愈，但一般愈后不再复发。

【Histopathology】

Mild acanthosis, focal parakeratosis, and extravasation of erythrocytes into the epidermis can be revealed under microscopy. Spongiosis may be present in acute cases and accompanied by a perivascular infiltrate of lymphocytes.

【组织病理】

轻度棘层增厚，灶性角化不全及红细胞外渗入表皮。急性病例可有海绵形成，血管周围有淋巴细胞浸润。

【Diagnosis and Differential Diagnosis】

Diagnosis of pityriasis rosea should always be made based on its typical clinical features, and a skin biopsy should only be carried out to confirm the diagnosis when necessary. The condition should be distinguished from nummular eczema, tinea corporis, secondary syphilis, drug eruption, psoriasis, and seborrheic dermatitis, etc.

【诊断与鉴别诊断】

根据典型临床表现不难诊断，必要时可进行病理活检协助诊断。本病应与盘状湿疹、体癣、二期梅毒、药疹、银屑病、脂溢性皮炎等疾病进行鉴别。

【Treatment】

In general, treatment for patients with mild symptoms is unnecessary, but oral antihistamines and topical glucocorticoids may be prescribed to treat the symptoms. In severe cases with generalized lesions, a short course of systemic glucocorticoids can

【治疗】

症状轻者无需特殊处理，瘙痒明显者可口服抗组胺药或局部外用糖皮质激素缓解瘙痒；对于严重的全身泛发的患者可以短程系统应用糖皮质激素，特别

be of considerable help, especially when combined with UVB therapy, which is beneficial for resolving the eruptions and speeding the progress of the disease.

是联合照射 UVB 能促进皮损的消退,缩短病程。

Section Five Pityriasis Alba

第五节 白色糠疹

Pityriasis alba is also known as pityriasis simplex. This is a common skin disease which occurs mostly in children and is characterized by round or oval, scaly hypopigmented patches on the face.

白色糠疹(pityriasis alba)又称为单纯糠疹,是一种好发于儿童的常见皮肤病,以面部圆形或椭圆形鳞屑性色素减退斑为特征。

【Etiology】

The cause of pityriasis alba is unknown. Malnutrition, vitamin deficiency, and exposure to sunlight may be triggers for this disease.

【病因】

病因尚不清楚,营养不良、维生素缺乏和日晒均可诱发本病。

【Clinical Manifestations】

This condition is mostly seen in children, but young adults may also be affected occasionally. Both sexes are affected with approximately equal frequency. The onset usually occurs in spring, and subsides in summer or autumn. Typical lesions are white or light pink, round to oval, hypopigmented patches appearing on the face, upper arms, neck, or shoulders. The patches vary in size, but are normally a few centimeters in diameter, with ill-defined borders and usually flat edges, covered by a few fine bran-like scales (Fig. 13-14). Pityriasis alba is usually asymptomatic except for a few patients which exhibit a mild pruritus. The course tends to be chronic and the lesions can resolve spontaneously after months or years, but relapses do occur occasionally.

【临床表现】

好发于儿童,青壮年亦可发病,无性别差异,与季节有一定关系,多在春天起病,夏秋后消退。皮损为好发于面部、上臂、颈或肩部,白色或淡粉红色的卵圆或圆形的色素减退斑,斑片大小不等,通常数厘米大小,边界不清楚,边缘一般无高起,上覆少量细小糠状鳞屑(图 13-14),一般无自觉症状,部分患者可有轻度瘙痒。病程慢性,经数月或更长时间自行消退,但可复发。

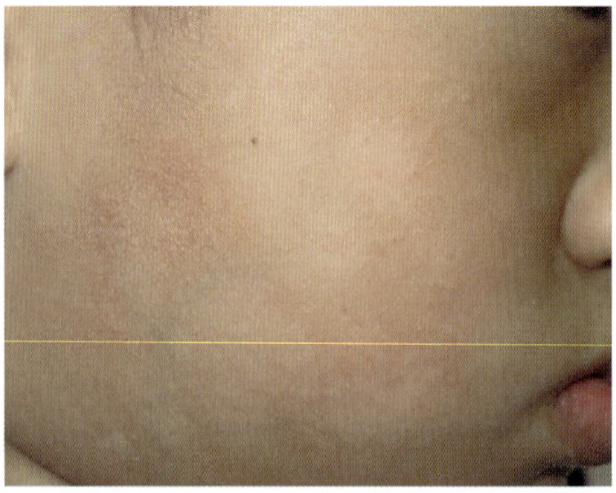

Fig. 13-14 Pityriasis alba(图 13-14 白色糠疹)

【Diagnosis and Differential Diagnosis】

The diagnosis of pityriasis alba is often based on the typical clinical manifestations. It should be distinguished from vitiligo and nevus anemicus.

【诊断与鉴别诊断】

根据典型临床表现诊断不难。本病应与白癜风和贫血痣鉴别。

【Treatment】

No special treatment is required as the disease tends to be resolved once the season changes. Vitamin B complex can be helpful. Topical emollient and 5% sulfur ointment are recommended. 0.03%-0.1% tacrolimus ointment speeds the resolution of rashes.

【治疗】

皮损可自行消退，无须处理。随着季节的改变此病可以自愈。可口服复合B族维生素，亦可局部外用润滑剂、5%的硫黄软膏。有报道0.03%～0.1%他克莫司软膏可以加速皮损消退。

Section Six　Lichen Planus

第六节　扁平苔藓

Lichen planus is an acute or chronic, recurrent, pruritic, inflammatory cutaneous disease. It is characterized by small, polygonal, violaceous, flat-topped papules occurring predominantly on the wrists, ankles, and mouth.

扁平苔藓(lichen planus)是一种急性或慢性、复发性、瘙痒性、炎症性皮肤病，典型皮损为小的多角形紫红色扁平丘疹，常累及腕部、踝部及口腔。

【Etiology and Pathogenesis】

The exact cause of lichen planus remains unknown, but immunologic factors appear to be important. Chronic viral infections (e.g., chronic hepatitis C infection), stress, anxiety, allergic reactions to medications (such as for the treatment of hypertension, coronary heart diseases, arthritis), and even some autoimmune diseases (e.g., vitiligo, chronic graft-versus-host disease, malignant tumors) have all been implicated as etiological factors of lichen planus. However, to date, none of them provides a satisfactory explanation for the certain antigens that trigger immune response and lead to the histopathological changes observed. A sufficient number of patients with lichen planus report a positive family history, indicating the existence of a genetic predisposition for this disease in the general population.

【病因及发病机制】

病因不明。免疫因素可能起重要作用。慢性病毒感染(如慢性丙型肝炎)，压力，精神紧张，对治疗高血压、冠心病和关节炎的药物的过敏反应，一些自身免疫性疾病(白癜风、慢性移植物抗宿主病反应、恶性肿瘤等)均可为扁平苔藓的发病因素。但迄今为止，还没有令人满意的解释来阐明某种抗原触发的免疫反应引起的相应的组织学改变。有相当数量的患者具有家族史，表明可能与遗传因素有关。

【Clinical Manifestations】

The lesions commonly affect the flexural surfaces of the extremities, the mouth, and the genital mucous membranes. The typical lesions of lichen planus are elevated, violaceous, polygonal, flat-topped papules (Fig. 13-15). Lesions begin as pinpoint papules and expand to 0.5-1.0 cm sized plaques, and larger lesions may be seen on rare occasions. Examining the surface of the plaques reveals grayish-white punctate or reticular streaks (Wickham striae) that are best seen by applying a drop of mineral oil to the surface. Lesions can appear abruptly or gradually. The small papule tends to heal, leaving a prominent dark black or brownish hyperpigmentation, which can persist for a long period.

Nail changes are present in 5%-10% of patients. Pterygium of the nail is characteristic for nail lichen planus. Longitudinal grooving, onycholysis, ridging, splitting, and a characteristic midline fissure are some of the manifestations of nail lichen planus (Fig. 13-16). The mucous membranes, especially the oral mucosa, are

【临床表现】

本病多累及四肢屈侧、口腔和生殖器黏膜。典型皮损可表现为高起的紫红色多角形扁平丘疹(图13-15)，损害开始为针头大小的丘疹，以后扩展至0.5～1.0 cm大小的斑块，偶尔可见较大的损害。其表面可见白色小点或网状白色条纹(Wickham纹)，用一滴矿物油滴于皮损表面能更好显示此特点。皮损可突然出现或逐渐形成。小丘疹愈合后可遗留暗黑色或暗褐色色素沉着，持续较长时间。

有5%～10%的病例有甲的损害，翼状胬肉的形成是甲扁平苔藓的特征，甲扁平苔藓可表现为甲纵沟、甲剥离、甲皱嵴、甲分裂和特征性甲中线裂纹(图13-16)。黏膜，尤其是口腔黏膜常受到侵

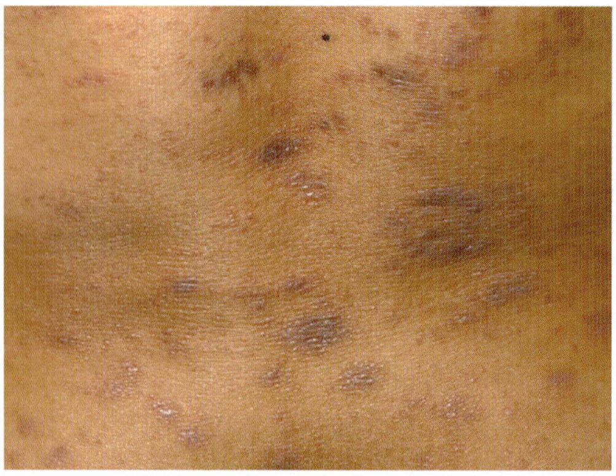

Fig. 13-15 Lichen planus(图 13-15 扁平苔藓)

frequently affected. Oral lesions may be reticulate (Fig. 13-17), atrophic, or ulcerative (erosive).

犯。口腔损害可为网状(图 13-17)、萎缩或溃疡(糜烂)。

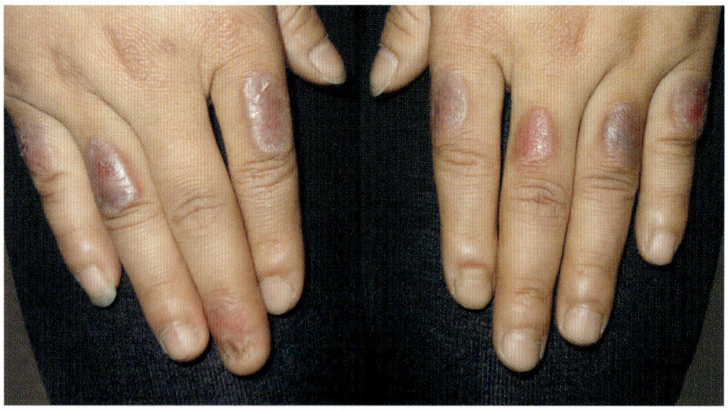

Fig. 13-16 Lichen planus-nail involved
(图 13-16 扁平苔藓-累及指甲)

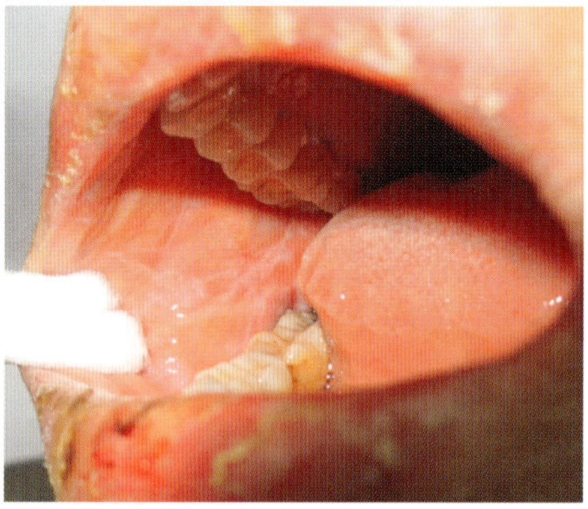

Fig. 13-17 Lichen planus-oral lesions
(图 13-17 扁平苔藓-口腔损害)

For acute lichen planus, the lesions will usually subside after several weeks to months. But some patients have a chronic, recalcitrant course with several episodes over a span of years. Patients with oral mucous membrane involvement are usually difficult to cure.

急性扁平苔藓患者的病程可持续数周或数月,但部分患者呈慢性、顽固病程,并可在数年内反复发作。口腔黏膜的皮损较难治愈。

There are several important clinical variants that have been described, such as acute generalized lichen planus, chronic localized lichen planus, hypertrophic lichen planus, lichen planus atrophicans, bullous lichen planus, pigmented lichen planus, and lichen planus-lupus erythematosus overlap syndrome, etc.

通常临床将此病分为多种亚型,如急性泛发性扁平苔藓、慢性局限性扁平苔藓、肥厚性扁平苔藓、萎缩性扁平苔藓、大疱性扁平苔藓、色素性扁平苔藓、扁平苔藓-红斑狼疮重叠综合征等。

【Histopathology】

The histopathological changes are distinctive for this disease. The diagnostic features are: ① hyperkeratosis, wedge-shaped hypergranulosis, irregular acanthosis, liquefaction degeneration of the basal cells, and necrotic and apoptotic keratinocytes (colloid bodies, Civatte bodies) in the lower part of the epidermis; ② a solid band of infiltrates mainly composed of lymphocytes, histiocytes, and some melanophages in the upper dermis; ③ colloid bodies and melanophages in dermal papilla.

【组织病理】

组织病理改变具有特征性,表现为:①角化过度,颗粒层楔形增厚,不规则棘层增厚,基底细胞液化变性,表皮下部可见坏死和凋亡的角质形成细胞(胶样小体,Civatte 小体);②真皮上部淋巴细胞和组织细胞呈致密带状浸润,并可见部分噬色素细胞;③真皮乳头层可见胶样小体及噬黑素细胞。

【Diagnosis and Differential Diagnosis】

A distinct rash together with histopathological features are sufficient for the diagnosis of lichen planus.

Once lichen planus lesions become confluent, atopic dermatitis, psoriasis, and chronic eczema must be ruled out. Chronic oral or vulva lichen planus may be clinically indistinguishable from leukoplakia. Widespread erosive lesions of lichen planus occurring in the oral cavities should be differentiated from candidiasis, carcinoma, aphthous ulcerations, pemphigus, cicatricial pemphigoid, and chronic erythema multiforme with extensive erosive lesions.

【Treatment】

There is no specific therapy for lichen planus. Although this disease appears to be self-limiting, therapy may promote a more rapid resolution of the lesions and symptoms, as described below.

(1) Topical therapy: topical glucocorticoid ointment alone for skin lesions, or followed with 0.05% tretinoin cream for mucosal lichen planus may be beneficial. Topical tacrolimus ointment has also proven effective in oral lichen planus.

(2) Systemic therapy: a short course of oral glucocorticoids (prednisone 40-60 mg/d) or retinoids may be prescribed in severe cases. Dose should be tapered after the lesions have been controlled. Chloroquine, hydroxyl chloroquine, dapsone, and immunomodulators such as transfer factor may be considered. Oral antihistamines, particularly those with sedative effects, are helpful in controlling the symptoms of severe itching.

(3) Phototherapy with UVB or PUVA may be effective.

【诊断与鉴别诊断】

根据皮损特征，结合组织病理变化不难诊断。

扁平苔藓的皮损融合时需与特应性皮炎、银屑病、慢性湿疹等相鉴别，持久的口腔或外阴扁平苔藓有时在临床上很难与黏膜白斑相鉴别，口腔广泛的糜烂性损害需要与念珠菌病、癌肿、阿弗他溃疡、天疱疮、瘢痕性类天疱疮和慢性多形性红斑（有广泛的糜烂性损害）相鉴别。

【治疗】

本病尚无特效治疗方法，虽然本病为自限性，但采用以下综合治疗常可加快皮损的愈合和症状的改善。

（1）局部治疗　可局部用糖皮质激素软膏，黏膜的扁平苔藓在局部应用糖皮质激素后，外用 0.05%的维甲酸软膏效果较好。外用他克莫司软膏对口腔扁平苔藓有效。

（2）系统治疗　皮损严重者可口服糖皮质激素（泼尼松 40～60 mg/d）或维A酸类药物，皮损减轻后应逐渐减量。也可用氯喹、羟氯喹、氨苯砜及免疫调节剂如转移因子，口服抗阻胺药特别是有嗜睡副作用的可以减轻瘙痒。

（3）UVB 或 PUVA 光疗　有一定疗效。

Section Seven　Pityriasis Rubra Pilaris

Pityriasis rubra pilaris (PRP), also known as pityriasis pilaris, is a rare chronic inflammatory skin disease characterized by scaling erythema and small follicular papules.

【Etiology and Pathogenesis】

The cause of PRP is unknown, although it can be classified into genetic and acquired forms, with the former type usually being associated with a positive family history. The onset of the disease begins in infancy or childhood with an autosomal dominant inheritance pattern. However, in sporadic cases, the onset starts in adulthood and one hypothesis states that pityriasis rubra pilaris may be related to vitamin deficiency, keratinization disorder, or endocrine disturbance.

第七节　毛发红糠疹

毛发红糠疹（pityriasis rubra pilaris）又称为毛发糠疹，是一种罕见的慢性炎症性皮肤病。其典型皮损为鳞屑性红斑、毛囊性小丘疹。

【病因及发病机制】

本病病因不明。可分为遗传型和获得型，前者有家族史，在婴儿期或儿童期发病，可能与常染色体显性遗传有关。后者常为散发，于成人期发病。可能与维生素缺乏、角化障碍及内分泌紊乱等有关。

【Clinical Manifestations】

The condition is characterized by grayish-white scaling erythema that then coalesces into red-orange scaly patches. Usually, the lesions begin on the scalp, spreading rapidly to the face and other parts of the body. The characteristic lesions are light red or reddish brown, pinhead to milium-sized acuminated follicular papules with a horny plug (including an embedded hair) at the center of the papules and scaly erythema. As the disease progresses, more follicular papules will appear and cluster together, finally giving rise to a gooseflesh-like appearance. The eruption has a predilection for the sides of the neck, the extensor surfaces of the extremities, and the trunk (Fig. 13-18(a)(b)(c)). Once it appears on the dorsal aspect of the proximal phalanges, PRP diagnosis can be made.

Koebner's phenomenon may sometimes be seen. In severe cases, the lesions can spread all over the body developing into erythroderma. Characteristic small islands of normal skin within the erythema can be seen. The patients may present hyperkeratosis of the palms and soles (Fig. 13-18(d)). The nails may be yellowish-brown, rough, thickened, or brittle. Patients may feel different degrees of pruritus, dryness, or burning sensations. The course of PRP is chronic.

【临床表现】

本病初起为表面覆有灰白色鳞屑的红斑，继而融合成红黄色鳞屑状斑片，皮损常先累及头皮、很快扩展到面部和身体其他部位。特征性皮损为毛囊性小丘疹和鳞屑性红斑，丘疹为针头至粟粒大，淡红色或红褐色，顶端尖锐，其中央顶端有一黑色角质小栓，通常有一根头发嵌入角栓中心。随着病情进展，毛囊性丘疹逐渐增多，密集成片，呈鸡皮样外观，多分布在颈侧、四肢的伸侧和躯干(图 13-18(a)(b)(c))。尤其发生在第 1、2 指节背面，为本病特有的症状，具有诊断意义。

有时可有同形反应。病情严重时，皮疹可泛发全身发展为红皮病。红斑间可见到特征性的正常小皮岛。患者可出现掌跖角化过度(图 13-18(d))。指(趾)甲可呈黄褐色，粗糙增厚，变脆等。自觉症状有不同程度的瘙痒、干燥及灼热感。病程为慢性。

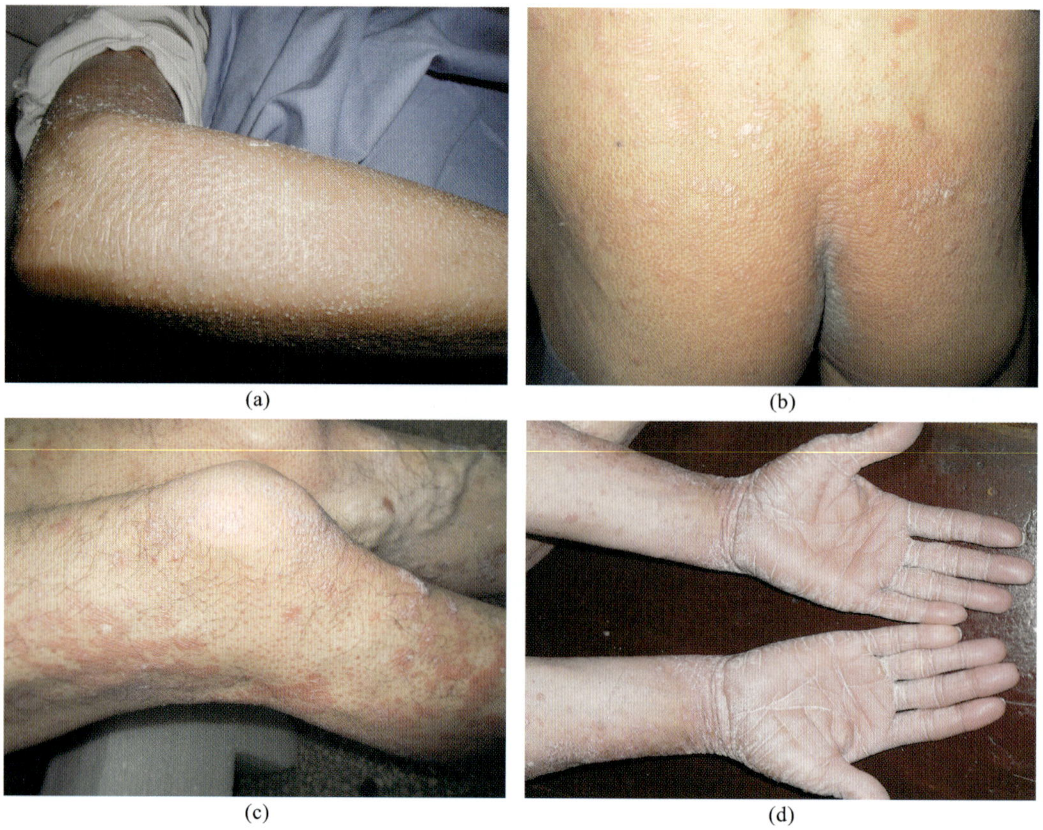

(a) (b) (c) (d)

Fig. 13-18　Pityriasis rubra pilaris(图 13-18　毛发红糠疹)

【Histopathology】

Epidermal hyperkeratosis, follicular plugging, focal parakeratosis at the follicular orifice, mild irregular acanthosis, and liquefaction degeneration of basal cells can all be seen histopathologically. The inflammatory infiltrate in the dermis is composed of mononuclear cells and is generally mild.

【组织病理】

表皮角化过度，在毛囊口处有角质栓和灶性角化不全，棘层轻度不规则增厚，基底细胞轻度液化变性。真皮有单核细胞浸润，但一般较轻。

【Diagnosis and Differential Diagnosis】

The diagnosis of PRP is usually based on the characteristic appearance of the lesions, and may be confirmed by biopsy if necessary. Differential diagnosis includes psoriasis, lichen planus, and seborrheic dermatitis, etc.

【诊断与鉴别诊断】

根据皮损特征不难诊断，必要时可行活检明确诊断。本病应与银屑病、扁平苔藓、脂溢性皮炎等疾病相鉴别。

【Treatment】

There are no specifically effective treatments for this disease. The lesions may improve with topical urea cream or tretinoin ointment, but will not be curable. Topical glucocorticoids can be used if pruritus is severe. Oral vitamin A, tretinoin, methotrexate, and PUVA are effective.

【治疗】

本病尚无特效疗法，局部给予尿素乳膏或维 A 酸软膏可好转，但不可治愈。如果瘙痒严重，可局部用糖皮质激素控制。口服维生素 A、维 A 酸、甲氨蝶呤和 PUVA 等治疗有效。

Section Eight　Lichen Nitidus

第八节　光泽苔藓

Lichen nitidus is a rare chronic inflammatory skin disease of unknown etiology. It is characterized by numerous tiny, shiny, skin-colored or light whitish or pink papules that tend to be localized. The natural clinical course of lichen nitidus is self-limiting.

光泽苔藓(lichen nitidus)是一种罕见的、病因不明的、慢性炎症性皮肤病。其典型皮损为大量微小的、有光泽的、肤色或淡白色或粉红色局限性丘疹，病程为自限性。

【Etiology and pathogenesis】

The cause of lichen nitidus is still unknown. The lesions may be related to lichen planus or tuberculosis, but this has not been proven.

【病因及发病机制】

本病病因不明，曾经认为与扁平苔藓、结核病有关，尚缺乏确切的论据。

【Clinical Manifestations】

Lichen nitidus is commonly seen in children and young adults. The lesions are generally confined to the abdomen, the chest, genitalia, and the flexor aspects of the extremities, presenting with many 1-2 mm sized, shiny, skin-colored or light whitish or pink, flat or dome-shaped uniform papules that tend to cluster in groups (Fig. 13-19). The lesions are usually asymptomatic although protracted pruritus may occur. This is a self-limiting condition that usually resolves in a year; however, the natural course for the individual patient is unpredictable.

【临床表现】

本病多见于小孩和青年。皮损常累及腹部、胸部、生殖器和四肢屈侧。典型皮损为大量 1～2 mm、有光泽的、肤色或淡白色或粉红色、扁平或圆形的丘疹，小丘疹形状规则，密集成簇(图 13-19)。皮损通常无症状，偶有顽固性痒。本病常在一年内自愈，病程自限，但不可预测。

【Histopathology】

The histopathology of lichen nitidus is significant for a diagnosis. The typical histopathological changes are focused on dermal papillae that contain a dense granulomatous infiltrate

【组织病理】

光泽苔藓具有特征性组织病理表现。真皮乳头变宽，有组织细胞、淋巴细胞和噬黑素细胞的致密浸润，可见多核

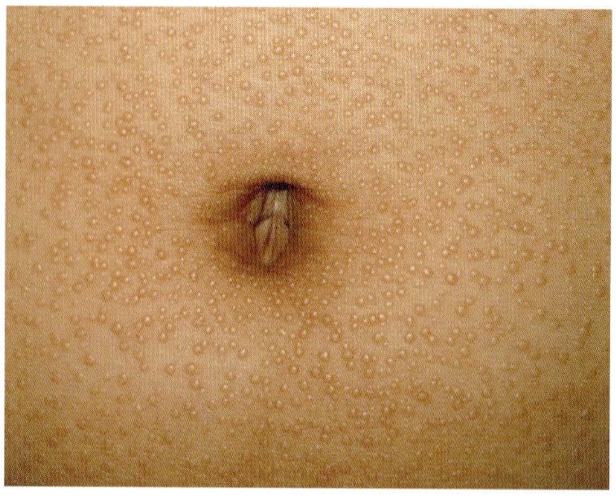

Fig. 13-19 Lichen nitidus(图 13-19 光泽苔藓)

composed of histiocytes, lymphocytes, melanophages, and multinucleated giant cells. With thinning of the overlying epidermis and downward extension of the rete ridges at the interface of the infiltrate, a typical 'claw clutching a ball' may present.

巨细胞，浸润部位呈现肉芽肿性改变。损害上方的表皮变薄，而浸润的两侧的表皮嵴向下向内延伸，形成特征性的“抱球”状。

【Diagnosis and Differential Diagnosis】

Given the typical lesions and histopathological features, a diagnosis is not difficult for lichen nitidus. However, the condition should be distinguished from lichen planus, verruca plana, etc.

【诊断与鉴别诊断】

根据皮损特征，结合组织病理变化易于诊断。本病应与扁平苔藓、扁平疣等疾病相鉴别。

【Treatment】

As lichen nitidus is asymptomatic and self-limiting, treatment is often unnecessary. Topical glucocorticoids may be applied if pruritus persists. Other reported treatments include systemic glucocorticoids, retinoids, PUVA, and dinitrochlorobenzene.

【治疗】

由于本病通常无症状，皮损可自动消退，故常不治疗。如果持续性瘙痒，可局部用糖皮质激素控制。有报道系统用糖皮质激素、维 A 酸类药物、PUVA 及二硝基氯苯等治疗有效。

Section Nine Lichen Striatus

第九节 线状苔藓

Lichen striatus is a chronic, self-limiting, inflammatory skin disease with an unknown etiology. It is characterized by small polygonal papules in a linear arrangement.

线状苔藓(lichen striatus)是一种病因不明、自限性、慢性炎症性皮肤病。其典型皮损为线状排列的多角形小丘疹。

【Etiology and Pathogenesis】

The cause of lichen striatus is still unknown. The reported endemic pattern of outbreaks and their tendency to occur in spring or summer suggest a viral cause, but this has not been proven.

【病因及发病机制】

本病病因不明，有报道地方性暴发，并且多暴发于春季或夏季，提示可能与病毒感染有关，尚缺乏确切依据。

【Clinical Manifestations】

Lichen striatus usually affects children aged 5-15 years, but may occasionally appear in infants and adults. Female patients outnumber males by roughly 2 to 1. Onset is usually sudden. The lesions are characterized by numerous discrete, 1-2 mm sized, light red or flesh-colored, flat or dome-shaped papules, which are covered with minimal white-grey scales. The uniform papules cluster and form linear bands following Blaschko's lines. The bands are 0. 2-

【临床表现】

本病好发于 5～15 岁儿童，婴儿及成人偶可见，女孩发病率高于男孩，比例约为 2∶1，多突然发病。典型皮损为大量散在的、1～2 mm 的、淡红色或肉色的、扁平或圆形的丘疹，上覆少量灰白鳞屑。小丘疹形状规则，密集成簇，随后融合成线条状，沿 Blaschko 线分布，线条宽

2.0 cm in width, either continuous or interrupted (Fig. 13-20).

0.2～2.0 cm，可连续或间断(图 13-20)。

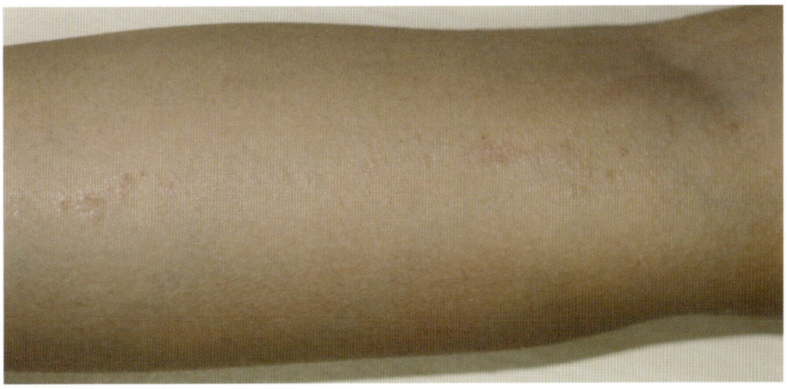

Fig. 13-20　Lichen striatus(图 13-20　线状苔藓)

The lesions usually involve only unilateral extremities, but the trunk or face may be involved as well. Nail involvement can occur with nail plate thinning, longitudinal ridging, splitting, and nail bed hyperkeratosis. Lesions are usually asymptomatic, but itching is possible. Most lesions may resolve spontaneously within months.

皮损常仅累及四肢的一侧，但躯干、面部也偶可发疹。指甲受累可出现甲板变薄、甲纵嵴、分裂、甲床角化过度。皮损通常无症状，偶可出现瘙痒，多数情况下皮损可在数月内自行消失。

【Diagnosis and Differential Diagnosis】

The diagnosis of lichen striatus is straightforward given the typical clinical features. The disease should be distinguished from linear epidermal nevus, linear lichen planus, linear psoriasis, lichen simplex chronicus, verruca plana, and other similar diseases.

【诊断与鉴别诊断】

根据典型临床表现易于诊断。本病应与线状表皮痣、线状扁平苔藓、线状银屑病、慢性单纯性苔藓、扁平疣等疾病相鉴别。

【Treatment】

Lesions usually resolve spontaneously, so treatment is seldom required. Topical 0.1% tretinoin ointment or glucocorticoid cream may help patients with severe pruritus or resistant lesions.

【治疗】

本病多可自愈，无需治疗。瘙痒显著或皮损顽固者可局部外用 0.1%维 A 酸软膏或糖皮质激素霜。

Section Ten　Erythroderma

第十节　红　皮　病

Erythroderma is also known as exfoliative dermatitis (ED). It is a rare and severe skin disease that is characterized by diffuse redness and desquamation involving more than 90% of the entire surface of the body.

红皮病(erythroderma)也称为剥脱性皮炎(exfoliative dermatitis)，是一种少见的以全身 90%以上皮肤弥漫性潮红、脱屑为特征的严重的皮肤疾病。

【Etiology and Pathogenesis】

The mechanism (s) responsible for the development of erythroderma is (are) unknown. It may be a reaction to underlying cutaneous disorders aggravated by inadequate treatment or some other source of irritation such as atopic dermatitis, psoriasis, eczema, or even pityriasis rubra pilaris. Some systemic or topical drugs such as penicillin, sulfonamides, phenytoin sodium or other barbiturates, allopurinol, or carbamazepine have also been associated with erythroderma. There are also cases where erythroderma is accompanied by malignant tumors such as cutaneous T-cell lymphoma, leukemia, or other internal

【病因及发病机制】

红皮病的发生机制还不清楚，可继发于其他皮肤病(如特应性皮炎、银屑病、湿疹、毛发红糠疹等)，多由治疗不当或其他刺激引起；某些药物(如青霉素、磺胺类、苯妥英钠或巴比妥类、别嘌醇和卡马西平等)内用或外用也可引起；某些恶性肿瘤(如皮肤 T 细胞淋巴瘤、白血病、内脏恶性肿瘤等)临床上也可出现红皮病改变；部分患者无确切病因，称为特发性红皮病。

malignancies. For the patients without distinct primary disorders, the disease is named as idiopathic erythroderma.

【Clinical Manifestations】

Erythroderma can be divided into acute erythroderma and chronic erythroderma according to the clinical condition and prognosis.

(1) Acute erythroderma: the onset is acute with prominent systemic symptoms such as high fever, malaise, splenomegaly, hepatomegaly, and lymphadenopathy. The lesions present initially as clustered patches and maculopapules spread over most areas of the body. Maculopapules resembling morbilliform or scarlatiniform rashes rapidly increase in number and coalesce to form an intense edematous erythema (Fig. 13-21), particularly on the face and extremities. The desquamation appears as either fine bran-like flakes or as large scaly sheets, which in turn may present as glove- or sock-like scales when the palms or soles are involved. Hair loss and nail shedding are also seen in some patients. Erosions and exudations in the oral cavity, vulva, and intertriginous regions are often accompanied with intense pruritus. Usually the course subsides in 1-2 months, leaving hyperpigmentation.

(2) Chronic erythroderma: patients often present with chronic diffuse infiltrative erythema and swelling skin covered with bran-like scales on the surface (Fig. 13-22). The extensive erythema and scaling may result in profound physiological changes. A marked increase in blood flow to the skin and consequent increased heat loss from the body and dysfunction of temperature regulation may cause patients to have chills and temperature fluctuations. Repeated desquamation may also result in a large amount of protein loss, hypoalbuminemia, ketoacidosis, secondary infections, gastrointestinal dysfunction, cardiovascular disorder, endocrine disturbance, etc.

【Diagnosis and Differential Diagnosis】

The presence of diffuse redness followed by a generalized scaly skin lesion gives a strong diagnostic clue for erythroderma. However, it is impossible to find the causative factors in some cases. Erythroderma should be distinguished from Sézary syndrome (SS), which is a primary cutaneous T-cell lymphoma, characterized by a triad of generalized erythroderma, superficial lymphadenopathy, and the presence of atypical T lymphocytes with cerebriform nuclei (Sézary cells) in the skin, lymph nodes, and peripheral blood. The histopathological features in SS are similar to those in mycosis fungoides (MF); there are some Sézary cells in the upper dermis, similar to MF cells. Epidermotropism and Pautrier microabscesses may also be observed.

【临床表现】

根据病情和预后可分为急性红皮病和慢性红皮病。

(1) 急性红皮病　发病急骤。伴有高热，全身乏力，肝、脾、淋巴结肿大等。皮损初为泛发的密集斑片、斑丘疹，呈麻疹样或猩红热样，迅速增多，融合成全身弥漫性潮红、水肿(图13-21)，以面部、肢端显著，伴有大量脱屑，呈细糠状或大片状，掌跖部可呈手套或袜套样脱屑，甚至出现脱发、甲脱落，口腔、外阴及皱褶部位可出现糜烂、渗出。常伴有剧烈瘙痒。经过1～2个月后皮肤逐渐恢复正常，遗留色素沉着。

(2) 慢性红皮病　慢性红皮病表现为慢性弥漫性浸润性红斑、肿胀，表面附糠状鳞屑(图13-22)。广泛的红斑和脱屑可导致显著的生理性改变。皮肤血流量增加可导致过多热量丢失，体温调节失衡，患者可伴有畏寒、低热和高热交替。反复脱屑后蛋白质大量丢失导致低蛋白血症、酮症酸中毒、继发感染、消化道功能障碍、心血管病变、内分泌失调等。

【诊断与鉴别诊断】

根据典型的弥漫性皮肤红斑和泛发性脱屑的临床表现本病不难诊断，但有时寻找原因相当困难。应与Sézary综合征(SS)鉴别，后者是一种原发于皮肤的T细胞淋巴瘤，其特征为红皮病、全身浅表淋巴结肿大、皮肤和淋巴结及外周血中有脑回状的不典型T细胞(称为Sézary细胞)组成的三联症。SS的组织学改变与MF相似，真皮上部有多少不等的Sézary细胞，与MF细胞形态相似，可见亲表皮现象和Pautrier微脓肿。

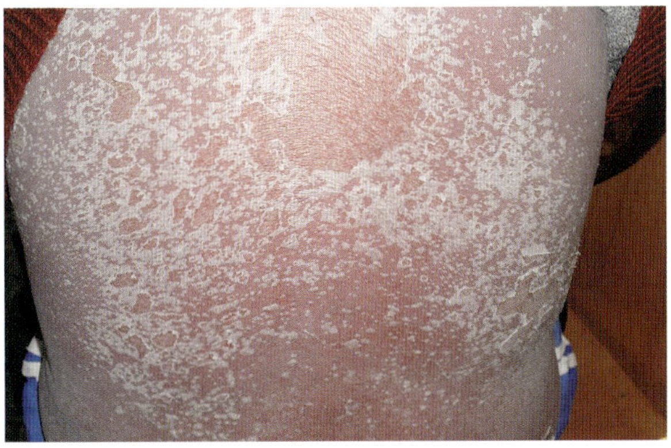

Fig. 13-21　Acute erythroderma
（图 13-21　急性红皮病）

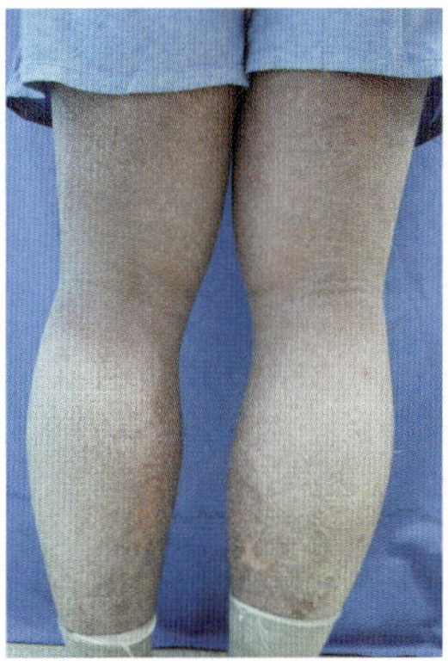

Fig. 13-22　Chronic erythroderma
（图 13-22　慢性红皮病）

【Treatment】

Medical history should be taken carefully to rule out causative factors that might need to be avoided. After the underlying primary disease has been identified (e. g. , tumor), effective treatment of the primary disease should proceed immediately.

(1) Topical therapy: the principle for selecting topical drugs is the avoidance of further irritation to the fragile skin lesions. The most common choices here are plant oils, zinc oxide oil, silicone cream, and low concentration and low-potency glucocorticoid creams, especially when the affected area is limited. A wet compress with 3% boric acid solution can be applied to exudation areas.

(2) Systemic therapy: patients with acute erythroderma often require treatment with supportive measures such as nutrient supplements and fluid and electrolyte balancing, which usually will require admission. The prescribed therapy will depend on the patient's pre-existing condition (s). For example, acitretin and cyclosporine can be helpful in psoriatic erythroderma and isotretinoin in erythroderma caused by pityriasis rubra pilaris. A severely erythroderma (other than psoriatic erythroderma) will often necessitate systemic glucocorticoid therapy. In adults, oral prednisone 40-60 mg can be given once daily and the dosage should be regularly adjusted according to the condition of the disease. Also, the physician should be alert for adverse reactions of the glucocorticoids. Oral antihistamines may be administered in patients with severe pruritus. Antibiotics may be suggested for patients with secondary infections.

【治疗】

应密切结合病史查找原因，重视病因治疗，针对原发病进行治疗，有明确诱因者应尽早去除，如确诊肿瘤者应积极治疗原发病。

（1）局部治疗　外用药物应无刺激性，常用植物油、氧化锌油、硅油霜或低浓度和低效糖皮质激素霜（小面积外用），以减轻症状。局部渗出者可用 3% 硼酸液湿敷。

（2）系统治疗　急性红皮病患者，应加强支持疗法，及时补充营养，维持水、电解质平衡；应根据不同的原发病进行针对性治疗，如阿维 A 酯和环孢素对银屑病性红皮病有效；异维 A 酸对毛发红糠疹（PRP）引起的红皮病有效；多数严重患者需要使用糖皮质激素（除外银屑病性红皮病），如成人剂量为泼尼松 40～60 mg/d 口服，并根据病情调整剂量，同时应注意不良反应。瘙痒明显者可口服抗组胺药；合并感染时给予抗感染治疗。

Yu-xue GAO（高玉雪）

Chapter Fourteen Dermatoses Resulting from Physical Factors

第十四章 物理因素引起的皮肤病

Section One Sunburn

第一节 日 晒 伤

Sunburn, also called solar dermatitis, is an acute inflammatory reaction caused by excessive exposure to sunlight.

日晒伤(sunburn),也称为日光性皮炎,是对过度日光照射产生的一种急性炎症反应。

【Etiology and Pathogenesis】

Sunburn is mainly caused by overexposure to ultraviolet B (UVB, wavelength from 290 to 320 nm) light, which covers a portion of the solar spectrum. Some chemical mediators such as prostaglandins, histamine, serotonin, kinin, and nitric oxide may play important roles in the pathogenesis of this skin disorder.

【病因及发病机制】

绝大多数日晒伤由中波紫外线(UVB,波长 290～320 nm)所致。前列腺素、组胺、血清素、激肽及一氧化氮等化学介质在其发病中可能起重要作用。

【Clinical Manifestations】

The exposed areas of the skin develop circumscribed erythema within several hours after sun exposure (Fig. 14-1). The erythema is usually accompanied by tenderness. In severe cases, blisters may occur, which may become confluent in even more severe cases. Sunburn symptoms are most prominent in the 12-24 hours following the exposure, and gradually resolve with desquamation and pigmentation in a few days; however, the pigmentation may persist for months. Edema may occur in the extremities and face. Severe, systemic symptoms such as chills and fever can occur on occasion.

【临床表现】

光辐射后数小时,被暴露部位产生境界清楚的红斑(图 14-1)。红斑后发生触痛,严重时形成水疱,可融合。日晒伤症状在照射后 12～24 h 最严重,之后逐渐好转。数天内常发生脱屑和色素沉着。某些情况痊愈后色素沉着可持续数月。水肿常出现于四肢和面部。全身症状可能出现,比如寒战和发热。

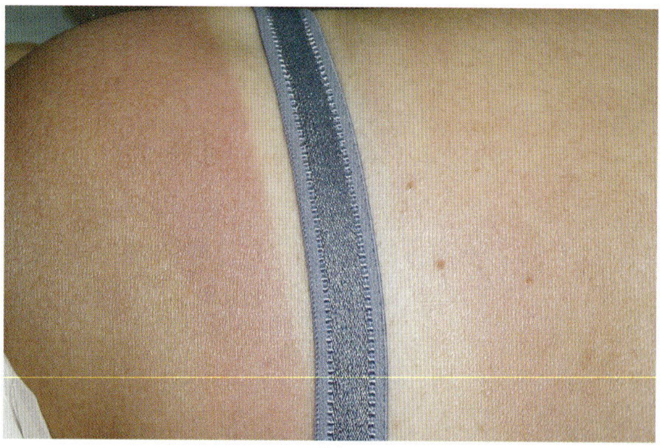

(a)

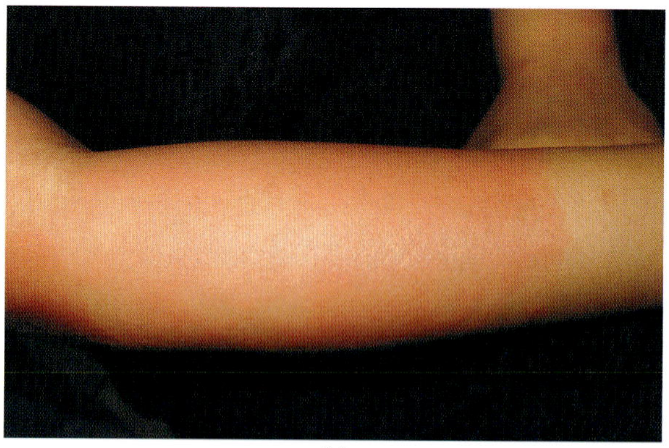

(b)

Fig. 14-1 Sunburn(图 14-1 日晒伤)

【Histopathology】

Apoptotic keratinocytes, epidermal edema, or spongiosis in the prickle cells layer, or even necrotic keratinocytes and subepidermal blistering can be seen in histological sections. In the dermis, it is also possible to observe swelling of the endothelial cells of the blood vessels and perivascular inflammatory infiltration composed mainly of lymphocytes.

【组织病理】

病理上可见凋亡的表皮细胞、表皮棘细胞层水肿或海绵变性,甚至有表皮细胞的坏死和表皮下水疱。真皮血管内皮肿胀,血管周围有淋巴细胞为主的炎症细胞浸润。

【Prevention and Treatment】

Further avoidance of strong sunlight is recommended. Proper sunscreen helps prevent sunburn, but is of little use as a therapeutic agent. Treatment in severe cases involves cool wet compresses and glucocorticoid ointments. Oral antihistamines and non-steroidal anti-inflammatory drugs are also helpful when systemic symptoms are present.

【预防和治疗】

避免日晒。遮光剂能有效防止日晒伤。冷敷和糖皮质激素软膏有效。当出现全身症状时，应口服抗组胺药和非甾体类抗炎药。

Section Two　Polymorphous Light Eruption

第二节　多形性日光疹

【Etiology and Pathogenesis】

Polymorphous light eruption (PLE) is a photosensitivity disorder induced by both UVA and UVB exposure, with UVA being the predominant contributor in most cases. The condition is caused by a delayed-type hypersensitivity reaction to sunlight.

【病因及发病机制】

多形性日光疹(polymorphous light eruption, PLE)是一种光敏性疾病，由紫外线引起，包括宽谱 UVB 和 UVA，大多数 PLE 由 UVA 所导致。它被认为是一种光引起的迟发型变态反应。

【Clinical Manifestations】

PLE is characterized by intermittent and relapsing photosensitivity. It occurs most often in spring. Young women between the ages of 10-30 are the most commonly affected. The lesions usually appear hours to days after sun exposure. Affected areas include any that are exposed to sunlight, such as the face, the V area of the chest, the neck, the extensor forearms, and the back of the hands. Rashes are usually polymorphic; however a single morphologic pattern may be observed in all affected areas for an individual patient. Pruritic papular and papulovesicular rashes are present in most patients. No scarring remains after resolution (Fig. 14-2). However, plaque-like, vesicular, bullous, or more complicated patterns may sometimes be seen. Usually, the condition is not accompanied by systemic symptoms.

【临床表现】

PLE 以间歇性反复发作的光敏性皮肤症状为特点。最常发生于春季，10～30 岁年轻女性好发。常于暴露日光后数小时到几天内发病。发病部位包括面、胸前"V"形区、颈、前臂伸侧和手背。皮疹呈多形性，但每个个体皮疹形态常是一致的。皮疹通常为丘疹和丘疱疹，伴痒，消退后不留瘢痕(图 14-2)；有时呈斑块样、水疱、大疱，或者混合皮损。PLE 很少伴发全身症状。

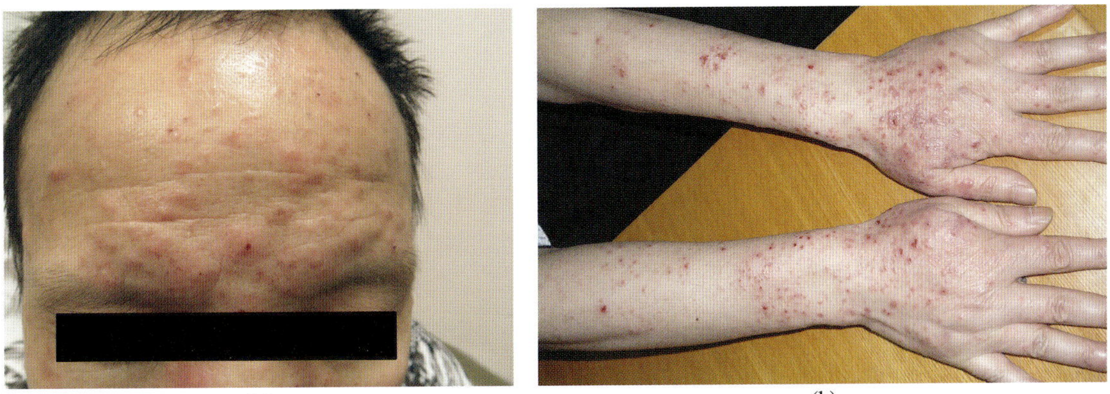

(a)　　(b)

Fig. 14-2　Polymorphous light eruption

(图 14-2　多形性日光疹)

【Diagnosis and Differential Diagnosis】

Any photosensitive disease with unknown cause and lack of

【诊断与鉴别诊断】

所有原因不明和缺乏其他光敏性疾

typical symptoms for other photosensitive diseases should be considered as PLE. In addition, each patient with PLE must be carefully evaluated to rule out other photosensitive diseases, such as lymphocytic infiltration of Jessner, lupus erythematosus, and solar urticaria.

病特有症状的光敏性疾病应考虑为PLE。应考虑与以下几种疾病相鉴别：Jessner淋巴细胞浸润症、红斑狼疮、日光性荨麻疹和其他光敏性皮肤病。

【Prevention and Treatment】

Mild PLE can be managed by total avoidance of ultraviolet exposure, for example using barrier protection or broad-spectrum sunscreens with high SPF number. Prophylactic therapy with low-dosage broad-or narrow-band UVB or PUVA is extremely beneficial. Oral antimalarial therapy has been recommended for prophylactic use in chronic severe cases. Antihistamines may be useful for pruritus. Systemic glucocorticoids may also be necessary to control the symptoms. For patients with very severe symptoms, azathioprine or cyclosporin may be effective.

【预防和治疗】

轻症PLE可采用避免紫外线照射、使用屏障保护及高SPF的宽谱遮光剂的方法。预防性的低剂量宽波或窄波UVB或PUVA治疗非常有效。预防性口服抗疟药提倡用于慢性严重病例。抗组胺剂可用于止痒；必要时可内用糖皮质激素；对于严重的病例，硫唑嘌呤或环孢素常有效。

Section Three　Chronic Actinic Dermatitis

第三节　慢性光化性皮炎

Chronic actinic dermatitis is an immunologically mediated lichenoid eczematous skin disorder, which usually occurs on sun exposed sites with a slow and intractable progress. Males are predominantly affected.

慢性光化性皮炎(chronic actinic dermatitis)是表现在曝光部位的免疫介导的、慢性进展性、苔藓样湿疹样皮肤改变，男性多见。

【Etiology and Pathogenesis】

The exact etiology of the disease is unclear. Solar exposure may elicit the production of intrinsic antigens that lead to the disease, in which the type Ⅳ delayed hypersensitivity reaction might play a role in the pathogenesis.

【病因及发病机制】

病因尚不完全清楚。日光照射诱导的内源性抗原可能导致该病的发生，属Ⅳ型变态反应。

【Clinical Manifestations】

Sun exposed sites such as scalp, face, neck, chest, arms, and dorsum of the hands are most often involved. Typical lesions manifest as eczematous, lichenified patches, or confluent plaques. The lesions are usually pruritic. If carefully observed, nasolabial folds, submental chin, or other skin creases are spared due to lower exposure (Fig. 14-3).

【临床表现】

头皮、面颊、颈部、胸部、手臂、手背等日光暴露部位最易受累。典型皮损为湿疹样、苔藓样的斑片或融合斑块，伴有瘙痒。仔细观察会发现鼻唇沟、下颌或皮肤皱褶部位因不易受光而表现正常(图14-3)。

【Diagnosis and Differential Diagnosis】

A correct diagnosis is reached by history, typical clinical manifestations, and histological features in combination with a photo patch test. Conditions that need to be differentiated from chronic actinic dermatitis include drug eruption, photo-allergic contact dermatitis, cutaneous T-cell lymphoma, and connective tissue diseases.

【诊断与鉴别诊断】

正确的诊断需要病史采集、典型的临床表现和组织学表现；必要时，结合光敏感试验。需要鉴别的疾病包括药疹、变应性光接触性皮炎、皮肤T细胞淋巴瘤和结缔组织病。

【Prevention and Treatment】

Photoprotection is the key for prevention of this disease.

【预防和治疗】

日光防护最为重要。患者应当外涂

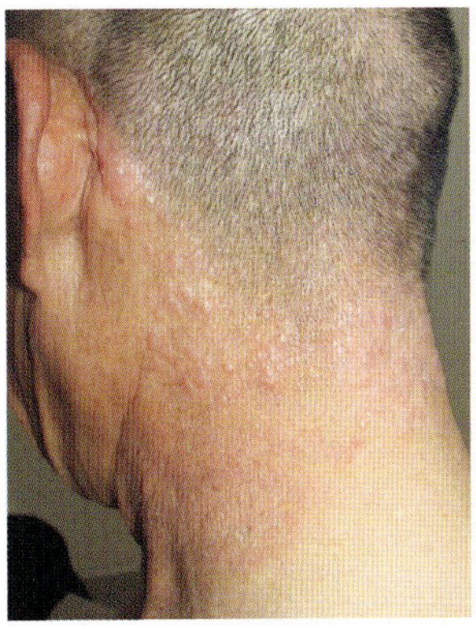

Fig. 14-3　Chronic actinic dermatitis(图 14-3　慢性光化性皮炎)

Patients are asked to apply a broad-spectrum sunscreen with SPF 30 or more. Long-sleeve shirts, umbrellas or hats are also advised. The first line of treatment is topical corticosteroid or calcineurin inhibitors. Systemic treatment is used for widespread or recalcitrant conditions, for example oral corticosteroids for several weeks (0.5-1.0 mg/(kg·d)). Other immunosuppressive agents such as cyclosporine, azathioprine, and mycophenolate mofetil can also be used.

SPF 不小于 30 的宽谱遮光剂。户外活动时可以穿长袖衣服、用遮阳伞。一线治疗一般外用糖皮质激素或钙调磷酸酶抑制剂有效。对严重泛发的病例，可以口服糖皮质激素(0.5～1.0 mg/(kg·d))。其他免疫抑制剂，如环孢素、硫唑嘌呤、麦考酚酸吗乙酯也有效。

Section Four　Miliaria

第四节　痱

Miliaria is caused by the retention of sweat as a result of occlusion of eccrine ducts and pores. According to the level at which obstruction occurs in the sweat ducts, it can be classified into miliaria crystallina, miliaria rubra, miliaria pustulosa, miliaria profunda.

痱子(miliaria)是由于外泌汗腺导管和开口闭塞导致汗液潴留而形成，根据汗腺导管受阻碍的位置分为白痱、红痱、脓痱、深痱。

【Etiology and Pathogenesis】

The pathogenesis of miliaria is not completely understood. It has been suggested that some polysaccharides block the sweat delivery to the skin surface and thus interfere with the excretion of the sweat glands. The retained sweat may leak into the tissue around the sweat ducts causing the characteristic rashes. Miliaria commonly arises in hot and humid conditions.

【病因及发病机制】

痱子的完整发病机制不详，通常认为是因某些多糖物质阻塞了汗液的排出，导致汗腺不能正常分泌。蓄积的汗液流入汗腺导管的邻近组织，引起发疹。痱子易发生于湿热环境。

【Clinical Manifestations】

(1) Miliaria crystallina: characterized by uniform, superficial transparent, minute clear vesicles with no inflammatory reaction (Fig. 14-4). The blockage of sweat is located within or directly under the horny cell layer. This is usually an asymptomatic, self-limiting eruption that resolves in one to a few days, leaving some thin, white scales following the drying out of the vesicles.

(2) Miliaria rubra: the most commonly encountered form of miliaria, in which obstruction causes leakage of sweat into the

【临床表现】

(1) 白痱(miliaria crystallina)　特征是大小一致、浅表透明、细小清亮和无炎症反应的水疱(图 14-4)，它由角质细胞层或角质细胞层下部的汗液潴留引起。水疱迅速干涸、变薄，产生白色鳞屑。皮疹无症状，有自限性。通常一至数日愈合。

(2) 红痱(miliaria rubra)　痱子中最常见的类型，由于汗管的堵塞引起汗

deeper layers of the epidermis, provoking a local inflammatory reaction and giving rise to discrete erythematous papules and papulovesicles (Fig. 14-5). It is often accompanied by flushing, prickling, burning and itching. The most commonly affected sites are the trunk, extensor surfaces of the extremities, the neck region and axillary fossae.

液积聚在表皮的下部,并导致局部炎症反应,表现为散在分布的红色丘疹和丘疱疹(图 14-5),常伴有红晕、刺痛、灼热和瘙痒,最常累及的部位是躯干、四肢伸侧、颈部和腋下。

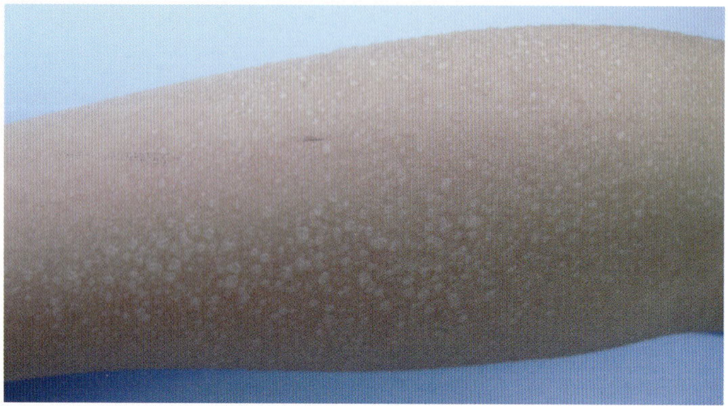

Fig. 14-4　Miliaria crystallina(图 14-4　白痱)

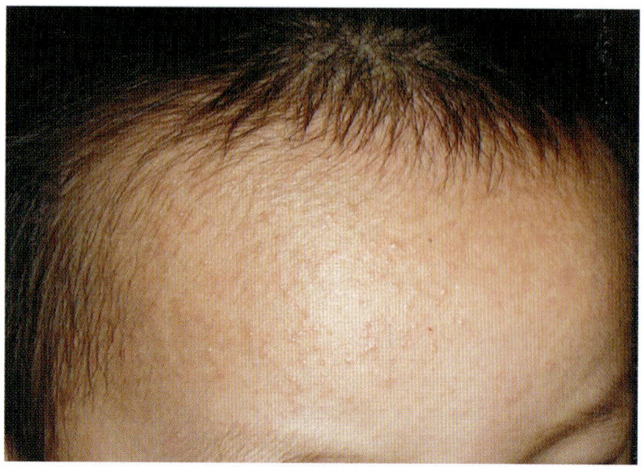

Fig. 14-5　Miliaria rubra(图 14-5　红痱)

(3) Miliaria pustulosa: usually develops from some other dermatitis and frequently occurs after miliaria rubra. The contents of the pustules are usually sterile.

(4) Miliaria profunda: the most severe form of miliaria, generally occurs as a complication of repeated episodes of miliaria rubra. The obstruction of sweat ducts is located deep in the upper dermis, causing the sweat to leak between the different layers of skin. The rash tends to exhibit as multiple flesh-colored, deep-seated, white papules with little pruritus.

(3) 脓痱(miliaria pustulosa)　多因其他皮炎诱发,常由红痱发展而来。脓疱内容物通常是无菌的。

(4) 深痱(miliaria profunda)　此型是痱子中最严重的,常发生于严重的红痱多次发作之后。汗腺导管在真皮浅层受损,导致汗液在皮肤各层间渗漏。皮损表现为多发、正常肤色、深在性的白色丘疹,一般不痒。

【Prevention and Treatment】

The only truly effective prevention or treatment for miliaria is avoidance of activities that induce further sweating. General measures, which should be recommended for all patients, include avoiding high temperatures and humid environments. Frequent soothing and cooling baths, followed by calamine lotion or a bland emollient are very helpful. Finally, clinicians should be alert for secondary infection.

【预防和治疗】

痱子唯一真正有效的预防和治疗是防止进一步出汗,避免高温和潮湿。在舒缓、清凉的沐浴之后使用炉甘石洗剂或温和的润滑剂有效。此外,还应避免继发感染。

Section Five　Chilblains (Perniosis)

第五节　冻　疮

【Etiology and Pathogenesis】

Chilblains are principally caused by prolonged exposure to cold and moisture, superimposed on poor peripheral blood circulation. Precipitating factors include dystrophy, anemia, hyperhidrosis, focal sepsis, hormonal changes and systemic diseases. Small arteries and veins become constricted because of the repetitive cold stimuli, and this triggers local inflammation, since vasoconstriction provokes

【病因及发病机制】

长期暴露于寒冷和潮湿,加之末梢血液循环较差是冻疮(chilblains)的主要发病因素。其他诱因包括营养不良、贫血、出汗过度、灶性脓毒症、激素异常及系统性疾病。由于局部反复受寒冷的作用,小动脉和静脉收缩,炎症形成。血管

tissue anoxia, and decreased muscular activity will further decrease the local blood supply.

收缩引起组织缺氧，肌肉活动减少进一步减少血液供应。

【Clinical Manifestations】

Chilblains are characterized by recurrent, localized, inflammatory erythematous swelling, usually tender, and often itchy dermatoses. They usually occur in early winter or early spring. Chilblains commonly involve hands, feet, auriculae and cheeks. Children are more likely to be affected. The lesions appear as itchy, red-purple edematous erythema and the color of the lesions tends to disappear when the erythema is compressed. Itching and burning symptoms are often intensified when entering a warm room. Blistering and ulcerations can develop in severe cases (Fig. 14-6).

【临床表现】

受冷后反复发作的局限性、炎症性红斑和肿胀，常伴触痛、瘙痒为特征表现，好发于初冬、早春季节。冻疮主要发生于手、足、耳部和面颊，多见于儿童。皮损为水肿性紫红斑，按之褪色，暖后灼热并瘙痒。严重时可发生水疱和溃疡(图 14-6)。

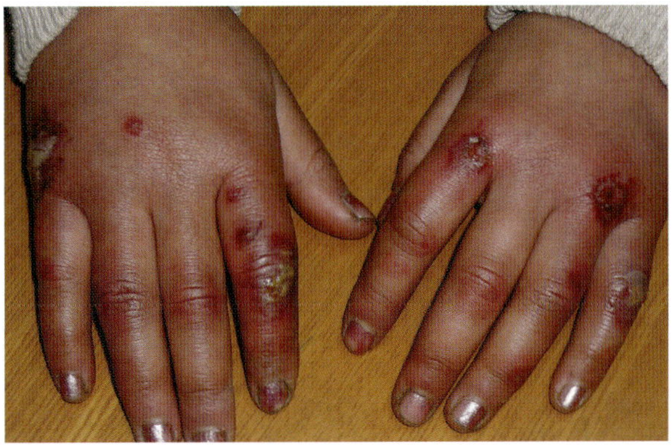

Fig. 14-6　Chilblains(图 14-6　冻疮)

【Prevention and Treatment】

Keeping warm and avoiding exposure to cold and dampness are important in preventing chilblains. Massaging gently with warm oil is helpful in improving blood circulation, and it has been suggested that orally administered vasodilators such as nifedipine and nicotinic acid are effective.

【预防和治疗】

避免暴露于湿冷环境，受冻部位保暖，用温热的油剂轻轻按摩有助于促进血液循环。口服硝苯地平、烟酸等血管扩张剂有效。

Section Six　Erythema Ab Igne

第六节　热激红斑

【Etiology and Pathogenesis】

Erythema *ab igne* (Latin, "from fire") is caused by chronic repeated exposure to moderate heat from an external heat source and especially from infrared radiation. Histological changes are similar to those seen in solar elastosis, in which elastic fibers of the dermis are increased. Although the livedo-like eruptions are present macroscopically, there is no sign of pathological vasculitis under microscopy.

【病因及发病机制】

长时间反复暴露于热，特别是红外线照射是热激红斑(erythema *ab igne*)的主要发病原因。组织学特征为真皮中弹力纤维增加，病变与光化性弹力纤维病所见相似。虽然表现为青斑样发疹，但病理上未见血管炎。

【Clinical Manifestations】

Erythema *ab igne* is characterized by reticular telangiectasia and pigmented dermatosis (Fig. 14-7), which results from

【临床表现】

热激红斑是一种特征性网状毛细血管扩张和色素沉着的皮肤病(图 14-7)，

persistent exposure to excessive heat that is not high enough to induce a burn reaction. The erythema patch is most commonly seen on women's legs. A red rash appears at first, which may be associated with a marked inflammatory reaction and which may be followed by pigmentation. Bulla formation also occurs on occasion. The lesions tend to fade gradually once the external heat source is removed; however the hyperpigmentation can be persistent in some cases.

通常因长期持续暴露于高温下，但又未致烧伤而引起，最常发生于妇女腿部。最早期改变为红斑，可能伴随相当明显的炎症改变，之后色素沉着，水疱有时形成。当病因消除后，病变逐渐消失，但有时留下持久性色素沉着。

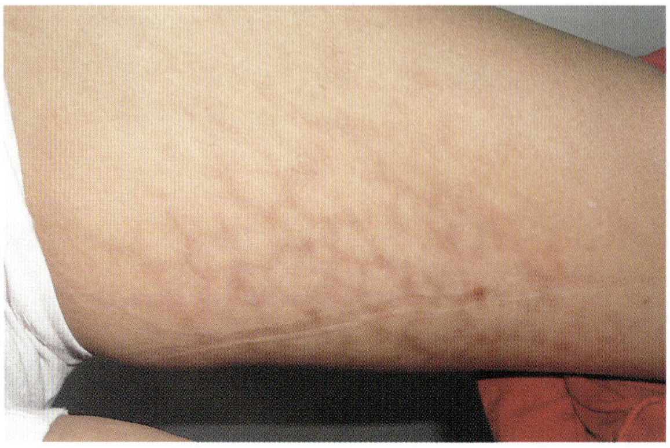

Fig. 14-7　Erythema *ab igne*(图 14-7　热激红斑)

【Treatment】

Hypothyroidism needs to be excluded. The topical use of bland emollients is helpful. It has been suggested that 5-fluorouracil cream could eliminate the dyskeratotic keratinocytes.

【治疗】

需要排除甲状腺功能低下，使用温和的润肤剂有效，可采用5-氟尿嘧啶霜去除角化不良的角质细胞。

Section Seven　Clavus (Corns) and Callus

第七节　鸡眼和胼胝

【Etiology and Pathogenesis】

Clavus (corns) and callus are both thickenings of the skin due to repeated heavy pressure and friction.

【病因及发病机制】

鸡眼(clavus)和胼胝(callus)均系长期压迫和摩擦引起角质细胞层增厚。

【Clinical Manifestations】

(1) Clavus or corns: a localized, cornified, conical thickening with the base on the surface and the apex pointing inward, which most commonly occurs on the forepart of the soles and also can be seen on the dorsa of the toes and heels. The lesions appear to be roughly the size of a soybean or bigger with a shiny surface and clear border (Fig. 14-8). Tenderness is obvious.

(2) Callus: localized, proliferative thickening of the epidermal horny cell layers. Usually these occur symmetrically on the palms and soles. The lesions appear as a waxy yellowish plaque with smooth surface and an obscure border (Fig. 14-9). In contrast to clavus, there is almost no tenderness.

【临床表现】

(1) 鸡眼　局限性、角质化、圆锥形的增厚物，其基底部在表面，尖端朝内，最常发生于足跖前部，也可见于趾背及足跟。皮损如黄豆大或更大，表面被磨平、有光泽，境界清楚(图14-8)。触痛明显。

(2) 胼胝　局限性、增生性增厚的表皮角质细胞层。主要对称发生于掌跖。皮损为蜡黄色、表面光滑、边界不清的斑块(图14-9)。与鸡眼不同，胼胝几乎无触痛。

【Differential Diagnosis】

Plantar clavus must be differentiated from plantar warts. Once

【鉴别诊断】

足底鸡眼需要与跖疣相鉴别。削去

the keratin on the surface is peeled off, one could see the wart extends deeply into the dermal papillae evidenced by the blood vessels that become visible. In contrast, the clavus stops at the cornified layer with a clear horny core.

表面角质后可明显看到，跖疣延伸至真皮乳头，其中有血管存在，而鸡眼则有清晰的角质核心。

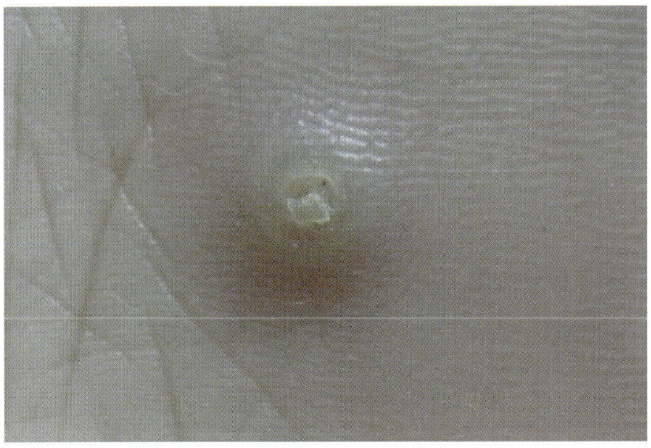

Fig. 14-8　Clavus(图 14-8　鸡眼)

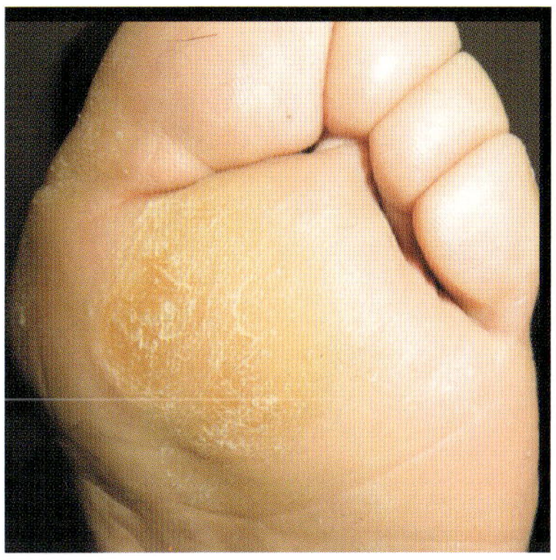

Fig. 14-9　Callus(图 14-9　胼胝)

【Prevention and Treatment】

Alleviating pressure and lessening friction through corrective footwear is of primary importance. Salicylic acid ointment can be applied to help with the removal of the thickening of the horny cell layer.

【预防和治疗】

矫正穿鞋以减小压迫或摩擦最重要。应用水杨酸软膏去除增厚的角质细胞层。

Section Eight　Radiodermatitis

第八节　放射性皮炎

Radiodermatitis is a mucocutaneous disease caused by various types of ionizing radiation. It can be divided into acute and chronic forms based on the time of presentation following radiation exposure. The lesions occur quickly after exposure in the acute form, but appear later in the chronic form.

放射性皮炎(radiodermatitis)是由各种电离辐射照射引起的皮肤黏膜损伤，可分为急性放射性皮炎和慢性放射性皮炎，前者受到照射后皮损迅速发生，后者皮损发生较晚。

【Etiology and Pathogenesis】

The severity of the cutaneous lesions varies with the source of ionizing radiation. The most susceptible target of radiation is intracellular DNA. As a result, cell function is impaired because of DNA damage or DNA synthesis inhibition. The effects of ionizing radiation on the cells are determined not only by the amount of radiation and the intensity (radiation rate) one receives, but also by the sensitivity of individual cells.

【病因及发病机制】

各种类型的电离辐射均可使皮肤产生不同程度的反应。放射性损伤的主要靶目标为细胞内 DNA。DNA 损伤及 DNA 合成抑制导致细胞功能缺失。离子辐射对细胞的影响取决于放射量、放射强度(照射率)和细胞敏感性。

【Clinical Manifestations】

(1) Acute radiodermatitis: the symptoms of radiodermatitis vary with the amount of irradiation, the sites exposed, and the age of the patient. Typically, when an "erythema dose" (the minimal single dose that produces an observed erythema) is given, initial erythema occurs within a latent period of up to 24 hours and disappears in 2-3 days. Subsequently, the second phase of lesions appears which includes edematous erythema, hyperpigmentation,

【临床表现】

(1) 急性放射性皮炎　症状根据放射量、位置、患者年龄不同而多种多样。当皮肤受到"红斑剂量"(导致可见红斑产生的单次最小剂量)的离子辐射时，经过 24 h 的潜伏期，初始红斑产生，并在 2～3 天后消失，二期损害随后发生。可有水肿性红斑、色素沉着、萎缩、毛细血管

atrophy and telangiectasia (Fig. 14-10), sometimes accompanied with pain. The skin turns dark after desquamation. Intractable ulcer and burn-like symptoms can be observed when a large amount of radiation (usually greater than 10 Gy)is received.

(2) Chronic radiodermatitis: commonly caused by a small amount of repetitive fractionated radiation, which often occurs on the site where radiation therapy has been repeatedly performed or on the skin of roentgenologists and radiation technicians. It can be classified into four stages: atrophy (dry, thin and smooth skin, accompanied by hyperpigmentation, hypopigmentation, alopecia, and telangiectasia, usually occurring 6 months later) (Fig. 14-11); keratinization (subcutaneous fibrosis, thickening); intractable ulceration (especially in areas of high moisture and post-trauma) and cancer (occurring up to 15 years later).

扩张(图 14-10),伴疼痛。脱屑后皮肤常呈暗黑色。顽固难治性溃疡和烧伤样表现常由大于 10 Gy 的大剂量放射所导致。

(2) 慢性放射性皮炎　通常由于长期反复接受小剂量放射线辐射所致,常见于反复接受放射性治疗的部位,也可见于 X 线科医师和技师。慢性放射性皮炎可见四个阶段:萎缩(皮肤干燥、细薄、光滑、伴色素沉着、色素减退、脱发、毛细血管扩张,通常发生于 6 个月之后)(图 14-11)、角化(皮下组织纤维化、增厚)、难治性溃疡(尤其在潮湿和创伤部位)、癌变(发生于 15 年后)。

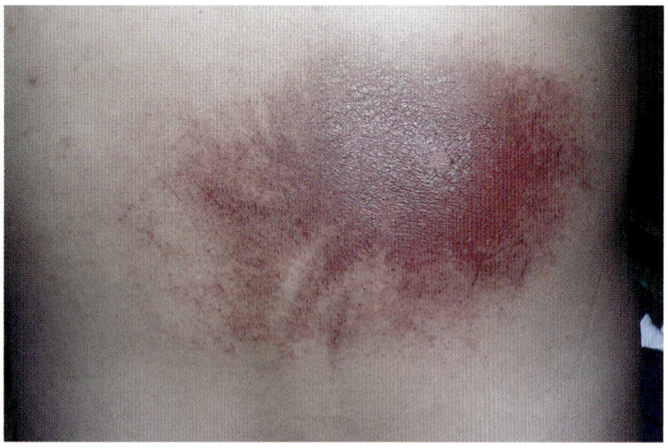

Fig. 14-10　Acute radiodermatitis
(图 14-10　急性放射性皮炎)

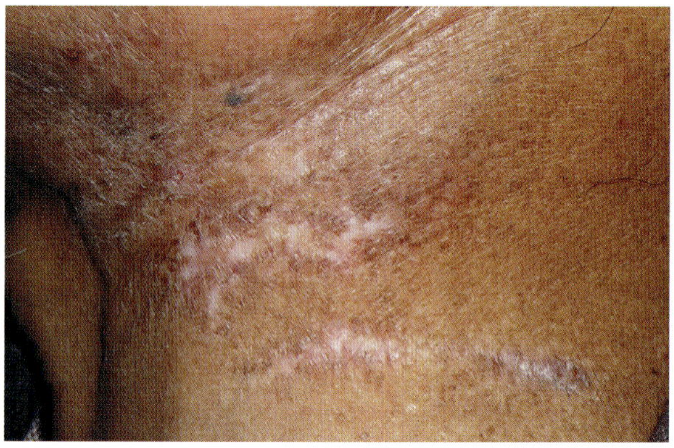

Fig. 14-11　Chronic radiodermatitis
(图 14-11　慢性放射性皮炎)

【Prevention and Treatment】

(1) Acute radiodermatitis: local stimulation should be avoided. Clean carefully with mild soap and water, and then use emollients. The low potent glucocorticoid creams such as hydrocortisone may help to relieve some symptoms.

(2) Chronic radiodermatitis: early removal of precancerous keratoses and ulcerations can prevent cancer development. A biopsy should be performed whenever necessary.

【预防和治疗】

(1) 急性放射性皮炎　应避免局部刺激,可用温和的肥皂和水仔细清洗,然后使用润肤剂。温和的糖皮质激素霜,特别是氢化可的松,可减轻症状。

(2) 慢性放射性皮炎　早期切除癌前角化病和溃疡可预防癌症发生,必要时应进行活检。

Section Nine　Rhagadia Manus and Pedis

Rhagadia manus and pedis is dry or chapped skin of the hands and feet.

第九节　手足皲裂

手足皲裂(rhagadia manus and pedis)是由各种原因引起的手足部皮肤干燥和皲裂。

【Etiology and Pathogenesis】

Internal factors: the skin of the palms and soles has predisposition for cracking because it is relatively thick with no hair follicles or sebaceous glands. Rhagadia is more likely to occur

【病因及发病机制】

内因:掌跖部皮肤较厚,无毛囊和皮脂腺,受摩擦变得更厚而失去弹性,加之冬季低温、干燥,易产生皲裂。

whenever the elasticity of the skin is impaired. Examples include skin dryness due to lower temperatures in winter, and skin thickening produced by repeated friction.

External factors: ① frequent friction; ② contact with strong acids, bases, or organic solvents; ③ cold, dry weather; ④ association with other dermatoses, such as chronic eczema, tinea manus and pedis, palmoplantar hyperkeratosis, ichthyosis, etc.

外因：①经常摩擦；②接触强酸、碱或有机溶剂；③寒冷、干燥天气；④伴发其他皮肤病，如慢性湿疹、手足癣、掌跖角皮症、鱼鳞病等。

【Clinical Manifestations】

It most commonly occurs in winter. The most frequently affected sites are on the palmar and plantar surface of the hands and feet when they are subjected to friction or pressure. The condition usually occurs along the natural lines of flexion known as the dermatoglyphics (Fig. 14-12). According to the depth of involvement, rhagadia is divided into three levels. In level one the fissures involve only the epidermis, without hemorrhage and pain; at level two the fissures reach the superficial dermis, accompanied with mild pain, but without hemorrhage; at level three they reach the dermis and subcutaneous tissue, with accompanying hemorrhage and pain.

【临床表现】

好发于冬季，多见于掌跖或经常受摩擦、牵拉的部位，皮损多沿皮纹方向发生(图 14-12)。根据皲裂的深浅程度分为三度：一度仅达表皮，无出血、疼痛；二度达真皮浅层，伴轻度疼痛，无出血；三度达真皮及皮下组织，伴出血和疼痛。

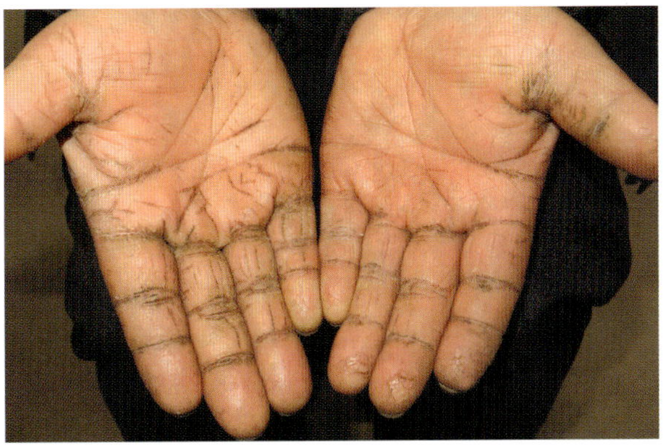

Fig. 14-12　Rhagadia manus and pedis(图 14-12　手足皲裂)

【Prevention and Treatment】

In order to prevent rhagadia, frequent soaking in warm water and soothing with a moisturizing cream is helpful. Avoid excess friction and contact with acid, base and organic solvents. The treatment for underlying diseases such as eczema and tinea manus and pedis may also help. External usage of 15% urea, salicylic acid or tretinoin ointments is usually effective. If the *corneum* is excessively thick, it may be shaved with a blade after being soaked.

【预防和治疗】

常用温水浸泡手足，外用有滋润作用的油脂。减少局部摩擦。避免接触酸、碱和有机溶剂。积极治疗湿疹、手足癣等基础疾病。外用 15% 尿素软膏、水杨酸或维 A 酸软膏，效果良好。如果角质过厚，可在浸泡后用刀片削薄增厚的角质层。

Lan ZHANG (张岚), Xing-hua GAO (高兴华)

Chapter Fifteen Congenital and Hereditary Dermatoses and Primary Immunodeficiency Disorders

第十五章 先天性和遗传性皮肤病及原发性免疫缺陷病

Section One Ichthyosis

第一节 鱼 鳞 病

【Etiology】

Ichthyosis constitute a heterogeneous group of skin diseases characterized by adherent (i. e., 'fish-like') scaling. Although phenotypic similarities exist, the genotypical entities for each subtype are distinct.

Ichthyosis vulgaris is characterized by a deficiency of profilaggrin, a main component of keratohyalin granules.

Recessive X-linked ichthyosis is associated with a deficiency in the microsomal enzyme-steroid sulfatase (STS).

A subgroup of patients with lamellar ichthyosis has been recognized and associated with mutations, deletions, and insertions of the gene that encodes transglutaminase 1.

Mutations of one or more of the genes that encode lipoxygenase-3, 12(R)-lipoxygenase, and loricrin have been identified in a subgroup of patients with congenital ichthyosiform erythroderma.

Mutations of genes for keratin 1 and keratin 10 have been identified in patients with congenital bullous ichthyosiform erythroderma.

【病因】

鱼鳞病(ichthyosis)是以附着性鳞屑为特征的一组皮肤病。虽然临床表现类似,各个疾病亚型的致病基因并不相同。

寻常型鱼鳞病的特征是缺乏丝聚蛋白原,后者是透明角质颗粒的重要组成部分。

X-连锁隐性遗传鱼鳞病的发病是由于一种微粒体酶——类固醇硫酸酯酶的缺乏所致。

转谷氨酰胺酶1基因的突变、缺失或者插入与一部分板层状鱼鳞病患者的发病有关。

编码脂氧合酶-3,12(R)-脂氧合酶以及兜甲蛋白的一个或多个基因缺陷与部分先天性鱼鳞病样红皮病发病有关。

角蛋白1和角蛋白10基因突变与先天性大疱性鱼鳞病样红皮病发病有关。

【Clinical Manifestations】

Ichthyosis vulgaris is an autosomal dominant disorder. Scaling begins in early childhood, often within the first few months or years of life. Areas most severely involved are the extensor surfaces of the extremities, in which the scales are fine, white, and resemble barley flakes. Scaling on the trunk is usually less pronounced, while flexural areas and the face are normally spared (Fig. 15-1). The skin over the palms and soles is thickened with apparent ridges and grooves and exhibits some degree of hyperkeratosis. The chance of developing atopic disorders is higher among patients with ichthyosis vulgaris.

Recessive X-linked ichthyosis can only be inherited genetically by males. The skin appears normal at birth, and starts to peel throughout the body during the first month of life. Cutaneous lesions are frequently brown and larger than those occurring in ichthyosis vulgaris. The scales are seen particularly on the trunk,

【临床表现】

寻常型鱼鳞病(ichthyosis vulgaris)是一种常染色体显性遗传性皮肤病,发病于出生后数月至数年内。皮损为白色细碎糠状鳞屑,以四肢伸侧为重,躯干部受累较轻(图15-1)。曲侧和面部常无累及。掌跖部皮纹更加明显,甚至表现为轻度的掌跖角化。患者发生特应性疾病的概率较高。

X-连锁隐性遗传鱼鳞病(recessive X-linked ichthyosis)仅累及男性。患者出生时皮肤正常,常在出生后一个月内出现泛发性鳞屑。相对于寻常型鱼鳞病,本型病情更加严重,皮损为褐色大片

extremities, and the posterior neck, sparing the palms and soles. The flexures and face are rarely affected (Fig. 15-2). Corneal opacities are seen in female carriers and in about 50% of affected patients by slit-lamp examination. A connection with testicular cancer has been documented, but remains quite rare.

鳞屑。以躯干、四肢以及后颈部为重，掌跖常无累及，面部与其他曲侧部位较少受累(图 15-2)。裂隙灯检查发现女性携带者以及 50%的患者可以出现角膜混浊。偶有睾丸癌发病的报道。

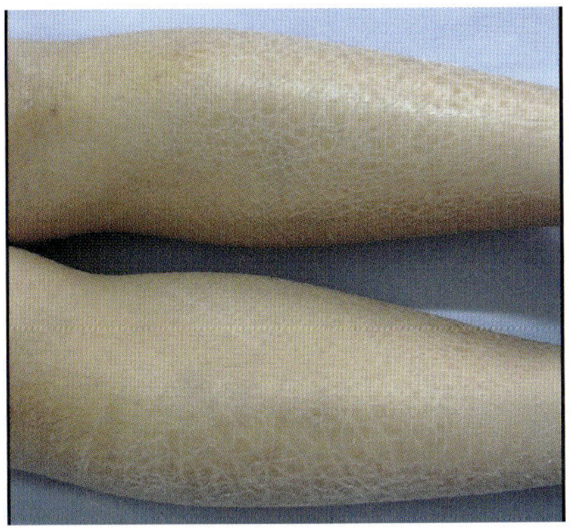

Fig. 15-1 Ichthyosis vulgaris
(图 15-1 寻常型鱼鳞病)

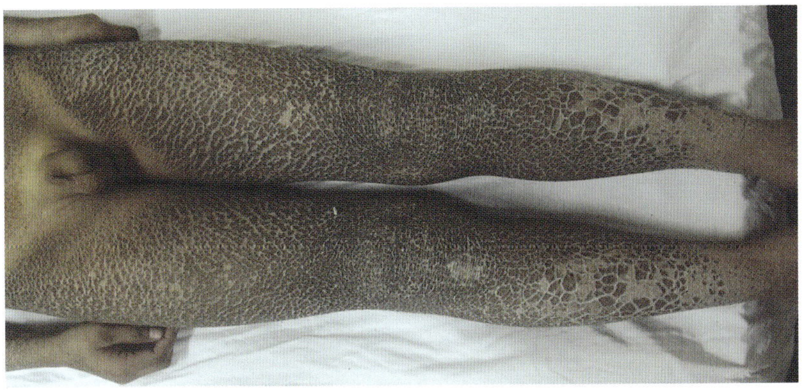

Fig. 15-2 Recessive X-linked ichthyosis
(图 15-2 X-连锁隐性遗传鱼鳞病)

Lamellar ichthyosis is inherited as an autosomal recessive trait. However, an autosomal dominant variant has recently been reported. At birth an infant with the disease is often encased in a collodion-like membrane, which may be shed within the first 2-3 weeks of life to reveal a mild erythroderma with generalized scaling. The scales over the entire body are large, grayish brown, strikingly quadrilateral, free on the edges and adherent in the center. In severe cases, the scales may be so thick that they resemble armor plate. Nail dystrophy and hair involvement may be observed in some cases. In addition, severe ectropion and eclabium are usually evident and characteristic in the diagnosis.

板层状鱼鳞病(lamellar ichthyosis)为常染色体隐性遗传性皮肤病，近来有也有常染色体显性遗传模式的报道。患儿出生时身体包被一层“火棉胶”样薄膜，2～3 周后薄膜脱落，皮损为轻度红皮病样外观，伴有泛发鳞屑。患者全身覆盖灰褐色大片状四方形鳞屑，中央黏着，边缘游离。重者鳞屑可厚如铠甲样。患者的指甲与头发可以受累，此外，严重的睑外翻和唇外翻具有特征性。

Congenital non-bullous ichthyosiform erythroderma has an autosomal recessive mode of inheritance. A collodion membrane is often present at birth. After shedding, the infant presents with an intense generalized erythroderma. Initially, small, white, coarse scales may cover the entire body, becoming thicker and darker over time, particularly in the case of scales involving the legs. Mild ectropion, eclabium, and palmoplantar keratoderma can be implicated. The risk for developing skin cancer is higher for this type of ichthyosis than for others.

先天性非大疱性鱼鳞病样红皮病(congenital non-bullous ichthyosiform erythroderma)为常染色体隐性遗传性皮肤病。患儿出生时身体包被一层“火棉胶”样薄膜，薄膜脱落后，皮损为重度红皮病样外观。最初，全身有细小的白色粗糙鳞屑，随着病程的延长，鳞屑逐渐变厚，颜色加深，尤其以腿部为著。患儿可伴有轻度的睑外翻、唇外翻以及掌跖角化。本型患儿发生皮肤癌变的概率较高。

Congenital bullous ichthyosiform erythroderma is a rare disease. It is inherited as an autosomal dominant mode, yet a high frequency of spontaneous mutations has been detected. The bullae usually appear at birth or shortly thereafter followed by formation of generally thickened, warty scales all over the body. As the scales are shed to leave a tender erythroderma appearance, a new bout of

先天性大疱性鱼鳞病样红皮病(congenital bullous ichthyosiform erythroderma)发病率极低。虽然有常染色体显性遗传的报道，本病仍以自发性突变为主要发病模式。出生时或出生后不久，患儿全身即可起大疱，随后为厚的疣

blisters and scales occurs on the healed areas. The erythema and blisters may become less apparent with age, and in these cases verruciform scales are more likely to develop, especially in flexural and intertriginous areas (Fig. 15-3).

状鳞屑替代。鳞屑脱落后皮损呈轻度红皮病样外观,创面修复后可有新的水疱以及鳞屑的形成。随着年龄的增长,红斑、水疱皮损逐渐减轻,代之以疣状鳞屑,此时曲侧以及间擦部位受累显著(图 15-3)。

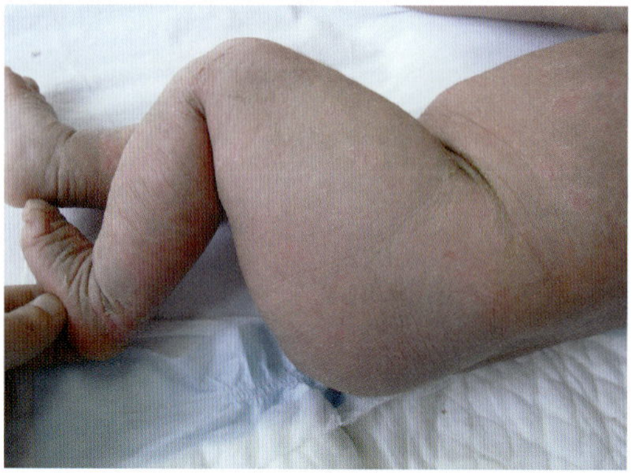

Fig. 15-3　Congenital bullous ichthyosiform erythroderma(图 15-3　先天性大疱性鱼鳞病样红皮病)

【Laboratory Findings】

Histological examination of a specimen from the involved skin in ichthyosis vulgaris reveals mild to moderate hyperkeratosis and a thin or absent granular cell layer. Under electron microscopy, those keratohyalin granules are seen to be poorly developed.

Recessive X-linked ichthyosis is characterized by a raised serum cholesterol sulfate and a lack of steroid sulfatase. Also, increased mobility of low density and very low density lipoproteins can be found by lipoprotein electrophoresis. This type of ichthyosis shows compact hyperkeratosis and variations in the granular cell layer, which may be normal, thickened, or thinned under light microscopy. Occasionally, a slight acanthosis and a perivascular infiltrate dominated by lymphocytic cells may be seen.

Histologic findings of acanthosis and marked hyperkeratosis are characteristics of lamellar ichthyosis. Epidermal proliferative activity is somewhat increased.

Epidermal turnover rates are increased in congenital ichthyosiform erythroderma. Histologically, hyperkeratosis, focal parakeratosis, and acanthosis are easily revealed. Under electron microscopy, conspicuous lipid droplets in the prickle cell layer may be seen and small and dysmorphic lamellar bodies in the granular layer are increased.

The histological features of congenital bullous ichthyosiform erythroderma are known collectively as epidermolytic hyperkeratosis. Massive hyperkeratosis, papillomatosis, and acanthosis are accompanied by thickened granular cell layer. Irregular eosinophilic intracytoplasmic keratohyalin granules may also be seen within the

【实验室检查】

光镜下,寻常型鱼鳞病组织病理表现为轻至中度角化过度,颗粒层变薄或消失。电镜下,透明角质颗粒形成不良。

X-连锁隐性遗传鱼鳞病患者的特征性改变为血清胆固醇硫酸盐水平高于正常,并伴有类固醇硫酸酯酶缺陷。脂蛋白电泳显示低密度脂蛋白以及极低密度脂蛋白电泳迁移率增加。光镜下,本病表现为致密角化过度,颗粒层的厚度可以正常、增厚或变薄。偶见轻度棘层肥厚以及血管周围淋巴细胞浸润。

板层状鱼鳞病的组织病理学特征为显著角化过度以及棘层肥厚。表皮增殖能力有所增强。

先天性鱼鳞病样红皮病的表皮周转速率加快。组织学上,可见角化过度、局灶性角化不全以及棘层肥厚。电镜下,棘层内可见明显的脂肪滴,颗粒层内有数目增多的小而异形的板层小体。

先天性大疱性鱼鳞病样红皮病的组织学特征是表皮松解性角化过度,可见重度的角化过度、乳头瘤样增生以及棘层肥厚伴有颗粒层增厚。颗粒层细胞中可见不规则形状的嗜酸性透明角质颗

granular cell layer. Intercellular edema above suprabasal keratinocytes is so prominent that it may lead to intraepidermal blister formation.

粒。表皮基底层以上显著细胞间水肿，最终可以导致表皮内大疱的形成。

【Diagnosis and Differential Diagnosis】

The diagnosis of ichthyosis can be made based on clinical features and laboratory findings.

The following features of ichthyosis vulgaris permit distinction from other types of ichthyosis.

(1) From recessive X-linked ichthyosis: complete absence from flexural areas, absence of corneal opacities, palmar-plantar involvement, small white scales, normal steroid sulfatase activity, and normal serum lipoprotein electrophoresis.

(2) From lamellar ichthyosis: not present at birth, complete absence from flexural areas, no ectropion or eclabium, and no erythroderma.

(3) From congenital bullous ichthyosiform erythroderma: complete absence from flexural areas, no blistering, and having histopathologic features that do not match those of congenital bullous ichthyosiform erythroderma.

(4) From acquired ichthyosis: onset in childhood, as well as family history.

【诊断与鉴别诊断】

鱼鳞病根据临床特征以及实验室检查一般均可明确诊断。

寻常型鱼鳞病可借如下几点与其他类型相鉴别。

(1) 与X-连锁隐性遗传鱼鳞病鉴别　无曲侧受累、无角膜混浊、掌跖部受累，鳞屑小而呈白色，类固醇硫酸酯酶活性正常，血清脂蛋白电泳正常。

(2) 与板层状鱼鳞病鉴别　出生时不发病，无曲侧受累，无睑外翻和唇外翻，无红皮病表现。

(3) 与先天性大疱性鱼鳞病样红皮病鉴别　无曲侧受累，无大疱形成，具有寻常型鱼鳞病的组织学特征。

(4) 与获得性鱼鳞病鉴别　幼年发病，具有家族史。

【Treatment】

Emollients such as urea ointment and alpha hydroxy acid (e.g., lactic acid) ointment may be effective in the treatment of ichthyosis vulgaris and recessive X-linked ichthyosis.

As for lamellar ichthyosis and congenital ichthyosiform erythroderma, collodion babies should be kept in a humid environment, and the membrane should not be manually debrided. Emollients and alpha hydroxy acid may be of some help.

Treatment for congenital bullous ichthyosiform erythroderma is often not successful. The keratolytic agents used in other forms of ichthyosis are usually too irritating for fragile neonate skin. Since secondary bacterial infection can promote the formation of the bullae, bacterial culture of the samples from the blisters and erosions should be carried out and oral antibiotics administered when necessary.

【治疗】

润泽剂如尿素软膏、α-羟基酸制剂如乳酸软膏对于寻常型鱼鳞病以及X-连锁隐性遗传鱼鳞病有一定的治疗作用。

对于板层状鱼鳞病以及先天性鱼鳞病样红皮病，初生的火棉胶儿应置于湿润的环境，其身上的薄膜不应人为剥除。上述外用药物对于这两型鱼鳞病也有一定的治疗效果。

先天性大疱性鱼鳞病样红皮病的治疗较为困难。适用于其他类型鱼鳞病的角质松解剂对于该型患儿过于刺激。除此之外，继发感染在患儿大疱形成的过程中具有重要促进作用，因此大疱以及糜烂面应做细菌培养，必要时口服抗生素。

【Prognosis】

Ichthyosis vulgaris and recessive X-linked ichthyosis are likely to improve with age, provided the patient survives. Residence in a mild moist climate may help.

Collodion babies with lamellar ichthyosis or congenital

【预后】

寻常型鱼鳞病以及X-连锁隐性遗传鱼鳞病的病情会随着年龄的增长逐渐减轻。居住于湿润的环境对于患者病情的稳定及消退有一定作用。

板层状鱼鳞病以及先天性鱼鳞病样

ichthyosiform erythroderma may die of sepsis or electrolyte imbalance. In addition, elderly patients suffering from congenital bullous ichthyosiform erythroderma may encounter a similar fate.

红皮病患儿常因败血症或电解质平衡紊乱而死亡。此外,年龄较大的先天性大疱性鱼鳞病样红皮病患者也常因同样的原因死亡。

Section Two　Keratosis Pilaris

第二节　毛发角化病

【Etiology】

The cause of keratosis pilaris is unknown.

【病因】

毛发角化病(keratosis pilaris)的病因不明。

【Clinical Manifestations】

Keratosis pilaris has an autosomal dominant mode of inheritance. The onset age is most often in the first 2 decades with a peak during adolescence. The follicular keratotic papules are discrete and asymptomatic, occurring predominantly over the extensor extremities (Fig. 15-4). The face, trunk and buttocks can also be affected.

【临床表现】

毛发角化病为常染色体显性遗传性疾病,发病年龄多在20岁以前,青春期为其发病高峰。皮损为四肢伸侧互不融合的毛囊角化性丘疹(图15-4),一般无自觉症状。面部、躯干及臀部也可受累。

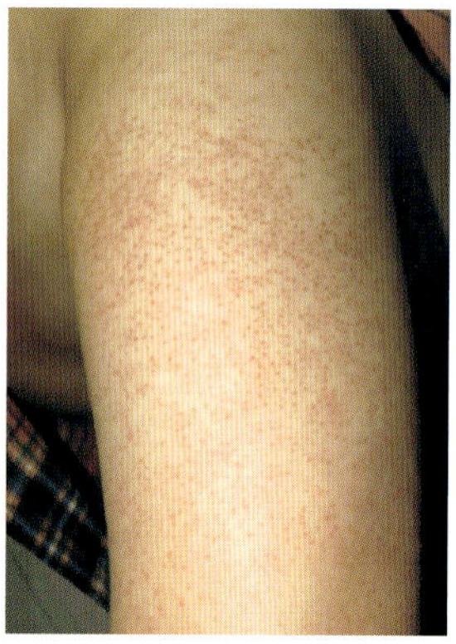

Fig. 15-4　Keratosis pilaris(图15-4　毛发角化病)

Keratosis pilaris atrophicans has a predilection for the face, which shows atrophy, scarring, and alopecia on the skin involved.

萎缩性毛发角化病好发于面部,常伴有萎缩、瘢痕以及脱发。

【Histopathology】

Histological examination (though rarely necessary) reveals that the dilated follicles are filled with a keratotic plug and one or more distorted hair shafts.

【组织病理】

组织学上(虽然并非必须做)可见扩张的毛囊,内含毛囊角栓、单根或数根变形的毛干。

【Diagnosis and Differential Diagnosis】

The diagnosis of keratosis pilaris can be based on its distinctive clinical features and histopathological findings.

Phrynoderma, which is related to vitamin and nutritional deficiencies, may present with similar follicular hyperkeratosis. However, the follicles afflicted with phrynoderma are apt to be surrounded by a halo of erythema. When the erythema is generally distributed, pityriasis rubra pilaris must be precluded in differentiation diagnosis.

【诊断与鉴别诊断】

毛发角化病根据临床特征以及组织病理检查一般均可明确诊断。

蟾皮病的临床表现与毛发角化病类似,前者的发病与维生素缺乏或营养障碍有关。有时毛囊周围绕以红斑,当红斑泛发时,要和毛发红糠疹鉴别。

【Treatment】

Emollients such as urea ointment applied after bathing may be effective. Preparations containing tretinoin are an alternative.

【Prognosis】

The condition improves during summer months.

Section Three　Keratosis Follicularis (Darier's disease)

【Etiology】

The gene for keratosis follicularis (also known as Darier's disease) has recently been identified as ATP2A2, located on chromosome 12q23-24.

【Clinical Manifestations】

Keratosis follicularis is a rare disorder, inherited as an autosomal dominant mode. The lesions are characterized by pruritic, greasy brown, keratotic papules and plaques found on the seborrheic areas such as the scalp, ears, face, neck, upper trunk (Fig. 15-5 to Fig. 15-7). There is mild involvement of the flexures in a majority of patients.

【治疗】

治疗可以选用润泽剂如尿素软膏，在洗澡后使用，也可使用维 A 酸制剂。

【预后】

本病在夏季病情可以缓解。

第三节　毛囊角化病(Darier病)

【病因】

毛囊角化病(keratosis follicularis)，又称为 Darier 病(Darier's disease)，其致病基因为 ATP2A2，定位于 12q23-24。

【临床表现】

毛囊角化病较为罕见，是一种显性遗传性疾病。皮损为油腻性、棕褐色角化性丘疹或斑块，多分布于脂溢性区域(头皮、耳部、面部、颈部以及躯干上部)(图15-5至图 15-7)，患者可自觉瘙痒。多数患者曲侧受累较轻。

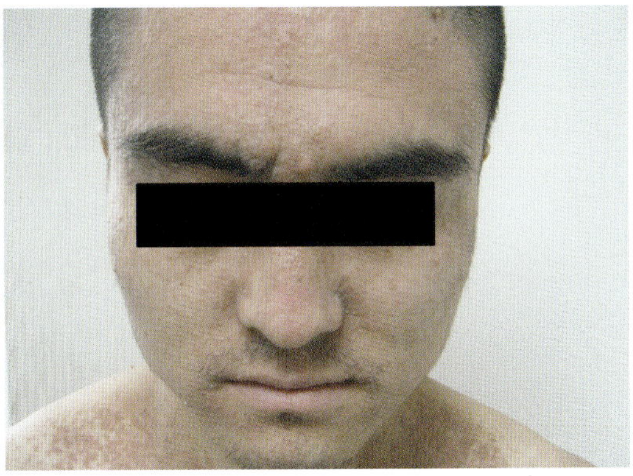

Fig. 15-5　Keratosis follicularis-face
(图 15-5　毛囊角化病-面部)

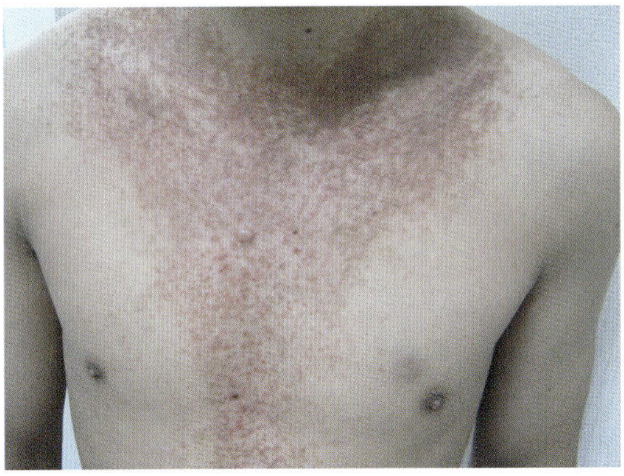

Fig. 15-6　Keratosis follicularis-chest
(图 15-6　毛囊角化病-胸)

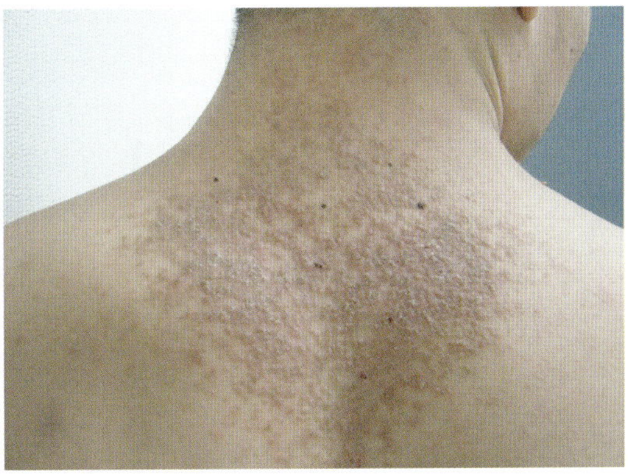

Fig. 15-7　Keratosis follicularis-back(图 15-7　毛囊角化病-背)

The hands are affected in most patients. Punctate keratoses with focal disruptions of skin ridges on the palms and soles are characteristic features for keratosis follicularis.

Nail changes provide important diagnostic clues. Typically, longitudinal white or red streaks can be seen, some of which terminate in a small nick on the free margin.

The mucous membranes can also be affected sometimes, with small white papules on the hard palate of the oral cavity. Ocular lesions, particularly affecting the cornea, are seen in most patients.

大多数患者均有手部受累,典型皮损为掌跖部点状掌跖角皮症伴有局限性皮嵴中断。

甲的改变具有特征性,表现为甲板上纵行分布的白色或红色条带,有一些终止于甲板游离缘的小缺口。

黏膜也可累及。口腔黏膜皮损为硬腭部小的白色丘疹。大多数患者的眼睛尤其是角膜出现损害。

【Histopathology】

Skin biopsies provide diagnostic value here. Foci of suprabasal clefts contain characteristic acantholytic keratinocytes, and dyskeratotic cells (corps ronds and grains) can be revealed histologically. A thickened parakeratotic *stratum corneum* over these lacunae is also commonly seen.

【组织病理】

组织学检查具有特征性。基底层上局灶性表皮内裂隙形成,其内有棘层松解和角化不良细胞(圆体和谷粒)。裂隙上方角质层增厚,可出现角化不全。

【Diagnosis and Differential Diagnosis】

The diagnosis of keratosis follicularis can be made based on clinical features and its distinctive histological findings.

Keratosis follicularis must be differentiated from seborrheic dermatitis, warty dyskeratoma, and Hailey-Hailey disease. Skin biopsy is usually helpful. A similar histologic picture may be seen in Grover's disease, but clinical manifestations differ in the two diseases.

【诊断与鉴别诊断】

毛囊角化病根据临床特征以及组织病理检查一般均可明确诊断。

毛囊角化病必须要与脂溢性皮炎、疣状角化不良瘤及家族性良性慢性天疱疮相鉴别,组织病理可资鉴别。毛囊角化病与暂时性棘层松解性皮病组织学类似,但两者临床表现不同。

【Treatment】

Patients should avoid excessive sun exposure. Topical tretinoin cream and oral retinoids may ameliorate the symptoms in severe cases.

【治疗】

患者应避免过度日晒。外用维 A 酸软膏或口服维 A 酸制剂对病情严重者的缓解有一定帮助。

【Prognosis】

This condition tends to become more severe with age.

【预后】

随着年龄的增长,本病会逐渐加重。

Section Four Keratosis Palmaris *et* Plantaris

第四节　掌跖角皮症

【Etiology】

Keratosis palmaris *et* plantaris consists of a large group of conditions, which can be divided into two subtypes. The first subtype involves the skin only, while the second type has a much broader spectrum of ectodermal defects beyond skin lesions. Here we discuss only the former subtype.

Palmoplantar keratoderma is an autosomal dominant inherited disease. Recently mutations in the keratin 9 gene have been linked to epidermolytic palmoplantar keratoderma (EPPK).

Also, mutations in keratin 1 and keratin 2 genes have been identified in patients with diffuse palmoplantar keratoderma.

【病因】

掌跖角皮症(keratosis palmaris *et* plantaris)包括一组疾病,通常可以分为两大类:一类仅有皮肤受累,另一类同时还有许多外胚叶发育不良的表现。本节仅讨论前者。

掌跖角皮症是一种常染色体显性遗传性疾病,角蛋白 9 基因突变导致表皮松解性掌跖角皮症发生。

弥漫性掌跖角皮症发病与角蛋白 1 和角蛋白 2 基因突变有关。

Mutations in desmoglein-1 and desmoplakin have been associated with patients who have striate palmoplantar keratoderma.

However, the genetic basis for punctate palmoplantar keratoderma has not yet been conclusively identified.

条纹状掌跖角皮症发病与桥粒芯糖蛋白-1 和桥粒斑蛋白基因突变有关。

点状掌跖角皮症的发病原因不明。

【Clinical Manifestations】

【临床表现】

Epidermolytic palmoplantar keratoderma is inherited as an autosomal dominant condition. The lesions are characterized by symmetrical well-demarcated yellowish keratoderma bordered by an erythematous margin and diffusely affecting the palms and soles.

Diffuse palmoplantar keratoderma is inherited as an autosomal dominant trait, but recently the possibility of an autosomal recessive variant has been reported. Lesions are characterized by diffuse hyperkeratosis involving the palms and soles as well as the ventral surfaces of the fingers and toes (Fig. 15-8, Fig. 15-9).

表皮松解性掌跖角皮症为常染色体显性遗传性疾病。皮损为掌跖部弥漫分布的界限清楚的角化性斑片，呈黄色，周围绕以红色的边缘。

弥漫性掌跖角皮症为常染色体显性遗传性疾病，近来也有隐性遗传的报道。皮损为掌跖部以及指（趾）腹侧弥漫分布的角化过度性损害（图 15-8，图 15-9）。

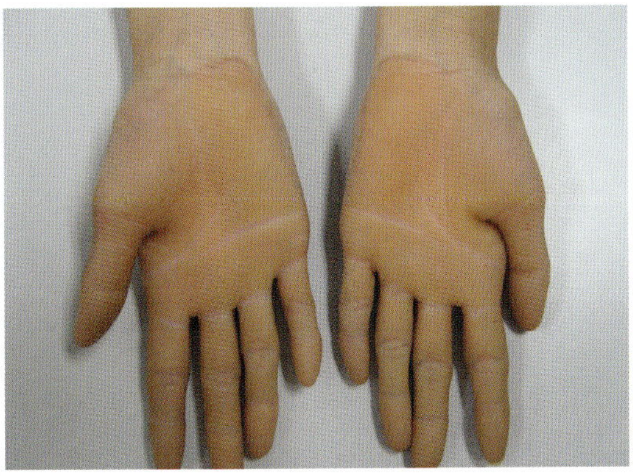

Fig. 15-8　Diffuse palmoplantar keratoderma-hands
（图 15-8　弥漫性掌跖角皮症-手）

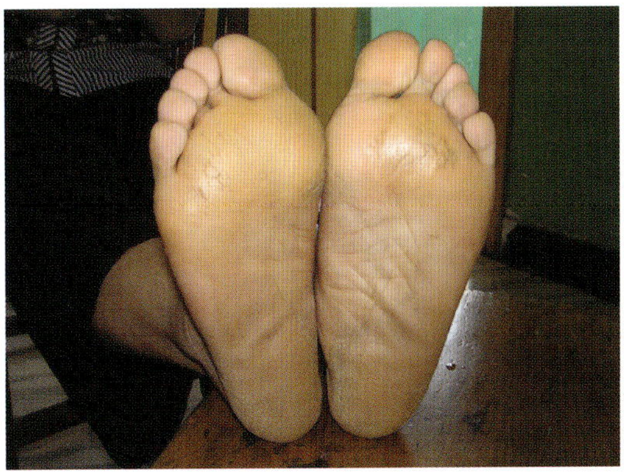

Fig. 15-9　Diffuse palmoplantar keratoderma-feet
（图 15-9　弥漫性掌跖角皮症-足）

Striate palmoplantar keratoderma has an autosomal dominant mode of inheritance. Linear bands of keratoderma on the palmar aspects of the palms and fingers, and island-like areas of hyperkeratosis on the soles of the feet, are typically seen. Abnormalities of the nails, teeth and hair may be observed as well.

Punctate palmoplantar keratoderma is also characterized by an autosomal dominant mode of inheritance (compare to preceding paragraph) although the genes responsible have not yet been identified. Small, discrete, yellow-brown, depressed keratotic lesions are seen on the palms, soles, and ventral aspects of fingers and toes. Lesions are usually asymptomatic, occasionally presenting with pain or burning. Keratosis of punctata of the palmar creases (KPPC) is a variant of punctate palmoplantar keratoderma in which the lesions are confined to the palmar and digital creases, but soles of the feet and heels may occasionally be involved as well.

条纹状掌跖角皮症为常染色体显性遗传性疾病。手掌和手指的掌侧可见条带状分布的角化过度性皮损，足跖部也可见岛屿状的类似损害。可见指（趾）甲、牙齿以及毛发的异常。

点状掌跖角皮症为常染色体显性遗传性疾病，但其致病基因还不清楚。掌跖以及指（趾）的腹侧可见散在分布的黄色至棕褐色小的深在角化性损害。皮损一般无自觉症状，偶有疼痛或烧灼感。手掌皱褶部点状角化过度症是本病的一种变型，皮损局限于手掌以及手指的皱褶部位，有时足跖和足踵部也可受累。

【Histopathology】

Under light microscopy, epidermolytic palmoplantar keratoderma is characterized by hyperkeratosis, papillomatosis, hypergranulosis, and acanthosis accompanied by the features of epidermolytic hyperkeratosis.

Diffuse palmoplantar keratoderma is characterized by marked hyperkeratosis, hypergranulosis, acanthosis, and widened and elongated epidermal ridges. In the recessive variant, the hyperkeratosis is even more marked than in the dominant form and the epidermis shows prominent psoriasiform hyperplasia.

Striate palmoplantar keratoderma is characterized by massive hyperkeratosis, hypergranulosis, and acanthosis. Dark-staining granular and filamentous material within the prickle cell layer, accompanied by slightly separated keratinocytes, has also been described.

Punctate palmoplantar keratoderma is characterized by marked hyperkeratosis areas, underneath which the epidermis exhibits punctate depressions.

【Diagnosis】

The diagnosis of keratosis palmaris *et* plantaris can be made based on clinical features, histological examination, and detection of the mutated genes.

【Treatment】

Topical application of keratolytic agents may soften the skin and provide some curative value when combined with oral synthetic retinoids.

【Prognosis】

Trauma or manual labor may exacerbate the disorder, and both should be avoided. There is a greatly increased risk of dermatophyte infections in patients with diffuse palmoplantar keratoderma.

Section Five　Inherited Epidermolysis Bullosa

【Etiology】

Inherited epidermolysis bullosa (EB) refers to a large group of unrelated mechanobullous diseases in which the skin and the mucous membranes sometimes easily form blisters due to external trauma.

The disease can vary in severity from life-threatening to minimal. It can be divided into four subtypes: simplex, hemidesmosomal, junctional, and dystrophic.

【组织病理】

光镜下，表皮松解性掌跖角皮症表现为角化过度、乳头瘤样增生、颗粒层增厚、棘层肥厚伴有特征性的表皮松解性角化过度。

弥漫性掌跖角皮症组织学上表现为显著角化过度、颗粒层增厚、棘层肥厚以及增宽延长的表皮嵴。表现为隐性遗传模式的弥漫性掌跖角皮症组织学上角化过度更加明显，表皮呈银屑病样增生改变。

条纹状掌跖角皮症表现为角化过度、颗粒层增厚以及棘层肥厚，偶见棘细胞内深染的颗粒状或细丝状物质伴有轻度角质形成细胞松解。

点状掌跖角皮症病理学特征为显著的角化过度，其下方的表皮凹陷。

【诊断】

掌跖角皮症根据临床特征、组织病理学检查以及突变基因的检测一般均可明确诊断。

【治疗】

外用角质剥脱剂可以缓解症状，也可口服合成的维 A 酸制剂。

【预后】

创伤以及体力劳动会加重本病病情，应尽量避免。弥漫性掌跖角皮症患者发生浅表感染的概率增高。

第五节　遗传性大疱性表皮松解症

【病因】

遗传性大疱性表皮松解症(epidermolysis bullosa, EB)包括一组疾病，本病在轻度外伤后，容易在皮肤甚至黏膜上形成水疱。

EB 可以是致命性的，病情也可很轻微。目前分为四型：单纯性 EB、半桥粒性 EB、交界性 EB 及营养不良性 EB。

EB simplex is associated with mutations in the genes of keratin 5 or keratin 14.

Hemidesmosomal EB is associated with gene mutations that encode hemidesmosomal proteins such as plectin, BP180 and the α6 and β4 integrin subunits.

Junctional EB results from laminin-5 gene mutations while dystrophic EB is associated with type Ⅶ collagen gene mutations.

单纯性 EB 发病与角蛋白 5 或角蛋白 14 基因突变有关。

半桥粒性 EB 发病与编码半桥粒蛋白（网蛋白、BP180 以及整合素的 α6 和 β4 亚单位）的基因突变有关。

交界性 EB 发病与层粘连蛋白-5 基因突变有关，营养不良性 EB 发病与Ⅶ型胶原蛋白基因突变有关。

【Clinical Manifestations】

(1) Five subtypes of EB simplex (EBS) are now recognized, and all of them have an autosomal dominant mode of inheritance.

Localized EB simplex of the hands and feet (Weber-Cockayne) is the most common form of EBS, in which lesions are confined to the palms and soles. The skin is mechanically rather fragile and tends to form clear blisters (Fig. 15-10). Usually the lesion heals without any scarring or postinflammatory hyperpigmentation. The condition may be aggravated during warmer months or when patients' skin undergoes excessive mechanical stimulation. Hyperhidrosis may also accompany this type of EBS.

【临床表现】

(1) 目前认为单纯性 EB(EBS)有五种亚型，遗传模式均为常染色体显性遗传。

局限于手足部位的 EBS（Weber-Cockayne 型）是最常见的一型。皮损局限于掌跖部位，皮肤脆性增加，水疱内容物清亮（图 15-10），一般愈后不伴有瘢痕和炎症后色素沉着。病情在高温季节以及患者接受过度机械刺激时加重。本病可伴有多汗症。

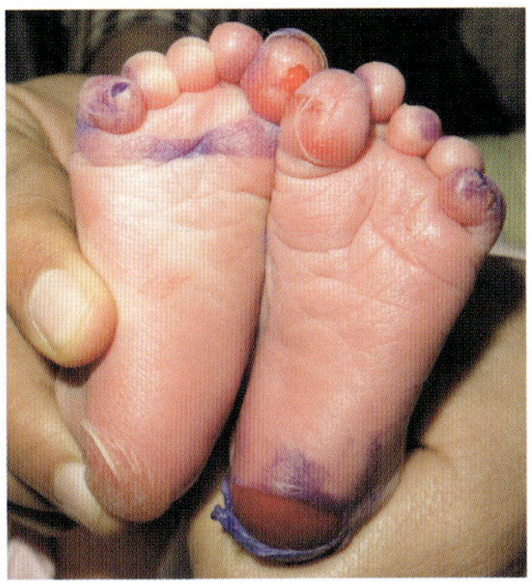

Fig. 15-10　Localized EB simplex of the hands and feet (Weber-Cockayne)
（图 15-10　局限于手足部位的 EBS（Weber-Cockayne 型））

In the case of EB simplex (Koebner), blisters are usually seen all over the patient's body, but will appear predominantly on the flexural aspects of the extremities. The blisters usually heal without scarring, atrophy, or milia. Like most forms of EB, EB simplex (Koebner) often worsens during the summer months. Nail and tooth involvement (e. g., nail dystrophy or hypodontia or anodontia) is rare, and systemic involvement is not apparent.

EB simplex herpetiformis (Dowling-Meara) is characterized by a herpetiform grouping of blistering. Lesions are usually present at birth. Milia formation is common, and nail dystrophy and palmoplantar keratoderma may also be seen (Fig. 15-11, Fig. 15-12). Hypodontia and anodontia have also been described with this type of EBS. Seasonal variation is not apparent, though.

Koebner 型 EBS 患者全身各处均可发病，尤以四肢的曲侧为重。水疱愈合后一般无瘢痕、萎缩和粟丘疹。同其他类型的 EB 一样，本型夏季病情加重。一般无甲（如甲营养不良）、牙齿（如牙齿发育不全或无牙）以及系统的受累。

疱疹样 EBS（Dowling-Meara 型）皮损为疱疹样簇集分布的水疱。出生时即可发病。可见粟丘疹、甲营养不良以及掌跖角皮症（图 15-11，图 15-12）。也有牙齿发育不全以及无牙症的报道。本病季节性变化不明显。

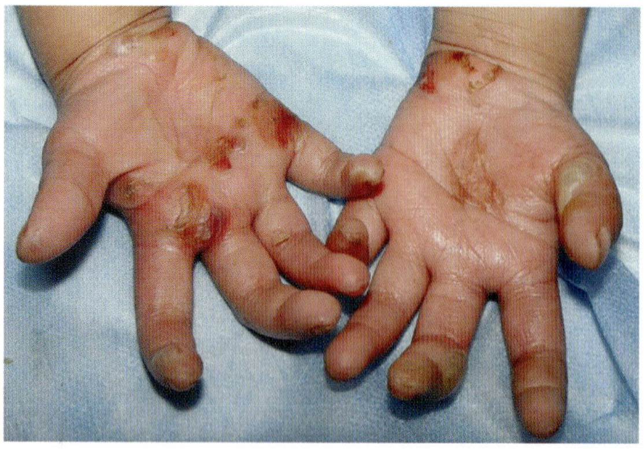

Fig. 15-11 EB simplex herpetiformis (Dowling-Meara)-hands
(图 15-11 疱疹样 EBS(Dowling-Meara 型)-手)

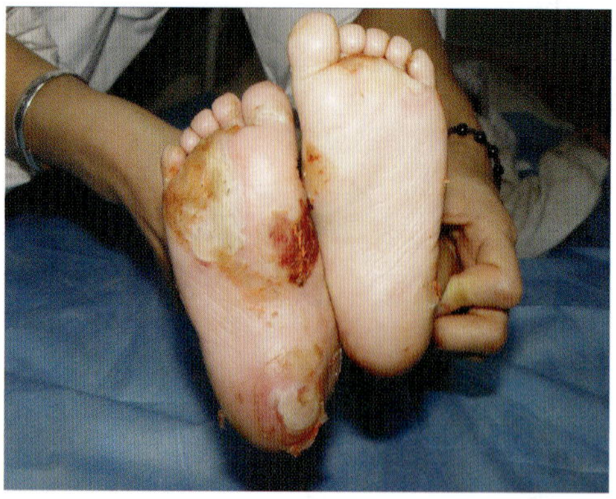

Fig. 15-12 EB simplex herpetiformis (Dowling-Meara)-feet
(图 15-12 疱疹样 EBS(Dowling-Meara 型)-足)

EB simplex with mottled pigmentation has similar skin lesions as the Dowling-Meara variant, but with the addition of mottled or reticulate pigmentation, particularly in the neck and trunk. Punctate keratoderma on the palms and warty hyperkeratotic lesions involving the hands, elbows, and knees may also be seen.

伴斑驳色素沉着的 EBS 的皮损除了与疱疹样 EBS(Dowling-Meara 型)类似之外,还可有网状或斑状色素沉着,尤其以颈部和躯干为重。手掌部可发生点状角皮症,手、肘以及膝有疣状角化性损害。

Patients with EB simplex superficialis present blisters, erosions, and crusts that spare the palms and soles in most cases. Atrophic scarring, nail dystrophy, and milia may be seen as well. The site of epidermal cleavage differs from other EB simplex variants: it is subcorneal rather than intrabasal.

表浅性 EBS 的皮损为水疱、糜烂、结痂,掌跖部常不受累。可见萎缩性瘢痕、甲营养不良和粟丘疹。本型的水疱位置与其他型 EBS 不同,水疱位于角质层下而不是基底层内。

(2) Hemidesmosomal EB includes three variants.

(2) 半桥粒性 EB 包括 3 种亚型。

Generalized atrophic benign EB has an autosomal dominant mode of inheritance. Patients present with multiple blisters and erosions, followed by mild scarring and widespread cigarette paper-like atrophy. Lesions are also characterized by alternating macules of varying size and shape of both hyper-and hypopigmentation. Nails, teeth, hair, and eyes may also be involved.

泛发型萎缩性良性 EB 的遗传模式为常染色体显性遗传。皮损为大量的水疱、糜烂伴有轻度的瘢痕以及广泛分布的香烟纸样萎缩。形状及大小各异的色素沉着和色素脱失斑是其特征。指(趾)甲、牙齿、毛发以及眼睛均可受累。

The inheritance of EB together with late-onset muscular dystrophy is autosomal recessive. Generalized blisters and erosions appearing at or shortly after birth with muscular dystrophy or myasthenia gravis will be inevitable in this case. Patients also suffer from atrophic scarring, milia, nail dystrophy or anonychia, alopecia, and oral lesions.

迟发型肌肉营养不良性 EB 为常染色体隐性遗传性疾病。出生时或出生后不久,患者即可泛发大疱以及糜烂,最终出现肌肉营养不良或重症肌无力。患者也可出现萎缩性瘢痕、粟丘疹、甲营养不良或无甲症、脱发以及口腔损害。

EB with pyloric atresia is a rare variant. Patients are at risk of urethrovesical junction obstruction with fibrosis and aplasia cutis congenita in addition to pyloric atresia.

伴有幽门闭锁的 EB 极为罕见。患者除发生幽门闭锁之外,还可伴有输尿管膀胱连接点纤维性阻塞以及先天性皮肤发育不全。

(3) Junctional EB includes four variants, all of which have autosomal recessive modes of inheritance.

(3)交界性 EB 包括 4 种亚型,遗传模式均为常染色体隐性遗传。

Patients with junctional EB-Herlitz present at birth with blisters and erosions accompanied by scarring and atrophy. Healing with the formation of hypertrophic granulation tissue is a

Herlitz 型交界性 EB 患者出生时即可有大疱以及糜烂面伴有瘢痕和萎缩。愈后形成增生性肉芽组织是本病的特征

distinctive sign. This is particularly common around the mouth, eyes and nares, sides of the neck, trunk and nails.

性损害。尤其以口腔、眼、鼻孔周围、颈侧部、躯干以及甲周围显著。

Junctional EB-non-Herlitz is associated with a mutation of the laminin-5 gene. The clinical features are similar to those in generalized atrophic benign EB, described above.

非 Herlitz 型交界性 EB 发病与编码层粘连蛋白-5 基因突变有关。其临床表现与泛发型萎缩性良性 EB 一致。

In patients with junctional EB-inversa, generalized blisters and erosions present at birth or develop in early infancy, and are usually confined to inverse sites such as the axillae and groin as the disease progresses. The lesions may be accompanied by atrophic scarring, and nails may be dystrophic or absent in this type of EB.

反向性交界性 EB 患者的皮损在出生时或婴儿早期发生，表现为泛发的水疱和糜烂面，伴萎缩性瘢痕，甲可有营养不良或缺失。随着病程的延长，皮损多局限于皱褶部位，如腋窝和腹股沟。

In patients with junctional EB-late onset (or progressive), lesions do not present until late childhood. Blisters and erosions affect the hands, elbows, knees, and feet. Nails may be dystrophic or absent, and enamel hypoplasia is characteristic.

迟发型(进行性)交界性 EB 的发病年龄为儿童后期。皮损为累及手、肘、膝以及足的大疱和糜烂面。甲可有营养不良或缺失，牙釉质发育不全具有一定特征性。

(4) Nine subtypes of dystrophic EB are now recognized.

(4) 营养不良性 EB 包括 9 种亚型。

Dominant dystrophic EB includes the Cockayne-Touraine and Pasini variants. Generalized blisters are seen at birth that may be accompanied by alopecia, milia, atrophic scarring, and dystrophic or absent nails. The Pasini type is a more severe condition with albopapuloid lesions. In contrast, the lesions of Cockayne-Touraine type are more limited in extent and severity, and lack albopapuloid lesions.

显性遗传性营养不良性 EB 包括 Cockayne-Touraine 型和 Pasini 型。患者出生时即有泛发水疱。可伴有脱发、粟丘疹、萎缩性瘢痕、甲营养不良或无甲。Pasini 型病情更加严重，并可见白色丘疹样皮损。Cockayne-Touraine 型病情较轻，分布的范围更加局限，无白色丘疹样皮损。

Recessive dystrophic EB-Hallopeau-Siemens is more severe than its autosomal dominant counterpart. Blisters and erosions are present at birth, and Nikolsky's sign is positive. In some cases, milia, atrophy, scarring, growth retardation, and pseudosyndactyly of the hands and feet may be observed (Fig. 15-13). The nails, teeth, eyes, and mucous membranes are often severely affected. Squamous cell carcinoma and melanoma may be seen in this variant.

Hallopeau-Siemens 型隐性遗传性营养不良性 EB 症状比显性遗传性营养不良性 EB 更加严重。水疱和糜烂面出生时即可发生，尼氏征阳性。可有粟丘疹、萎缩、瘢痕、发育迟滞以及手足的假性并指(趾)(图 15-13)。指甲、牙齿、眼睛以及黏膜受累严重。患者可能并发鳞状细胞癌以及黑素瘤。

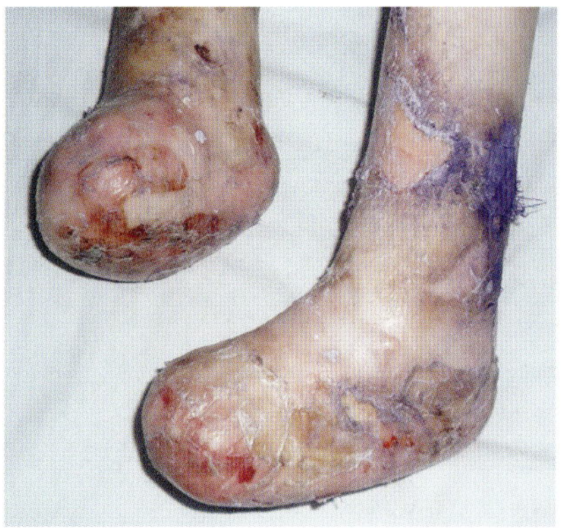

Fig. 15-13　Recessive dystrophic EB-Hallopeau-Siemens

(图 15-13　Hallopeau-Siemens 型隐性遗传性营养不良性 EB)

Recessive dystrophic EB-non-Hallopeau-Siemens is similar to the Hallopeau-Siemens variant except that the extracutaneous lesions are less severe and the risk of developing cutaneous squamous cell carcinoma is lower.

非 Hallopeau-Siemens 型隐性遗传性营养不良性 EB 临床特征与 Hallopeau-Siemens 型类似，但皮肤外症状较轻，发生鳞状细胞癌的概率更低。

Dominant dystrophic EB-pretibial is a mild variant. Lesions are localized and typically symmetrical and usually present in early childhood. Blisters and erosions accompanied by atrophic scarring and milia are seen particularly on the pretibial region and dorsal aspects of the feet. The forearms and trunk may also be involved. An autosomal recessive variant of this type has recently been described.

显性遗传性胫前型营养不良性 EB 病情较轻，皮损局限且对称性分布。一般在儿童早期发病，为分布于胫前或足背部的水疱、糜烂伴有萎缩性瘢痕和粟丘疹。前臂和躯干也可受累。近来也有常染色体隐性遗传模式的报道。

Dystrophic EB-pruriginosa includes dominant and recessive variants. Nodular prurigo-like nodules are seen against a background of blisters, milia, and albopapuloid lesions (Fig. 15-14). Nail dystrophy may be seen.

痒疹型营养不良性 EB 包括显性遗传和隐性遗传两种遗传模式。在水疱、粟丘疹以及白色丘疹样损害的基础上可见结节性痒疹样皮损(图 15-14)，可见甲营养不良。

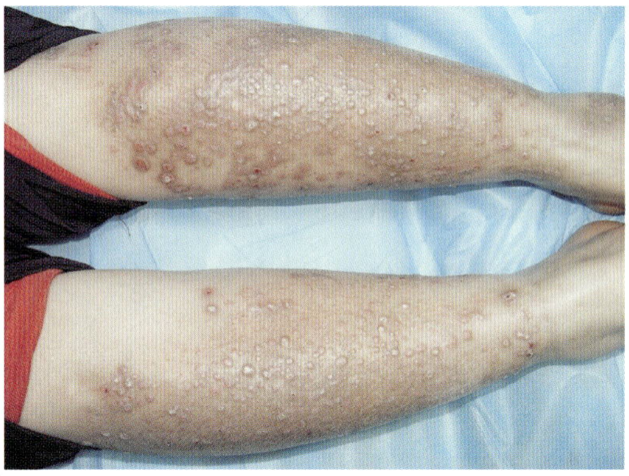

Fig. 15-14　Dystrophic EB-pruriginosa(图 15-14　痒疹型营养不良性 EB)

Dystrophic EB-inversa has an autosomal recessive mode of inheritance. Lesions are found particularly on the flexural sites, including the inguinal regions, axillae, neck, and lower back. Severe oral and esophageal involvement is a characteristic sign for this type.

反向型营养不良性 EB 为常染色体隐性遗传。皮损多局限于皱褶部位，如腹股沟、腋窝、颈部以及下背部。重度的口腔以及食道受累具有特征性。

Dystrophic EB-centripetalis is an autosomal recessive variant. Widespread blisters are present at birth; however, the distribution becomes acral in adulthood. Lesions show a characteristic centripetal spread.

向心型营养不良性 EB 为常染色体隐性遗传。出生时皮损为广泛分布的大疱，但成年后皮损局限于肢端，呈特征性的向心性分布。

Dystrophic EB-acral has an autosomal dominant mode of inheritance. Lesions at birth or in early childhood often affect limb extremities. Blisters and erosions may cease after childhood.

肢端型营养不良性 EB 为常染色体显性遗传性疾病。皮损在出生时或儿童早期出现，多局限于肢端部位。儿童期后水疱和糜烂可能不再发生。

Transient bullous dermolysis of the newborn includes dominant and recessive variants. The disease is a self-limiting condition. Blisters usually resolve within the first 2 years and heal with mild atrophy, milia and scarring.

新生儿暂时性大疱性皮肤松解症包括常染色体显性和隐性遗传两种模式。本病具有自限性，水疱多在 2 岁以内自愈，留有轻度萎缩、粟丘疹以及瘢痕。

【Laboratory Findings】

In EB simplex variants, the cell-free blister is intraepidermal in location. By direct immunofluorescent antigen mapping, laminin-5, type Ⅳ collagen, and keratin are found along the floor of the blister. Under electron microscopy, the level of cleavage is deep within the basal keratinocytes, just above the level of the hemidesmosome.

In EB simplex superficialis, the clefting is located at the upper epidermis just beneath the *stratum corneum*.

The histological features for hemidesmosomal EB are not distinctive, and show cell-free subepidermal blisters similar to those in other variants. The site of cleavage is through the hemidesmosome under electron microscopy.

Junctional EB are also characterized by subepidermal blistering, usually not accompanied by substantial inflammatory cell infiltrate. The site of cleavage is through the lamina lucida with this type of EB under electron microscopy. Antigen BP230 can be found in the roof of the blister, while laminin-5 and type Ⅳ collagen are present along the floor of the blister by direct immunofluorescent antigen mapping.

The histological features of dystrophic EB are similar to those of the junctional or hemidesmosomal variants. The site of cleavage is through the lamina densa under electron microscopy. By direct immunofluorescent antigen mapping, BP230, laminin-5 and type Ⅳ collagen are present along the floor of blisters.

【Diagnosis and Differential Diagnosis】

The diagnosis of inherited epidermolysis bullosa can be made based on clinical features, family history, histological examination and detection of the mutated gene.

In occasional cases the lesions of EB resemble aplasia cutis or bullous impetigo. Cell-free subepidermal blisters may be seen in a variety of conditions including EB acquisita, bullous cutaneous amyloidosis, and porphyria cutanea tarda.

【Treatment】

The patient should avoid trauma for all forms of EB. When bullae arise, they should be punctured and the collapsed blister top left intact to serve as a protective covering. The use of topical antibiotics may decrease the frequency of secondary bacterial infection. Nutritional support is also of critical importance. Split-thickness skin grafts have been shown to be useful in treating non-healing cutaneous defects.

【实验室检查】

单纯性 EB 水疱位于表皮内，疱内无细胞成分。免疫荧光显示层粘连蛋白-5、Ⅳ型胶原以及角蛋白均位于水疱的底部。电镜下，裂隙位于基底层角质形成细胞下部，位置高于半桥粒。

表浅性 EBS 水疱位于上表皮即角质层下。

半桥粒性 EB 的组织病理无特征性，表现为表皮下水疱，疱内无细胞成分。电镜下，裂隙位于半桥粒。

交界性 EB 组织病理为表皮下水疱，一般不伴有大量的炎症细胞浸润。电镜下，裂隙位于透明板。免疫荧光显示，BP230 位于水疱顶壁，层粘连蛋白-5 和Ⅳ型胶原位于水疱底部。

营养不良性 EB 的组织病理学改变与交界性或半桥粒性 EB 类似。电镜下，裂隙位于致密板。免疫荧光显示，BP230、层粘连蛋白-5 和Ⅳ型胶原位于水疱底部。

【诊断与鉴别诊断】

遗传性大疱性表皮松解症根据临床特征、家族史、组织学检查以及突变基因的检测一般均可明确诊断。

有时 EB 的皮损需要与皮肤发育不全或大疱性脓疱病相鉴别。表皮下疱不伴有细胞成分的疾病还有获得性大疱性表皮松解症、大疱性皮肤淀粉样变以及迟发性皮肤卟啉病。

【治疗】

所有类型的 EB 都应避免外伤。出现水疱时，可将其挑破，但要保留疱壁作为创面的保护层。局部应用抗生素可以降低继发感染的发生。营养支持对于患者很重要。分层皮肤移植术对于难以愈合的创面具有一定的治疗效果。

【Prognosis】

EBS tends to have periods of exacerbation, but as time passes blistering decreases considerably. As for the three other variants of EB, however, the severe subtypes have a high mortality.

【预后】

单纯性 EB 在一定时期内会有病情加重,但随着病程的延长,皮损可逐渐减轻。对于其他三型 EB,某些严重的亚型有较高的致死性。

Section Six　Familial Benign Chronic Pemphigus(Hailey-Hailey Disease)

第六节　家族性良性慢性天疱疮(Hailey-Hailey 病)

【Etiology and Pathogenesis】

With regard to the pathogenesis of familial benign chronic pemphigus (Hailey-Hailey Disease), a few theories have been proposed. One is that an overall defect of keratinocyte adhesion is caused by a gene mutation in a calcium pump protein-ATP2C1 located at chromosome 3q21-24.

【病因及发病机制】

家族性良性慢性天疱疮(familial benign chronic pemphigus)或 Hailey-Hailey 病(Hailey-Hailey Disease)的发病机制有多种解释,其中之一是定位于染色体 3q21-24 上的编码钙泵蛋白的特异性基因 ATP2C1 突变,导致角质形成细胞的黏附功能的缺陷。

【Clinical Manifestations】

Familial benign chronic pemphigus is an autosomal dominant disorder. Vesicles and bullae arising on normal or erythematous skin are soon replaced by erosions, crusts and scaly plaques. Superinfection is a frequent complication. Sites of predilection are the intertriginous areas such as the armpits, groin and perianal regions (Fig. 15-15). The upper trunk, scalp and extremities may also be involved. Lesions may be itchy or painful, and symptoms may be aggravated by movement. Symptoms often improve or even disappear during winter, but tend to worsen in summer.

【临床表现】

家族性良性慢性天疱疮的遗传模式为常染色体显性遗传。在正常皮肤或红斑的基础上,可发生水疱、大疱,很快皮损被糜烂、结痂或者鳞屑性斑块替代。皮损处常发生浅表感染。病变好发于皱褶部位,如腋窝、腹股沟和肛周(图 15-15),躯干上部、头皮以及四肢也可受累。患者可自觉瘙痒或疼痛,运动可能加重症状。病情一般夏季加重,在冬季减轻甚至消失。

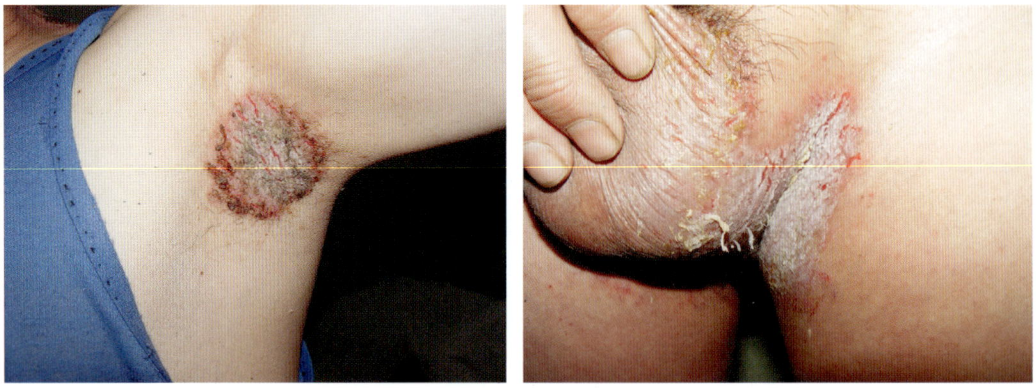

(a)　(b)

Fig. 15-15　Familial benign chronic pemphigus

(图 15-15　家族性良性慢性天疱疮)

【Histopathology】

The histopathology changes consist of suprabasal clefting and

【组织病理】

组织病理学特征为几乎累及表皮全

acantholysis in the greater part of the overlying epidermis. Typically, the acantholysis is incomplete, and the cells retain some connections, giving the appearance of a "dilapidated brick wall". Dermal changes include papillary edema and superficial perivascular lymphohistiocytic infiltrates.

层的裂隙形成伴有棘层松解。本病的棘层松解并不完全，细胞之间还有一定的联系，形成一种"塌砖墙"样外观。真皮的改变为真皮乳头水肿，浅层血管周围有淋巴组织细胞浸润。

【Diagnosis and Differential Diagnosis】

【诊断及鉴别诊断】

The diagnosis of familial benign chronic pemphigus can be made based on clinical features, familial history and histopathological changes.

家族性良性慢性天疱疮根据临床特征、家族史、组织病理学改变一般均可明确诊断。

Chronic bacterial or fungal infection of intertriginous areas, pemphigus vulgaris, pemphigus vegetans, and keratosis follicularis must be differentiated from familial benign chronic pemphigus.

本病应与皱褶部位的细菌或真菌感染、寻常型天疱疮、增殖型天疱疮以及毛囊角化病相鉴别。

【Treatment】

【治疗】

In general, if a secondary infection is promoted by the lesions, appropriate therapy should be instituted. Systemic antibiotic treatment may be of some help. Some patients benefit from glucocorticoids creams when they are used to minimize the ordinarily severe inflammation. Regarding the chronic vegetating lesions, surgical removal with subsequent skin grafting may be of value.

如果皮损处发生继发感染，可以用外用药进行对症处理。系统应用抗生素对病情缓解也有一定帮助。如果皮损处炎症反应较重，也可使用糖皮质激素制剂。对于慢性增殖性损害，可以进行外科手术切除后植皮。

【Prognosis】

【预后】

The disease tends to run a benign but protracted course. In some patients, the condition improves with age.

本病为良性病变，病程较长。在部分患者中，随着年龄的增长，病情可以逐渐减轻。

Section Seven　Neurofibromatosis

第七节　神经纤维瘤病

【Etiology】

【病因】

Neurofibromatosis is classified into 8 subtypes (NFⅠ-NFⅧ). The genes that are responsible for NFⅠ have been located at chromosome 17, chromosome 19 and chromosome 22q; and the genes for NFⅡ have been mapped to chromosome 22.

神经纤维瘤病(neurofibromatosis, NF)分为8型(NFⅠ-NFⅧ)。NFⅠ致病基因定位于17号、19号染色体以及22号染色体长臂。NFⅡ的致病基因定位于22号染色体。

【Clinical Manifestations】

【临床表现】

The typical clinical features of neurofibromatosis include *café-au-lait* spots, neurofibromas, axillary freckling (Fig. 15-16), and Lisch nodules.

神经纤维瘤病的临床特征包括咖啡牛奶斑、神经纤维瘤、腋窝部雀斑(图15-16)以及Lisch小体。

Café-au-lait spots are flat, light-brown patches, usually 2-5 cm in diameter. Lesions may be distributed anywhere on the integument, but are seen particularly on unexposed areas.

咖啡牛奶斑为扁平、浅褐色斑片，直径为2～5 cm。皮损可见于体表各处，但以非暴露部位为主。

Neurofibromas are soft, skin colored tumors which can be pushed down into the panniculus by light pressure with the finger and spring back when released. They range in number from a few isolated tumors to hundreds in a single patient. Most of the tumors

神经纤维瘤为柔软的肤色肿瘤，轻压肿块，病变可呈疝囊样形成凹陷，松开手指后可恢复原状。肿瘤数量可为几个到几百个。其体积一般较小，偶有直径

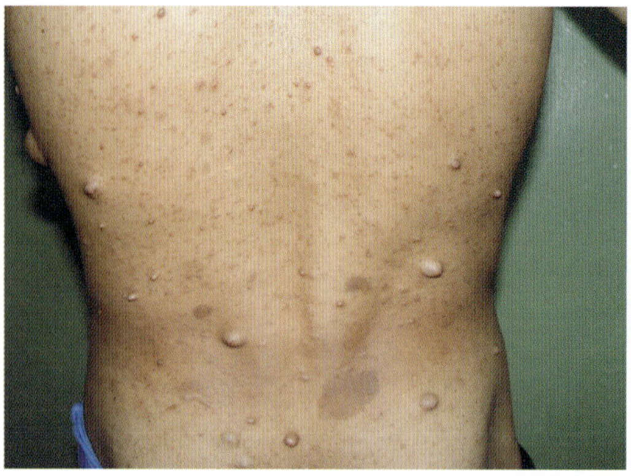

Fig. 15-16　Neurofibromatosis type Ⅰ(图 15-16　Ⅰ型神经纤维瘤病)

are small, but occasionally a single neurofibroma may measure 10-20 cm in diameter. These large neurofibromas are called plexiform neurofibromas.

为 10～20 cm 的巨大肿块,后者称为丛状神经纤维瘤。

Axillary freckling is found in approximately 20 percent of patients. This finding is highly pathognomonic for neurofibromatosis. Lisch nodules are pigmented iris hamartomas.

腋窝部雀斑发生于大约 20％的神经纤维瘤病患者,是本病的特征性病变。Lisch 小体是色素性虹膜错构瘤。

The conditions that are frequently associated with neurofibromatosis can be categorized as neurologic, skeletal, or endocrinal abnormalities.

神经纤维瘤病还可累及多个脏器,导致神经系统、骨骼系统、内分泌系统疾病。

The clinical features of NF Ⅰ manifest all the characteristics described above. NF Ⅱ or "central" neurofibromatosis is more strongly associated with a positive family history but exhibits fewer skin lesions and no Lisch nodules. Most patients with this type of neurofibromatosis develop bilateral acoustic neuromas.

Ⅰ型神经纤维瘤病包括上述所有临床特征。Ⅱ型神经纤维瘤病也被称为"中央型",皮损较少,无 Lisch 小结,但多发生双侧听神经瘤,家族史阳性。

NF Ⅲ is characterized by a positive family history, skin lesions and central nervous system tumors. Lisch nodules may or may not be present. NF Ⅳ or "variant" neurofibromatosis may or may not have a positive family history or central nervous system tumors but presents as neurofibromas and *café-au-lait* spots.

Ⅲ型神经纤维瘤病具有阳性家族史、皮肤病变以及中枢神经系统肿瘤,可伴或不伴有 Lisch 小结。Ⅳ型神经纤维瘤病也被称为"变异型",患者出现神经纤维瘤和咖啡牛奶斑,可伴或不伴有阳性家族史和中枢神经系统肿瘤。

NF Ⅴ, or "segmental" neurofibromatosis is characterized by unilateral segmental distribution of neurofibromas and *café-au-lait* spots. This type of neurofibromatosis is associated with a negative family history and the absence of Lisch nodules. The common presentation of NF Ⅵ is multiple *café-au-lait* spots with no neurofibromas whatsoever.

Ⅴ型神经纤维瘤病也被称为"节段型",单侧节段性分布的神经纤维瘤和咖啡牛奶斑是其特征。患者常无家族史,不伴有 Lisch 小结。Ⅵ型神经纤维瘤病表现为多发的咖啡牛奶斑,但无神经纤维瘤。

NF Ⅶ or "late onset" neurofibromatosis is characterized by the development of neurofibromas at or after age 30. NF Ⅷ is a heterogeneous group that includes all clinical types that do not fit into any of the seven subtypes described above.

Ⅶ型神经纤维瘤病也被称为"迟发型",患者发病年龄在 30 岁或 30 岁以后。临床特征与上述 7 型均不相符的归为Ⅷ型神经纤维瘤病。

【Histopathology】

【组织病理】

The histological findings for *café-au-lait* spots are that the

咖啡牛奶斑的病理特征为黑素细胞

number of melanocytes is increased, and the function of melanocytes is also promoted, evidenced by the enlarged melanosomes.

The histological feature of neurofibromas is a well defined but unencapsulated dermal or subcutaneous lump. It consists of loosely arranged spindle cells with scant, pale cytoplasm and elongated wavy nuclei. Scattered inflammatory cells, particularly mast cells within or throughout the tumor, are a prominent feature for diagnosis. Positive staining with S-100 can be seen in 30%-50% of the cells. Variable positivity for CD34 staining is seen in some individuals.

数目增多，功能活跃，含有较大的黑素小体。

神经纤维瘤的组织病理学特征为真皮或皮下的境界清楚的无包膜团块。其内可见胞质淡染的梭形细胞，细胞核扭曲伸长。瘤体内可见散在炎症细胞浸润，尤其是肥大细胞具有一定特征性。S-100染色可有30%～50%的细胞呈阳性着色，CD34的阳性率不一。

【Diagnosis】

The diagnostic criteria of the National Institute of Health (NIH) of America for type Ⅰ neurofibromatosis require patients to have at least two conditions as listed below:

(1) 6 or more *café-au-lait* spots of a diameter greater than 5 mm in children under 6 years, or greater than 15 mm in older individuals.

(2) 2 or more neurofibromas of any type, or one plexiform neurofibroma.

(3) Freckling in the axillary or inguinal regions.

(4) An optic nerve glioma.

(5) 2 or more Lisch nodules.

(6) A distinctive osseous lesion such as dysplasia of the sphenoid bone or thinning of the cortex of long bones, with or without pseudoarthrosis.

(7) A first-degree relative with NFⅠ.

The same standard applies for type Ⅱ neurofibromatosis, but the patient must also exhibit one or both of the following:

(1) Bilateral eighth nerve tumors as demonstrated by CT or MRI.

(2) History of a first-degree relative with NF Ⅱ and either unilateral eighth nerve mass or two of the following: neurofibroma, meningioma, glioma, schwannoma, or juvenile posterior subcapsular lenticular opacity.

【诊断】

美国国立卫生研究院制订的Ⅰ型神经纤维瘤病的诊断标准如下，符合其中的两条或两条以上即可诊断。

(1) 6个或以上的咖啡牛奶斑，6岁以前直径大于5 mm，6岁以后直径大于15 mm。

(2) 2个或以上任何类型的神经纤维瘤，或一个丛状神经纤维瘤。

(3) 腋窝或腹股沟部位的雀斑。

(4) 视神经胶质瘤。

(5) 2个或以上的Lisch结节。

(6) 独特的骨骼损害，如蝶骨发育不良、长骨皮质细化、伴有或不伴有假关节。

(7) 一级亲属患有符合上述标准的Ⅰ型神经纤维瘤病。

具备下述一项即可诊断Ⅱ型神经纤维瘤病。

(1) CT或核磁共振成像诊断双侧听神经瘤。

(2) Ⅱ型神经纤维瘤病的一级亲属和单侧听神经瘤或下列疾病中的任何两种，如神经纤维瘤、脑膜瘤、神经胶质瘤、神经鞘瘤或青少年型后囊下晶体混浊。

【Differential Diagnosis】

Isolated *café-au-lait* spots can be seen in normal individuals. The spots are usually less than 15 mm in size and do not contain large melanosomes. *Café-au-lait* spots are also seen in Albright's syndrome, tuberous sclerosis, and ataxia telangiectasia.

【鉴别诊断】

孤立分布的咖啡牛奶斑可见于正常人，一般直径小于15 mm，不含有大的黑素小体。咖啡牛奶斑还可见于Albright综合征、结节性硬化症以及共济失调性毛细血管扩张。

【Treatment】

Some neurofibromas may be removed surgically. The patients

【治疗】

神经纤维瘤可以手术切除。患者必

must also be ruled out for tumor development within the central nervous system or other life threatening disorders.

须排除中枢神经系统肿瘤或其他危及生命的疾病。

【Prognosis】

The number of neurofibromas and pigmented spots may increase with age. Some neurofibromas may become neurofibrosarcomas and metastasize later. Also, other tumors and endocrine abnormalities may occur in some cases.

【预后】

随着年龄的增长，神经纤维瘤和咖啡牛奶斑的数量会增加。一些神经纤维瘤会演变为神经纤维肉瘤并可发生转移。其他肿瘤或内分泌疾病也可发生。

Section Eight　Incontinentia Pigmenti

第八节　色素失禁症

【Etiology】

Incontinentia pigmenti is an X-linked dominant inherited skin pigmentation disorder. It is caused by mutations of the gene mapped to the Xq11 and Xq28 loci.

【病因】

色素失禁症(incontinentia pigmenti)为 X 连锁显性遗传性皮肤色素性疾病。致病基因定位于 Xq11 和 Xq28。

【Clinical Manifestations】

Incontinentia pigmenti is a rare disorder with a striking female bias, with affected males usually dying in utero. Typically, the condition has three stages.

【临床表现】

色素失禁症多见于女性，男性往往在胎儿期死亡。本病一般分为 3 期。

In stage Ⅰ, erythema and linear vesiculation on the trunk and extremities are apparent at birth or during the first 2 weeks of life (Fig. 15-17). On average, this stage is completely resolved by the 4th month.

第一期，出生时或出生后 2 周内躯干和四肢可见红斑以及线状分布的水疱(图 15-17)。本期一般持续 4 个月。

Stage Ⅱ consists of hyperkeratotic verrucous papules and plaques that are most frequently found on the extremities. The hyperkeratotic lesions develop at the sites of earlier blistering (Fig. 15-18). This stage appears during the 2-6 weeks of life and usually resolves by the 6th month.

第二期皮损为分布于四肢的角化性疣状丘疹或斑块，角化性损害发生于原水疱的部位(图 15-18)。本期出生后 2～6 周出现，一般持续 6 个月。

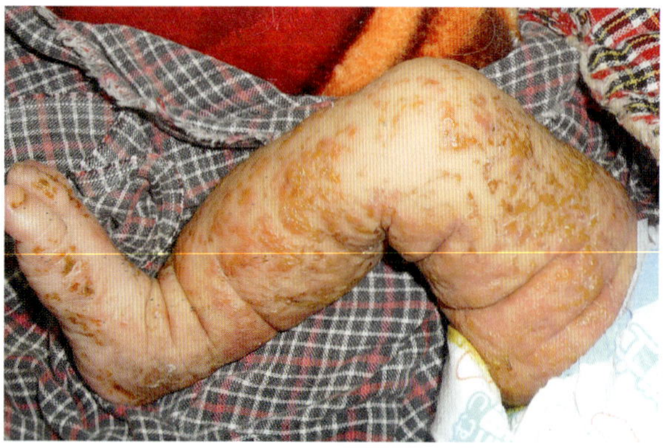

Fig. 15-17　Incontinentia pigmenti-stage Ⅰ

(图 15-17　色素失禁症-第一期)

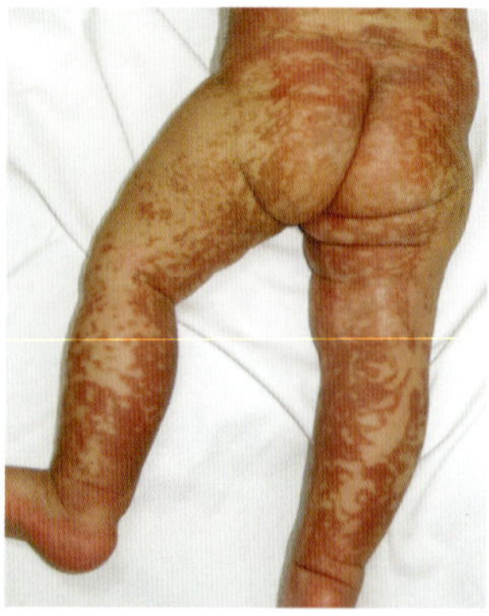

Fig. 15-18　Incontinentia pigmenti-stage Ⅱ

(图 15-18　色素失禁症-第二期)

Stage Ⅲ is the pathognomonic stage of the disorder, and usually occurs between 12 and 26 weeks after birth. The brown to slate-gray pigmentation appears as splashes, streaks and whorls on the torso and extremities (Fig. 15-19). The nipples are typically

第三期的病变具有诊断价值，多在出生后 12～26 周出现。皮损为褐色至蓝灰色的色素沉着，呈斑点状、条纹状或漩涡状分布于躯干和四肢(图 15-19)。

hyperpigmented and involvement of the groin and axillae is characteristic.

乳头、腋窝及腹股沟的色素沉着具有特征性。

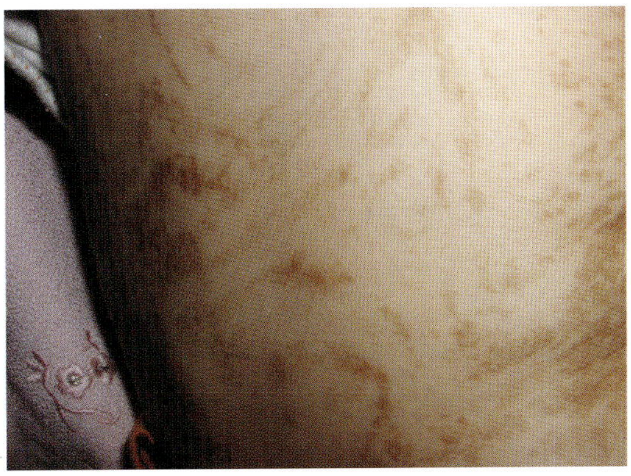

Fig. 15-19 Incontinentia pigmenti-stage Ⅲ
(图 15-19 色素失禁症-第三期)

Other cutaneous changes include patchy alopecia at the vertex of the scalp, onychodystrophy, subungual tumors, and palmoplantar hyperhidrosis. The teeth, eyes, bones and the central nervous system can also be involved.

其他皮损包括头顶部片状脱发、甲营养不良、甲下肿瘤以及掌跖多汗症。牙齿、眼睛、骨骼以及中枢神经系统均可受累。

【Histopathology】

【组织病理】

Histological examination of the lesions in stage Ⅰ shows eosinophilic spongiosis. A chronic inflammatory cell infiltrate dominated by eosinophils may also be present within the dermis.

第一期色素失禁症的组织病理特征是表皮内的嗜酸性海绵水肿。真皮内也可见以嗜酸性粒细胞为主的慢性炎症细胞浸润。

The lesions in stage Ⅱ reveal hyperkeratosis, acanthosis, papillomatosis and focal dyskeratosis. Histological features from the lesions in stage Ⅲ are characterized by marked pigmentary incontinence, numerous melanophages in the superficial dermis, and liquefaction degeneration of the basal cell layer.

第二期皮损的病理特征为角化过度、棘层肥厚、乳头瘤样增生以及局灶性角化不良。第三期皮损的病理特征为显著的色素失禁，真皮浅层可见大量的噬黑素细胞，表皮基底层细胞液化变性。

【Diagnosis and Differential Diagnosis】

【诊断与鉴别诊断】

The diagnosis of incontinentia pigmenti can be made based on clinical features and histopathological findings.

色素失禁症根据临床特征、组织病理一般均可明确诊断。

Incontinentia pigmenti may be confused with incontinentia pigmenti achromians (also named hypomelanosis of Ito) because both conditions produce congenital neurologic defects. However, the typical cutaneous pigmentary changes in the latter are not preceded by vesicular or verrucous lesions.

色素失禁症应与无色素性色素失禁症(Ito 色素减少症)鉴别。两者均具有类似的先天性神经系统缺陷。但后者出现色素沉着以前常缺乏水疱以及疣状皮损。

【Treatment and Prognosis】

【治疗和预后】

There is no specific treatment for incontinentia pigmenti. The pigmentation usually disappears by age 20.

本病无特殊治疗。色素沉着通常在 20 岁时消退。

Section Nine　Tuberous Sclerosis

【Etiology】

Tuberous sclerosis is associated with mutations of two separate genes: the TSC1 gene located at 9q34 and the TSC2 gene located at 16p13.

【Clinical Manifestations】

Angiofibromas on the face (previously termed Pringle adenoma sebaceum) are the characteristic lesions for this disease, and appear as smooth, dome-shaped, pink or reddish brown papules and nodules. Lesions are located particularly in the butterfly area of the face (Fig. 15-20).

Facial angiofibromas begin to develop in the centrofacial area within the first 2 years of life. The lesions may appear as a mild erythema on the cheeks and forehead at first, later turning into the signature papules or papulonodules, which may then coalesce to form plaques.

3 types of hypomelanotic macules can be observed in tuberous sclerosis. Although the most common type is the polygonal macule, the lance-ovate macule and "confetti" macules are more characteristic for tuberous sclerosis (Fig. 15-21).

第九节　结节性硬化症

【病因】

定位于 9q34 的 TSC1 和定位于 16p13 的 TSC2 与结节性硬化症(tuberous sclerosis, TS)发病有关。

【临床表现】

面部血管纤维瘤(以往称为 Pringle 皮脂腺腺瘤)是本病特征性皮损，为表面光滑的、圆顶形、粉红色或红棕色丘疹或结节，多见于面部蝶形区(图 15-20)。

面部血管纤维瘤于出生后头 2 年在面部中央出现。早期可为面颊和前额的轻度红斑，后演变为粉红色至红棕色的丘疹或丘疹结节，聚集成斑块。

结节性硬化症可见 3 种色素减退斑，最常见的一种是多角形斑，矛状卵圆形斑和"五彩纸屑样"斑较少见，但是更具有特征性(图 15-21)。

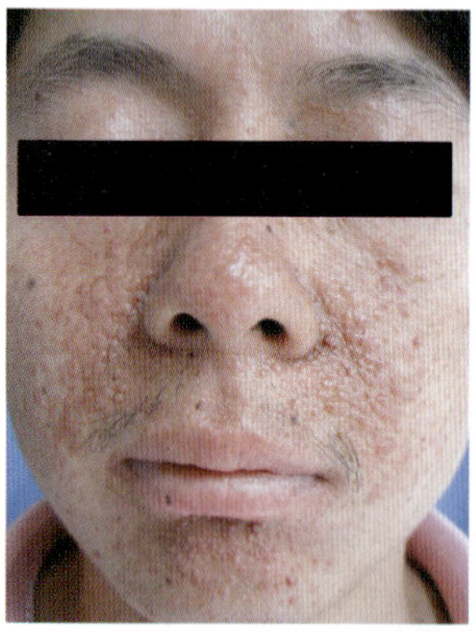

Fig. 15-20　Tuberous sclerosis-facial angiofibromas
(图 15-20　结节性硬化症-面部血管纤维瘤)

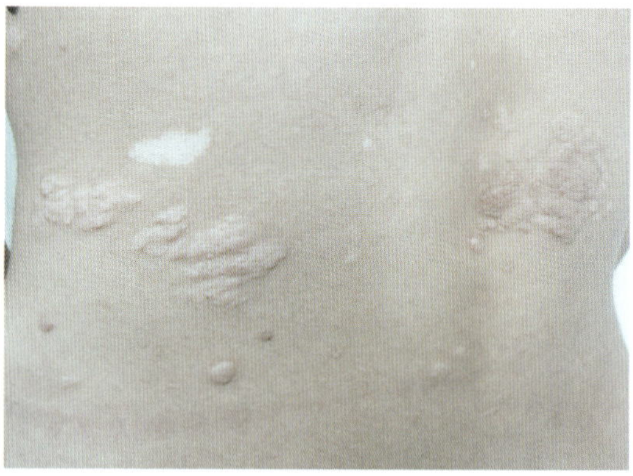

Fig. 15-21　Tuberous sclerosis-hypomelanotic macules and shagreen patch
(图 15-21　结节性硬化症-色素减退斑和鲛鱼皮样斑)

A characteristic lesion on the trunk is the shagreen (leather) patch, which occurs most commonly in the lumbosacral area, starting around the age of 2 years old. This is a skin-colored plaque that can extend to 10 cm in diameter and often has an uneven surface. The pigskin-like appearance of the lesion is pathognomonic, and is caused by prominent, slightly elevated follicular openings (Fig. 15-21).

Periungual fibromas (Fig. 15-22) and gingival fibromas also can be seen in tuberous sclerosis patients.

躯干特征性皮损是鲛鱼皮样(鲨革)斑，通常分布在腰骶部，常发生于 2 岁左右。临床可见此皮损为肤色，可至 10 cm 大小，表面粗糙不平。其特点为猪皮样外观的皮损表面有突起的毛囊开口(图 15-21)。

结节性硬化症患者还可以出现甲周纤维瘤(图 15-22)和牙龈纤维瘤。

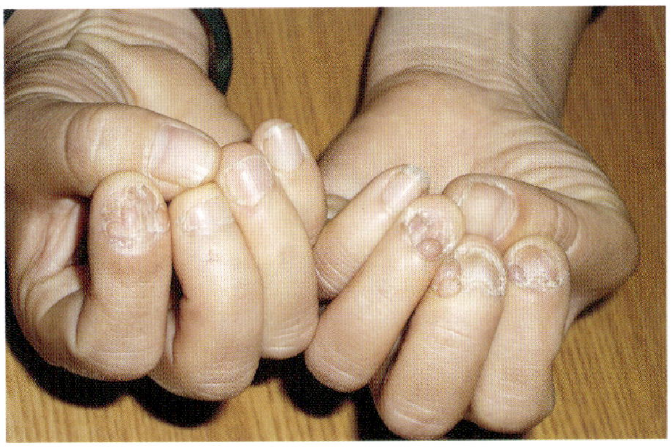

Fig. 15-22 Tuberous sclerosis-periungual fibromas
(图 15-22 结节性硬化症-甲周纤维瘤)

Retinal lesions are present in about half of the individuals with tuberous sclerosis. 40% of these cases suffer from retinal hamartomas and another 40% have retinal depigmentation.

接近一半的结节性硬化症患者有视网膜病变，其中视网膜错构瘤和视网膜脱色各占40%。

In approximately 70% of affected infants, infantile spasms may be observed. These spasms begin at about 3 months of age. Patients with tuberous sclerosis are at high risk to develop mental retardation or neuropsychiatric disturbances.

大约70%的新生儿可以发生婴儿性痉挛，症状多出现于3月龄时。智力障碍以及精神症状在患者的发病率较高。

Cardiac rhabdomyomas, multiple bilateral angiomyolipomas, and asymptomatic pulmonary lymphangioleiomyomatosis have also been seen in patients with tuberous sclerosis.

本病患者还可发生心脏横纹肌瘤、多发性双侧血管肌脂肪瘤和无症状肺淋巴管平滑肌瘤。

【Laboratory Findings】

【实验室检查】

The histological feature of angiofibromas of the face consists of an irregular proliferation of fibrous tissue and blood vessels. In older lesions, the adnexae become surrounded and compressed by concentric lamellae of collagen.

面部血管纤维瘤的组织学特征是不规则增生的纤维组织和血管。陈旧的皮损中，附属器周围可见成层的胶原组织包绕。

The hypomelanotic macules reveal either normal or diminished numbers of melanocytes. However, the impaired melanogenesis is easily seen under electron microscopy.

色素减退斑病理上可见正常或数目减少的黑素细胞。超微结构显示黑素形成障碍。

The shagreen patch is a collagenoma, in which the dermis is replaced by broad bundles of fibrous tissue with diminished or absent elastic fibers. Similar to collagenoma, the periungual fibromas are fibrous tissue hamartomas.

鲛鱼皮样斑是一种胶原瘤，真皮被大量条束状纤维组织替代，其内弹性纤维减少或缺如。与之类似，甲周纤维瘤是一种纤维组织错构瘤。

Multiple calcified subependymal nodules along the ventricular surface can be seen in CT scans in over 80% of children under the age of 2 years with tuberous sclerosis. Subependymal giant cell astrocytomas and multiple cortical tubers can also be detected by neuroimaging (e. g. ,MRI) in the majority of patients.

CT扫描发现80%的2岁以下患儿可沿室膜表面出现多发室管膜下钙化结节。大多数病例经影像学检查(如磁共振成像)也可发现室管膜下巨细胞性星形细胞瘤和多皮质瘤。

Cardiac rhabdomyomas, which can be detected prenatally by MRI, are found in over 80% of infants with tuberous sclerosis.

80%的结节性硬化症患儿发生的心脏横纹肌瘤，可以在产前用MRI检查到。

Arrhythmias, especially Wolff-Parkinson-White syndrome, can be detected by ECG.

心电图检查发现患者可伴有心律失常，尤其是预激综合征。

【Diagnosis】

(1) Major features:

Facial angiofibromas or forehead fibrous plaque;

Non-traumatic ungual or periungual fibromas;

Hypomelanotic macules (3 or more);

Shagreen patch (connective tissue nevus);

Multiple retinal nodular hamartomas;

Cortical tubers;

Subependymal nodules;

Subependymal giant cell astrocytoma;

Renal angiomyolipoma;

Cardiac rhabdomyoma, single or multiple;

Lymphangioleiomyomatosis.

(2) Minor features:

"Confetti" macules;

Multiple randomly distributed pits in dental enamel;

Gingival fibromas;

Retinal achromic patch;

Cerebral white matter radial migration lines;

Multiple renal cysts;

Hamartomatous rectal polyps;

Bone cysts;

Non-renal hamartoma.

(3) Definite tuberous sclerosis:

Patients with either 2 major features or 1 major feature plus 2 minor features.

(4) Probable tuberous sclerosis:

Patients with 1 major plus 1 minor feature.

(5) Possible tuberous sclerosis:

Patients with either 1 major feature or 2 or more minor features.

【Differential Diagnosis】

Idiopathic guttate hypomelanosis (IGH) may resemble the "confetti" macules of tuberous sclerosis; however, IGH is an acquired disorder that tends to appear on the shins and extensor forearms of elderly patients.

The differential diagnosis for facial angiofibromas includes primarily acne vulgaris and multiple trichoepitheliomas. The lesions of acne vulgaris occur predominantly during puberty and contain comedones. These lesions are apt to resolve over a period of weeks. By contrast, trichoepitheliomas are often less inflammatory; nevertheless, a skin biopsy will usually be necessary in order to reach a conclusive diagnosis.

【诊断】

(1) 主要标准

颜面血管纤维瘤或前额纤维斑块;

非外伤性的甲或甲周纤维瘤;

色素减退斑(3 个或以上);

鲨革斑(结缔组织痣);

多发性视网膜结节错构瘤;

皮质瘤;

室管膜下结节;

室管膜下巨细胞性星形细胞瘤;

肾血管肌脂肪瘤;

心肌横纹肌瘤,单个或多发;

淋巴管平滑肌瘤。

(2) 次要标准

"五彩纸屑样"斑;

多发散在牙釉质凹陷;

牙龈纤维瘤;

视网膜色素脱失斑;

脑白质径向迁移;

多发肾囊肿;

错构瘤直肠息肉;

骨囊肿;

非肾脏性错构瘤。

(3) 确诊结节性硬化症

任意 2 个主要标准或 1 个主要标准加 2 个次要标准。

(4) 很可能的结节性硬化症

1 个主要标准和 1 个次要标准。

(5) 可能的结节性硬化症

任意 1 个主要标准,或 2 个及 2 个以上次要标准。

【鉴别诊断】

特发性点状白斑(IGH)也类似于结节性硬化症的"五彩纸屑样"斑。但 IGH 是后天获得性的,常见于老年人小腿和前臂伸侧皮肤。

面部血管纤维瘤首先需要与痤疮和多发性毛发上皮瘤鉴别。痤疮皮损主要见于青春期,含有粉刺,可在几周内消退。毛发上皮瘤皮损常无明显炎症,但往往需要活检以明确诊断。

A congenital smooth muscle hamartoma may present during infancy as a firm, hyperpigmented plaque that often resembles a shagreen patch or as a congenital melanocytic nevus. However, smooth muscle hamartomas are characterized histologically by numerous randomly arranged intradermal bundles of smooth muscle rather than collagen.

先天性平滑肌错构瘤可以在婴儿期出现,表现为坚实的色素加深的斑块而与鲨革斑或者先天性黑素痣类似。但平滑肌错构瘤的病理特点为有大量杂乱排列的平滑肌束而不是胶原束。

【Treatment】

The management of tuberous sclerosis consists of genetic counseling, use of anticonvulsants to control seizures, cutaneous cosmetic surgery to remove facial angiofibromas, and a thorough medical evaluation with close follow-up to detect and treat any associated medical conditions.

【治疗】

本病的治疗包括遗传咨询、应用抗癫痫药控制疾病发作、皮肤美容手术去除面部血管纤维瘤,以及对相关疾病进行检查并进行针对性治疗。

【Prognosis】

Even though the disorder is often progressive, it is nevertheless manageable and compatible with long-term survival.

【预后】

尽管本病呈进行性发展,但患者可进行一定程度的治疗并有较长的生存期。

Jin-gang AN(安金刚)

Section Ten Primary Immunodeficiency Diseases

第十节 原发性免疫缺陷病

Primary immunodeficiency disease(PID) refers to a heterogeneous group of genetic disorders that are characterized by compromised or absent function of one or more components of the immune system. In recent years an increasing number of PIDs have been identified, and the disease is now considered not as rare as was once believed.

原发性免疫缺陷病(primary immunodeficiency disease, PID)指一类一种或几种免疫功能低下或缺失的基因遗传疾病。近年来,深入研究使越来越多的PID病例被发现,因此此类疾病并不像之前认为的罕见。

PIDs are broadly classified into two categories:the disorders of innate immunity (e. g. , phagocyte and complement disorders) or of adaptive immunity (i. e. , T-cell, B-cell or combined immunodeficiencies).

PID大致分为固有免疫缺陷(吞噬和补体系统异常)或适应性免疫缺陷(T细胞、B细胞或联合免疫缺陷)。

【Etiology】

PID results from defects in immune system development and/or function. Insufficient or absent function of one or more components of the immune system will lead to repeated, severe and intractable infections.

The human immune system is typically categorized into innate immunity and adaptive immunity. The innate immune system, also known as the nonspecific immune system, represents the first line of defense against potentially invading organisms. The innate system is mainly composed of eosinophils, monocytes, macrophages, natural killer cells, toll-like receptors (TLRs), and complement system. Failure of the innate system to respond to a given pathogen delays the onset of the immune response and may worsen outcomes

【病因学】

PID由免疫系统发育或功能缺陷所致。一种或几种免疫成分功能低下或缺失导致少见的反复、严重、难治愈的感染。

人类免疫系统包括固有免疫和适应性免疫。固有免疫也称为非特异性免疫,是防御微生物入侵的一线机制。固有免疫系统主要由嗜酸性粒细胞、单核巨噬细胞、自然杀伤细胞,toll样受体(TLRs)及补体系统构成。固有免疫识别病原缺陷将延迟免疫反应,使感染恶化。

of infection.

The adaptive or specific immune system is charged with attacking the specific invaders. It consists of highly specialized cells called T-cells and B-cells. These cells can be programmed to recognize specific foreign antigens very precisely and have the potential to generate immunological memory. B-cells mediate humoral immunity while T-cells govern cell-mediated immune responses. Defects occurring at any stage of T/B-cell development, differentiation and maturation lead to immunodeficiency disease. Since B-cell-mediated antibody production requires intact T-cell function, most T-cell defects lead to combined (i. e., B-and T-cell) immunodeficiency disease.

适应性免疫或特定免疫系统主要攻击特定的入侵者，由 T 细胞和 B 细胞组成，二者可以精确识别外源性抗原并产生记忆性免疫。B 细胞介导体液免疫，而 T 细胞介导细胞免疫。发生在 T/B 细胞发育、分化及成熟任一阶段缺陷都可导致免疫缺陷病发生。由于 B 细胞介导抗体产生需要完整的 T 细胞功能，因此，多数 T 细胞缺陷可导致联合(B 细胞和 T 细胞)免疫缺陷病。

【Clinical Manifestations】

Increased susceptibility to infection and persistent infections are the most signs of PID. In addition, some PID cases may involve particular organs due to autoimmune and granulomatous disease, such as gastrointestinal complications and an enhanced risk of malignancy (e. g., lymphoma and carcinoma). Underdevelopment of the facial or skeletal system may occur in certain PID cases.

The International Union of Immunological Societies defines 9 classes of PID for a total of over 120 conditions based on the part of the immune system that is affected:

Ⅰ: Combined T-and B-cell immunodeficiencies
Ⅱ: Predominantly antibody deficiencies(B-cell)
Ⅲ: Other well-defined immunodeficiency syndrome
Ⅳ: Diseases of immune dysregulation
Ⅴ: Congenital defects of phagocyte number, function, or both
Ⅳ: Defects in innate immunity
Ⅶ: Autoinflammatory disorder
Ⅷ: Complement deficiencies
Ⅸ: Unknown (idiopathic)

The main PIDs with skin involvements are described briefly as follows:

(1) Severe combined immunodeficiency (SCID): included in type Ⅰ of PID. It usually presents within the first year of life with chronic diarrhea and even death. Patients often suffer repeatedly from severe bronchopulmonary infections by opportunistic pathogens (bacteria, *Candida albicans*, *Pneumocystis jiroveci*, or virus), neurological defects and skin rashes. Therefore slow growth and inadequate gain weight is a common symptom. These infections can cause death and children rarely live past the age of 2 without treatment. Currently, bone marrow transplantation (BMT) is a curative.

(2) Hyper-IgE syndrome (HIES): included in type Ⅲ PID,

【临床表现】

对感染易感性增强或持久性感染是多数 PID 的表现。此外，自身免疫和肉芽肿会导致特定器官受累，例如胃肠并发症和肿瘤易患性(淋巴瘤和癌)。面部发育异常及骨骼系统受累也可发生在特定 PID。

根据受累的免疫成分不同，国际免疫联合会认定 9 类 PID，共有超过 120 种病症。

Ⅰ: T 细胞-B 细胞联合免疫缺陷
Ⅱ: 优势抗体缺陷(B 细胞)
Ⅲ: 其他明确免疫缺陷综合征
Ⅳ: 免疫调控异常性疾病
Ⅴ: 先天性吞噬细胞数目、功能缺陷
Ⅵ: 固有免疫缺陷
Ⅶ: 自身炎症性疾病
Ⅷ: 补体缺陷
Ⅸ: 未定类(特发性)

以下将对具有皮肤受累的主要 PID 做简要阐述。

(1) 严重联合免疫缺陷 (severe combined immunodeficiency, SCID) 归于Ⅰ型 PID，患者常幼年即出现慢性腹泻、1 岁内早逝，发生肺支气管严重复发机会性感染(细菌感染、白色念珠菌感染、耶氏肺孢子虫感染或病毒感染)、神经系统缺陷及皮疹。由于多重感染，患儿生长发育缓慢。SCID 引发的感染可致患者多在 2 岁内死亡。SCID 可通过骨髓移植(BMT)治愈。

(2) 高 IgE 综合征 (hyper-IgE

this is a phagocyte defect disorder resulting from a mutation in the signal transducer and activator of transcription 3 (STAT3). It is characterized by high serum IgE levels, eosinophilia, recalcitrant eczema, and recurrent skin or lung infections. Other manifestations, such as a characteristic facial appearance, scoliosis, retained primary teeth, joint hyperextensibility, or bone fractures following minor traumas and craniosynostosis may occur but are not directly related to immunity (Fig. 15-23 to Fig. 15-27). Elevated IgE is the hallmark of HIES. An IgE level greater than 2000 IU/mL is often considered diagnostic for HIES.

syndrome)(HIES)　归于Ⅲ型PID，是一类STAT3基因突变诱发吞噬细胞缺陷引起的疾病，主要特征为高IgE和嗜酸性粒细胞、顽固性湿疹、反复皮肤和肺部感染，而特殊面容、脊柱侧突、乳牙滞留、关节过伸、轻创后骨折、颅缝早闭则是高IgE综合征非免疫学表现(图15-23至图15-27)。血清中IgE升高是HIES的标志，IgE高于2000 IU/mL考虑本病诊断。

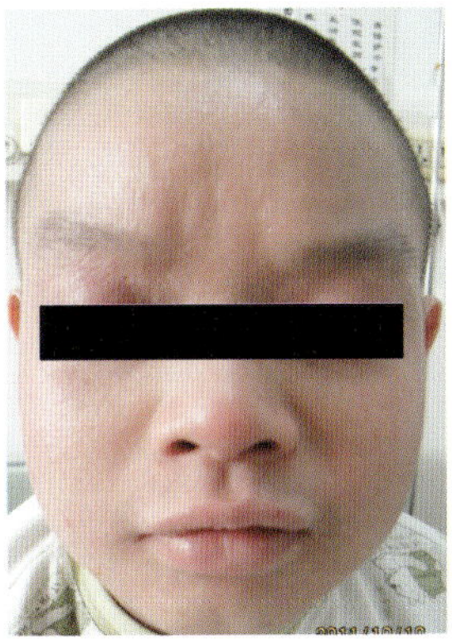

Fig. 15-23　Hyper-IgE syndrome-special facial expression

(图15-23　高IgE综合征-患者特殊面容)

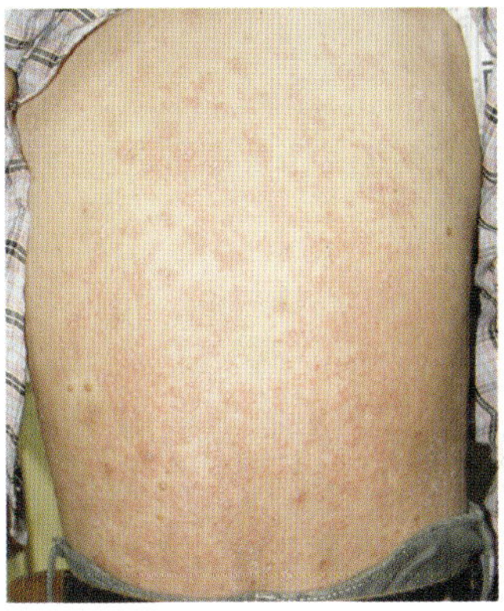

Fig. 15-24　Hyper-IgE syndrome-recalcitrant eczema-like lesions

(图15-24　高IgE综合征-顽固性湿疹样皮损)

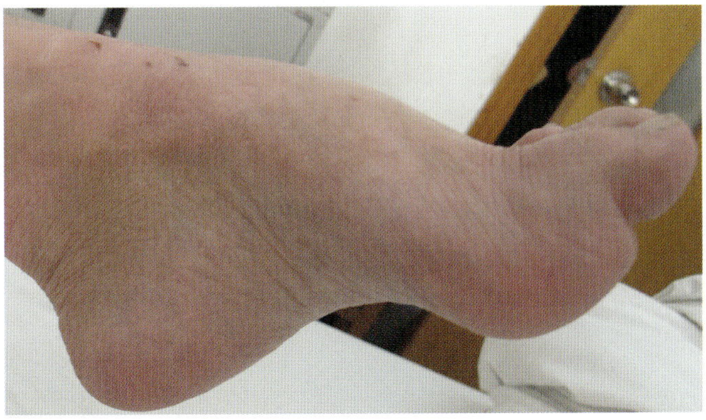

Fig. 15-25　Hyper-IgE syndrome-skeletal dysplasia

(图15-25　高IgE综合征-骨骼发育异常)

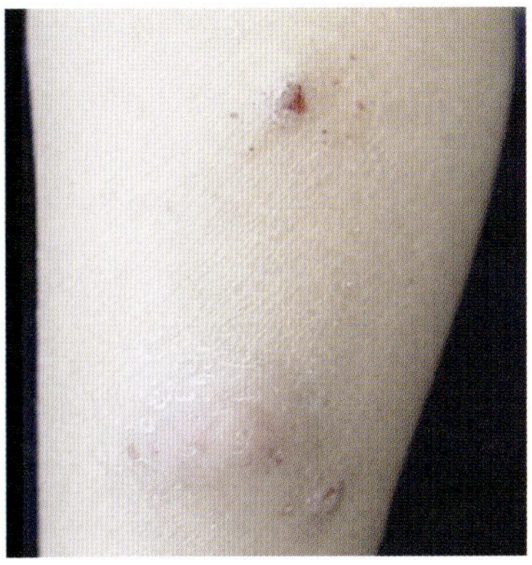

Fig. 15-26　Hyper-IgE syndrome-multiple furuncles

(图15-26　高IgE综合征-多发疖肿)

(3) Wiskott-Aldrich syndrome (WAS), also called the eczema-thrombocytopenia-immunodeficiency syndrome and described in type Ⅲ of PID, is a rare X-linked recessive disease characterized by eczema (Fig. 15-28), thrombocytopenia, immune deficiency, and bloody diarrhea (secondary to the thrombocytopenia).

(3) Wiskott-Aldrich综合征(Wiskott-Aldrich syndrome, WAS)　又称湿疹-血小板减少-免疫缺陷综合征，也归于Ⅲ型PID，是一种罕见的X连锁隐性遗传病，临床表现为湿疹(图15-28)、血小板减少、免疫缺陷及血样腹泻(继发于血小板减少)。

WAS occurs in males only. The first signs of WAS are usually petechiae and bruising, resulting from a low platelet count. Spontaneous nose bleeds and bloody diarrhea are common. Eczema

WAS仅见于男性，首发症状为因血小板减少引起的瘀点和瘀伤。自发性鼻出血及血样腹泻也常见。患儿生后一个

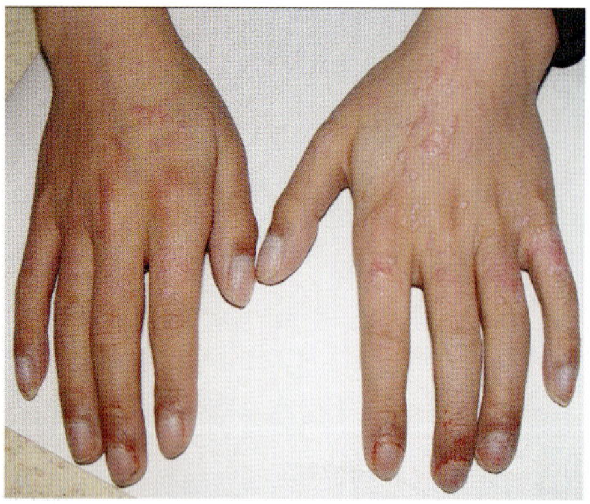

Fig. 15-27　Hyper-IgE syndrome-multiple verruca plana on the hands

(图 15-27　高 IgE 综合征-手部多发扁平疣)

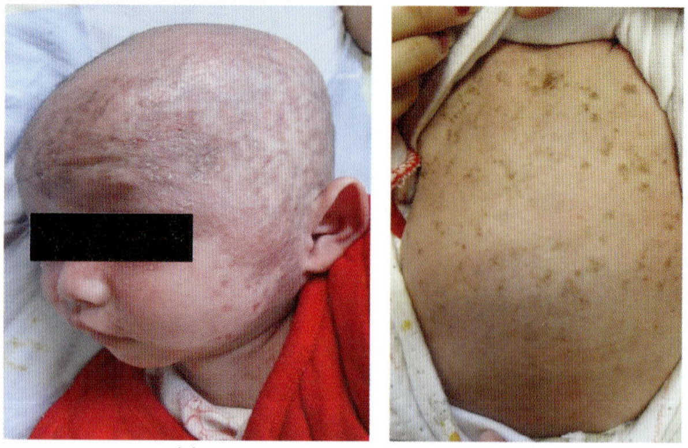

(a)　(b)

Fig. 15-28　Wiskott-Aldrich syndrome-eczema-like lesions

(图 15-28　Wiskott-Aldrich 综合征-湿疹样皮损)

develops within the first month of life. Recurrent bacterial infections take place by 3 months. Splenomegaly is a common finding. The majority of WAS children develop at least 1 autoimmune disorder, and cancers (mainly lymphoma and leukemia) develop in up to one third of patients. Immunoglobulin M (IgM) levels are reduced while IgA and IgE are elevated, and IgG levels can be normal, reduced, or elevated.

月即出现湿疹,三个月时会出现反复细菌感染。脾大较为常见,多数患儿出现至少一种自身免疫性疾病,1/3 患者出现肿瘤(主要为淋巴瘤及白血病)。免疫球蛋白 M(IgM)降低,IgA 和 IgE 升高,而 IgG 水平可升高、正常或降低。

(4) Ataxia telangiectasia (A-T) is also described in type Ⅲ of PID. It is caused by a mutation in the A-T gene, which encodes a protein that is crucial for cell cycle control and DNA repair. A-T disease is characterized by progressive cerebellar ataxia, oculocutaneous telangiectasia, combined immunodeficiency of humoral and cellular immune systems, and a predisposition towards malignancy.

Symptoms most often appear first in early childhood. The patients appear drunk when walking, standing still or sitting. Later, they develop distorted speech (oculomotor apraxia) and dysphagia. Some are at high risk for infections (e. g., respiratory tract infection, ear infections, sinusitis, bronchitis, and pneumonia). Telangiectasia can also appear on sun-exposed areas of skin, such as the face and ears. A-T patients can exhibit early signs of aging such as graying of the hair, vitiligo and warts. But only a small number of patients develop a chronic inflammatory skin disease (granulomas). People with A-T have a greatly increased risk for cancer, particularly lymphoma and leukemia. On the other hand, patients may have a low amount of lymphocytes (especially T lymphocytes) or low levels of immunoglobulins (IgG, IgA, IgM or IgG subclasses), which may paralyze the immune system, leading to an absence of immune response to vaccines or infections.

(4) 共济失调伴毛细血管扩张(ataxia telangiectasia, A-T)　归于Ⅲ型 PID,由 A-T 基因突变引起,此基因编码蛋白参与细胞周期调控及 DNA 修复。表现为进行性小脑共济失调伴眼皮肤毛细血管扩张,合并体液及细胞免疫缺陷,并易发生肿瘤。

症状常在儿童早期出现,患者在走路、站立及坐时表现类似醉酒样,之后发展为动眼失调、发音失真及出现吞咽问题。有些患者易发生感染(呼吸道、耳、鼻窦、支气管、肺等)。毛细血管扩张可发生在皮肤曝光部位如面部及耳部。A-T 可引起早老特征如灰白头发、白癜风及病毒疣,少数患者可出现慢性炎症性皮肤病如肉芽肿。患者罹患肿瘤风险增高,尤其是淋巴瘤和白血病。患者可出现淋巴细胞减少(尤其 T 细胞)、低免疫球蛋白血症(IgG, IgA, IgM 或 IgG 亚型),对感染或疫苗不应答。

(5) Blau syndrome (BS) has been described in type Ⅶ of PID

(5) Blau 综合征(Blau syndrome,

that is caused by NOD2 gene mutations, which result in NF-κB activation and excessive inflammation. Multiple organs can be involved. BS is characterized by the clinical triad of granulomatous dermatitis, symmetric arthritis and recurrent uveitis with onset below 4 years of age.

BS) 归于Ⅶ型 PID，由 NOD2 基因突变所致炎症因子 NF-κB 激活引发过度炎症反应，可累及多个脏器。BS 常在 4 岁内发病，特征表现为非干酪性肉芽肿累及关节、皮肤、眼葡萄膜。

Blau arthritis manifests as a polyarticular synovitis and tenosynovitis, typically affecting peripheral joints especially wrists, knees, ankles, and proximal interphalangeal joints of the hands (Fig. 15-29).

BS 关节炎表现为多关节滑膜炎和腱鞘炎，主要累及外周关节如腕、膝、踝及近端指关节(图 15-29)。

Skin rashes often appear as the first symptom. BS has various skin manifestations but generalized erythematous maculopapular rashes with fine scale are the most frequent, and are easily misdiagnosed as atopic dermatitis, or ichthyosis vulgaris. Later the exanthema may exhibit a "dirty' scaly appearance. In addition, multiple, firm, subcutaneous nodules and pinhead-sized, lichenoid, yellow to brown papules typically appearing in clusters or even coalescent may sometimes be seen (Fig. 15-30).

皮损常最早出现。BS 有多种临床表现，泛发的、小的、红色鳞屑性斑丘疹最常见，并常被误诊为特应性皮炎或鱼鳞病，后期皮疹可呈污秽的鳞屑样外观。多发、质韧皮下结节，成簇或融合的针头大小苔藓样黄棕色丘疹也可见到(图 15-30)。

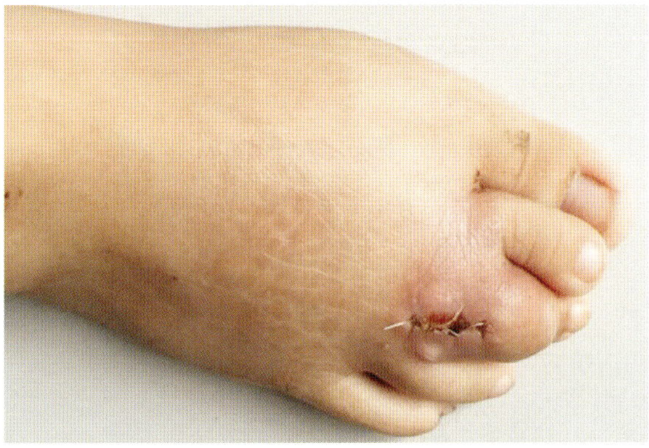

Fig. 15-29 Blau syndrome-joint involvement
(图 15-29 Blau 综合征-关节受累)

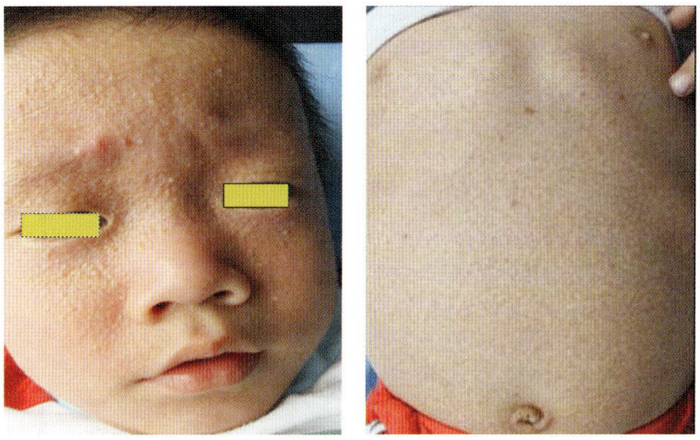

(a) (b)

Fig. 15-30 Blau syndrome-lichenoid lesions
(图 15-30 Blau 综合征-苔藓样皮损)

Uveitis, another common symptom of BS, presents as an insidious granulomatous iridocyclitis and may evolve into a severe panuveitis with multifocal choroiditis. It is usually bilateral and associated with an increased risk of visual morbidity.

葡萄膜炎，另一种 BS 常见症状，表现为肉芽肿型后房虹膜睫状体炎，可进展为合并有多病灶脉络膜炎的严重全葡萄膜炎。常双侧发生，伴有视力不全的风险。

BS usually affects multiple organs and multiple body sites. The presence of fever and cardiovascular, neurological, renal, intestinal and other system involvement has been documented. Non-caseating granulomatous inflammatory infiltrate ane characteristic histopathological features of BS (Fig. 15-31).

BS 伴发多脏器、多部位受累，发热，心血管、神经、肾脏、肠道和其他器官受累有过报道。非干酪坏死型肉芽肿性炎性浸润是 BS 组织病理学特征(图 15-31)。

(6) Chronic mucocutaneous candidiasis described in type Ⅲ of PID is one common phagocyte defect and often presents in childhood with recurrent infections. The fungus may cause mouth infections (thrush)and infections of the scalp, skin, and nails which

(6) 慢性皮肤黏膜念珠菌病(chronic mucocutaneous candidiasis) 归于Ⅲ型 PID，是一类常见吞噬缺陷性疾病，常发生于儿童期，表现为反复、难以治疗的鹅

are difficult to treat. A disfiguring crusted, thick and exudative rash may cover the face and scalp. Usually, this disorder is chronic, but it does not affect life span.

口疮及头部、皮肤、指(趾)甲的真菌感染。特殊的皮损为面部及头皮覆盖厚痂并有渗出斑疹。病程趋慢性,但不影响寿命。

(7) Complement deficiencies belong to type Ⅷ PID, accounting for less than 1% of all PID cases. The complement system plays an important part in defense against microorganisms. Genetic defects of C1q, C1r/s, C2, C4, and C3 are associated with autoimmune diseases, whereas deficiencies in C5, C6, C7, C8, and C9 increase susceptibility to infections (Fig. 15-32). Deficiencies in the complement cascade can lead to severe infections and autoimmune diseases such as systemic lupus erythematosus (SLE), and episodes of angioedema.

(7) 补体缺陷病(complement deficiencies) 所占比例低于 1%,归于Ⅷ型 PID。补体系统在防御微生物感染中发挥重要作用。补体 C1q、C1r/s、C2、C4 和 C3 基因缺陷与自身免疫性疾病相关,而 C5、C6、C7、C8、C9 基因缺陷导致感染易感性(图 15-32)。补体系统缺陷可导致严重感染和自身免疫性疾病如系统性红斑狼疮(SLE)及血管性水肿。

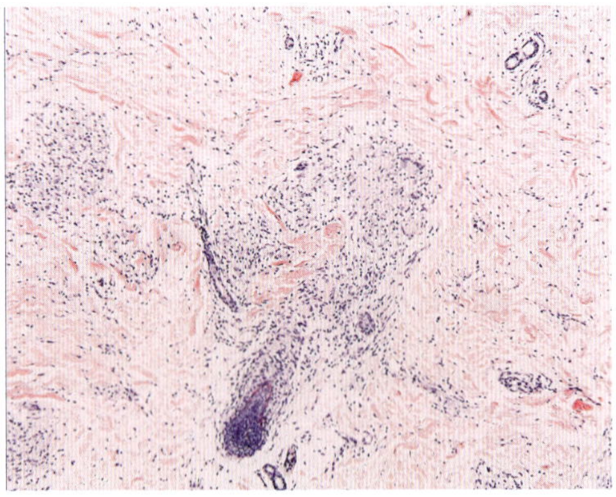

Fig. 15-31 Blau syndrome-epithelioid granuloma histopathologically

(图 15-31 Blau 综合征-组织病理呈上皮样肉芽肿)

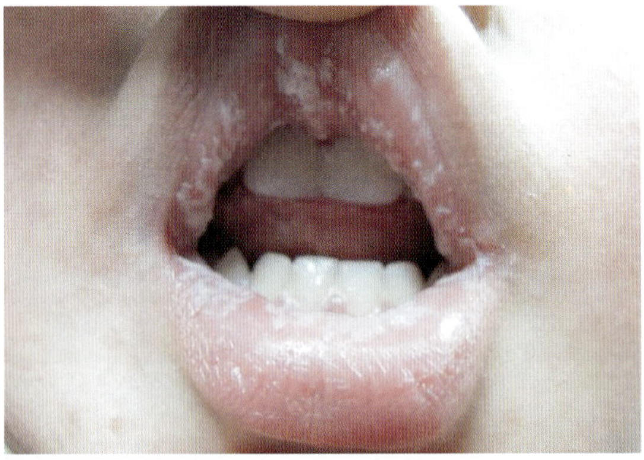

Fig. 15-32 Complement deficiencies-recalcitrant oral candidal infection

(图 15-32 补体缺陷-顽固性口腔念珠菌感染)

【Laboratory Test】

The first line of laboratory tests should include complete blood count and immunoglobulin (IgG, IgA and IgM) level measurements. However, normal T/B-cell numbers or serum immunoglobulin levels would not exclude the possibility of T/B-cell defects. Further investigations of T/B-cell function may be warranted in such cases.

Some immune tests may be chosen based upon the suspected disorders, for example, T lymphocyte transformation test; flow cytometry analysis of subgroups of T-cells, natural killer cells and monocytes; quantitative measurement of serum immunoglobulin (Ig) levels by protein electrophoresis; assessment of serum specific antibody titers in response to vaccine antigens; neutrophil function assays; stimulation assays for cytokine responses; and complement studies.

The histological findings of granuloma in skin biopsy have been described in patients with ataxia telangiectasia (AT), severe combined ID (SCID), combined variable ID (CVID), unclassified

【实验室检查】

基本实验检测包括全血细胞计数及免疫球蛋白(IgG, IgA 和 IgM)水平检测。然而,正常的 T/B 细胞计数或血清中免疫球蛋白水平并不能排除 T/B 细胞缺陷可能,需要进一步检测 T/B 细胞功能。

其他深入的检测依赖于怀疑的疾病种类,如 T 细胞增殖实验,流式细胞仪检测 T 细胞亚群、NK 细胞和单核细胞,蛋白电泳检测免疫球蛋白亚型,评估针对疫苗的血清特定抗体滴度,中性粒细胞功能检测,细胞因子激发实验及补体系统检测。

皮损组织学表现为肉芽肿改变可见于以下 PID:共济失调伴毛细血管扩张(AT)、重症联合免疫缺陷(SCID)、普通

combined ID (UCID), chronic granulomatous disease, Wiskott-Aldrich syndrome, and X-linked hypogammaglobulinemia.

可变免疫缺陷(CVID)、未定类联合免疫缺陷(UCID)、慢性肉芽肿病、Wiskott-Aldrich综合征和X连锁低丙球蛋白血症。

【Diagnosis and Differential Diagnosis】

Prompt diagnosis and early treatment are critical for improving patient outcomes. In fact, many PIDs present as "routine" infections. PIDs should be suspected in patients with recurrent sinus, ear infections or pneumonias within 1 year, persistent thrush or skin abscesses, poor response to a prolonged use of antibiotics, or a family history of PID. The diagnosis of specific PID is based on the clinical features and necessary laboratory tests for the immune system.

A secondary immune deficiency disease occurs when the immune system is compromised due to some external factor. Examples of these external causes include HIV, chemotherapy, severe burns or malnutrition. Therefore, the cause of the immune deficiency-possibly encompassing other diseases, drug treatment, or exposure to toxins-must be excluded before a diagnosis of PID will be possible.

【诊断及鉴别诊断】

PID的早期诊断和治疗对提高患者预后很重要。实际上,许多PID被认为是常规感染,但如果患者表现为1年内反复肺部、耳、鼻窦感染,持续性鹅口疮和皮肤脓肿,长期抗生素治疗效果不佳,或有PID家族史应考虑PID可能。特定类型PID的诊断依赖于临床特征和必要的与免疫相关的实验室检查。

外界因素抑制免疫系统可导致继发免疫缺陷病,如HIV感染、化疗、严重烧伤及营养不良。诊断PID,需要排除继发原因(如其他疾病或药物诱发,或暴露于环境毒素等)。

【Treatment】

The treatment of PID depends on the type of defect (e.g., phagocyte disorder or complement deficiency). Antifungal or antibiotic prophylaxis, cytokine replacement, vaccinations and/or bone marrow transplant may be required for improvement on occasion. The mainstay of treatment for antibody-deficiency disorders patients is Ig replacement. Severe disorders such as SCID require prompt and definitive therapy for immune reconstitution (e.g., hematopoietic stem cell transplantation or bone marrow transplant). Patients with innate immunodeficiency disorders often present with unusual or refractory infections. Reduction of exposure to pathogens and prophylactic antibiotics are recommended in most situations.

Furthermore, some specific immunodeficiency disorders may lead to carcinoma. Radiation and chemotherapeutic drugs should be avoided during treatment, these being particularly toxic for people with ataxia telangiectasia.

【治疗】

PID的治疗取决于免疫缺陷的类型(如吞噬异常或补体缺陷等),需要预防性使用抗真菌和抗细菌药物、细胞因子替代、疫苗及骨髓移植。抗体缺陷病主要采用免疫球蛋白替代治疗,严重免疫缺陷病如SCID需尽快采用血液干细胞移植或骨髓移植来重建免疫等。先天性免疫缺陷患者常表现为不常见或难以治疗的感染,因此很多时候需要注意减少对病原暴露和预防性使用抗生素。

此外,特定的免疫缺陷可诱发肿瘤,在治疗时,需要注意避免使用放疗和一些化疗药物,如对于共济失调伴毛细血管扩张患者可引起特殊的毒害。

Song-mei GENG(耿松梅)

Chapter Sixteen Cutaneous Vascular Diseases

Section One Allergic Purpura

Allergic purpura is a special type of cutaneous small-vessel vasculitis also known as Henoch-Schönlein purpura. The typical symptoms include multiple palpable purpura appearing predominately on the lower legs, often accompanied by joint pain, abdominal pain and renal abnormalities.

【Etiology and Pathogenesis】

The exact cause of this disease is unknown. However, the condition often develops after respiratory tract infection, such as viral and streptococcal infections of the throat, or after allergic reactions to some drugs and certain foods. It has been suggested that the immune complex, which comprises heterogenetic antigens together with antibodies (mainly IgA), leaves deposits on the walls of blood vessels, and these then induce an immune reaction resulting in leakage of red blood cells into the interstitial spaces of the tissues. This damage to the blood vessels (it is suggested) lead to purpura lesions on the skin and may lead to other symptoms when the blood vessels in the joints or kidneys are involved.

【Clinical Manifestations】

Allergic purpura occurs at all ages, but mainly in children. Purpura, abdominal pain, arthralgia and kidney involvement are the classic symptoms of Henoch-Schönlein purpura. The cutaneous lesions manifest as palpable purpura and typically appear on the distal extremities, thighs and buttocks, but may be seen anywhere on the body (Fig. 16-1). Gastrointestinal involvement often presents as abdominal pain, vomiting and bleeding that may vary from occult to bloody or black stools. Joint involvement is mainly manifested by migratory arthralgia and edema in the large joints of the lower limbs; however, upper limb joints can be affected as well. Joint pain can be the first symptom for some patients. Renal involvement in most patients is generally mild and self-limiting, presenting either as mild proteinuria or hematuria (which should not persist). Only 2% of patients develop persistent kidney damage.

【Laboratory Findings】

Elevated antistreptolysin O (ASO) may be detected in those individuals with streptococcal infections. Hematuria and proteinuria are shown in patients who have kidney vasculitis. Other non-

第十六章 皮肤血管性疾病

第一节 过敏性紫癜

过敏性紫癜(allergic purpura)是一种特殊类型的皮肤小血管炎，又称为 Henoch-Schönlein 紫癜(Henoch-Schönlein purpura)，是一种主要发生于下肢，可伴有关节症状、消化道症状或肾脏症状的可触及性紫癜的皮肤病。

【病因及发病机制】

本病病因不明，发病前多有上呼吸道感染等症状，常见的是病毒或链球菌咽炎。药物及食物也可诱发本病。这些异种抗原与诱导机体产生的抗体(主要是 IgA)结合后形成的免疫复合物沉积于血管壁诱发机体免疫反应，导致红细胞渗出到组织间隙，从而形成临床可见的皮肤紫癜或其他症状(如关节、肾血管受累时)。

【临床表现】

过敏性紫癜可发生于任何年龄，但主要见于儿童。过敏性紫癜的主要表现为皮肤紫癜、腹痛、关节痛及肾脏受累。皮损表现为可触及的紫癜，主要发生于双小腿、股和臀部，也可广泛分布(图 16-1)。胃肠道的受累常见症状包括腹痛、呕吐和肠胃出血，胃肠道出血可表现为隐血便、大量鲜血便和黑便。关节受累主要表现为侵犯下肢大关节的游走性关节痛及下肢水肿，上肢关节也可受累，部分患者以关节痛为首发症状。肾脏受累大部分病变较轻，表现为轻度的蛋白尿和血尿并且有自限性(不会迁延)，但有 2%的患者会发展为迁延的肾脏损害。

【实验室检查】

链球菌感染引起患者 ASO 升高。肾脏受累的患者可出现血尿和蛋白尿。其他非特异性表现包括血清中 IgA 和

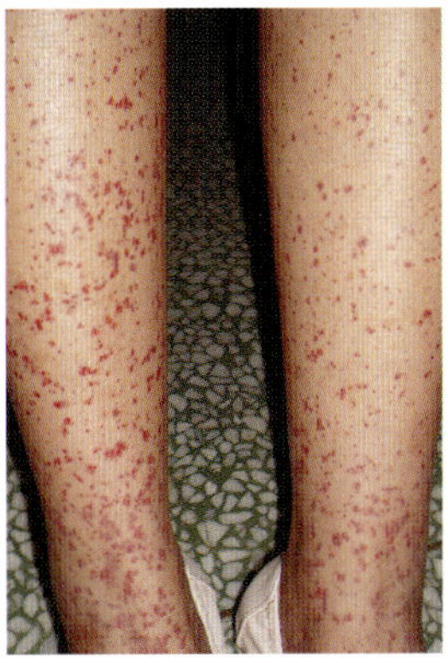

Fig. 16-1　Allergic purpura(图 16-1　过敏性紫癜)

specific findings for Henoch-Schönlein purpura are raised levels of serum IgA and IgE.

IgE 水平可升高。

【Histopathology】

Under microscopy, a typical leukocytoclastic vasculitis can be revealed in affected cutaneous small vessels. IgA, C3 and fibrins deposition on the walls of the blood vessels will show under direct immunofluorescence.

【组织病理】

皮损组织病理检查显示典型皮肤小血管的白细胞碎裂性血管炎，直接免疫荧光检查可见真皮血管周围和血管壁中IgA、C3 和纤维素沉积。

【Diagnosis and Differential Diagnosis】

The diagnosis is based on the combination of the symptoms and laboratory findings. It is necessary to distinguish Henoch-Schönlein purpura from other diseases that cause purpura and vasculitis involving cutaneous small vessels. The differential diagnosis is fairly straightforward, as the majority of purpura related diseases have no palpable purpuric lesion. But, given that other diseases may also cause leukocytoclastic vasculitis, a histological examination is necessary in order to make that distinction.

【诊断与鉴别诊断】

根据典型的临床表现和实验室检查，过敏性紫癜可以诊断。本病需和其他紫癜性皮肤病及其他累及皮肤小血管的血管炎相鉴别，但其他疾病引起的紫癜不是可触及性紫癜。组织学上还需和其他白细胞碎裂性血管炎鉴别。

【Treatment】

The majority of patients can benefit from supportive therapy since this disease is usually self-limiting. Removal of inducing factors should be the first priority, and symptomatic measures, including bed rest and elevation of the affected limbs, are of help. The administration of antispasmodics, antibiotics, anti-inflammatory drugs, and systemic glucocorticoids generally leads to the resolution of an acute process.

【治疗】

本病常为自限性，治疗以支持治疗为主。首先应去除诱因，注意卧床休息，并抬高患肢。应用解痉药、抗生素和抗炎药物，系统应用糖皮质激素对急性过程常有效。

【Prognosis】

Henoch-Schönlein purpura is normally a benign disease with a good prognosis and resolves within 6-16 weeks in most cases. However, 5%-10% of patients can develop chronic or recurrent purpura.

【预后】

大部分患者病程 6～16 周，预后良好。但有 5%～10%患者的病情呈持续性或复发性。

Section Two　Allergic Cutaneous Vasculitis

Allergic cutaneous vasculitis is not a single disease, but a group of conditions that represent as leukocytoclastic vasculitis of the capillaries, micro veins and the micro arteries following a deposit of circulating immune complexes on the walls of these blood vessels.

【Etiology and Pathogenesis】

Allergic cutaneous vasculitis results from the destruction of small blood vessels caused by circulating immune complexes deposited on the walls of these vessels, which in turn activate their corresponding complements. As a result, various inflammatory mediators are produced that further damage the endothelial cells of the blood vessels. The causes are unknown for the majority of patients, but possible causative factors are infection, autoimmune connective tissue diseases, cancer, drugs, and other chemicals.

【Clinical Manifestations】

The skin lesions are usually located on the legs, and in severe cases will spread to the buttocks, arms, ankles, feet, trunk, and face. Typically, polymorphic skin lesions appear at the same time, consisting of palpable purpura, erythema, papules, wheal, blisters and bullae, pustules, hemorrhagic blisters, nodules and ulcerations, which usually last 1-4 weeks (Fig. 16-2). The eruption often occurs in episodes at irregular intervals. Pruritus or burning is a common complain for most patients. Systemic manifestations of allergic cutaneous vasculitis including abdominal pain and gastrointestinal tract bleeding, arthralgia and/or arthritis, renal abnormalities and symptoms of nervous system can sometimes accompany the skin lesions. Hyperpigmentation or atrophic scars may occur after the regression of the skin lesions.

第二节　变应性皮肤血管炎

变应性皮肤血管炎(allergic cutaneous vasculitis)并不是一种独立的疾病，它是一种由多种病因引起的循环免疫复合物所致累及毛细血管、微静脉和微动脉的白细胞碎裂性血管炎。

【病因及发病机制】

变应性皮肤血管炎是免疫反应引起的，循环免疫复合物沉积于皮肤小血管管壁，这些复合物激活补体产生炎性介质，导致血管内皮损伤。大部分患者原因不明，可能的致病因子有感染、自身免疫性结缔组织疾病、肿瘤、药物及其他化学品。

【临床表现】

皮损主要侵犯小腿，病情较重者也可广泛分布于臀部、前臂、踝部、双足、躯干和面部。皮损典型者为多形性，主要表现为可触及的紫癜、红斑、丘疹、风团、水疱和大疱、脓疱、血疱、结节、溃疡等(图 16-2)。皮损常间歇性发作，间隔时间不规则，每次持续 1～4 周。患者常诉皮损有瘙痒或灼痛感，有的患者可有腹痛和胃肠出血、关节疼痛和/或关节炎、肾脏受累及神经系统等表现。皮损消退后可留下色素沉着或萎缩性瘢痕。

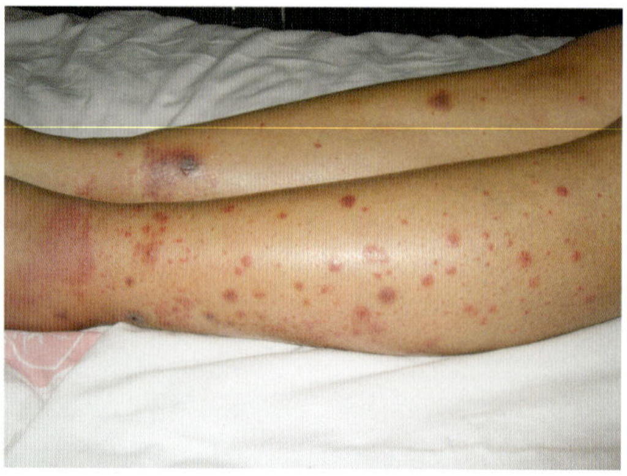

Fig. 16-2　Allergic cutaneous vasculitis(图 16-2　变应性皮肤血管炎)

【Laboratory Findings】

White blood cell counts in peripheral blood may not undergo

【实验室检查】

外周血白细胞一般无明显变化，有

any marked change, but can be elevated on occasion. Anemia may also occur in severe cases. The erythrocyte sedimentation rate may be elevated and the level of serum complements often decreases. Hematuria and proteinuria can be found when blood vessels in kidneys are involved.

时可升高，严重者有贫血，血沉增快，血清补体下降。肾脏受损可出现血尿和蛋白尿。

【Histopathology】

Skin biopsy shows typical leukocytoclastic vasculitis in the capillaries, micro veins and micro arteries in the superficial and middle dermal layers.

【组织病理】

皮损病理检查显示主要侵犯真皮浅中部毛细血管、微静脉和微动脉的白细胞碎裂性血管炎。

【Diagnosis】

The diagnosis is primarily based on the clinical manifestations that develop after exposure to particular medications or infections or other triggers as reported in the patient's history. Again, confirmation may be obtained from laboratory findings and histological examination of skin lesions.

【诊断】

当患者有使用特定的药物史、感染史或其他诱因，结合临床表现可以初步诊断；而确诊则需要结合实验室检查和皮损组织病理检查。

【Differential Diagnosis】

Allergic cutaneous vasculitis is not a single disease. It is necessary to differentiate it from other leukocytoclastic vasculitis such as allergic purpura.

【鉴别诊断】

变应性皮肤血管炎并不是一独特的疾病，须和其他白细胞碎裂性血管炎（如过敏性紫癜）相鉴别。

【Treatment】

Treatment is aimed at reducing inflammation, and allowing the natural healing process to proceed. Thus, symptomatic measures, including bed rest, elevation of or applying mild heat to the affected limbs are all helpful. Exposure to the causative medication or other antigens (infectious agents) if known, should be terminated. Oral nonsteroidal anti-inflammatory drugs (NSAIDs), diaminodiphenylsulfone (DDS), colchicine and/or thalidomide may be used to reduce inflammation of the blood vessels. In severe cases, treatment with systemic glucocorticoids or immunosuppressants may be necessary.

【治疗】

治疗的目标是减轻炎症和缩短自然病程。对症处理（如卧床休息、抬高患肢和保暖）常有帮助。若患者是由感染、药物或其他原因诱发，要去掉诱因。口服非甾体类抗炎药（NSAIDs）、氨苯砜（DDS）、秋水仙碱和反应停可有效减轻患者症状。对于有严重系统症状者，系统应用糖皮质激素或免疫抑制剂有效。

【Prognosis】

The prognosis for allergic cutaneous vasculitis varies among individuals, ranging from a mild, self-limiting illness to a serious or even fatal disorder. Allergic vasculitis usually goes into remission over time, but about 50% of patients may experience an acute course. On occasion, people will also have repeated episodes, and about 1.9% of patients fail to ultimately recover from this disorder.

【预后】

变应性皮肤血管炎预后各不相同，从轻微的自限性到严重的致命性都可发生。大多数患者预后良好，约 50% 的患者表现为临床急性过程，有些患者表现为慢性病程或复发和缓解交替。大约 1.9%的患者死于严重的系统性疾病。

Section Three　Nodular Vasculitis

Nodular vasculitis is a chronic recurrent lobular panniculitis mixed with fat septa vasculitis that appears as painful or tender purple-colored nodules on the lower legs of women usually of age 30-60.

第三节　结节性血管炎

结节性血管炎（nodular vasculitis）是一种主要累及青中年女性（一般为 30～60 岁）下肢的疼痛或触痛的紫红色硬结的慢性复发性小叶性脂膜炎伴有脂肪

间隔的血管炎。

【Etiology and Pathogenesis】

The exact cause of nodular vasculitis is unknown. However, some cases may be closely associated with tuberculosis infection. To date, immune complexes and delayed hypersensitivity to endogenous or exogenous antigens have been considered as etiological factors. The inducing factors for such immune response in some patients are infectious agents such as *Mycobacterium tuberculosis*, *Streptococcus* and hepatitis C virus and drug interactions. It should be kept in mind, however, that the promoters for this condition are unclear in some cases.

【病因及发病机制】

结节性血管炎的确切病因尚不明确,部分患者与结核病感染有着非常密切的关系。目前认为是一种针对内源性抗原或外源性抗原的免疫复合物型和迟发型变态反应导致的皮肤病。导致这种免疫反应的诱发因子包括感染(如结核杆菌、链球菌和丙型肝炎病毒)和药物,部分患者诱发因素尚不清楚。

【Clinical Manifestations】

Nodular vasculitis mainly affects young or middle aged women; men are less often affected. The nodules are usually found on the extensor surfaces of the lower legs but they may also occur on the shins, feet, ankles, thighs and upper limbs. The lesions include infiltrative erythema and subcutaneous indurated nodules which are painful, symmetrically distributed, diffuse and elevated (Fig. 16-3). The nodular lesions can be aligned as a circular array on occasion. The nodules usually last for 1-2 months. The nodules may erupt at irregular intervals over months or years and sometimes will be accompanied by ulceration. Most nodules heal slowly to leave scars or hyperpigmentation macules.

【临床表现】

本病好发于青中年女性,男性少见。结节主要累及小腿屈侧,也可发生于胫前、足、踝、大腿和上肢,表现为疼痛性、弥漫性对称性分布的、隆起浸润性红斑和皮下硬结(图 16-3),部分患者皮损可表现为环状排列的结节,硬结在 1～2 个月内可消退。皮损常反复发作数月或数年,有时伴有溃疡,多数结节愈合较慢,常留有瘢痕和色素沉着斑。

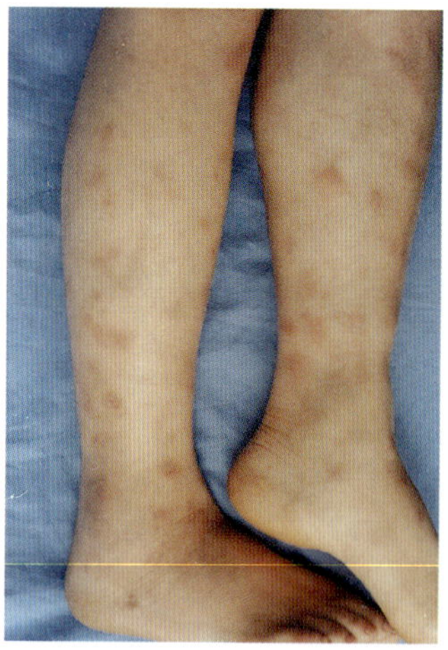

Fig. 16-3　Nodular vasculitis(图 16-3　结节性血管炎)

【Laboratory Findings】

Laboratory examination typically reveals no special markers. The erythrocyte sedimentation rate may elevate at the acute stage and ASO titer may increase in a few cases. Occult tuberculosis should be excluded by tuberculin skin test, chest X-ray and PCR detection of tubercle bacillus DNA extracted from the skin lesions.

【实验室检查】

实验室检查无特殊发现,急性期血沉可以增快,少数病例 ASO 升高。皮肤结核菌素实验、胸片和 PCR 检测皮损的结核杆菌 DNA 可帮助发现是否有结核杆菌感染。

【Histopathology】

Biopsies of cutaneous lesions show mixed septal and fat lobular inflammation and necrosis of the fat lobules. Granulomatous infiltrations are composed mainly of giant cells and epithelioid cells. Meanwhile, a heavy inflammatory infiltrate of neutrophils, lymphocytes and histiocytes surrounds the affected vessels that either become necrotic on the vessel wall or form intraluminal thromboses. Tuberculous granulomas will also be seen in typical cases caused by *M. tuberculosis*.

【组织病理】

皮损病理检查显示脂肪间隔和小叶改变，脂肪小叶坏死和多核巨细胞、上皮样细胞浸润形成的肉芽肿。血管累及时可见大量的中性粒细胞、淋巴细胞和组织细胞浸润，血管壁坏死和血管内栓塞。由结核杆菌引起的典型病例可见结核性肉芽肿。

【Diagnosis】

When the typical clinical manifestations, laboratory findings and biopsies of cutaneous lesions described above occur in one patient, nodular vasculitis can be diagnosed.

【诊断】

当患者出现上述典型临床表现、实验室检查和组织病理检查特点，结节性血管炎可以诊断。

【Differential Diagnosis】

Unfortunately, the histologic features are not specific for this disease. Also, these pathological manifestations will vary depending on the age of the lesion at the time of the biopsy, and the condition can overlap with other forms of panniculitis as well, such as erythema nodosa, cutaneous polyarteritis nodosa, thrombophlebitis migrans and other forms of vasculitis. It is also necessary to exclude infective causes of panniculitis, particularly mycobacterial and fungal infections.

【鉴别诊断】

本病的组织学特征常无特异性。其病理改变根据皮损取材的时间而不同，因而与其他的脂膜炎（如结节性红斑、皮肤结节性多动脉炎、游走性血栓性静脉炎和其他血管炎）有重叠。此外，此病还必须排除由感染，特别是分枝杆菌和真菌感染引起的脂膜炎。

【Treatment】

Bed rest is needed above all. Antituberculosis therapy should be given in any case caused by *M. tuberculosis*. Oral potassium iodide is effective in about 50% of cases. Oral NSAIDs, colchicine and diaminodiphenylsulfone (DDS) are also helpful and systemic glucocorticoid therapy is used for severe cases.

【治疗】

患者应卧床休息。若患者是由结核杆菌感染诱发，应进行抗结核治疗。饱和碘化钾溶液对 50%的患者有效，口服 NSAIDs、秋水仙碱和氨苯砜（DDS），系统应用糖皮质激素对病情严重患者有效。

【Prognosis】

The prognosis is good if treated properly in most cases. Usually each episode runs its course in 3-6 weeks, but recurrences are not unheard of, especially if the underlying infection is still present.

【预后】

大多数患者经过适当的处理后预后良好，发作期为 3～6 周，可有复发，特别是潜在性感染仍然存在时。

Section Four　Behçet's Disease

Behçet's disease was originally described as a syndrome of recurrent oral and genital ulcerations with associated uveitis. The new definition recognizes this condition as a systemic vasculitis illness, which affects the skin and mucous membranes, joints, central nervous system as well as vascular, respiratory, gastrointestinal, and urogenital systems.

第四节　白　塞　病

白塞病（Behçet's disease）又称为复发性口腔和生殖器溃疡伴眼葡萄膜炎综合征。目前认为该疾病为系统性的血管炎疾病，可侵犯皮肤黏膜、关节、中枢神经系统以及血管、呼吸、胃肠道及泌尿生殖道系统。

【Etiology and Pathogenesis】

The precise etiology and pathogenesis of this disease is unknown. Epidemiological evidence indicates that genetic and environmental factors are both associated with the occurrence of this disease, and the pathogenic manifestations are derived from vascular injury and autoimmune reaction. Behçet's disease is strongly correlated with HLA-B5、HLA-B12、HLA-B27, and particularly with HLA-B51. It has been reported that heat shock proteins and anticardiolipin antibodies might play an important role in the pathogenesis of Behçet's disease. However, the underlying antigen that leads to these changes remains elusive. Immune reaction to bacteria, especially to hemolytic *Streptococcus* and viruses, has been suggested as a promoter for this condition.

【病因及发病机制】

本病的确切病因和发病机制仍不清楚，流行病学证据表明遗传和环境因素与本病的发生有关，致病机制包括血管损伤和自身免疫反应。白塞病的发病与人类白细胞抗原 HLA-B5、HLA-B12、HLA-B27，特别是与 HLA-B51 有关。有报道热休克蛋白和抗心磷脂抗体被认为在发病机制中起到重要作用。诱发这些改变并最终导致该病发生的潜在抗原仍然未知，对细菌(特别是溶血性链球菌)、病毒的免疫反应被认为是疾病发生的始动因子。

【Clinical Manifestations】

Behçet's disease shows male predominance and most commonly presents in young adults, with a peak incidence of onset in the third decade. Recurrent oral ulcer is the primary symptom (Fig. 16-4). These ulcers may develop anywhere in the oral cavity, pharynx, or larynx. The ulcers are painful and usually regress spontaneously in 2 weeks, although they can persist for much longer in some cases.

【临床表现】

本病好发于男性，最常见于青年人，21～30 岁为高发年龄。复发性口腔溃疡是主要特征(图 16-4)，可见于口腔及咽喉各处，溃疡有疼痛，常在 2 周或更长的时间内自行消退。

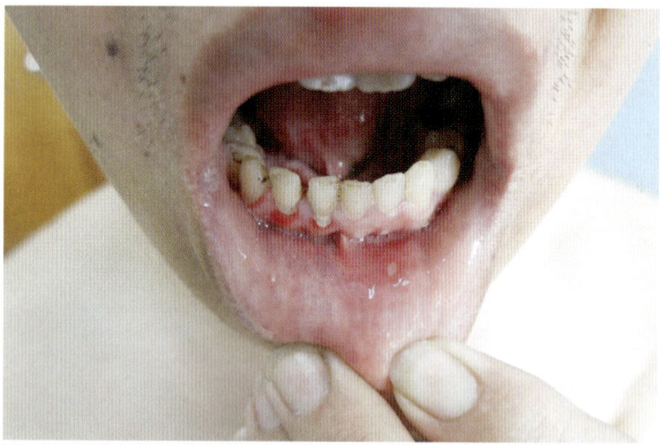

Fig. 16-4 Behçet's disease-recurrent oral ulcer(图 16-4 白塞病-复发性口腔溃疡)

Cutaneous lesions are common and recurrent. Patients may develop erythema nodosa-like lesions (Fig. 16-5), acneiform papules, pustules, furuncles, pyoderma, thrombophlebitis or Sweet's syndrome-like features. The development of sterile pustules at sites of mild skin trauma such as injection sites is known as positive "pathergy test" or "pathergy response", and is relatively common (Fig. 16-6).

皮肤损害常见，多反复发生，可表现为结节性红斑样皮损(图 16-5)、痤疮样丘疹、脓疱、疖、脓皮病、血栓性静脉炎和 Sweet's 综合征样皮损。皮肤注射等微创处可发生无菌性脓疱，即针刺试验(同形反应)阳性(图 16-6)。

Genital lesions that occur usually on the scrotum, penis, vulva and vagina are similar in appearance to those of the oral mucosa. Bilateral ocular lesions of anterior uveitis, posterior uveitis with hypopyon and vitritis can be observed in the majority of the cases

好发于男性阴囊、阴茎及女性外阴、阴道的生殖器损害与口腔黏膜损害类似。大多数患者可见双侧眼部受累，双眼前葡萄膜炎、后葡萄膜炎伴前房积脓

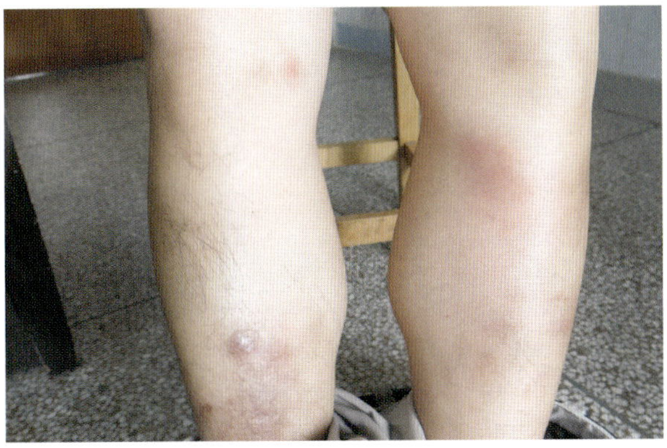

Fig. 16-5　Behçet's disease-erythema nodosa-like lesions
(图 16-5　白塞病-结节性红斑样皮损)

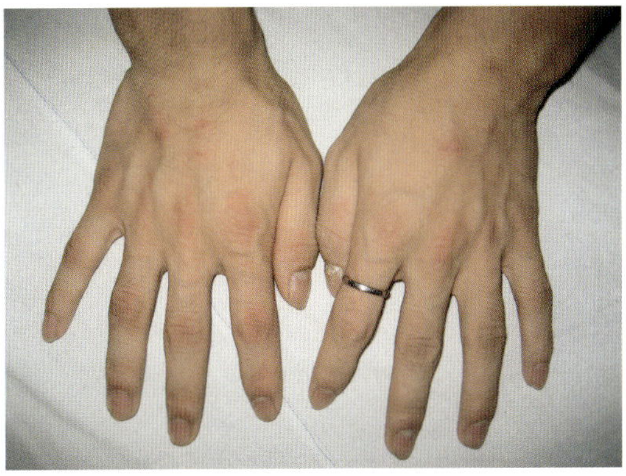

Fig. 16-6　Behçet's disease-positive pathergy test
(图 16-6　白塞病-针刺试验阳性)

and have all been said to be pathognomonic.

Joint involvement is common and usually affects knees, ankles, elbows and wrists. The affected joints are swollen, red, painful and tender, but joint deformities do not develop under normal circumstances.

The vascular diseases in Behçet's disease may take the form of either thrombo-occlusive diseases or vasculitis with obvious symptoms. Respiratory involvement presents as dyspnea, coughing and chest pain in some patients. When the gastrointestinal tract is affected, abdominal pain and bleeding or perforation of the intestine may also present. Involvement of the central nervous system occurs in up to 25% and kidney involvement occurs in up to 55% of all the cases.

【Laboratory Findings】

Anemia of different degrees or intensities may be found in some patients. Blood work shows increased white blood cells (especially neutrophils) and erythrocyte sedimentation rate. The high levels of CRP and immunoglobulins are commonly seen in Behçet's patients. More than 80% of Asian patients are positive for the HLA-B51 genetic marker. Pathergy test is positive in 70% of patients.

【Histopathology】

The underlying pathological features of the biopsied skin lesion in Behçet's disease are vasculitis and perivascular inflammatory infiltrates affecting all sizes of blood vessels in the dermis and subcutaneous tissue. A blood-vessel-centric neutrophilic infiltration with neutrophil fragmentation and extravasation of erythrocytes can be seen. Thrombosis and necrotic vessels may or may not be found. However, the dominant cells in perivascular infiltrates are lymphocytic infiltration for an old lesion.

和玻璃体炎是特征性的损害。

关节受累常见，主要侵犯膝、踝、肘和腕关节，表现为关节红肿、疼痛和压痛，但通常不发生关节畸形。

血管受累可表现为血栓闭塞性疾病和症状明显的血管炎。部分患者可有肺部受累的症状，表现为呼吸困难、咳嗽、胸痛等。胃肠道受累可表现为疼痛、出血或肠穿孔。高达25%的患者有中枢神经系统病变，55%的患者有肾损害。

【实验室检查】

部分患者可有不同程度的贫血，白细胞(特别是中性粒细胞)升高，血沉增快，CRP、免疫球蛋白升高。80%以上亚洲患者HLA-B51阳性。70%的患者针刺试验阳性。

【组织病理】

皮损病理检查显示累及真皮及皮下组织中各种大小血管的血管炎和血管周围炎性浸润，可见以血管为中心的中性粒细胞浸润，伴有白细胞碎裂和红细胞溢出，伴或不伴血栓形成和坏死，陈旧皮损表现为血管周围淋巴细胞浸润为主。

【Diagnosis】

The diagnostic criteria for Behçet's disease issued by the International Study Group in 1990 are summarized in Tab. 16-1.

【诊断】

1990 年国际研究小组制订的白塞病诊断标准总结于表 16-1。

Tab. 16-1　Behçet's disease: diagnostic criteria(表 16-1　白塞病的诊断标准)

Criterion(标准)	Definition(定义)
Recurrent oral ulcer(复发性口腔溃疡)	Minor aphthous, major aphthous, or herpetiform ulcer observed by physician or patient, and recurrent at least 3 times in 1 12-month period(医师或患者观察到 1 年内至少反复发作 3 次轻微的或较重的口疮性或疱疹性溃疡)
Plus two of(加上以下两个表现)	
Recurrent genital ulcer(复发性生殖器溃疡)	Aphthous ulcer or scarring, observed by physician or patient(医师或患者观察到生殖器复发性口疮性溃疡或瘢痕)
Eye lesions(眼部损害)	Anterior uveitis, posterior uveitis or cells in vitreous on slit lamp examination; or retinal vasculitis observed by ophthalmologist(眼科医师观察到有前、后葡萄膜炎,或裂隙灯检查玻璃体内可见细胞;或视网膜血管炎)
Skin lesions(皮肤损害)	Erythema nodosum, pseudofolliculitis or papulopustular lesions; or acneiform nodules observed by physician, patient not on corticosteroid treatment(结节性红斑、假性毛囊炎或丘脓疱疹,非糖皮质激素性痤疮样结节(医师或患者观察到))
Positive pathergy test(针刺试验阳性)	Read by physician at 24-48 hours(由医师 24~48 h 判断结果)

From the "McKee P, et al. Pathology of the skin with clinical correlation. P793".

【Differential Diagnosis】

It is necessary to differentiate Behçet's disease from other diseases that also present as oral ulcers, folliculitis, infections, erythema nodosum, connective tissue diseases, neutrophilic and lymphocytic vasculitis.

【鉴别诊断】

本病须和其他原因所致的其他口腔溃疡性疾病、毛囊炎、感染、结节性红斑、结缔组织病、中性粒细胞性血管炎、淋巴细胞性血管炎相鉴别。

【Treatment】

Mild mouthwashes should be prescribed when oral lesions occur. Sucralfate suspension was found to decrease pain and shorten the healing time for Behçet's oral and genital ulcers. Oral colchicine, thalidomide, dapsone and NSAIDs are also effective in many cases. However, systemic glucocorticoids, methotrexate, azathioprine, cyclophosphamide, cyclosporine, tacrolimus and TNF-α monoclonal antibody or TNF-α antagonist should be reserved for severe refractory cases.

【治疗】

当有口腔损害时,可用温和的漱口液,硫糖铝混悬液用于口腔和生殖器溃疡,可减轻疼痛和缩短愈合时间。口服秋水仙碱、沙利度胺、氨苯砜和 NSAIDs 有效。系统性糖皮质激素、甲氨蝶呤、硫唑嘌呤、环磷酰胺、环孢素、他克莫司和 TNF-α 单克隆抗体或 TNF-α 拮抗剂可用来治疗严重顽固病例。

【Prognosis】

Prognosis of Behçet's disease varies with patients. In most cases the outcome is benign, but a chronic course or a pattern of relapses and remissions may be seen in some patients. In cases where the respiratory and/or central nervous systems are involved, the prognosis in general is poor.

【预后】

白塞病预后各不相同,大多数患者预后良好,有些患者表现为复发和缓解交替。呼吸和中枢神经系统受累的患者预后不良。

Section Five　Pigmentary Purpuric Dermatoses

Pigmentary purpuric dermatoses encompass a number of clinical syndromes characterized by orange/brown pigmentation,

第五节　色素性紫癜性皮病

色素性紫癜性皮病(pigmentary purpuric dermatoses)是一组以橙黄色或

interspersed with fine pinpoint purpura.

褐色色素沉着斑，其间散在细小针尖大小的紫癜为临床特征的疾病。

【Etiology and Pathogenesis】

At present our understanding of the pathogenesis of this disease is still incomplete. The precise causes for the disease is unclear. However, in some patients the possibility of an altered immune response to different antigens may contribute to the pathogenesis. For example, drugs and food additives can cause this condition on occasion and gravity and elevated venous pressure seemed to be inducers for its development. Also, some clinical signs of pigmentary purpuric dermatoses can also be observed in rheumatoid disease or in certain specific types of mycosis fungoides.

【病因及发病机制】

本病的确切病因和发病机制不明，目前认为患者免疫应答的异常改变在色素性紫癜性皮病的发病过程中起到很重要的作用。重力和静脉压升高是重要的诱发因素，偶可由药物和食物添加剂引起。也可发生于类风湿疾病或可能是特殊类型蕈样肉芽肿的表现。

【Clinical Manifestations】

Pigmentary purpuric dermatoses occur most frequently in the lower extremities of middle-aged men. It can manifest as progressive pigmented purpuric dermatoses, pigmentary purpuric lichenoid dermatitis, purpura annularis telangiectodes, itching purpura, and lichen aureus, etc. These disorders may display overlapping clinical and histological features.

Progressive pigmented purpuric dermatoses, also known as Schamberg's disease, is characterized by purpura and petechiae with conspicuous pigmentation. The lesions are pinpoint-sized, reddish or golden brown puncta resembling grains of red pepper, arranging in irregularly shaped patches on the lower legs. The most common sites are around the lower shins and ankles (Fig. 16-7). The lesions are seldom itchy.

Pigmentary purpuric lichenoid dermatitis or Gougerot-Blum syndrome: it is characterized by minute, rust-colored lichenoid papules that tend to fuse into plaques of various hues (Fig. 16-8). Males are also predominant for this type of disease, and predominantly affected locations include the legs, thighs, or lower trunk. The lesions are commonly asymptomatic and seldom itchy.

Purpura annularis telangiectodes or Majocchi's disease: here the lesions tend to be discrete and annular, varying from one to several centimeters in diameter, and are associated with telangiectasias. The central part of these lesions gradually fades so that the central involution and the peripheral extension form circular or semicircular (target-like) concentric rings. The eruption begins on the lower extremities and then spreads up to the legs and

【临床表现】

色素性紫癜性皮病好发于中年男性的下肢，它包括进行性色素性紫癜性皮病、色素性紫癜性苔藓样皮炎、毛细血管扩张性环状紫癜、瘙痒性紫癜和金黄色苔藓等一组疾病。这些疾病在临床和组织学上的特征可互相重叠。

进行性色素性紫癜性皮病(progressive pigmented purpuric dermatoses)：又称为Schamberg's病(Schamberg's disease)，其特征性的表现为紫癜和瘀斑，伴有明显的色素沉着，主要在小腿部表现为针尖大小的淡红色或金黄褐色辣椒粉样损害构成的不规则斑片，好发于小腿胫部下段和踝部(图16-7)。皮损很少瘙痒。

色素性紫癜性苔藓样皮炎(pigmentary purpuric lichenoid dermatitis)或Gougerot-Blum综合征(Gougerot-Blum syndrome)：其特征为铁锈色苔藓样小丘疹，易融合成不同颜色的斑块(图16-8)，好发于男性的小腿、大腿和躯干下部，常无症状，偶有瘙痒。

毛细血管扩张性环状紫癜(purpura annularis telangiectodes)或Majocchi's病(Majocchi's disease)：皮损往往呈环状散在分布，直径从一厘米到数厘米不等，伴有毛细血管扩张。皮损中央逐渐褪色，而向周围扩展成环状、半环状、靶形或同心圆状。损害从下肢远端开始，

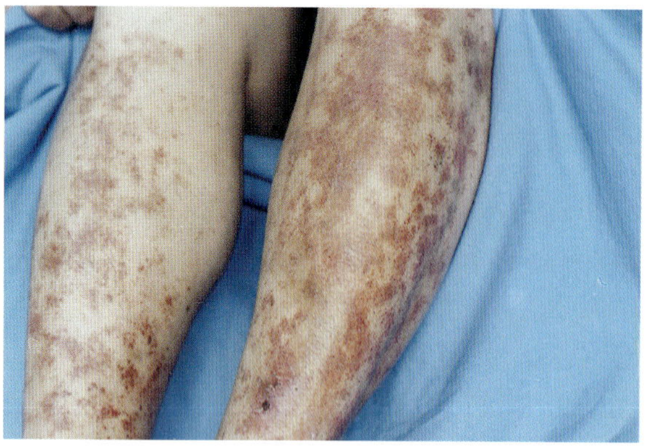

Fig. 16-7　Progressive pigmented purpuric dermatoses
(图 16-7　进行性色素性紫癜性皮病)

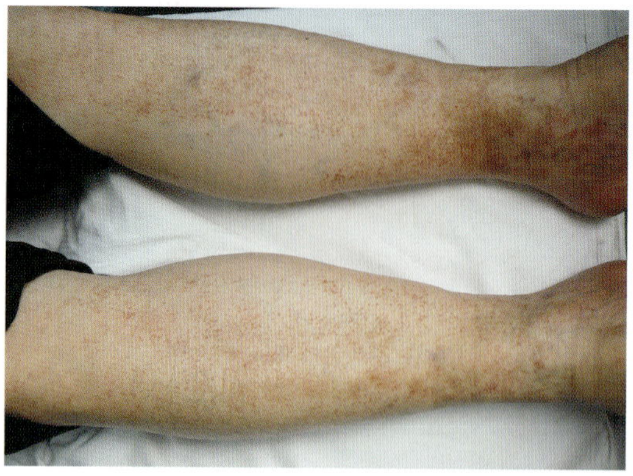

Fig. 16-8　Pigmentary purpuric lichenoid dermatitis
(图 16-8　色素性紫癜性苔藓样皮炎)

may extend onto the trunk and arms. The lesions are commonly asymptomatic.

Itching purpura: the lesions are widely distributed orange macules. The itching is usually severe. It commonly begins on the dorsal surface of the feet or ankles, and soon spreads upward to the thighs, buttocks, trunk and arms.

Lichen aureus: often expressed as solitary light red to brown patches or plaques with a golden yellow tone mixture. Usually the skin lesions are otherwise asymptomatic.

【Histopathology】

All variants share similar histopathological features. Biopsies of cutaneous lesions show superficial perivascular lymphocytic infiltrates with extravasation of erythrocytes. However, a small amount of neutrophils may be found in the infiltration. As the lesions evolve, hemosiderin deposits may become more pronounced.

【Diagnosis】

When the typical clinical manifestations and histopathogical findings described above occur, especially in a middle-aged man, pigmentary purpuric dermatoses should be diagnosed.

【Differential Diagnosis】

The features of superficial perivascular lymphocytic infiltrate with extravasation of erythrocytes and hemosiderin deposits are non-specific findings. The differential diagnosis of pigmentary purpuric dermatoses includes other forms of perivascular lymphocytic infiltrates and lymphocytic capillaritis.

【Treatment】

Bed rest is recommended for all patients. Topical application of glucocorticoids is the preferred effective for relief of itching or obvious erythema, which can also be suppressed by PUVA or narrow band UVB. In addition, pentoxifylline has been reported to be effective in some cases. Agents to reinforce blood vessels (e. g. ,

可扩展到小腿、躯干和臂部，一般无症状。

瘙痒性紫癜(itching purpura)：皮损为广泛分布的橘黄色斑疹，常常伴有明显的瘙痒。皮损先发生在足背或踝部，很快扩展至大腿、臀部、躯干和上肢。

金黄色苔藓(lichen aureus)：常表现为下肢孤立的淡红色至棕色斑片或斑块，可伴有金黄色色调，皮损常无症状。

【组织病理】

所有的临床类型有相似的组织病理改变。皮损病理检查显示真皮浅层淋巴细胞浸润和红细胞外溢，偶有少量中性粒细胞浸润。随着损害的发展，含铁血黄素的沉着变得更突出。

【诊断】

当患者特别是中年男性出现上述典型临床表现和实验室检查，色素性紫癜性皮病可以诊断。

【鉴别诊断】

表浅血管周围淋巴细胞浸润、红细胞外溢和含铁血黄素沉积不是特异性改变。色素性紫癜性皮病需和其他血管周围淋巴细胞浸润和淋巴细胞性毛细血管炎的疾病相鉴别。

【治疗】

首先要注意休息。针对有瘙痒或较明显红斑者局部应用糖皮质激素有效，PUVA 和窄波 UVB 有较好的疗效。有报道己酮可可碱有效。增强血管壁的药物(如维生素 C 和芦丁片)有效。

vitamin C, rutoside) are also effective.

【Prognosis】

Pigmentary purpuric dermatoses have a good prognosis in most cases. However, in some patients the disease might be persistent or recurrent.

【预后】

大部分患者预后良好。但有部分患者的病情呈持续性或复发性。

Section Six　Polyarteritis Nodosa

Polyarteritis nodosa (PN) is a rare, segmental, necrotizing vasculitis affecting small and medium-sized arteries of multiple systems. This disease is a syndrome with many triggering causes and associated with many other diseases. PN is further classified into systemic and cutaneous varieties.

第六节　结节性多动脉炎

结节性多动脉炎(polyarteritis nodosa)(PN)是一种罕见的、多系统的血管炎，表现为累及中小动脉为主的节段坏死性血管炎。本病是由多种诱因所致并与许多疾病有关的一种综合征，可以分为系统型和皮肤型结节性多动脉炎。

【Etiology and Pathogenesis】

The etiology of PN is unknown. PN has been suggested to be an immune-complex mediated disease on the basis of serum immune-complex levels, immunofluoresence and ultrastructural evidence. Possible antigens include hepatitis B virus surface antigens and cryoglobulins. The hepatitis C virus, parvovirus, bacterial infection (e. g., *Streptococcus*), and drug hypersensitivity have also been associated with PN in some reports. Furthermore, this condition has also been associated with other diseases such as SLE, inflammatory bowel disease, familial Mediterranean fever, and hairy cell leukemia.

【病因及发病机制】

本病病因不明。血清免疫复合物水平、免疫荧光和超微结构的研究提示本病是由免疫复合物介导的。可能的抗原有乙肝病毒表面抗原和冷球蛋白。有报道结节性多动脉炎还与丙型肝炎病毒、细小病毒及细菌(如链球菌)感染和药物过敏有关。本病还可伴随于系统性红斑狼疮、炎症性肠病、家族性地中海热、毛细胞性白血病等疾病。

【Clinical Manifestations】

Typical PN is a multisystem disease. It most frequently occurs in male patients aged 30-60. Patients commonly present with constitutional symptoms including pyrexia, weight loss and anorexia.

Lower limbs are most frequently affected. The skin lesions include palpable subcutaneous nodules of 1-2 cm in diameter, purpura, livedo, and ulcers that tend to align with the network of superficial arteries. Tenderness may be present. Vesicular and pustular lesions are also occasional features. Arthralgias and myalgia involving the legs (and other parts of the body on occasion) are often present, usually asymmetrically.

Both peripheral and central nervous system involvement are often encountered, presenting as numbness, paresthesias, wrist or foot drop, confusion, and delirium. Cerebrovascular episodes are a rare complication. Involvement of the kidneys is also very common, producing symptoms including microscopic hematuria, proteinuria and hypertension. Renal failure is the most common cause of death in this disease. When the gastrointestinal tract is affected, nausea,

【临床表现】

典型的结节性多动脉炎是一种多系统疾病，好发于30～60岁，男性多见。一般有发热、体重下降和纳差等全身症状。

皮损好发于下肢，包括可触及的直径1～2 cm的皮下结节、紫癜、青斑和与表浅动脉平行分布的溃疡，触痛明显。还可见水疱形成和脓疱样皮损，关节痛和肌痛常见，通常不对称，主要累及下肢。

外周神经系统和中枢神经系统均可受累，可表现为麻木、感觉异常、腕或足下垂、精神错乱和谵妄等，脑血管意外是一种少见并发症。肾脏受累常见，可表现为血尿、蛋白尿和高血压，肾功能衰竭是常见的死亡原因。胃肠受累表现为恶心、呕吐和腹痛。心血管受累可表现为

vomiting and abdominal pain may appear. The manifestations for cardiac involvement include pericarditis, arrhythmias and myocardial infarction. Finally, men are likely to suffer from orchitis.

心包炎、心律失常和心肌梗死。男性较易出现睾丸炎。

In addition to typical systemic PN, cutaneous PN has also been described (where only the skin is affected). There are no significant differences in cutaneous manifestations between cutaneous PN and systemic PN. The former is a relatively benign variant, and serious visceral involvement is never a feature.

除典型的系统型结节性多动脉炎外,还有皮肤型结节性多动脉炎(只累及皮肤)的报道。皮肤型和系统型结节性多动脉炎的皮肤损害无明显差别,是一种相对良性的类型,不会发生严重的内脏损害。

【Laboratory Findings】

Laboratory investigations often reveal anemia, leukocytosis and a raised ESR. Diminished serum complement levels may be detected. Cryoglobulins are positive in some patients. Proteinuria and hematuria may be observed in some cases.

【实验室检查】

实验室检查一般显示贫血、白细胞增多、血沉增快,血清补体下降,冷球蛋白偶尔阳性,蛋白尿及血尿。

【Histopathology】

Biopsies of cutaneous lesions show features of typical leukocytoclastic vasculitis, accompanied by swelling in the tunica media of small and medium-sized arterial walls, fibrinoid degeneration, and neutrophilic cellular infiltration. In cutaneous PN, these findings occur in the arteries located in the deep dermal layer or subcutaneous fat layer, but occur in almost all the nutrient arteries in systemic PN. Immune complex deposition may be found in affected blood vessels; also C3 and IgM deposit can be indicated by direct immunofluorescence.

【组织病理】

皮损组织病理检查显示典型的白细胞碎裂性血管炎。中动脉和小动脉管壁中膜层肿胀、纤维素样变性和中性粒细胞浸润。在皮肤型结节性多动脉炎中,这种病理改变可见于真皮深部和皮下脂肪组织中的动脉,在系统型结节性多动脉炎中,几乎所有的营养动脉都可发生上述改变。直接免疫荧光可见免疫复合物及 C3 和 IgM 沉积于血管壁。

【Diagnosis】

PN can be diagnosed by clinical features, laboratory findings and histopathological assessments of the skin lesions. Since other vasculitis may show similar histological features, clinical examination, serological, and histological results should be carried out rigorously to render a diagnosis that can be considered definitive.

【诊断】

结节性多动脉炎的诊断依赖临床特征、实验室检查和皮损活检。因为其他血管炎有类似的组织学改变,只有密切结合临床、血清学和组织学检查才能做出明确诊断。

【Differential Diagnosis】

It is necessary to differentiate PN from cutaneous small-vessel vasculitis, erythema nodosa, erythema induratum, cryoglobulinemia and SLE.

【鉴别诊断】

结节性多动脉炎需和皮肤小血管血管炎、结节性红斑、硬红斑、冷球蛋白血症和系统性红斑狼疮相鉴别。

【Treatment】

The patients should have bed rest and elevate the effected leg. Administration of vasodilators, NSAIDs and dapsone are effective. Systemic glucocorticoids may be administered orally on a temporary basis during any acute aggravation stage. Glucocorticoids, cyclophosphamide, methotrexate, and other immunosuppressive

【治疗】

患者应卧床休息并抬高患肢。应用血管扩张剂、NSAIDs 和沙利度胺有效。疾病的急性进展期可短期系统口服糖皮质激素。对于系统型结节性多动脉炎患者,有必要应用糖皮质激素或环磷酰胺

drugs are all effective for systemic PN.

【Prognosis】

The prognosis of cutaneous PN is in general good. The skin lesions can be healed in a few weeks. However, the condition may persist and recur over a span of years. By contrast, the prognosis of systemic PN is poor due to severe multiple system and visceral involvements.

及甲氨蝶呤等免疫抑制药物。

【预后】

皮肤型结节性多动脉炎通常预后良好，皮损数周内可愈合，但可持续存在或多年后复发。由于严重的内脏受累，系统型结节性多动脉炎预后不良。

Section Seven　Livedoid Vasculopathy

Livedoid vasculopathy is a chronic recurrent thrombotic disease of the skin. It is also known as livedo vasculitis, atrophie blanche, segmental hyalinizing vasculitis, mainly involving small blood vessels in the dermis of young to middle-aged women.

第七节　青斑样血管病

青斑样血管病(livedoid vasculopathy)又称青斑样血管炎(livedo vasculitis)、白色萎缩(atrophie blanche)、节段型透明性血管炎(segmental hyalinizing vasculitis)，为主要累及年轻到中年女性的真皮小血管的慢性复发性血栓性皮肤疾病。

【Etiology and Pathogenesis】

The cause of the disease is unclear, the chronic venous insufficiency and the increase of the capillary pressure being the main pathogenic factors. Immunoglobulin and complement depositions in the vascular wall indicate that some immune response may also contribute to the pathogenesis. In addition, trauma may play a role in the occurrence of skin lesions.

【病因及发病机制】

本病病因不清，慢性静脉功能不全和毛细血管流体压力增加是主要致病因素。血管壁内免疫球蛋白和补体沉积说明免疫机制参与了发病过程。此外，外伤在皮损发生中可能起一定的作用。

【Clinical Manifestations】

The disease occurs mainly in young and middle-aged women, but men may suffer from it as well. The lesions commonly occur at the lower legs and feet, especially the ankles, while the forearms and hands are less frequent affected. Early lesions are purpuric and blister, then painful and continuous excavating ulcer appear afterwards. In some patients, livedo reticularis may clearly display around the ulcers. The formation of star shaped ivory white atrophic scar can be seen once the ulcer heals, and may be accompanied by telangiectasia and hyperpigmentation due to hemosiderin deposits(Fig. 16-9).

【临床表现】

本病好发于青中年女性，男性也可发生。主要累及小腿和足部，特别是踝部。也可见于前臂和手部。早期表现为紫癜样皮损，可发生水疱，随后发生疼痛性、持续性的穿凿性溃疡，部分患者溃疡周围有明显网状青斑，溃疡愈合后形成星状象牙白色萎缩性瘢痕，周边可有毛细血管扩张及含血铁黄素沉积导致的色素沉着(图 16-9)。

【Laboratory Findings】

No obvious abnormalities are likely in laboratory tests. For patients with underlying diseases such as anti-phospholipid antibody syndrome, protein C deficiency, hepatitis C virus hepatitis and fibronogenolytic disorder, corresponding abnormalities of laboratory tests may reflect these diseases.

【实验室检查】

一般实验室检查无明显异常，与抗磷脂抗体综合征、蛋白 C 缺乏症、丙型病毒性肝炎、纤维蛋白溶解异常等疾病相关的青斑样血管病患者可出现相应的实验室检查异常。

【Histopathology】

The typical pathological features for this disease are vascular endothelial cell proliferation, fibrinoid degeneration on the vascular

【组织病理】

特征性病理表现为真皮浅中层小血管内皮细胞增生，管壁纤维素样变性，管

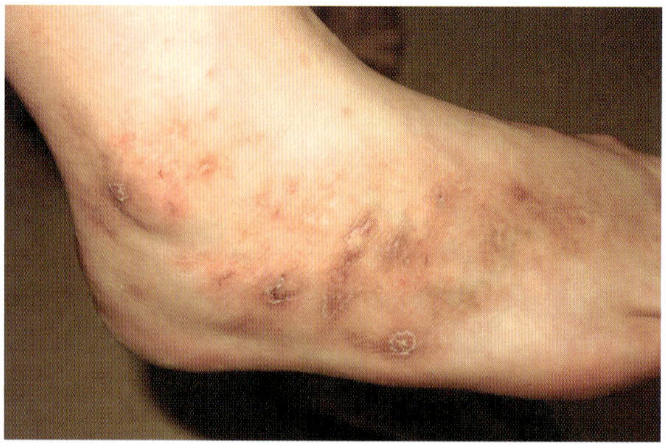

Fig. 16-9　Livedoid vasculopathy(图 16-9　青斑样血管病)

wall, fibrin embolism and thrombosis within the lumen of the vessels, perivascular lymphocyte infiltration and extravasation of red blood cells in the superficial and middle dermis.

腔内纤维蛋白栓塞和血栓形成，血管周围淋巴细胞浸润及红细胞外渗。

【Diagnosis】

The diagnosis can be made based on the typical clinical manifestations and histopathological changes.

【诊断】

根据典型临床皮损及组织病理改变可诊断。

【Differential Diagnosis】

This disease should differentiate from the other diseases with inflammatory reticulate purpura. Primary and secondary high coagulation status should also be excluded. Skin lesions appearing on other parts of the body are necessary to differentiate from DLE and Degos' disease.

【鉴别诊断】

需与引起炎性网状紫癜的其他疾病鉴别，还应排除原发性和继发性高凝状态。发生于身体其他部位皮损要与盘状红斑狼疮、恶性萎缩性丘疹性皮病等相鉴别。

【Treatment】

The medicines that can inhibit platelet thrombus formation or which can stimulate endogenous fibrinolytic activity such as aspirin, dipyridamole and heparin sodium (Hepudiod) are effective for most patients. Available vasodilators such as low molecular dextran are also helpful. Other drugs including tripterygium, dapsone, niacin, nicotinamide and guanethidine are also good alternatives.

【治疗】

抑制血小板血栓形成或刺激内源性纤维蛋白溶解活性的药物如阿司匹林、双嘧达莫、肝素钠(海普林)等可使大部分患者病情缓解；同时可用血管扩张剂如低分子右旋糖酐等，也可用雷公藤类药物，其他治疗包括氨苯砜、烟酸、胍乙啶和烟酰胺。

Si-yuan CHEN(陈思远)

Chapter Seventeen　Nutritional Diseases

第十七章　营养性疾病

Section One　Niacin Deficiency (Pellagra)

第一节　烟酸缺乏症（糖皮病）

Niacin deficiency (pellagra) is a chronic nutritional disease resulting from a niacin (vitamin B3) deficiency or from a deficiency of its precursor amino acid, tryptophan. The term pellagra is derived from the Italian words "pelle agra" meaning rough skin. Pellagra is clinically characterized by a classic triad of symptoms: dermatitis, diarrhea, and dementia.

烟酸缺乏症（niacin deficiency）（糖皮病，pellagra）是因缺乏烟酸（维生素B3）或其前体氨基酸——色氨酸而引起的一种慢性营养性疾病。糖皮病（pellagra，注：中文曾用音译"陪拉格"）这个术语源于意大利语"pelle agra"，表示粗糙的皮肤。它在临床上以皮炎、腹泻和痴呆组成的经典的三联征为特征。

【Etiology and Pathogenesis】

【病因及发病机制】

Niacin (nicotinic acid) is a water-soluble vitamin, also known as vitamin B3 or historically as vitamin PP. Both niacin and its natural derivative niacinamide (nicotinamide) can be readily absorbed by the stomach in a sodium-dependent manner, and the latter can be converted into niacin in the body. Niacin is critical for numerous biochemical reactions and is one of the essential components of coenzyme Ⅰ (the oxidized form of nicotinamide adenine dinucleotide (NAD)) and coenzyme Ⅱ (the reduced form of nicotinamide adenine dinucleotide phosphate (NADP)). Niacin is thus necessary for a number of redox reactions including glycolysis, pentose biosynthesis, protein and amino acid metabolism, fatty acid metabolism, pyruvate metabolism, glycerol metabolism, ATP generation, tissue respiration, and detoxification. Therefore, any niacin deficiency (pellagra) will affect almost all cellular functions in multiple organs, and will produce a variety of clinical manifestations.

烟酸（尼克酸）是一种水溶性维生素，也被视为维生素 B3 或维生素 PP。烟酸和其天然衍生物烟酰胺（尼克酰胺）很容易在胃部以钠依赖的形式吸收。烟酰胺在体内可转化为烟酸。作为生命所必需的氧化还原反应中辅酶Ⅰ（尼克酰胺腺嘌呤二核苷（NAD）的氧化形式）和辅酶Ⅱ（尼克酰胺腺嘌呤二核苷磷酸盐（NADP）的还原形式）的基本成分，烟酸为多种生化反应所必需。它作为重要的辅酶发挥功能，参与了糖酵解、戊糖代谢、蛋白质及氨基酸代谢、脂肪酸代谢、丙酮酸代谢、甘油代谢、ATP 生成、组织呼吸和解毒。烟酸缺乏引起糖皮病。由于多种器官中几乎所有细胞功能因烟酸缺乏而受影响，糖皮病的临床表现呈多样性。

Niacin can be obtained either directly from the diet or synthesized from dietary tryptophan. Fish, meat, poultry, eggs and nuts are rich sources of niacin. Cereals, rice and milk also contain great amounts of niacin. Besides preformed niacin, approximately 60 mg of dietary tryptophan can be converted into 1 mg of niacin in the presence of vitamins B2 and B6. Thus, deficiency of either vitamins B2 or B6 may also promote the development of pellagra in malnourished people.

烟酸可从膳食中直接获取，也可由膳食性色氨酸合成而来。鱼、肉、禽、蛋和坚果是烟酸的丰富来源。谷物、大米和牛奶也含有大量的烟酸。除了已形成的烟酸，大约 60 mg 膳食性色氨酸在维生素 B2 和 B6 存在的情况下在体内可转化为 1 mg 烟酸。因此，维生素 B2 和 B6 中的某一种缺乏在营养不良的人中也可促使糖皮病发生。

In general, primary type pellagra is a result of inadequate dietary intake of niacin and/or its precursor, tryptophan, which is one of the essential amino acids. Secondary pellagra occurs when adequate quantities of niacin are present in the diet, but the intake,

原发性糖皮病可因膳食中烟酸和/或其前体，必需氨基酸中的色氨酸的不足而引起。继发性糖皮病可发生于膳食中烟酸含量足够，但因其他疾病或状态，

absorption and/or processing of the niacin suffer some interference due to the presence of other diseases or conditions, such as anorexia nervosa, prolonged diarrhea, chronic colitis, severe ulcerative colitis, regional ileitis, Hartnup's syndrome (i. e., impaired absorption of tryptophan), chronic alcoholism, hepatic cirrhosis, carcinoid syndrome, tuberculosis of the gastrointestinal tract and certain medications (e. g., isoniazid, 5-fluorouracil and 6-mercaptopurine).

如神经性厌食症、慢性腹泻、慢性结肠炎、严重的溃疡性结肠炎、节段性回肠炎、Hartnup 综合征(色氨酸吸收功能受损)、慢性酒精中毒、肝纤维化、类癌综合征、胃肠道结核和某些治疗(如异烟肼、5-氟尿嘧啶和 6-巯基嘌呤)等干扰了烟酸的摄取、吸收和/或处理。

Primary pellagra is still an endemic disease in some areas of some developing countries such as Africa and Asia due to dietary deficiencies of niacin or tryptophan. Sporadic cases of pellagra may occur in chronic alcoholics, drug users, psychiatric patients, and patients with other intestinal malabsorption problems.

在非洲和亚洲的发展中国家的某些地区,因膳食缺乏烟酸或色氨酸,糙皮病仍有区域性发生。其散发病例也可见于慢性酒精中毒者、对毒品依赖者、精神病患者和肠道吸收不良的患者。

【Clinical Manifestations】

【临床表现】

Pellagra is clinically characterized by symmetric photosensitive skin eruptions, gastrointestinal manifestations, and neurologic and psychiatric disturbances. The symptoms of pellagra are well-known to specialists and are usually referred to as pellagra's "4D's": dermatitis, diarrhea, dementia, and, very occasionally, when untreated, death.

糙皮病在临床上以对称性光敏感性皮损、胃肠道表现、神经及精神功能紊乱为特征。其著名的症状通常被记作糙皮病的"4 个英文字母 D":皮炎(dermatitis),腹泻(diarrhea),痴呆(dementia),未治疗时可发生(尽管很少发生)死亡(death)。

The classic triad of pellagra symptoms consists of dermatitis, diarrhea and dementia, but the symptoms do not have to appear in any consistent order. Early symptoms of pellagra include lassitude, weakness, loss of appetite, mild digestive disturbances (nausea, vomiting, epigastric discomfort, abdominal pain and increased salivation), psychiatric or emotional distress (anxiety, irritability, or depression) and photosensitivity. Skin lesions may be the earliest sign in some cases but gastrointestinal and neurologic symptoms can occur without skin lesions. Gastrointestinal involvement is quite common in pellagra, in which mucosal inflammation and atrophy may appear in most parts of the gastrointestinal tract. Approximately, 50% of cases suffer from gastritis, achlorhydria, low levels of duodenal enzymes, and diarrhea. In severe cases, anorexia and malabsorptive diarrhea may result in severe malnutrition that eventually will lead to cachexia. Neurologic abnormalities, including muscle weakness, headaches, paraesthesias, attacks of fainting, seizures, dementia, depression, apathy, hallucinations, and psychosis are more likely to manifest in later stages of pellagra.

糙皮病的经典三联征由皮炎、腹泻和痴呆组成。这些症状并不按此顺序出现。糙皮病的早期症状包括疲倦、虚弱、食欲减退、轻度消化道功能紊乱(如恶心、呕吐、上腹部不适、腹痛及唾液分泌增加)、精神或情感紧张(如焦虑、易怒和抑郁)和光敏感。皮损在一些病例可为最早的体征。胃肠道和神经系统表现可不伴有皮损而发生。胃肠道受累在糙皮病中很常见。黏膜炎症和萎缩累及大部分胃肠道。胃炎、胃酸缺乏症、十二指肠分泌酶的水平降低和腹泻可发生于约 50%的病例。厌食症和吸收障碍性腹泻可引发营养不良状态并最终导致恶病质。在糙皮病晚期,神经系统表现尤为突出,包括肌肉无力、头痛、感觉异常、晕厥、癫痫、痴呆、抑郁、淡漠、幻觉和精神错乱。

It is difficult to diagnose pellagra in the absence of cutaneous findings, which are often characteristic. Three types of skin lesion are seen in dermatitis associated with pellagra as follows: ①photosensitive eruptions; ② perineal lesions; ③ seborrheic dermatitis-like eruptions on the face.

糙皮病的皮损常具有特征性,在无皮损时,很难诊断糙皮病。三种类型的皮损见于糙皮病的皮炎:① 光敏感性皮疹;②会阴部皮损;③面部脂溢性皮炎样皮疹。

A bilaterally symmetrical photosensitive eruption in areas exposed to sunlight (the face, neck, upper chest, extensor arms, and the dorsa of the hands) is the most common characteristic for this disease (Fig. 17-1), and usually worsens in spring and summer. It begins as erythema and swelling with an acute or intermittent onset, accompanied by itching, burning or pain sensations. In severe cases, vesicles or bullae may occur and sometimes exudation may be seen. Pellagra may resemble sunburn in its early phase, but the suntan process develops more slowly than for regular sunburn. Initial bright well-demarcated erythema gradually turns cinnamon or brown in color. After several phototoxic reactions due to re-exposure to sunlight at the same site, the affected skin area thickens with scaling and hyperpigmentation, especially in areas over bony prominences.

在曝光部位(面、颈、上胸部、上肢伸侧和手背)的双侧对称性光敏感性皮疹,在糙皮病皮损中是最有特征性的(图17-1),常在春季和夏季加重。初起以红斑和肿胀的形式呈急性或间歇性发病,伴有瘙痒、烧灼感或疼痛。水疱或大疱可发生于严重病例,皮疹可变为渗出性的。糙皮病在初期与日晒伤相似,但与日晒伤时典型表现相比,其晒黑却缓慢发生。最初鲜亮的境界清楚的红斑逐渐变为肉桂色至棕色。在相同部位因反复曝光而发生多次光毒性反应后,出现受累皮肤增厚、脱屑和色素沉着。骨隆起部的皮肤增厚和色素沉着可更明显。

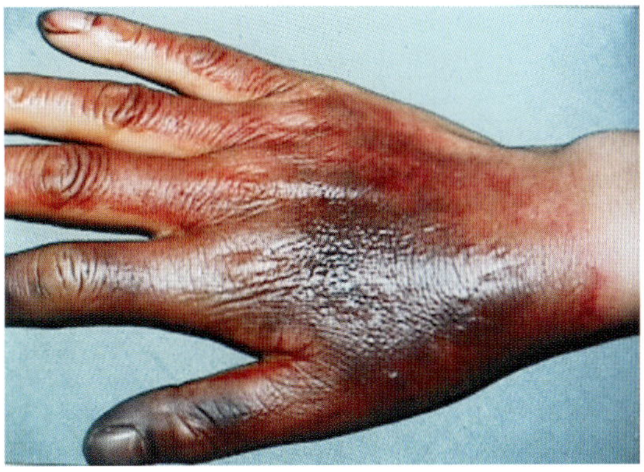

Fig. 17-1　Pellagra(图 17-1　糙皮病)

Perineal lesions are one of the common cutaneous lesions of pellagra, characterized by erythema and erosion in the scrotal and perineal areas. Painful fissures, ulcers, and atrophy may affect the mucous membranes of the mouth and vagina as well. Seborrheic dermatitis-like rash can be found in patients with pellagra. Usually a dull erythema appears on the face, with fine, powdery scales over follicular orifices. When an erythematous rash appears on the nasal bridge and extends to the cheeks, chins, and lips, it may resemble the "butterfly rash" of lupus erythematosus. Each facial eruption mentioned above often occurs concurrently with lesions found elsewhere. When the eruptions on the face spread into a broad band or collar around the neck, it is known as "Casal's necklace".

会阴部的皮损也见于糙皮病。阴囊及会阴部的糜烂和红斑常见。疼痛性裂隙、溃疡形成和萎缩可累及口腔及阴道的黏膜。糙皮病存在脂溢性皮炎样皮疹。不鲜亮的红斑发生于面部,伴有毛囊开口处纤细、粉末状的鳞屑。有时鼻梁部的红斑性皮疹扩展至颊、颏及唇部,与红斑狼疮的"蝶形红斑"相似。前述面部皮疹常与其他部位出现的皮损同时发生。皮疹可围绕颈部形成一条宽带或项圈,被称为"Casal 项链"。

【Laboratory Findings】

The definitive diagnosis of pellagra can be strongly suggested by low levels of serum niacin, tryptophan, NAD, and NADP. A combined urinary excretion of N'-methylnicotinamide and pyridone of less than 1.5 milligrams in 24 hours also indicates severe niacin deficiency. However, such chemical tests may not be available in

【实验室检查】

检测血清中烟酸、色氨酸、NAD 和 NADP 的水平降低可强烈提示糙皮病的诊断。尿中 24 h N'-甲基烟酰胺和吡啶的混合排泄量小于 1.5 mg 提示严重的烟酸缺乏。然而,医院和诊所中尚无实

most hospitals. Routine laboratory tests may display anemia, hypoproteinemia, elevated levels of serum calcium, decreased levels of serum potassium and phosphorus, abnormal liver function and increased serum porphyrin levels. Physical examination may reveal some changes in gastrointestinal and neurologic involvement. Unfortunately, the histopathological findings of dermatitis seen in pellagra are also nonspecific.

际可用的化学试验测量上述指标。常规实验室检查可显示糙皮病患者的贫血、低蛋白血症、血清钙水平升高、血清钾和磷水平降低、肝功能异常和血清卟啉水平增加。辅助检查也可显示糙皮病患者胃肠道和神经系统受累的某些变化。糙皮病的皮炎的组织病理学表现是非特异性的。

【Diagnosis】

Pellagra may be primarily diagnosed on the basis of the patient's history and clinical appearances. Detailed dietary habits and underlying diseases or conditions that may interfere with the intake, absorption and metabolism of niacin and previous treatments should be especially emphasized during the history taking. The clinical investigation should focus on the presence of the "3 D's" (diarrhea, dermatitis, and dementia), localization of the eruptions, and seasonal appearances. Routine laboratory examination described above may further support the conclusion of niacin deficiency even though these are not specific. Finally, therapeutic response to niacin supplementation in a patient with the typical symptoms and signs of pellagra should confirm the correct diagnosis.

【诊断】

糙皮病可根据患者的病史和临床表现做出诊断。在询问病史时应留意有关患者膳食和影响烟酸摄取、吸收和/或代谢的疾病或情况及治疗经过的详细信息。糙皮病的诊断应着重于"3个英文字母D"代表的症状(腹泻、皮炎、痴呆)、受累部位的局限性和季节性表现。上述实验室检查虽然为非特异性的,但可支持诊断。最终通过评价患者对增加烟酸量的治疗反应而确定诊断。

【Differential Diagnosis】

Pellagra should be differentiated from exogenous photosensitive dermatitis, polymorphous light eruption, porphyria cutanea tarda, porphyria variegate, chronic actinic dermatitis, and drug-induced pellagroid reactions. It may also need to be distinguished from kwashiorkor, a dietary protein deficiency seen in children. In addition, primary pellagra should be distinguished from secondary pellagra.

【鉴别诊断】

糙皮病需要与外源性光感性皮炎、多形日光疹、迟发性皮肤卟啉症、变异性卟啉症、慢性光化性皮炎和药物诱发的糙皮病样反应等鉴别。它还需要与蛋白营养不良(kwashiorkor)——见于儿童的一种膳食蛋白缺乏症相鉴别。原发性糙皮病应与继发性糙皮病区分开来。

【Prevention and Treatment】

Dietary treatment with a diet rich in niacin and/or tryptophan is essential to prevent the occurrence of pellagra, correct malnutrition and stop the progress of the disease. Typically, pellagra should respond well to oral administration of niacinamide or niacin 100-300 mg/d in 3 divided doses. Most physicians prefer niacinamide which is less likely to cause vasomotor disturbances in the acute phase. The dosage of niacinamide for an adult with pellagra is 100 mg orally every 6 hour until the major acute symptoms are resolved, followed by oral administration of 50 mg every 8-12 hour until the skin lesions subside completely. In severe cases with marked mental or gastrointestinal tract symptoms, 1 g of niacinamide should be administered intravenously 3 to 4 times daily. The dosage of niacinamide for children with pellagra is 10-50

【预防和治疗】

通过摄取烟酸和/或色氨酸含量丰富的膳食,可预防糙皮病,以及纠正其营养不良和阻止本病的进程。经典的糙皮病可对口服100～300 mg/d的烟酰胺或烟酸(分三次剂量服用)显示良好的治疗反应。医师们更喜欢用烟酰胺,因为它不引起血管舒缩功能失调。糙皮病急性期的成人剂量为每6 h口服烟酰胺100 mg,直至主要的急性症状消退,继而每8～12 h口服烟酰胺50 mg直至皮损痊愈。在具有显著精神症状或胃肠道症状的严重病例,可给予烟酰胺1 g 3～4次/天,最初常以静脉补充之。糙皮病的

mg PO, every 6 hour until symptoms resolve. Because such patients are often malnourished and have other vitamin deficiencies, provisions for a high-protein diet and a long-term administration of B-complex vitamins (particular B2 and B6) are usually needed for complete recovery. Regarding secondary pellagra, the underlying diseases or special conditions need to be identified and managed at the same time. Topical therapy with emollients may reduce the discomfort of the skin lesions.

儿童剂量为每 6 h 口服烟酰胺 10～50 mg 直至糙皮病的症状和体征消退。大多数糙皮病患者常有营养不良及其他维生素缺乏，需要同时给予高蛋白质膳食并长期使用 B 族维生素，特别是维生素 B2、B6 以改善之，从而达到完全康复。对于继发性糙皮病，其潜在疾病或特殊状态应予以查明和处置。使用滋润剂的局部疗法可缓解皮损的不适感。

【Prognosis】

If pellagra is diagnosed and treated appropriately, the prognosis is excellent. However, without treatment the condition will gradually worsen and soon develop severe complications, such as malnutrition and dehydration due to continued diarrhea, and secondary infections or neuropsychiatric complications, which may eventually lead to death.

【预后】

如果糙皮病被及时诊断和治疗，其预后良好。未治疗的糙皮病将逐渐发展并恶化。持续腹泻所致的严重营养不良和脱水以及继发感染或神经系统受累所致并发症最终可引起死亡。

Section Two　Zinc Deficiency and Acrodermatitis Enteropathica

Zinc deficiency may be either an inherited or an acquired disorder. Acrodermatitis enteropathica is a rare autosomal recessive disorder of zinc deficiency, affecting early infancy. It is characterized by the classic triad of clinical manifestations consisting of dermatitis, alopecia, and intractable diarrhea.

第二节　锌缺乏症与肠病性肢端皮炎

锌缺乏症可以是遗传性的或获得性的。肠病性肢端皮炎（acrodermatitis enteropathica）是一种少见的、累及婴儿早期的、常染色体隐性遗传性的锌缺乏疾病。皮炎、脱发和难治性腹泻组成的三联征是肠病性肢端皮炎的诊断特征。

【Etiology and Pathogenesis】

Zinc is one of the essential minerals and trace elements that is found in almost every cell in the human body, and is involved with numerous aspects of cellular metabolism. Zinc is a vital component of many metalloenzymes which are critical for protein and nucleic acid synthesis and for the maintenance of T-cell and NK cell function. The concentration of zinc in various compartments of the cells is closely regulated. 2 solute-linked carrier (SLC) gene families-ZnT (SLC30) and Zip (SLC39)-have been documented to transport zinc between compartments of cells. The two types of transmembrane proteins encoded by two gene families (ZnT and Zip) have opposite roles in cellular zinc homeostasis. ZnT transporters reduce intracellular zinc by either promoting zinc efflux from cells or zinc transport into intracellular vesicles, while Zip transporters increase intracellular zinc concentrations by promoting zinc influx into cells or zinc release from intracellular vesicles. 10 ZnT transporter genes and 15 Zip transporter genes have been identified in the human genome. The genetic defect in

【病因及发病机制】

锌是人体细胞中必需的矿物质和微量元素。细胞代谢的许多方面是锌依赖性的。锌是许多金属酶的重要成分，在蛋白质和核酸的合成及 T 细胞和 NK 细胞的功能方面具有重要作用。细胞内的锌的水平被精确调节。锌转运蛋白是由 2 个溶质连接载体（SLC）基因家族 ZnT（SLC30）和 Zip（SLC39）编码的跨膜蛋白。这两个基因家族 ZnT 和 Zip 在细胞内锌的动态平衡中具有相反的作用。ZnT 转运蛋白通过促进细胞中的锌外流或锌转运至细胞内小泡中而减少细胞内的锌。与此相反，Zip 转运蛋白通过促进锌的内流入细胞或锌从细胞内小泡中释出而增加细胞内的锌浓度。在人类存在着 10 种 ZnT 转运蛋白基因和 15 种 Zip 转运蛋白基因。肠病性肢端皮炎患者的

patients with acrodermatitis enteropathica have been mapped to 8q24 and the defective gene identified as SLC39A4, which encodes the zinc transporter Zip4. This tissue-specific zinc-regulated transporter is abundantly expressed in enterocytes that are responsible for dietary zinc absorption from the small intestine. Therefore, individuals with acrodermatitis enteropathica have severe zinc deficiency derived from a defect of zinc absorption in both the duodenum and jejunum.

遗传缺陷已被定位于染色体 8q24，其缺陷基因被鉴定为编码锌转运蛋白 Zip4 的 SLC39A4。Zip4 这种组织特异性锌调节的转运蛋白丰富地表达于肠上皮细胞，在从小肠中吸收膳食锌方面发挥作用。肠病性肢端皮炎患者存在着空肠和回肠锌吸收缺陷引发的严重锌缺乏。

【Clinical Manifestations】

Acrodermatitis enteropathica usually presents within days after an infant is bottle-fed or within days to weeks after weaning. However, some breast-fed infants may develop acrodermatitis enteropathica as a result of insufficient concentration of zinc in their mother's milk.

The typical clinical manifestations in acrodermatitis enteropathica are the triad of: ①dermatitis localized around the body orifices and on the extremities; ②diffuse alopecia; ③intractable diarrhea.

The dermatitis presents with sharply demarcated erythematous scaly patches or plaques which can become vesicular, bullous, pustular, or desquamative. The skin lesions often present on the extremities, anogenital and periorificial areas (Fig. 17-2). Angular cheilitis and stomatitis are common early manifestations, often followed by paronychia. Chronic skin lesions may resemble psoriasis, accompanied by nail dystrophy. Without treatment, erythematous and scaly lesions slowly evolve into erosions secondarily infected by bacteria and *Candida albicans*, and patients may develop alopecia and diarrhea. Growth retardation, mental depression or irritability, ophthalmic diseases, poor wound healing, anemia, photophobia, anorexia, delayed puberty, and hypogonadism in males may be seen in patients with acrodermatitis enteropathica.

【临床表现】

肠病性肢端皮炎通常见于婴儿期，可在对婴儿行人工喂养数天内发生，也可在母乳喂养的婴儿断奶后数天至数周内发生。一些母乳喂养的婴儿也可发生肠病性肢端皮炎，这是其母乳中锌浓度非常低的结果。

肠病性肢端皮炎的典型临床表现为三联征：①局限于人体腔口周围和肢端的皮炎；②广泛的脱发；③难治性腹泻。

皮炎表现为境界鲜明的红斑鳞屑性的斑片或斑块，可成为水疱性、大疱性、脓疱性或脱屑性皮损。皮损发生于肢端、肛门生殖器部位和腔口周围区域(图 17-2)。口角唇炎和口腔炎是常见的早期表现，继之以甲沟炎发生。慢性皮损可呈银屑病样，并伴有甲营养不良。如未经治疗，红斑鳞屑性损害缓慢发展为继发有细菌或白念珠菌感染的糜烂性损害，患者并可发生脱发和腹泻。生长延迟、精神抑郁或易兴奋、眼受累、伤口愈合不良、贫血、畏光、食欲减退、青春期发育延迟和男性性欲减退等可见于肠病性肢端皮炎的患者。

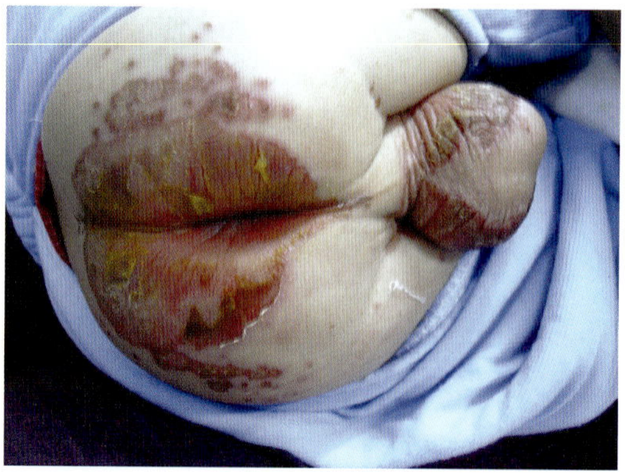

Fig. 17-2 Acrodermatitis enteropathica(图 17-2 肠病性肢端皮炎)

【Laboratory Findings】

Patient's age, serum albumin levels and inflammation may all affect zinc levels from time to time. Thus it is difficult to accurately determine the status of zinc deficiency. Zinc levels in the plasma, serum, urine, or hair appear to be of some value in determining the status of zinc levels for hypozincemia diagnosis. However, the zinc values obtained from different labs vary dramatically, especially in infants or children, and the values may even overlap with other disorders. Therefore, these results may sometimes be misleading. For example, serum zinc level of less than 50 μg/dL is suggestive but is by no means a diagnostic indicator for acrodermatitis enteropathica.

The second approach to determining body zinc status is to measure the activity or concentration of zinc-dependent enzymes, such as the measurement of alkaline phosphatase. Other methods include measuring the concentrations of zinc-regulated proteins such as erythrocyte metallothionein and serum albumin. Metallothionein levels may be reduced in cases of zinc deficiency. Serum albumin that can bind to zinc should also be tested since patients with hypoalbuminemia also have decreased zinc levels.

【Histopathology】

Skin lesions of acquired and hereditary zinc deficiency share similar or even identical histopathological presentations. Histopathological findings of the typical skin lesions of acrodermatitis enteropathica include confluent parakeratosis with variable neutrophils, hypogranulosis, psoriasiform epidermal hyperplasia with large pale keratinocytes in the upper spinous layer and scattered dyskeratotic cells. Vesicles or bullae also form above those large pale keratinocytes and under the cornified layer, accompanied by an inflammatory infiltrate in dermis. It must be remembered that the histopathological pattern is not specific for acrodermatitis enteropathica.

【Diagnosis】

The diagnosis of acrodermatitis enteropathica can be based on the history and clinical presentation, together with laboratory tests of serum or plasma zinc and histopathological features. Because of their general lack of precision, laboratory tests are usually only regarded as a supplement for the clinical based diagnostic approach in this condition. It is worthwhile to administer 3-30 mmol zinc/kg for 5 days in a trial of zinc supplementation to test the clinical response prior to the laboratory results. A positive response to the

【实验室检查】

年龄、血清白蛋白水平和炎症状态均可影响锌的水平。因此，准确地测量机体的锌的状况是困难的。初步测定一个人的血浆或血清、尿液和头发的锌的水平对确定低锌血症是必要的辅助手段。检测结果在不同的实验室有显著差异，特别是在婴儿和儿童中。检测值可与健康人或其他相似疾病有一定程度的重叠。因而对检测结果的解释容易出错。如小于 50 μg/dL 的血清锌水平对肠病性肢端皮炎是提示性的，而非诊断性的。

确定机体锌的状况的第二种途径是检测锌依赖性酶的活性或浓度。碱性磷酸酶是评价锌状况的一种易行可用的检测指标。其他方法包括检测锌调节蛋白如红细胞金属巯基组蛋白和血清白蛋白的浓度。前一种蛋白的浓度在锌缺乏症时可降低。循环中可结合锌的血清白蛋白也应检测，因为低白蛋白血症时锌水平将降低。

【组织病理】

获得性和遗传性锌缺乏症的皮损拥有相似或相同的组织病理学表现。肠病性肢端皮炎典型皮损取材的皮肤活检标本的组织病理学发现包括融合性角化不全伴有数量不等的中性粒细胞、颗粒层减少、银屑病样表皮增生伴有棘层上部大且苍白的角质形成细胞和散在的角化不良细胞、上述大且苍白的角质形成细胞上方的角层下水疱或大疱形成、真皮炎性浸润。总之，上述组织病理学表现并不是肠病性肢端皮炎所特有的。

【诊断】

肠病性肢端皮炎可根据其病史、临床表现并结合血清或血浆锌的实验室检测及组织病理特点进行诊断。实验室检测结果由于缺乏准确性因而仅可辅助临床诊断。当无预先的实验室检测结果时，在补锌治疗性试验时给予锌 3～30 mmol/kg，共 5 天，此疗法值得一试。对补锌的良好反应将可证实临床诊断。

zinc replacement will confirm the clinical diagnosis.

【Differential Diagnosis】

Acrodermatitis enteropathica needs to be distinguished from diffuse cutaneous candidiasis, diaper dermatitis, psoriasis, acrodermatitis continua, epidermolysis bullosa, acquired zinc deficiency and Olmsted syndrome. A comprehensive consideration of the patient's history, clinical manifestations, and necessary laboratory tests are all helpful for the differential diagnosis of acrodermatitis enteropathica.

【鉴别诊断】

肠病性肢端皮炎需与泛发性皮肤念珠菌病、尿布皮炎、银屑病、连续性肢端皮炎、大疱性表皮松解症、获得性锌缺乏症、Olmsted综合征等进行鉴别诊断。对病史、临床表现和必要的实验检查的综合考虑有助于对其鉴别诊断。

【Treatment】

The clinical manifestations of acrodermatitis enteropathica can be rapidly reversed by direct supplementation with zinc sulfate or gluconate in a daily dose of 1-2 mg/kg. Zinc replacement is an inexpensive, nontoxic and efficient therapy. In cases of acquired zinc deficiency, it is necessary to continue zinc supplementation for a short period, coupled with correction of the underlying conditions that may lead to the deficiency. In cases of acrodermatitis enteropathica, supplementation with zinc sulfate 3 mg/(kg · d) should be continued for a longer period and may be a lifelong requirement.

【治疗】

每日 1～2 mg/kg 的剂量直接补充硫酸锌或葡萄糖酸锌，肠病性肢端皮炎的临床表现可被迅速缓解。补锌治疗并不昂贵，是非毒性和有效的疗法。在获得性锌缺乏症的患者中，短暂的补锌治疗和改善潜在的健康条件是必要的。对肠病性肢端皮炎患者，补充 3 mg/(kg · d)硫酸锌应持续终生。

【Prognosis】

In general, prognosis of acrodermatitis enteropathica is good with zinc replenishment. Patients with acrodermatitis enteropathica should exhibit apparent therapeutic response to zinc supplementation.

【预后】

总体而言，经补锌治疗后，肠病性肢端皮炎预后良好。在肠病性肢端皮炎患者中，补锌疗法显示了明显的治疗反应。

Wei HE (何威)

Chapter Eighteen Metabolic Disorders and Endocrine Diseases

Section One Xanthomatosis

Xanthomatosis is a common fat (lipid) storage disorder that can affect many areas of the body such as the skin and tendons. It manifests as yellowish patches, papules, or nodules, sometimes referred to as xanthomas. This lipid metabolic disease is characterized by accumulations of lipid-laden macrophages/histiocytes and the localized deposition of lipoprotein in the tissue. The skin condition is often associated with a systemic disorder of lipid metabolism and can be accompanied by hyperlipaemia, atherosclerosis, and cardiovascular disease.

【Etiology and Pathogenesis】

The etiology and pathogenesis of xanthomatosis is complicated and still not fully determined. Under normal circumstances, most lipids combine plasma proteins to form plasma lipoproteins that are transported throughout the body. However, plasma lipoprotein concentrations must remain in a normal range; when the total level is higher than normal upper limits, the condition is called hyperlipoprotememia. Excessive deposition of lipoprotein in tissues such as the skin or tendons may be caused by either lipoprotein metabolic disorder or quantitative or structural changes in lipoprotein. Clinically, this condition can be divided into primary and secondary xanthomatosis. Primary xanthomatosis can be further divided into familial and non-familial types. The former is usually accompanied by certain levels of lipid metabolic disorder and systemic symptoms, while the latter often occurs sporadically, without any abnormal lipid metabolism or systemic symptoms. Secondary xanthomatosis usually results from diseases that cause lipid metabolic disorders or hyperlipidemia, such as hypothyroidism, nephrotic syndrome, diabetes mellitus, myeloma and lymphoma, etc.

【Clinical Manifestations】

Cutaneous xanthomas can present as one of the following common types.

(1) Tuberous xanthoma: tuberous xanthoma can occur at any age. The lesions vary in size and shape, from small papules of 0.5 cm in diameter to 5 cm wide firm round nodules. The lesions may be single or multiple, sometimes confluent, with a color ranging from yellowish orange to brownish yellow (Fig. 18-1). Most lesions are seen on the extensor aspects of the limbs and on areas that are frequently pressed or subjected to pressure, such as the elbows,

第十八章 代谢障碍与内分泌性疾病

第一节 黄 瘤 病

黄瘤病(xanthomatosis)是一种常见的脂质代谢障碍性疾病，是由于含有脂质的组织细胞和巨噬细胞浸润及脂蛋白局限型沉积，导致皮肤或肌腱出现黄色斑片、丘疹或结节的一组皮肤病。常伴全身脂质代谢紊乱，合并有血脂增高、动脉粥样硬化和心血管疾病等。

【病因及发病机制】

黄瘤病的病因和发病机制较为复杂，尚未完全清楚。正常情况下大部分血脂与血浆蛋白结合形成血浆脂蛋白而转运全身，血浆脂蛋白浓度高于正常值上限时称为高脂蛋白血症。当脂蛋白代谢发生障碍或含量增高或结构异常时，可导致脂蛋白在组织中沉积，如沉积于皮肤或肌腱中。本组疾病可分为原发性黄瘤病和继发性黄瘤病。前者又可分为家族性和非家族性两类，家族性者常有不同程度的血脂代谢障碍及系统表现，非家族性者常为散发，一般无血脂代谢障碍及系统表现。继发性黄瘤病是指由其他疾病引起血脂代谢障碍和血脂增高所致的黄瘤病，如甲状腺功能减退症、肾病综合征、糖尿病、骨髓瘤和淋巴瘤等。

【临床表现】

黄瘤病根据其临床表现，有如下常见的临床类型。

(1) 结节性黄瘤(tuberous xanthoma) 结节性黄瘤可发生于任何年龄，皮损形态和大小不等，可为直径为 0.5 cm 的丘疹到直径为 5 cm 的圆形坚实结节，单发或多发，可融合，呈橘黄色到棕黄色(图 18-1)，好发于四肢伸侧和容易受压的部位，如肘、膝关节和臀部。患者常伴血浆

knees and buttocks. Patients with tuberous xanthoma are often found to have metabolic abnormalities of plasma cholesterol and/or triglycerides or have hyperlipoprotememia, and the condition may be associated with atherosclerotic cardiovascular disease.

胆固醇和/或甘油三酯代谢异常、高脂蛋白血症，可伴发动脉粥样硬化性心血管疾病。

(2) Eruptive xanthoma: it appears as pinhead to match head sized, soft, yellowish papules with an erythematous base in sudden or rapid appearing in clusters. The lesions may be pruritic or tender on occasion and are most commonly located on the buttocks, shoulders and extensor surfaces of the extremities (Fig. 18-2). Patients with eruptive xanthoma are commonly found to have hyperchylomicronemia.

(2) 发疹性黄瘤(eruptive xanthoma) 皮损为针头到火柴头大小的柔软黄色丘疹，突然发生或迅速分批出现，基底有红晕，可伴有瘙痒和压痛，常以臀、肩及四肢伸侧多见(图 18-2)，患者常伴发高乳糜微粒血症。

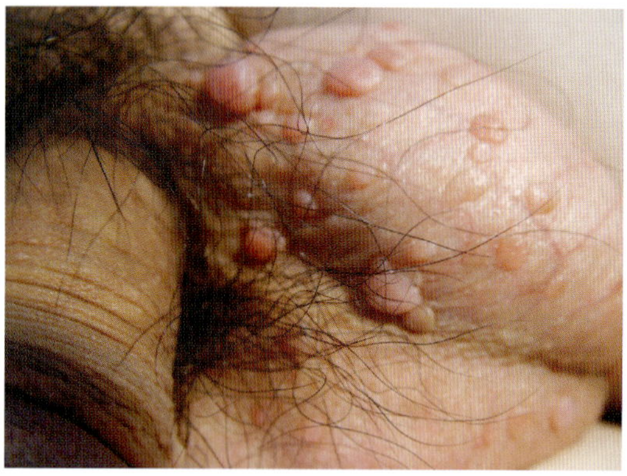

Fig. 18-1　Tuberous xanthoma(图 18-1　结节性黄瘤)

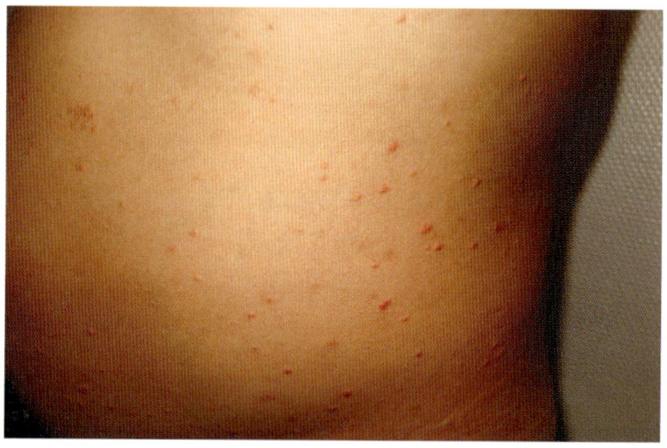

Fig. 18-2　Eruptive xanthoma(图 18-2　发疹性黄瘤)

(3) Plane xanthoma: it generally appears as slightly palpable papules or plaques, yellow to brownish yellow in color. The lesions may occur on any part of the body. When it presents as yellowish streaks following the distribution of creases on the palms or plaques on the eyelids, it is referred to as xanthoma striatum palmare (Fig. 18-3) or xanthelasma (Fig. 18-4) respectively.

(3) 扁平黄瘤(plane xanthoma) 皮损为稍高起的可触及的丘疹或斑块，呈黄色到棕黄色。扁平黄瘤可发生于身体任何地方，如发生于手掌纹的条状和眼睑的淡黄色斑块分别称为掌纹黄瘤(xanthoma striatum palmare)(图 18-3)和睑黄瘤(xanthelasma)(图 18-4)。

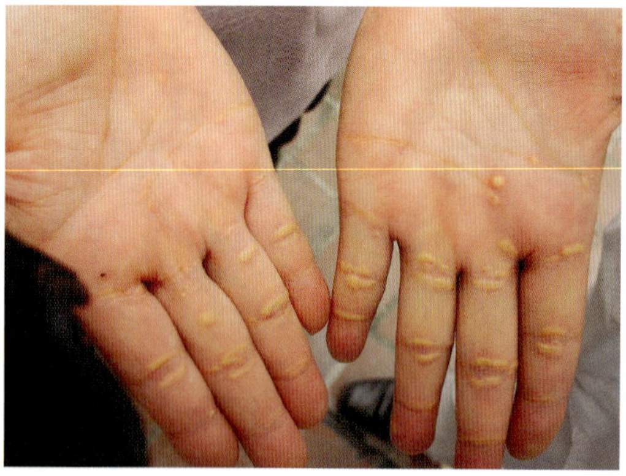

Fig. 18-3　Xanthoma striatum palmare(图 18-3　掌纹黄瘤)

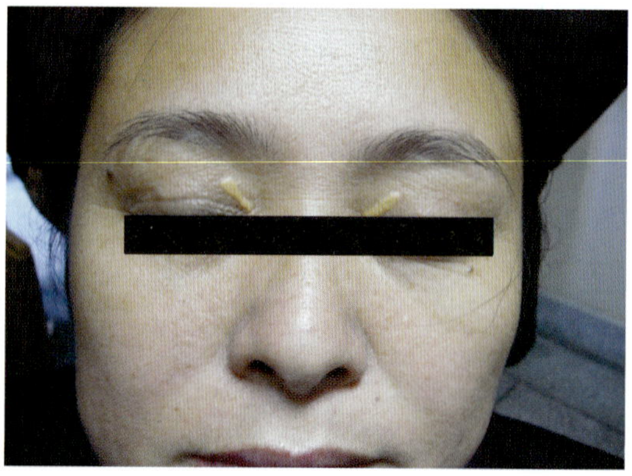

Fig. 18-4　Xanthelasma(图 18-4　睑黄瘤)

【Histopathology】

The histologic features are quite similar among all varieties of

【组织病理】

各型黄瘤的组织病理学表现基本相

xanthoma. Aggregation of foam cells in the dermis is commonly seen in the lesional areas of the skin. At the early stages of xanthoma, inflammatory cell infiltration and sometimes Touton giant cells may be found. Proliferation of fibroblast cells may be seen when lesions are at their catagenetic stage.

同,主要是在真皮中可见泡沫细胞,早期损害中可见炎症细胞浸润,有时可见Touton巨细胞。退行期皮损可见增生的成纤维细胞。

【Diagnosis and Differential Diagnosis】

The unique skin lesions and histopathological features will be helpful in diagnosis, but xanthoma should be differentiated from the following: various types of histiocytosis, Langerhans cell histiocytosis, juvenile xanthogrannloma, progressive nodular histiocytoma, verruca plana and steatocystoma multiplex, etc.

【诊断与鉴别诊断】

根据典型皮损的特点,结合组织病理学检查,一般可确诊。本病应与各种组织细胞增生症、朗格汉斯组织细胞增生症、幼年黄色肉芽肿、进行性结节性组织细胞瘤、扁平疣、多发性皮脂囊瘤等相鉴别。

【Treatment】

For a patient with hyperlipidemia, dietary control is recommended low in fat, cholesterol and sugar. Meanwhile, appropriate medicines for lipid disorders are necessary in order to decrease the LDL levels in some patients. Fulguration, laser ablation, or surgery may also be considered when the lesions are sufficiently localized.

【治疗】

患者如伴有高脂血症应控制饮食,给予低脂、低胆固醇、低糖饮食,同时服用降脂药物。如皮损范围较小可选用电灼、激光或外科手术等方法治疗。

Section Two Primary Cutaneous Amyloidosis

Amyloidosis is a group of diseases that caused by the deposition of amyloid protein in tissues or organs, thereby interfering in the function of these organs. Primary cutaneous amyloidosis is one type of amyloidosis and refers to a chronic skin disorder caused by accumulation of amorphous glycoproteins (amyloids) in the normal skin tissues or in the interstitial spaces, with an absence of other systemic disorders.

第二节 原发性皮肤淀粉样变

淀粉样变(amyloidosis)是指由于淀粉样蛋白沉积于组织或器官并导致功能障碍的一组疾病。原发性皮肤淀粉样变(primary cutaneous amyloidosis)属淀粉样变病的一型,是指组织病理学表现为淀粉样蛋白沉积于正常皮肤组织或组织间隙而不累及其他器官的一种慢性皮肤病。

【Etiology and Pathogenesis】

The etiology of primary cutaneous amyloidosis remains unclear. Amyloid displays as a homogeneous eosinophilic transparent glass-like material that is composed of 3 kinds of substances: amyloid fibril proteins, the amyloid P component, and the extracellular matrix. The amyloid precursors may originate from epidermal keratin escaping into the dermis by those degenerated epidermal cells, where they convert into amyloids, and lodge in the papillary layer of the dermis.

【病因及发病机制】

病因尚不完全清楚,淀粉样蛋白是一种嗜酸性均一的透明玻璃样物质,由淀粉样原纤维蛋白、淀粉样蛋白P和基质三种物质组成,目前已知本病的淀粉样物质来源于表皮中的角蛋白,由变性的表皮细胞逸入真皮中,并转化为淀粉样蛋白,沉积在真皮乳头内所致。

【Clinical Manifestations】

Several types of primary cutaneous amyloidosis have been described. The most common two variants are listed below.

(1) Lichen amyloidosis: this is also known as idiopathic keratin amyloidosis, and commonly affects middle-aged males. The skin lesions are usually seen on the anterior tibial area, the lateral side of

【临床表现】

临床上有不同的类型,以下两型为最常见。

(1) 苔藓性淀粉样变(lichen amyloidosis) 又称为特发性角蛋白性淀粉样变,以中年男性多见。皮损好发

the arm, and the back. In the early stages, the skin lesions manifest as pinhead sized brown spots that gradually become semiglobular, conical or polygonal papules that are firm, skin-colored, light-red or brown, and about 2 mm in diameter. Lichenification and hyperkeratosis can be found at the top of the papules. Bead-like (miniliformed) lesions along the dermatoglyphic linesoncalf and upper back are the typical manifestation (Fig. 18-5). The disease tends to be chronic and patients experience intense pruritus.

于胫前、臂外侧和背部，早期表现为针头大小的褐色斑点，后逐渐增大形成半球形、圆锥形或多角形丘疹，直径约为 2 mm，质硬，正常皮色，淡红或褐色，表面可见苔藓样变、角化过度等，小腿和上背部皮损可沿皮纹方向成念珠状排列，为本病的特征性皮损(图 18-5)。皮损发展缓慢，自觉剧烈瘙痒。

(2) Macular amyloidosis: this type most commonly appears in middle-aged females. The lesions are grey, blue or brown papules that tend to coalesce and give rise to a reticulated or wavy appearance, which is of some diagnostic value. The lesions are usually symmetrical, with preferences on the scapular area of the back, trunk, and extremities (Fig. 18-6). Patients may be asymptomatic or only suffer from mild pruritus. This type is often easily misdiagnosed as post-inflammatory pigmentation.

(2) 斑疹性淀粉样变(macular amyloidosis) 好发于中年女性，皮损为灰色、蓝色或褐色的点状色素斑融合而成，呈网状或波纹状，后者有诊断价值，对称分布于背部肩胛区、躯干和四肢(图 18-6)，一般无自觉症状或仅有轻度瘙痒。本型易误诊为炎症后色素沉着。

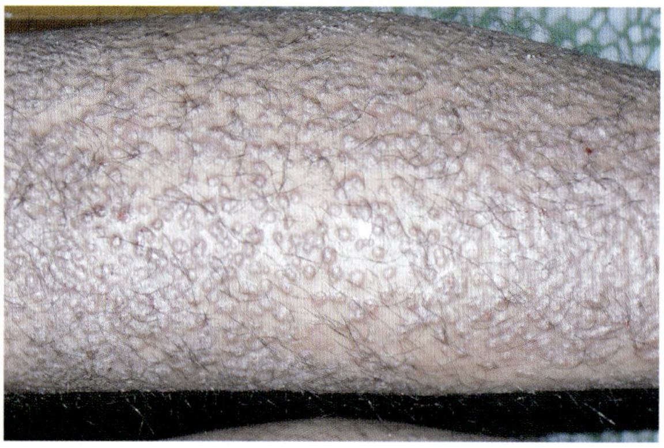

Fig. 18-5 Lichen amyloidosis(图 18-5 苔藓性淀粉样变)

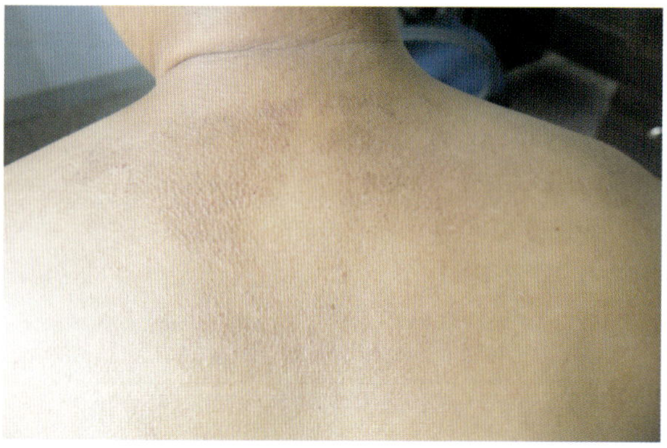

Fig. 18-6 Macular amyloidosis(图 18-6 斑疹性淀粉样变)

The two forms of cutaneous amyloidosis described above may also overlap or convert into each other on some occasions. Then the condition is known as mixed amyloidosis or biphasic amyloidosis.

上述两种皮损可同时存在或相互转变，称为混合型或双相型皮肤淀粉样变。

【Histopathology】

The histological changes are similar in all forms of cutaneous amyloidosis, characterized by focal and amorphic amyloid deposits in the dermal papilla and in the upper portion of the dermis. These amyloid proteins are visible as a eosinophilic non-structural glass-like substance under HE staining, reddish purple under crystal violet staining, and red under Congo red staining. However, the gold standard for diagnosing primary cutaneous amyloidosis is the presence of amyloid filaments in the lesional areas under electron microscopy.

【组织病理】

各型的组织病理变化表现相似，即真皮乳头处及真皮上部局灶性无定型淀粉样蛋白团块沉积。HE 染色淀粉样变蛋白为嗜酸性性无结构玻璃样物质，结晶紫染色呈紫红色，刚果红染色呈红色。电镜检查发现淀粉样蛋白细丝为诊断本病的金标准。

【Diagnosis and Differential Diagnosis】

The diagnosis of primary cutaneous amyloidosis can be made on the basis of its typical skin lesions and its characteristic

【诊断与鉴别诊断】

根据典型皮损，结合组织病理及电镜检查可确诊。本病应与慢性单纯性苔

pathological changes under both light and electron microscopy. Primary cutaneous amyloidosis should be differentiated from lichen simplex chronicus, lichen planus hypertrophicus, poikiloderma, and dermatomyositis and dyskeratosis congenita.

藓、肥厚性扁平苔藓、皮肤异色病、皮肌炎、先天性角化不良等相鉴别。

【Treatment】

As of today there are no specific treatments for primary cutaneous amyloidosis available. Avoidance of scratching or prolonged mechanical scratching with rough objects may interrupt the "itch-scratch-itch" cycle. Antihistamines can be beneficial for relief of the pruritus, and mild cases can be treated with topical high-potency glucocorticoids in occlusive dressings or with 0.1% tretinoin. Intralesional injection of triamcinolone acetonide is only used in patients with small skin lesions. Cryotherapy, dermabrasion, and a combination of potent topical corticosteroids with UVB or PUVA can be helpful alternatives for lichen amyloidosis.

【治疗】

本病尚无特效疗法，避免搔抓及用粗糙的物品长期机械性搔抓刺激皮肤，阻断"痒-抓-痒"的循环。瘙痒明显者应用抗组胺药可减轻病情，病情轻者可局部用高效糖皮质激素软膏封包、0.1%维A酸霜外用等，小片皮损可用曲安萘德等皮损内注射，可获疗效。苔藓样型可用冷冻或皮肤磨削术或外涂强效糖皮质激素制剂联合UVB或PUVA等治疗。

Section Three　Gout

Gout is a purine metabolic disease. It is an inflammatory condition of the articular cartilage, subcutis and kidneys, and is caused by the accumulation of urate crystals in tissues due to hyperuricemia (increased amount of uric acid in the blood) as a result of the long term of purine metabolic disturbance and/or decreased uric acid excretion.

第三节　痛　　风

痛风(gout)是一种嘌呤代谢性疾病，是由于长期嘌呤代谢紊乱和/或尿酸排泄减少，血尿酸增高引起组织损伤的一种炎症性疾病，各种原因产生的高尿酸血症，在组织中以尿酸盐结晶沉积导致沉积部位发生炎症反应，主要累及关节软骨、皮下、肾脏等器官。

【Etiology and Pathogenesis】

Uric acid is one product of purine metabolism. In the human body, it can be produced endogenously and exogenously. Endogenous uric acid mainly comes from the decomposition of tissue proteins, nucleic acids, and some of the associated auxiliary acids. Exogenous uric acid derives from food that contains purine components. Serum uric acid levels are determined by the balance between production and excretion; therefore, increased inserum uric acid levels are caused by excessive production and reduced excretion.

Gout can be categorized into primary and secondary types. Genetic factors may play a key role in the development of the primary type. Most patients with primary gout have inherited it as a dominant trait with a congenital purine metabolic abnormality, resulting in increased uric acid synthesis. By contrast, most cases of secondary gout are the consequence of decreased excretion of uric acid due to some other renal diseases. No matter what the causes of hyperuricemia are, abundant uric acid in the tissues will eventually

【病因及发病机制】

尿酸是嘌呤类化合物的代谢产物，人体尿酸来源可分为内源性和外源性。内源性尿酸主要来自组织蛋白、核酸和一些辅酸的分解代谢产物。外源性尿酸来自含嘌呤成分的食物。血清尿酸水平取决于其产生和排泄之间的关系，产生过多和排泄减少均可引起血清尿酸水平升高。

本病有原发性和继发性两类。原发性痛风与遗传因素相关，多数为显性遗传，由先天性嘌呤代谢紊乱引起，导致尿酸合成增加；继发性痛风常继发于各种肾病，使尿酸排泄减少。由于尿酸排泄减少或者生成增加，都能导致血中尿酸增高，从而以尿酸盐的形式沉积在组织中，引起局部炎症反应而产生痛风性关

trigger a local inflammatory reaction that manifests as gouty arthritis, renal stones, or skin lesions.

节炎、肾结石或皮肤损害等临床症状。

【Clinical Manifestations】

The disease occurs mostly in middle-aged and elderly men or in women mostly after menopause. Emotional factors, stress, diet, alcohol, drugs, and other factors may provoke the disease. Hyperuricemia appears rarely before puberty, and usually occurs earlier in males than in females. The first symptom of gouty arthritis is typically the sudden onset of one or more hot, red, swollen and painful joints. The first metatarsophalangeal joint is the most common initial site, and later the inflammatory reaction spreads to multiple joints but is often limited to the lower extremities, even in advanced cases. Tophi develop very often in patients with chronic gout. Tophi are the firm yellow or white papules or nodules in the cartilage or soft tissues that result from deposition of uric acid crystals (Fig. 18-7). The tophic lesions may be single or multiple and most commonly occur on the earlobe or the joints of the index finger. Renal colic may be severe in some cases, and is caused by the accumulation of uric acid crystals into the collecting ducts of the kidney.

【临床表现】

本病好发于中老年男性，女性多在绝经期后发病，情绪因素、应激、饮食不当、饮酒、药物等因素均可促发本病。高尿酸血症常于青春发育期后出现，男性发生比女性早，痛风性关节炎的首发症状常表现为突然发生的关节红、肿、热、痛，典型的惯发于第一跖趾关节，之后多关节也受累，常累及下肢关节。痛风石多发于慢性痛风患者，此时，尿酸盐沉积在软骨、软组织等处，表现为坚硬的、黄色或白色丘疹或结节(图 18-7)。典型痛风石局限在耳轮及食指关节，单发或多发；痛风石沉积于肾脏可出现剧烈肾绞痛，由于尿酸盐结晶沉淀在肾脏的集合管所致。

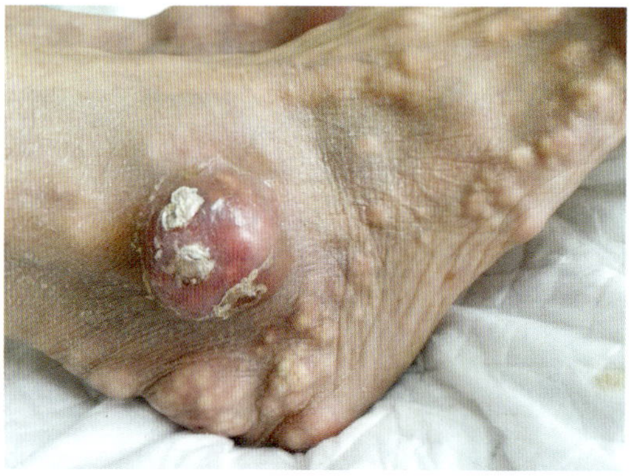

Fig. 18-7 Gout(图 18-7 痛风)

【Histopathology】

Some care is required for biopsy processing when gout tissues are involved, since the tissue specimens must be fixated with pure ethanol since sodium urate crystals will be destroyed by formaldehyde (formalin). Histopathologically, the clusters of urate crystals are of various sizes and are brownish in color, with clear margins in the subcutaneous layer. Around these crystals one may find infiltration by foreign body giant cells, hyperplasia of fibrous tissue and sometimes even calcification.

【组织病理】

组织样本仅用无水乙醇固定，以甲醛(福尔马林)固定会破坏尿酸钠结晶。HE 显示皮下有大小不等境界清楚的尿酸盐结晶，呈集束状，褐色，其周围有异物巨细胞浸润及纤维组织增生，沉淀物可钙化。

【Diagnosis and Differential Diagnosis】

According to the clinical manifestation of hyperuricemia,

【诊断与鉴别诊断】

根据临床症状、高尿酸血症、痛风石

discharge of gout stones, urate crystal exudation in synovial fluid, and histopathologic features, the diagnosis of gout can be confirmed. Gout should be differentiated from calcium pyrophosphate deposition diseases, tendinous xanthoma, multicentric reticulohistiocytosis, rheumatic arthritis, rheumatoid arthritis and Reiter's syndrome, etc.

排出物和滑膜液渗出尿酸盐结晶和组织病理表现即可以确诊。本病应与钙质沉着病、腱黄瘤、多中心性网状组织细胞增生症、风湿性关节炎、类风湿关节炎、Reiter综合征等相鉴别。

【Treatment】

Any patient with gout or with raised levels of uric acid should be investigated to ascertain the cause. In acute attacks, patients should have sufficient rest, avoid incentives, avoid foods with high purine content, be given plenty of water, and not drink alcohol in any quantity. Treatment with anti-inflammatory agents such as colchicine and indomethacin are effective in managing acute attacks and are generally well tolerated. However, physicians should be careful in their choice of diuretics that may inhibit renal tubular excretion. For chronic gout, probenecid and allopurinol will accelerate the excretion of uric acid.

【治疗】

所有痛风病患或血尿酸升高的患者应调查清楚原因。急性发作期应充分休息，避免诱因，少食含嘌呤高的食物，大量饮水，不饮酒。抗炎治疗，如秋水仙碱和吲哚美辛，常可用于急性发作，患者一般均能耐受，慎用抑制肾小管排泄的利尿剂。对慢性痛风患者，可用丙磺舒和别嘌呤醇以增加尿酸的排泄。

Section Four Calcinosis Cutis

第四节 皮肤钙质沉着症

Calcinosis cutis is a skin disorder wherein calcium and phosphate (hydroxyapatite) compounds are deposited in the skin. The condition has a variety of causes. The main clinical manifestations are firm papules, nodules, or lumps which upon bursting discharge a cheese-colored, oily, sand-like substance.

皮肤钙质沉着症(calcinosis cutis)是由于各种原因使钙和磷酸盐(羟磷灰石)复合物在皮肤组织中沉着所产生的疾病。临床主要表现为坚硬的丘疹、结节或肿块，破溃后排出奶酪色油状沙粒样物质。

【Etiology and Pathogenesis】

Based on the causative factors, calcinosis cutis can be divided into 4 major types.

(1) Dystrophic calcinosis cutis: calcium salts accumulate in the skin, subcutaneous tissue, muscles, and tendons, where there have been previous injuries or inflammations, or where the areas have become neoplastic or necrotic. The causes of this damage can be mechanical, chemical, infectious, or may arise from other factors. Usually the serum levels of both calcium and phosphate are within normal ranges.

(2) Metastatic calcinosis cutis: this type is caused by calciumorphosphorus metabolic abnormalities that lead to elevated serum calcium and phosphorus levels and the deposition of calcium salts in the normal skin, subcutaneous tissue and even in the internal organs. This condition is often a complication of hyperparathyroidism.

(3) Iatrogenic and traumatic calcinosis cutis: as the name(s) suggests, calcium salts were mistakenly introduced into the injured skin (iatrogenic) during a medical procedure, or the exogenous

【病因及发病机制】

皮肤钙质沉着症根据病因主要分为以下4种类型。

(1) 营养不良性皮肤钙质沉着症(dystrophic calcinosis cutis) 钙盐沉积于皮肤、皮下组织、肌肉和肌腱中，此型发生在组织损伤、炎症、肿瘤或坏死的皮肤组织，组织受损伤可能由物理、化学、感染或其他因素引起，患者血清钙、磷正常。

(2) 转移性皮肤钙质沉着症(metastatic calcinosis cutis) 此型是由于钙、磷代谢异常(血清钙、磷升高)而导致钙盐在正常皮肤、皮下组织甚至内脏器官沉着。常见于甲状旁腺功能亢进的患者。

(3) 医源性和损伤性皮肤钙质沉着症(iatrogenic and traumatic calcinosis cutis) 此型由于医疗操作过程中误将

calcium salts entered the pre-injured skin (traumatic), resulting in tissue calcification or calcium salt deposition at the damaged sites.

钙盐导入受损伤的皮肤中，或因外伤使外源性钙盐进入受伤皮肤内而引起损伤部位的组织钙化或钙盐沉着。

(4) Idiopathic calcinosis cutis: indicates an unknown cause for the calcium deposition in the skin, subcutaneous tissue and muscles. The patients have neither a calciumorphosphorus metabolic disorder (serum levels of calcium and phosphorus are normal) nor any history of injury. The lesions occur most commonly on the scrotum, in which the condition is called idiopathic scrotal calcinosis.

(4) 特发性皮肤钙质沉着症(idiopathic calcinosis cutis)　指患者既无钙磷代谢紊乱(血清钙、磷正常)，又无组织损伤，皮肤、皮下组织和肌肉发生原因不明的钙沉着，最好发于阴囊，称之为特发性阴囊钙质沉着症。

【Clinical Manifestations】

The signs and symptoms of calcinosis cutis vary with the underlying causes. Usually, the lesions begin as single or multiple, firm, whitish or yellowish papules, plaques or nodules (Fig. 18-8). These lesions may then enlarge, soften and later ulcerate on the surface, exuding a chalk-like creamy discharge composed of calcium phosphate and a small amount of calcium carbonate.

【临床表现】

不同病因引起的皮肤钙质沉着，其症状和体征都不一样。皮损表现为单个或多个质硬、白色或黄色的丘疹、斑块或结节(图18-8)，皮损可增大、变软、表面溃烂并流出具有特征性的石灰样、奶油样的物质，主要为磷酸钙和少量碳酸钙。

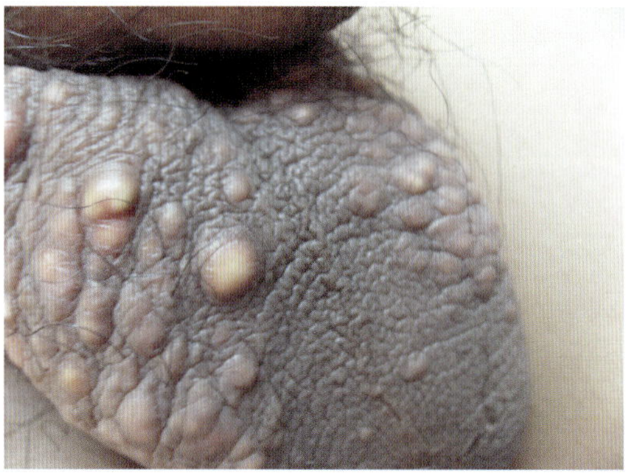

Fig. 18-8　Idiopathic scrotal calcinosis(图18-8　特发性阴囊钙质沉着症)

【Diagnosis】

The skin lesions, especially at the stage of ulceration, where they yield a chalk-like discharge, are characteristic for calcinosis cutis. Laboratory tests can be performed to determine the serum levels of calcium and phosphate and the possible underlying causative agents. Radiological examinations including plain film X-ray may also be used to demonstrate the extent of the tissue calcification. A skin biopsy may also be useful to confirm the diagnosis.

【诊断】

根据皮损的质地，特别是破溃后流出石灰样物质可确诊，通过实验室检查明确血清钙和磷的水平及可能原因，必要时进行X线摄片以明确组织钙化的范围。皮损组织病理检查可明确诊断。

【Treatment】

The underlying causes of calcinosis cutis should be identified and treated accordingly. Patients with hypercalcemia should be given a low calcium diet. By the same token patients with high phosphate levels in the blood should restrict their phosphorus intake. Solitary lesions can be removed by surgery. Medicines that

【治疗】

必须找出和明确引起皮肤钙质沉着症的原因并进行相关治疗。伴高血钙者，需限制钙的摄入，高血磷者应限制磷质的摄入。对于单个损害可考虑手术切除，药物治疗可选用糖皮质激素、丙磺

can help with symptomatic relief are glucocorticoids, probenecid, colchicine, sodium etidronate, and diphosphonates, etc.

舒、秋水仙碱、羟乙磷酸钠、二磷酸盐等以缓解症状。

Section Five　Myxedema

第五节　黏液性水肿

Myxedema includes a group of dysmetabolic diseases that stem from the deposition of mucopolysaccharides in the dermis and subcutis. These diseases are characterized by a non-pitting edema and can be divided into generalized myxedema, pretibial myxedema and lichen myxedematosus according to their clinical manifestations.

黏液性水肿(myxedema)是一种由于黏多糖沉积于真皮及皮下组织内，使皮肤产生特征性的非凹陷性水肿的代谢障碍性疾病，分为全身性黏液性水肿(generalized myxedema)、胫前黏液性水肿(pretibial myxedema)及黏液水肿性苔藓(lichen myxedematosus)三种。

1. Generalized myxedema

一、全身性黏液性水肿(generalized myxedema)

【Etiology and Pathogenesis】

Generalized myxedema is caused by hypothyroidism. As a result of low thyroxine levels and basal metabolic rate, mucin degradation in fibroblasts is affected throughout the body, leading to mucin deposits in the dermis and subcutis, producing a non-pitting edema all over the body.

【病因及发病机制】

本病是由于甲状腺功能减退，体内甲状腺素和基础代谢率降低，导致成纤维细胞降解黏蛋白障碍，使其沉积在真皮及皮下组织内，从而引起全身皮肤发生非凹陷性水肿等症状。

【Clinical Manifestations】

The condition may manifest as follows:

(1) Cretinism: the onset of symptoms is within weeks after birth. This is a systemic disease that is associated with multiple organs and systems especially the central nervous system, presenting as a developmental disorder (also known as retardation, but this term is somewhat out of favor). The patient has a low basal metabolic rate, feels cold, cries less and shows drowsiness, listlessness, anorexia, constipation, and slow response. With age the patient will display physical growth retardation, nonuniform dwarfism, a short neck, distended belly, a hoarse voice, hernia due to muscle separation and underdeveloped limbs. Apart from these considerable systemic symptoms, the skin shows a dry, non-pitting edema of sallow complexion with desquamation. Other body traits that are associated with cretinism include ocular hypertelorism, eyelid edema, a flat (bridge of the) nose, hypertrophiclips, odontiasis retardation, thick and brittle hairs. Mental development retardation and a lack of facial expression are characteristic, and the onset of normal activities such as climbing, sitting, standing and walking are all more delayed than in normal children.

【临床表现】

本病可有以下临床表现。

(1) 呆小病(cretinism)　出生后数周内出现症状，主要表现为全身特别是中枢神经系统发育障碍或迟缓，患儿基础代谢率低、怕冷、嗜睡、少哭、不活泼、食欲不振、便秘、反应迟钝。随着年龄增长会发现患儿体格发育迟缓、呈不均匀性矮小、颈短、腹膨胀，常有疝气。四肢粗短，哭声嘶哑。皮肤蜡黄、干燥脱屑，呈非凹陷性水肿。两眼距增宽、眼睑肿胀、鼻梁塌陷扁平、口唇肥厚、出牙迟缓、头发粗而脆。智力发育迟缓，表情淡漠，爬、坐、站、走都晚于正常儿。

(2) Juvenile myxedema: clinical manifestation varies according to the age of onset. Children with an early onset of the disease may have symptoms similar to cretinism, but less severe. While the onset of the disease is in elder children or adolescents, the

(2) 幼年黏液性水肿(juvenile myxedema)　临床表现随发病年龄而不同。幼小儿童发病者与呆小病相似但较轻。较大儿童或青春期发病者，大多与

symptoms are mostly similar to adult myxedema, but are usually accompanied by a different degree of growth restriction.

(3) Adult myxedema: patients often manifest with fatigue, poor appetite, weight gain, intellectual decline, low body temperature, facial expression apathy, edema and cutis laxa of the cheeks and eyelids, narrowed oculi rimae, and sometimes slightly protruding eyes. The face is pale and cold. Hypohidrosis may occur. As with cretinism, the skin is pale or of sallow complexion, dry, showing scaling, thickening (Fig. 18-9), and occasional cyanosis on the facial skin. Hair is thick, dry, brittle, and shedding diffusely; eyebrows are sparse, dry, thin and show hair loss on the outer edge; hair in armpits and pubic areas will also often fall off; beard is sparse, the nails become thin or thick, brittle, easy to crack with strips, and nails separation may occur. Teeth are sparse and fragile; muscle relaxation and muscle weakness are common. In severe cases, patients may suffer from bradycardia, cardiomegaly, pericardial effusion, and coma.

成人黏液性水肿相似,但一般伴有不同程度的生长受限。

(3) 成人黏液性水肿(adult myxedema) 疲困、胃口欠佳、体重增加、智力减退,体温低。面部表情淡漠、面颊及眼睑水肿和松弛下降、眼裂狭窄、有时有轻度突眼。面色苍白、冰冷、少汗。皮肤呈苍白或蜡黄色,干燥、脱屑、增厚(图 18-9),面部皮肤偶见发绀。头发粗、干、脆,弥漫脱落,眉毛外侧脱落、稀疏、干而细,腋毛和阴毛也常脱落,胡须稀少。指(趾)甲变薄或增厚、易脆、易裂和多横纹,可发生甲分离。牙齿稀疏易碎,可出现肌肉松弛无力。心动过缓、心脏扩大、心包积液,严重者可致昏迷。

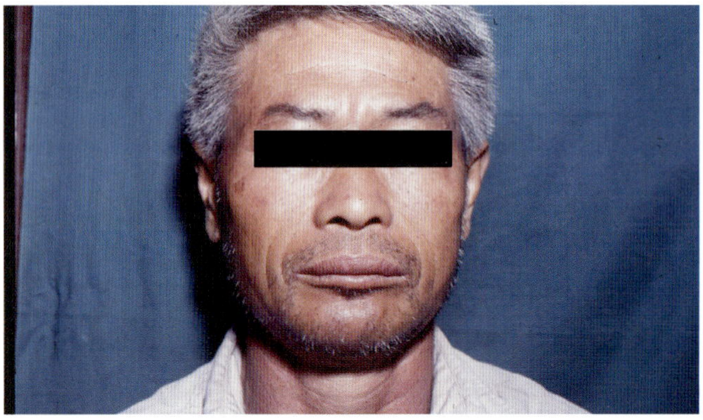

Fig. 18-9 Generalized myxedema(图 18-9 全身性黏液性水肿)

【Laboratory Findings】

The basal metabolic rates in patients with this condition fall below normal levels, being usually lower than 20%. Typically, the patients also have hypercholesterolemia and high serum levels of TSH. Anemia and abnormalities of hepatic and renal functions may sometimes be seen.

【实验室检查】

基础代谢率低于正常,常低于 20%,伴高胆固醇血症和促甲状腺素(TSH)水平明显增高,可有贫血及肝肾功能异常。

【Histopathology】

The epidermis can be normal or undergo hyperkeratosis. In severe cases, there may be slight swelling and separation between the collagen bundles in the dermis. Mucin deposits can be seen throughout the entire thickness of the skin.

【组织病理】

表皮可正常或有角化过度,在较严重时,真皮有轻度水肿伴胶原束分离,全层均有黏蛋白沉积。

【Diagnosis and Differential Diagnosis】

On the basis of those clinical symptoms, non-pitting edema of the skin, abnormal basal metabolism and mucin deposition in the histopathological slides, diagnosis of myxedema should easily be

【诊断与鉴别诊断】

根据患者的临床表现、皮肤有非凹陷性水肿、基础代谢异常、病理可见黏蛋白沉积可确诊。本病应与贫血、肾炎等

confirmed. However, the generalized myxedema should be differentiated from anemia and nephritis.

相鉴别。

【Treatment】

Thyroid tablets or levothyroxine sodium is effective in treating generalized myxedema. The dosage should begin with the smallest dose and then rise gradually until reaching the effective dose.

【治疗】

甲状腺片或左甲状腺素钠均有显著疗效，宜先从小剂量开始，逐渐加至耐受量。

2. Pretibial myxedema

Pretibial myxedema is also known as nodular myxedema, resulting from the local deposition of mucin that leads to solid and uplifted edematous plaques or nodules on the anterior tibial areas. This type of myxedema is an autoimmune disorder associated with hyperthyroidism.

二、胫前黏液性水肿

胫前黏液性水肿(pretibial myxedema)又名结节性黏液性水肿(nodular myxedema)，是由于黏蛋白局部沉积，导致胫前皮肤出现坚实隆起的水肿性斑块或结节，伴有甲状腺功能亢进的自身免疫性疾病。

【Etiology and Pathogenesis】

The etiology of pretibial myxedema remains unclear. In contrast to generalized myxedema, this disease is usually accompanied by symptoms of hyperthyroidism, such as an increased basal metabolic rate. As this condition is often accompanied by Graves' disease (an autoimmune problem that causes the thyroid gland to produce too much thyroid hormone), most researchers believe that pretibial myxedema arises from some autoimmune mechanism. Patients tend to have elevated serum levels of long-acting thyroid stimulator (LATS), which can be found in the skin lesions as well. Through the activation of lymphocytes, LATS promotes fibroblast proliferation that causes massive mucin deposits at local sites. However, the disease can also occur in patients with abnormal local blood circulation or lymph circulation, but in those cases it occurs without the accompanying hyperthyroidism.

【病因及发病机制】

病因尚未明确，与全身性黏液性水肿不同，患者常有基础代谢率显著增高等甲状腺功能亢进的症状。本病多伴发Graves病(一种甲状腺产生过多甲状腺激素的自身免疫性疾病)，目前多数专家认为该病是自身免疫性疾病的一种表现，患者血清中长效甲状腺刺激物(LATS)升高，在患者皮损中可检出LATS存在，LATS参与激活淋巴细胞，促使成纤维细胞增生，产生大量黏蛋白局部沉积。另外，本病亦可发生于局部血液循环或淋巴循环异常但无甲状腺功能亢进的患者。

【Clinical Manifestations】

The skin lesions begin on the anterolateral aspects of the lower legs, and then gradually spread to the thighs and dorsa of the feet. In some severe cases, pretibial myxedema can present at other sites of the body, such as the arms, shoulders, abdomen, neck, face and even the ears. The skin lesions of pretibial myxedema manifest as pink or yellow waxy plaques and nodules (Fig. 18-10). When the follicular orifices in the affected areas of the skin are dilated, the lesions take on a characteristic orange peel-like appearance. Beyond the damage to the skin, patients often have no distinct complaint. This disease can be divided into three types: localized, diffuse and elephantiasis (Fig. 18-11).

【临床表现】

皮损开始于双侧胫前下部，逐渐向大腿、足背发展，严重者可同时损害手臂、肩、腹、颈、面，甚至耳，皮损表现为粉红色或黄色的蜡样斑块和结节(图18-10)，皮损处毛囊口扩张可呈具有特征性的橘皮样外观，常无明显自觉症状。本病临床上可分为三型：①局限型；②弥漫型；③象皮病型(图18-11)。

【Laboratory Findings】

The basal metabolic rate can be normal, but serum IgA and IgG may be elevated.

【实验室检查】

基础代谢率可正常，血清中IgA、IgG增高。

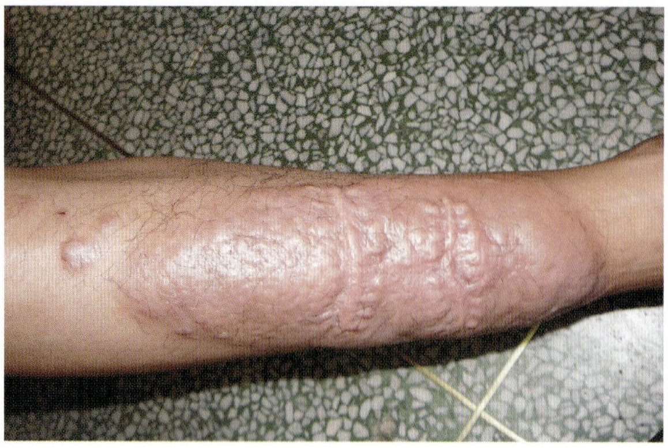

Fig. 18-10 Pretibial myxedema
(图 18-10 胫前黏液性水肿)

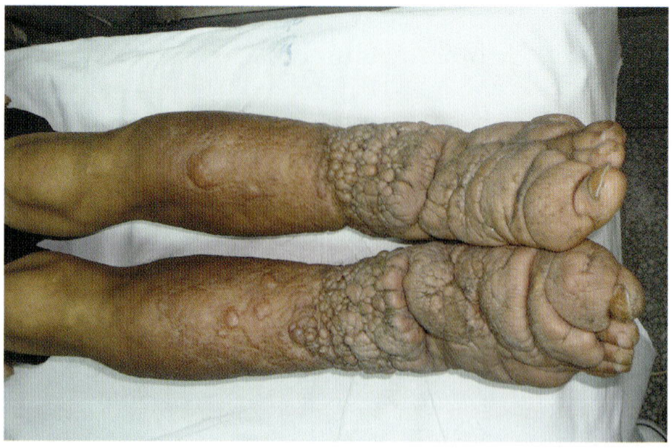

Fig. 18-11 Pretibial myxedema-elephantiasis variant
(图 18-11 胫前黏液性水肿-象皮病型)

【Histopathology】

The epidermis reveals hyperkeratosis, follicular plugs, flattened rete ridges, basal cell nuclear pyknosis, and dermo-epidermaljunction edema. The dermis is significantly thickened due to edema and large quantities of mucin deposits in the reticular dermis. Infiltration of lymphocytes, plasma cells and histiocytes around the blood vessels and the appendages can be found. Mucin deposition can be detected under Alcian blue staining.

【组织病理】

表皮角化过度,毛囊角栓,表皮棘变平,基底细胞核固缩,表皮-真皮交界处水肿。真皮网状层水肿及有大量黏蛋白沉积,真皮明显变厚,并见血管和附属器周围有淋巴细胞、浆细胞、组织细胞浸润,阿辛蓝染色可见黏蛋白沉积。

【Diagnosis and Differential Diagnosis】

The hyperthyroidism symptoms accompanied by the non-pitting edema on the pretibial area of the skin, the characteristic mucin deposits in the histopathological sections, the increased serum levels of IgA and IgG, and the normal basal metabolic rates will give a diagnosis of pretibial myxedema. However, pretibial myxedema should be differentiated from lichen simplex chronicus, lichen planus hypertrophicus, and lymphoedema.

【诊断与鉴别诊断】

根据患者有甲状腺功能亢进的表现,特别是胫前有非凹陷性斑块,组织病理有特征性改变及黏蛋白沉积,基础代谢正常而血清中 IgA、IgG 增高可确诊。本病应与慢性单纯性苔藓、肥厚性扁平苔藓、淋巴水肿等相鉴别。

【Treatment】

Treatment for pretibial myxedema is often carried out in conjunction with treatment for a concomitant thyroid disease, for example administering drugs that decrease thyroid stimulating hormone (TSH) levels in the body-if the thyroid is simply over-active-or which defeat the action of certain antibodies that stimulate the thyroid hyperactivity. At the same time thyroid function needs to be monitored closely during the treatment. A special regimen for the skin condition may not even be necessary if the case is a mild one, since symptoms in such cases may be self-resolving. On the other hand, patients with serious outbreaks of pretibial myxedema should be treated with oral or topical glucocorticoids, but the dosage and the course of treatment are likely to vary with the individual. Prednisone 30～40 mg/d can be used as an initial dose, gradually tapering off as the condition improves. Intralesional

【治疗】

本病患者应注意伴发的甲状腺疾病,进行相应的甲状腺功能检查和治疗(如仅仅是单纯的甲状腺功能亢进可采用降低体内甲状腺刺激素(TSH)的药物或对抗使甲状腺亢进的抗体)。部分轻型患者可自行消退。严重者可口服或局部应用糖皮质激素,要注意根据不同的个体,选择不同的剂量及疗程。常用泼尼松 30～40 mg/d,好转后逐渐减量。皮损肥厚明显者,可选用糖皮质激素皮损内注射。

injection of glucocorticoids is an alternative when the patients manifest thickening skin lesions.

3. Lichen myxedematosus

Lichen myxedematosus can be classified into generalized lichen myxedematosus (also known as scleromyxedema), localized lichen myxedematosus which includes discrete papular lichen myxedematosus, acral persistent popular mucinosis, self-healing popular mucinosis and papular mucinosis of infancy, and atypical or intermediate lichen myxedematosus. This form of myxedema is characterized by fibroblast proliferation and abundant mucin deposits in the dermis, which usually give those lichenoid papular eruptions.

三、黏液水肿性苔藓

黏液水肿性苔藓(lichen myxedematosus)包括泛发性黏液水肿性苔藓(又称硬化性黏液水肿)、局限性黏液水肿性苔藓(包括散在性丘疹性黏液水肿性苔藓、肢端持续性丘疹性黏蛋白病、自愈性丘疹性黏蛋白病、婴儿丘疹性黏蛋白病)和非典型或中间型黏液水肿性苔藓。本病是由于成纤维细胞增殖和黏蛋白大量沉积于真皮内,而引起皮肤出现苔藓样丘疹的皮肤病。

【Etiology and Pathogenesis】

The etiology of lichen myxedematosus is still uncertain. It is believed that the mucin deposits in the dermis are caused by the action of long-acting thyroid stimulator (LATS), which ultimately provoke fibroblast proliferation and increased mucin production.

【病因及发病机制】

本病病因尚不清楚。目前多认为是由于长效甲状腺刺激物(LATS)的作用,刺激成纤维细胞增多,使黏蛋白合成增加,导致大量黏蛋白沉积于真皮内而发病。

【Clinical Manifestations】

Patients are most likely to experience lichen myxedematosus between the ages of 30 and 50. The lesions manifest as skin colored or reddish lichenoid papules or nodules on the skin, and may cluster into groups (Fig. 18-12). Lesions often occur on the dorsa of the hands, the face, or on the arms and legs. The consequence of fusion lesions at the glabella and forehead may create some obvious wrinkles in the brow and forehead area to give a 'leontiasis' look. Mucosal involvement is rare for this disease. A majority of the patients are asymptomatic but some may experience fatigue or tiredness.

【临床表现】

本病好发于 30～50 岁的成年人。皮损表现为正常肤色或红色的苔藓样丘疹、结节,可成群分布(图 18-12)。皮损好发于手背、面部、手臂和小腿。不侵犯黏膜,在眉间及前额,融合的皮损造成明显的皱纹,状如“狮面”。一般无自觉症状,部分患者可有四肢无力和疲劳等。

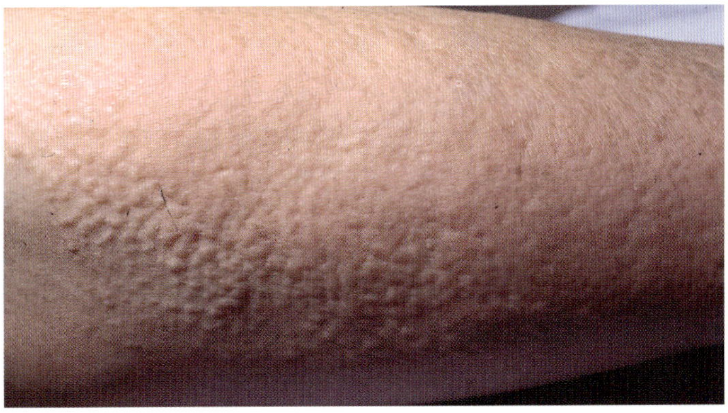

Fig. 18-12　Lichen myxedematosus(图 18-12　黏液水肿性苔藓)

【Laboratory Findings】

Increased serum levels of IgG and IgA may be found, but the

【实验室检查】

基础代谢正常,血清中 IgA、IgG

basal metabolic rate is normal.

增高。

【Histopathology】

The epidermis becomes thinner and basal cells are degenerated. A large quantity of mucin deposits are found in the dermis and fibroblasts are also increased. Perivascular infiltration of lymphocytes and histiocytes is evident.

【组织病理】

表皮变薄，基底细胞变性，真皮有大量黏蛋白沉积，成纤维细胞增多，血管周围淋巴细胞、组织细胞浸润。

【Diagnosis and Differential Diagnosis】

The diagnosis of lichen myxedematosus can be made from the lichenoid papules or nodules, the large quantities of mucin deposits seen under microscopy, and laboratory tests. Lichen myxedematosus should be differentiated from systemic scleroderma and localized cutaneous amyloidosis.

【诊断与鉴别诊断】

根据皮肤苔藓样丘疹、结节，组织病理见真皮大量黏蛋白沉积，实验室检查，可诊断。本病应与系统性硬皮病、局限性皮肤淀粉样变等相鉴别。

【Treatment】

No particular treatment is consistently effective for this form of myxedema. However, a few case reports indicate that topical tacrolimus may be of benefit for some patients with limited lesions.

【治疗】

本病尚无特效疗法。有报告指出部分患者皮损局限者，局部应用他克莫司治疗有一定的疗效。

Section Six Acanthosis Nigricans

第六节 黑棘皮病

Acanthosis nigricans is also known as keratosis nigricans or dystrophic papillaire *et* pigmentaire. Acanthosis nigricans is a skin condition characterized by hyperpigmented papillomatous hyperkeratosis and is found to affect mostly the neck, armpit, groin and other flexures of the skin.

黑棘皮病(acanthosis nigricans)又称为黑角化病(keratosis nigricans)、色素性乳头状营养不良(dystrophic papillaire *et* pigmentaire)。本病是一种以皮肤色素沉着及乳头状增生为特征，好发于颈、腋、腹股沟等皮肤皱褶处的疾病。

【Etiology and Pathogenesis】

The cause of acanthosis nigricans is still not well understood. Recently some have suggested that it may be related to the elevation of cytokines upon stimulations of keratinocytes and dermal fibroblasts at the cellular receptor level. The onset of the disease appears to be associated with insulin resistance in type Ⅱ diabetes mellitus. The current assumption is that elevated insulin levels may be responsible for a direct or indirect activation of the inflammatory mediators-for instance, tyrosine kinase growth factor receptors (epidermal growth factor receptor or fibroblast growth factor receptor)-for the ‘true’ root cause or causes. This inflammatory activation may in turn promote cellular proliferation via some as yet incompletely understood signaling transduction pathway and may facilitate the ultimate development of acanthosis nigricans.

【病因及发病机制】

本病病因及发病机制尚不清楚，目前已有文献报道，可能与在细胞受体水平上刺激角质形成细胞和真皮成纤维细胞引起细胞因子水平升高有关。本病患者的发病和胰岛素抵抗有密切关系，常与Ⅱ型糖尿病相关。现有理论推测其机制与胰岛素浓度的升高引起炎症介质的直接或间接激活有关，如酪氨酸激酶生长因子受体(表皮生长因子受体或纤维母细胞生长因子受体)通过某种目前尚未完全清楚的信号转导通路促进细胞的增生，并最终导致黑棘皮病。

Some insulin resistance mechanisms are related to genetic factors. For obese people, for example, in the early stages of the disease the insulin receptors might turn on sooner and more aggressively to compensate for a reduction in the number of

有些胰岛素抵抗与遗传有关，肥胖者最初可能是功能性受体的数量减少，但最终受体缺失呈优势。恶性黑棘皮病多数可能是由肿瘤分泌产物引起，这些

functional receptors, but the total number of functional receptors will eventually diminish to the point that no further compensation is possible. On the other hand, the majority of malignant acanthosis nigricans cases may be induced by tumor secretion products, which act on those cellular receptors when they have insulin-like activity. In addition, this disease can be induced by certain drugs (nicotinic acid or diethylstilbestrol) or autoimmune disorders.

肿物分泌产物作用于细胞受体水平，其有胰岛素样活性，此外，本病也可由药物(烟酸或乙烯雌酚)引起或是自身免疫现象。

【Clinical Manifestations】

Acanthosis nigricans can be categorized into 6 subtypes: malignant, familial, associated with syndromes, obesity associated, drug-induced, and nevoid acanthosis nigricans. The basic clinical features are similar in all forms of the disease.

【临床表现】

本病可分为恶性黑棘皮病(malignant acanthosis nigricans)、家族性黑棘皮病(familial acanthosis nigricans)、综合征性黑棘皮病(acanthosis nigricans associated with syndromes)、肥胖相关性黑棘皮病(obesity associated acanthosis nigricans)、药物诱导黑棘皮病(drug-induced acanthosis nigricans)、痣样黑棘皮病(nevoid acanthosis nigricans)等6型，其基本损害是相同的。

Acanthosis nigricans often starts with symmetric, brown thickening of the skin, which may gradually develop multiple small papillomatous or hyperkeratotic papules. The most common sites of involvement include the axillae, neck, groin, breasts, umbilicus and the dorsal surfaces of the fingers and toes.

初起皮损表现为对称、棕色增厚的皮肤，后皮损逐渐发展成细小的乳头瘤样或角化性丘疹。皮损好发在腋窝、颈、腹股沟、乳房、脐和指(趾)背侧。

(1) Malignant acanthosis nigricans: it commonly occurs in adults, and is usually associated with some internal malignancy, especially adenocarcinoma of the gastrointestinal and genitourinary tracts. This type should be strongly suspected when a non-obese man over 40 years old presents with acanthosis nigricans skin lesions.

(1) 恶性黑棘皮病(malignant acanthosis nigricans) 好发于成人，本型伴有内脏肿瘤，特别是胃肠道和泌尿生殖道腺癌。40岁以上非肥胖男性发生黑棘皮病时，要高度怀疑此类型。

(2) Familial acanthosis nigricans (benign acanthosis nigricans): this is a rare inherited disease with anautosomal dominant trait. The onset of the disease may occur at any age, but tends to be early, often during infancy, childhood, or adolescence. The skin lesion is generally not associated with visceral tumors (Fig. 18-13).

(2) 家族性黑棘皮病(familial acanthosis nigricans)(真性良性黑棘皮病) 本型为一种少见的常染色体显性遗传皮肤病。发病较早，可在任何年龄发病，如婴儿期、儿童期或青春期。一般不伴发内脏肿瘤(图18-13)。

(3) Acanthosis nigricans associated with syndromes: lesional manifestations of this type are part of some syndromes, such as Bloom's syndrome, ataxiatelangiectasis syndrome, Costello syndrome, MONFAN syndrome, etc.

(3) 综合征性黑棘皮病(acanthosis nigricans associated with syndromes) 本型为某些综合征的一种皮损表现，如Bloom综合征、共济失调性毛细血管扩张症、Costello综合征、MONFAN综合征等。

(4) Obesity associated acanthosis nigricans: it is also called pseudoacanthosis nigricans. This is the most common type of acanthosis nigricans, and is characterized by the absence of

(4) 肥胖相关性黑棘皮病(obesity associated acanthosis nigricans) 又称假性黑棘皮病(pseudoacanthosis

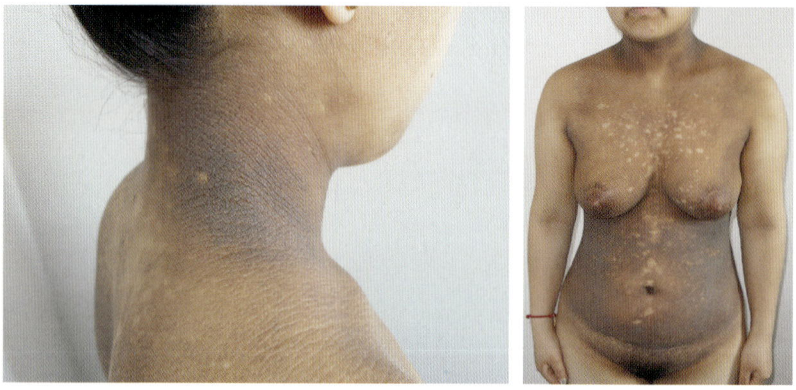

(a)　(b)

Fig. 18-13　Familial acanthosis nigricans(the same patient in (a) and (b))

(图 18-13　家族性黑棘皮病((a)和(b)中为同一患者))

malignant tumors, but may relate to obesity, endocrine disease, and insulin resistance. It occurs mostly in obese people, with or without endocrine disorders. It manifests as pale grey color and velvet-like thickening of the skin on the neck, armpits, and groin (Fig. 18-14).

nigricans),本型是最常见的一种,不伴有恶性肿瘤,与肥胖、内分泌疾病及胰岛素抵抗状况相关。多发生在肥胖者,伴有或不伴有内分泌紊乱。表现为颈部、腋窝、腹股沟淡灰色、天鹅绒样增厚的皮肤(图 18-14)。

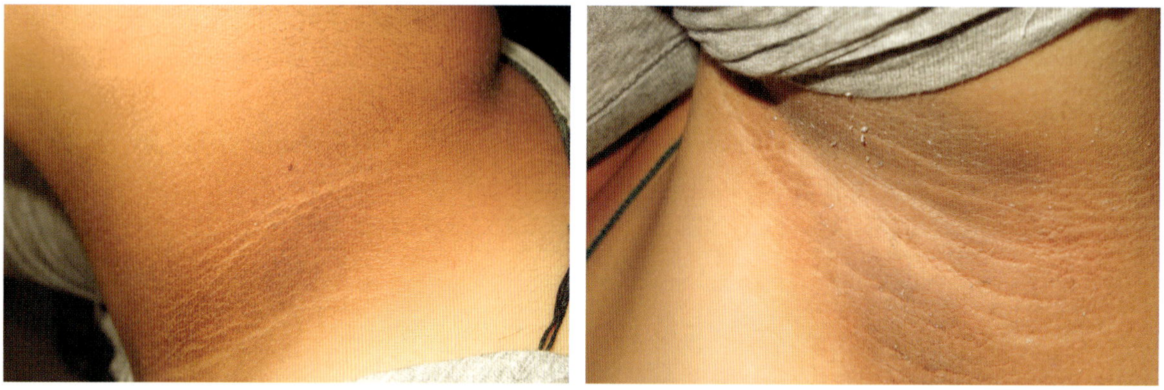

(a)　(b)

Fig. 18-14　Obesity associated acanthosis nigricans (the same patient in (a) and (b))

(图 18-14　肥胖相关性黑棘皮病((a)和(b)中为同一患者))

(5) Drug-induced acanthosis nigricans: some medications can also promote acanthosis nigricans. These include glucocorticoids, nicotinic acid, pituitary extracts, insulin, stilboestrol and oral contraceptives (Fig. 18-15).

(6) Nevoid acanthosis nigricans: also called unilateral acanthosis nigricans. This variety of acanthosis nigricans occurs as a unilateral, localized lesions without endocrine abnormalities.

(5) 药物诱导的黑棘皮病(drug-induced acanthosis nigricans)　某些药物,如糖皮质激素、烟酸、垂体浸出物、胰岛素、己烯雌酚、口服避孕药等,可诱发黑棘皮病(图 18-15)。

(6) 痣样黑棘皮病(nevoid acanthosis nigricans)　又称单侧黑棘皮病,本型不伴有内分泌异常,皮损较局限,呈单侧分布。

【Histopathology】

Histopathology reveals hyperkeratosis and papillomatosis without thickening effects at the basal cell layer. The dermal papillae extend

【组织病理】

表皮角化过度,乳头瘤样增生,不伴表皮生发层增厚,真皮乳头向上延伸呈

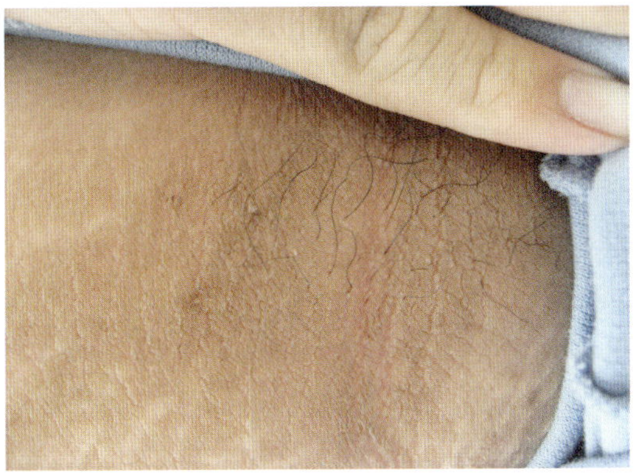

Fig. 18-15　Drug-induced acanthosis nigricans(图 18-15　药物诱导的黑棘皮病)

upwards to form finger-like projections. At the epidermal depressions filled with keratins, slight or moderate acanthosis are easily seen. Slight hyperpigmentation of the basal cell layer is often accompanied by pigment-laden macrophages in the papillary dermis. A mild perivascular lymphocytes infiltrate may be present.

手指状，在乳头凹陷处有轻度或中度棘层肥厚并充满角质，基底细胞层轻度黑素增多，真皮可见噬色素细胞，血管周围有少量淋巴细胞浸润。

【Diagnosis and Differential Diagnosis】

The characteristic skin hyperpigmentation and verrucous hyperplasia on the cervical, axillary, inguinal and other folded areas, in combination with histopathological features, lead to a straightforward diagnosis of this disease. However, the condition should in every case be carefully evaluated for benign or malignant entities, as malignant acanthosis nigricans is quite aggressive and can spread quickly in a short period of time. Furthermore, acanthosis nigricans should be differentiated from Addison's disease, confluent and reticulate papillomatosis, and keratosis follicularis.

【诊断与鉴别诊断】

根据颈、腋、腹股沟等皱褶部位皮肤色素增加和疣状增生等特点及组织病理检查，本病不难诊断。必须区分良性型或恶性型，恶性型具有侵袭性并可在短期内蔓延。本病应与下列各病相鉴别：Addison 病、融合性网状乳头瘤病和毛囊角化病。

【Treatment】

The goal of acanthosis nigricans treatment is to correct the underlying disease process and to remove or avoid any inducers. The benign type generally does not require treatment, although cosmetic surgery can be carried out if the skin lesions happen to affect the patient's appearance or quality of life. Also, keratolytics, podophyllin or 0.1% tretinoin gel can be applied topically. For cases accompanied by malignancy, visceral tumor detection should be carried out aggressively and early surgical treatment should be given.

【治疗】

寻找可能的致病因素，采取相应的治疗措施，良性型一般不需治疗，若皮损影响美观或患者的生活质量，可进行美容手术。局部外用角质松解剂、足叶草脂或 0.1% 维 A 酸凝胶。对恶性黑棘皮病应积极探查内脏肿瘤，早期手术治疗。

Hua ZHAO(赵华)

Chapter Nineteen　Dermatoses Caused by Disturbances of Pigmentation

第十九章　色素障碍性皮肤病

Section One　Vitiligo

第一节　白　癜　风

Vitiligo is a common acquired pigmentary disease of the skin and mucous membranes that characterized by depigmented macules or patches due to the lack of melanocytes. The white spots may be restricted focally or spread widely, but the color of the skin or mucous tissue around these spots is normal or hyperpigmented.

白癜风(vitiligo)是一种常见的获得性皮肤黏膜色素异常，表现为黑素细胞缺失所致的局限性或泛发性皮肤黏膜脱色性白斑，周边颜色正常或有色素增加。

【Etiology and Pathogenesis】

The etiology of this disease is unknown. The pathogenesis of vitiligo remains obscure but a number of hypotheses have been proposed to explain how the epidermal melanocytes are destroyed. These include neurogenic, self-destructed of the melanocytes, and autoimmune mechanisms. Some genetic trait may also contribute to this skin disorder since some cases do demonstrate a genetic predisposition. It may also be possible to conclude that the disease is caused by multiple factors that occur simultaneously during the pathogenesis of vitiligo.

【病因及发病机制】

本病的病因不明，发病机制尚不清楚，有几种学说来解释黑素细胞遭到破坏的原因，如神经精神学说、黑素细胞自毁学说和自身免疫学说以及遗传因素。本病很可能是由多种因素所致，几种机制可能同时发挥作用。

【Clinical Manifestations】

Vitiligo most often occurs in men and women aged 10 to 30; however, affected people can range from the newborns to the elders with a 1%-2% incidence rate for the entire population. Vitiligo is an acquired pigmentary disorder of the skin and mucous membrane that manifests by depigmented white patches surrounded by a normal or hyperpigmented border (Fig. 19-1). The patches are of various sizes and configurations. The hairs in the vitiliginous areas also turn white. In rare cases, the patches may have red inflammatory borders.

【临床表现】

白癜风初发年龄从刚出生的婴儿到老年人均有，但更常见发生于 10～30 岁的男性与女性。人群中的发病率为 1%～2%。白癜风是一种获得性皮肤黏膜色素异常，表现为黑素细胞缺失所致的局限性脱色性白斑，周边颜色正常或有色素增加(图 19-1)。白斑的大小和形状各异。白斑部位的毛发通常也为白色。白斑的周围偶见红色炎性边界。

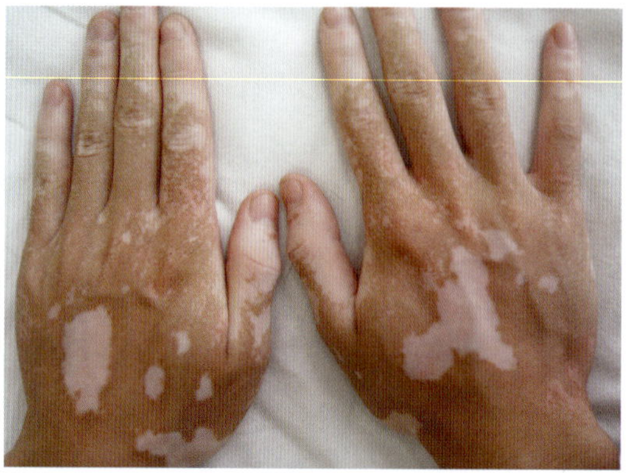

Fig. 19-1　Vitiligo(图 19-1　白癜风)

Vitiligo can be divided into 3 types: localized, generalized and

白癜风可分为局限型、泛发型和全

universal. The localized type can be further classified as focal, segmental, and mucosal. For the focal subtype, a single or a few depigmented spots are restricted at the same anatomical unit. In the segmental subtype, the spots are arranged along the cutaneous nerve segments, and the depigmented spots still do not stretch beyond the vertical midline of the body. Finally, as the name suggests, the mucosal subtype of vitiligo only presents depigmented spots in mucosal areas.

身型。局限型包括局灶型、节段型和黏膜型。局灶型表现为同一解剖部位单个或数个色素脱失斑，但不呈节段分布。节段型表现为沿皮神经节段支配的皮肤区域分布的节段性色素脱失斑，不超过身体中线。黏膜型表现为仅黏膜处的色素脱失斑。

The generalized type is further classified into the vulgaris, acral and mixed subtypes according to the affected body area. Vulgaris has a widespread distribution of the depigmented patches all over the body. By contrast, in the acral subtype the affected areas are confined to the extremities of the limbs, and periorifacial areas. The mixed subtype is reserved for cases where different types of pigment loss appear in one patient at same time. Finally, the condition known as universal vitiligo occurs when an individual suffers from complete or nearly complete depigmentation.

泛发型包括寻常型、肢端型和混合型。寻常型表现为广泛分布的散在色素脱失斑。肢端型侵犯指(趾)末端和面部腔口周围。混合型表现为几种不同类型白癜风混合存在。全身型白癜风是指全身皮肤均出现脱色。

【Histopathology】

Biopsies of cutaneous lesions show complete absence of melanocytes associated with total loss of epidermal pigmentation. Some lymphocytes or histiocytes or other inflammatory cells may be found in the papillary dermis biopsied from the periphery of the lesions.

【组织病理】

皮损组织病理检查显示黑素细胞及表皮色素明显减少直至全部缺失。皮损周围组织真皮乳头内可发现淋巴细胞和组织细胞等炎症细胞浸润。

【Diagnosis】

The clinical presentation is usually sufficient to confirm the diagnosis; histological examination of the skin biopsy would rule out other causes of pigment loss.

【诊断】

白癜风从临床表现一般就可以确立诊断。皮损组织病理检查可以排除某些其他原因引起的色素脱失。

【Differential Diagnosis】

The disease should be differentiated from guttate hypomelanosis, postinflammatory hypopigmentation, piebaldism, nevus depigmentosus, senile leukoderma and nevus anemicus.

【鉴别诊断】

本病需和点状色素减少症、炎症后色素减退、斑驳病、无色素痣、老年性白斑和贫血痣相鉴别。

【Treatment】

The treatment of vitiligo can be frustrating. Resolution by spontaneous repigmentation occurs in only 15%-20% of cases. The major concern is cosmetic. Topical glucocorticoids may be useful on focal or limited lesions, but the thinner skin areas of the face seem to respond best. The systemic application of glucocorticoids is only used for rapid control of the progress of vitiligo. 0.1% tacrolimus ointment is more effective for facial vitiligo. Topical tacrolimus ointment in combination with laser irradiation (308 nm) is also effective for local skin lesions. Narrowband ultraviolet, psoralen photochemotherapy, 308 nm excimer laser and focusing light therapy have certain curative effects on vitiligo.

【治疗】

白癜风治疗困难，仅有15%～20%的患者可发生自发性的色素恢复。治疗的目的主要是为了美容。局部应用糖皮质激素可能对局灶型或皮损较少的患者有效，面部皮肤较薄的部位反应最好。系统应用糖皮质激素仅用于快速控制白癜风的进展。局部外用免疫抑制剂，如0.1%的他克莫司软膏对面部白癜风有显著疗效。局部用他克莫司软膏联合波长为308 nm的激光照射，对局部皮损有显著疗效。窄波紫外线、补骨脂光化学

Surgical treatment can be considered for small lesions if the above methods are not effective. Alternatively, bleaching regimens may be considered when the affected area is more than 50% of the entire body surface area.

疗法、308 nm 准分子激光及聚焦微光疗都有一定的疗效。

如果上述方法无效，局限性皮损可手术治疗。如果皮损超过体表面积的50%，可以考虑用脱色方法治疗，使色素完全脱失。

Section Two Melasma

第二节 黄褐斑

Melasma is an acquired hypermelanosis occurring most commonly on women's faces and has an unknown etiology. Typically it presents as symmetrical hyperpigmented macules or patches.

黄褐斑(melasma)是一种常见的、好发于女性面部的、多对称发生的、原因不明的后天性色素沉着过度性疾病。

【Etiology and Pathogenesis】

Although no causative agent has been identified, clinical manifestations suggest a strong link between pathogenesis and female hormonal activity such as pregnancy, hormone replacement therapy, or the use of oral contraceptives. It is also closely associated with exposure to sunlight. Other supposed causative factors are photosensitizing medications, anticonvulsants, isotretinion, autoimmune thyroid disease, visceral tumors, liver disease and genetics. Some believe that cosmetics may be implicated in the development of melasma.

【病因及发病机制】

黄褐斑的确切发病原因仍不清楚。但临床表现显示其与女性激素异常(怀孕、激素替代疗法和口服避孕药)和日晒密切相关。据报道此病还与光敏性药物、抗惊厥药物、异维A酸、自身免疫性甲状腺疾病、内脏肿瘤、肝病和遗传有关，甚至与化妆品也有关。

【Clinical Manifestations】

Melasma is much more common in women (typically in their 30s) than in men. Approximately 90% of the cases are female, and only 10% are male. The light to dark brown hyperpigmented macules are usually distributed in the centrofacial and malar areas, with occasional involvement of the mandibular areas. The lesions can be confluent or punctuate with sharp edges (Fig. 19-2). A mild erythema may also be seen sometimes. No scales or subjective symptoms are manifest.

【临床表现】

黄褐斑好发于女性(特别是30多岁者)，男性少见，女性患者约占90%，而男性仅占报告病例的10%。皮损以面部中央和颧部最为常见，下颌部也可见受累。黄褐斑皮损的特点为不规则的浅褐色至深褐色、融合或散在的斑疹，边界清楚(图19-2)，有时可见轻度红斑，局部无鳞屑及主观症状。

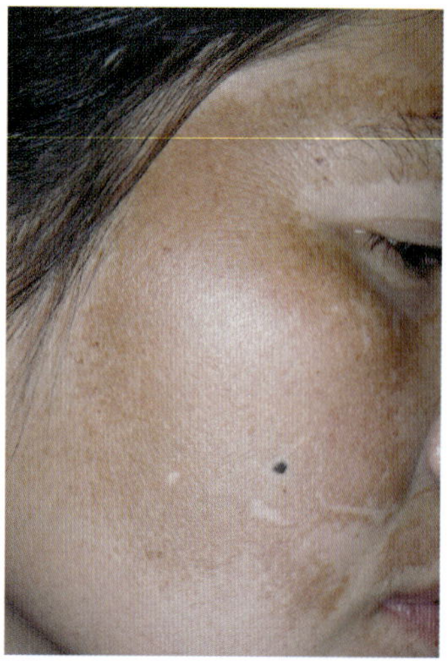

Fig. 19-2 Melasma(图 19-2 黄褐斑)

【Histopathology】

Histology typically shows increased melanin in the keratinocytes throughout the epidermal layers. The absolute number of melanocytes is normal or increased in the epidermis as well. Dermal melanin may be found in the melanophages which often congregate around small vessels in the superficial and mid papillary dermis to give a scattered pattern.

【组织病理】

皮损组织病理检查显示表皮各层角质形成细胞中黑素增加，表皮内黑素细胞数量正常或增加，真皮乳头层的上部和中部小血管周围聚集有散在的噬黑素细胞。

【Diagnosis】

Melasma can be diagnosed based upon the typical color and the location of the skin patches. Histological findings from biopsies of the lesions (as described above) may also be of help with differential diagnosis.

【诊断】

根据皮损的发病部位和典型颜色常可对黄褐斑做出诊断。皮损组织病理检查(如上述)有助于鉴别诊断。

【Differential Diagnosis】

The differential diagnosis of the lesions should include Riehl melanosis and poikiloderma of Civatte.

【鉴别诊断】

黄褐斑需和 Riehl 黑病变、Civatte 皮肤异色病等相鉴别。

【Treatment】

The best treatment for melasma is prevention. The key to preventing melasma is to avoid unnecessary exposure to sunlight and to apply sunscreen with broad-spectrum UVA protection whenever the patient is engaged in any outdoor activities. A combination of tretinoin cream, a bleaching cream containing 2%-4% hydroquinone, and a topical glucocorticoid cream may be useful in controlling some types of melasma. In severe cases, laser, cryotherapy, chemical peeling and even surgery may be applied to remove the dark pigment from the lesions, but one should be aware of the likelihood of scar formation, pigmentation and other side effects when these more aggressive treatments are used.

【治疗】

黄褐斑治疗的最好的方法是预防，其中最重要的是避免过度日晒和每天使用宽谱 UVA 遮光剂。联合应用维 A 酸霜、含有 2%～4%氢醌的脱色霜以及糖皮质激素霜对某些类型的黄褐斑常有效。激光、冷冻、化学剥脱，甚至手术方法治疗以去除比较深的色素，但要注意瘢痕形成及色素异常沉着等副作用。

Section Three　Freckles

第三节　雀　斑

Freckles are very common autosomal inherited skin conditions that are characterized by multiple uniform small brown marks arising on the face or other areas exposed to direct sunlight.

雀斑(freckles)是一种很常见的皮肤损害，常染色体显性遗传为特征，主要表现为面部或其他曝光部位均一的成群点状的褐色色素斑。

【Etiology and Pathogenesis】

Although the key element for freckle development has not been determined, clinical pictures indicated that the sunlight induces freckles since they become apparent when exposed to sunlight in summer, and are less perceptible in winter. Freckles are an inherited disorder that can be passed on to offspring as an autosomal dominant trait. In such cases, the lesions typically appear in the same locations as the parents.

【病因及发病机制】

雀斑的确切发病原因仍不清楚，但临床发现其明显与日光暴露直接有关，夏季皮损较冬季更明显。雀斑可遗传给后代，其后代可在类似部位发生相似的皮损，以常染色体显性遗传为特征。

【Clinical Manifestations】

The number of pigmented marks varies with the individual, and the condition is more often seen in females. Commonly, freckles first appear in childhood, increasing in number in adulthood, but generally become less noticeable as the person ages. The freckles are most commonly found on sun-exposed areas, such as the nose, cheeks, neck, shoulders and dorsa of the hands, and present as multiple, small, tanned macules, about 2 mm in diameter, with uniform pigmentation (Fig. 19-3).

【临床表现】

女性好发,雀斑常初发于儿童,皮损数目因人而异,成人期逐渐增多,老年后可消退,易发生于鼻、面颊、颈、肩和手背等日光暴露部位,主要表现为均一的成群的针头至粟粒(2 mm)大小、淡褐色至黑褐色点状斑(图 19-3)。

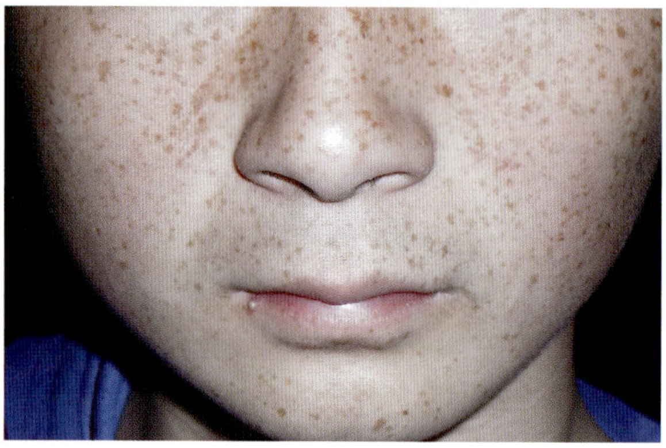

Fig. 19-3 Freckles(图 19-3 雀斑)

【Histopathology】

Histopathologically, the number of melanocytes in the lesions is normal or even diminished in the epidermis. However, the melanosomes are larger in size in affected areas than those in the surrounding normal skin ultrastructurally.

【组织病理】

皮损组织病理检查显示皮损处表皮的黑素细胞数量正常甚至减少,超微结构显示黑素小体比周围正常皮肤中的要大。

【Diagnosis】

Freckles can be diagnosed based upon the typical coloration and configuration of the skin spots. Biopsy is rarely necessary but the histological finding of lesion biopsy described above may help with definitive diagnosis.

【诊断】

雀斑可以根据其皮损的典型颜色和形态而诊断。活检并非必需,但皮损组织病理可以帮助进一步确诊。

【Differential Diagnosis】

The differential diagnosis includes lentigo simplex, centrofacial lentiginosis, Peutz-Jeghers syndrome and xeroderma pigmentosum.

【鉴别诊断】

本病必须和单纯性黑子、面正中黑子、Peutz-Jeghers 综合征和着色性干皮病相鉴别。

【Treatment】

Exposure to sunlight should be minimized and sunscreen with broad-spectrum UVA coverage may be used daily to prevent aggravation of the freckling due to sun exposure. Topical applications of compounds such as bleaching creams with 2%-4% hydroquinone, tretinoin, adapalene are effective and liquid nitrogen freezing are also available. Aggressive surgical options, such as Q-switched laser surgery, or chemical peeling, may also be attempted

【治疗】

避免日晒和每天使用宽谱 UVA 遮光剂,以防日晒而加重雀斑。局部应用含有 2%～4%氢醌的脱色霜、维 A 酸、阿达帕林和液氮冷冻有效。以上方法无效者可采用更激进的方法如调 Q 开关激光、化学剥脱。调 Q 开关激光治疗疗效肯定,但不能防止复发。

to make freckles less pronounced if the methods described above are not effective. Q-switched laser has definite clinical efficacy, but can't prevent the recurrence of the lesions.

Section Four Riehl Melanosis

Riehl melanosis is a common acquired hypermelanosis producing grey to brown pigmentation on the face.

【Etiology and Pathogenesis】

The exact etiology of Riehl melanosis remains unknown. However, there is a clear etiological link to long-term exposure to tar, asphalt, petroleum and petroleum derivatives, the cosmetic products containing mineral oil, alkanes, spices, antiseptics, surfactants, and sun exposure.

【Clinical Manifestations】

The condition can occur at any age, but primarily appears for the first time in middle-aged women. The commonly affected areas are the sun-exposed regions such as the forehead, malar and periauricular areas and sides of the neck. Typically, a diffuse, vaguely circumscribed grayish-beige-brown-sable pigmented patch appears on the face (Fig. 19-4). In most cases, erythema and itching precede to the pigmentation.

第四节 Riehl 黑变病

Riehl 黑变病(Riehl melanosis)是好发于颜面部的后天获得性灰褐色色素沉着性疾病。

【病因及发病机制】

本病的确切病因尚未完全确定。但明显与长期接触焦油、沥青、石油及其衍生物和含有矿物油及烃类化合物、香料、防腐剂、表面活性剂等的化妆品及日晒有关。

【临床表现】

本病任何年龄均可发生,好发于中年女性,皮损以前额、颧骨、耳前、耳后及颈部两侧的曝光部位明显,本病皮损表现为播散分布,边界不清的呈淡灰色、灰褐色、褐色、深褐色面部色素沉着斑(图 19-4)。大多数患者色素沉着前可出现红斑和瘙痒。

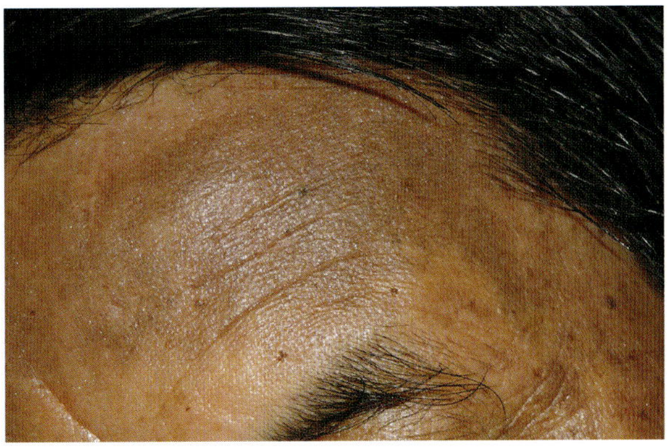

Fig. 19-4 Melanosis(图 19-4 黑变病)

【Histopathology】

Biopsies of cutaneous lesions show hydropic degeneration of basal cells, superficial perivascular inflammatory cell infiltrates composed of lymphocytes and histiocytes, variable numbers of melanophages and free melanin in the papillary dermis and superficial perivasculature.

【Diagnosis】

When the typical clinical manifestations and histological features described above occur in a patient, Riehl melanosis is diagnosed.

【组织病理】

皮损组织病理检查显示基底细胞液化变性,真皮浅层血管周围有淋巴细胞及组织细胞浸润,真皮乳头及浅层血管周围有噬黑素细胞及游离的黑素颗粒。

【诊断】

当患者出现上述典型临床表现,Riehl 黑变病可以诊断,皮损组织病理可以帮助进一步确诊。

【Differential Diagnosis】

Differentiation from melasma, Civatte poikiloderma, Addison's disease and other hypermelanoses is necessary.

【鉴别诊断】

本病必须和黄褐斑、Civatte 皮肤异色病、Addison 病及其他色素沉着性疾病相鉴别。

【Treatment】

Exposure to sunlight and long-term exposure to tar compounds should be avoided. A complete sun block with 2.5% titania or 5% paraminan should be used daily. Topical application of bleaching creams with 2%-4% hydroquinone and intravenous injection of vitamin C are also useful.

【治疗】

避免日晒和长期接触焦油类等化合物。每天应用含有 2.5%二氧化钛霜或 5%对氨苯甲酸防晒霜。局部应用含有 2%~4%氢醌的脱色霜和静脉注射维生素 C 可能有效。

Section Five Peutz-Jeghers Syndrome

Peutz-Jeghers syndrome is an autosomal dominant disease characterized by hyperpigmentation on perioral skin, lips, oral mucosa, distal extremities, and by the presence of gastrointestinal polyps.

【Etiology and Pathogenesis】

Peutz-Jeghers syndrome is considered an autosomal dominant inherited disease in which about 50% of patients have mutations on the LKB1 gene located on chromosome 19 (19p13.3). However, the remaining cases seem to occur sporadically.

【Clinical Manifestations】

Pigmented macules appear mostly at birth or in infancy, and tend to increase in number and size with age, fading gradually through adulthood. Typical lesions are flattened, asymptomatic, and blackish to brown macules 2-10 mm in diameter with sharply defined margins. They occur symmetrically on perioral skin, lips, oral mucosa, palms and soles (Fig. 19-5). Polyps appear later than the pigmented macules and can develop in any part of gastrointestinal tract, but most commonly in the jejunum, where they can occur singly, or in numbers greater than ten. These polyps may sometimes cause intussusception, intestinal obstruction, abdominal pain, diarrhea, melena and malnutrition.

【Histopathology】

Histologically, the pigmentation of basal cells is increased but the number of melanocytes is normal. Melanophages are revealed in the superficial layer of the dermis. No special histological features of the gastrointestinal polyps are noted compared to other regular gastrointestinal polyps. However the malignancy rates for these gastrointestinal polyps are 3%-25% according to the literature.

第五节 Peutz-Jeghers 综合征

Peutz-Jeghers 综合征(Peutz-Jeghers syndrome)是一种常染色体显性遗传性疾病，特点是口周、唇、口腔黏膜、四肢远端的色素沉着和胃肠道息肉。

【病因及发病机制】

Peutz-Jeghers 综合征是一种常染色体显性遗传性疾病。50%的患者中 19 号染色体(19p13.3)上 LKB1 基因发生突变引起本病。但是一半的患者是偶发病例。

【临床表现】

色素沉着斑出现于出生时和婴儿期，随着年龄增大，其数目和大小也增加，成人后可逐渐消退。表现为平的、无症状的、边界清楚、直径为 2~10 mm 大小的浅黑色或棕色的斑疹。它们对称发生于口周、唇、口腔黏膜和手足(图19-5)。息肉较色斑出现迟，可发生于胃肠道任何部位，但好发于空肠。息肉可为单发或 10 个以上的多发。它们可导致肠套叠、肠梗阻、腹痛、腹泻及黑便。还可伴发营养不良等。

【组织病理】

皮损组织学上表现为基底层色素增加，但黑素细胞数量正常，真皮浅层有噬色素细胞。胃肠道息肉与其他疾病所致的息肉无明显组织学特异性，但有报道息肉癌变率为 3%~25%。

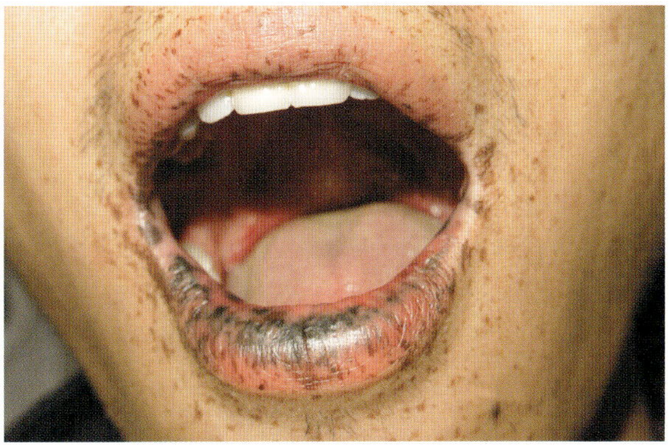

Fig. 19-5 Peutz-Jeghers syndrome(图 19-5 Peutz-Jeghers 综合征)

【Diagnosis】

The diagnosis is based on the typical clinical manifestations and histological features.

【Differential Diagnosis】

Differentiation from lentigo, Laugier-Hunziker syndrome and Cronkhite-Canada syndrome is necessary.

【Treatment】

Alexandrite laser therapy and dermabrasion are effective in reducing pigmentation. Endoscopic and surgical excision should be considered for the gastrointestinal polyps.

【诊断】

Peutz-Jeghers 综合征根据典型的临床表现和组织病理特征常易诊断。

【鉴别诊断】

本病必须和雀斑样痣、Laugier-Hunziker 综合征及 Cronkhite-Canada 综合征鉴别。

【治疗】

紫翠宝石激光治疗和皮肤磨削术对减轻色素沉着斑有效。胃肠道息肉可采用消化内镜或外科手术切除。

Si-yuan CHEN(陈思远)

Chapter Twenty Connective Tissue Diseases

第二十章 结缔组织疾病

Connective tissue disease refers to any pathogenic process which has connective tissues as its primary target. The disease tends to share many features with autoimmune diseases such as producing auto-antibodies specifically against connective tissues, and affecting multiple organs at the same time. In dermatological practice, these connective tissue inflammatory conditions may present as variety of skin lesions in different patients. Today, the diagnosis of connective tissue disease is based primarily on criteria established by the American College of Rheumatology, in which cutaneous lesions are also included. Therefore, the dermatologist's role in the diagnosis and treatment of connective tissue disease is quite important.

一般地讲，结缔组织疾病是指发病以结缔组织作为主要靶点的疾病。结缔组织疾病与自身免疫性疾病有某些共同点，表现在会产生针对自身结缔组织和多种器官特异性的自身抗体。在皮肤科，这些结缔组织疾病表现为在不同的患者具有各种不同的皮肤损害。结缔组织疾病的诊断主要依据美国风湿病协会制订的标准，标准中包括了皮损的表现。因此，皮肤科医师在结缔组织疾病的诊断和治疗中扮演了重要角色。

Section One Lupus Erythematosus

第一节 红斑狼疮

Lupus erythematosus (LE) is the diagnostic name for a closely connected group of conditions that produce a variety of systemic changes not limited to the skin. Two good examples of this are systemic lupus erythematosus (SLE) and neonatal lupus erythematosus. The term is also used for patients with localized cutaneous lesions such as those seen in discoid lupus erythematosus (DLE), lupus erythematosus profundus and subacute cutaneous lupus erythematosus (SCLE). Cutaneous LE may be subcategorized as acute, subacute, or chronic, with each subcategory having its own characteristic features (Tab. 20-1). Since acute cutaneous LE usually occurs as one manifestation of SLE, it will be discussed in the section on SLE. On the other hand, SCLE and chronic LE only involve the skin, and so are normally not able to meet the diagnostic criteria for SLE.

红斑狼疮(lupus erythematosus, LE)是对一些会引起各种系统性改变的疾病的诊断名称，不仅仅只限于皮肤损害，如系统性红斑狼疮(SLE)和新生儿红斑狼疮。它还包括可见局限性皮损的红斑狼疮，如盘状红斑狼疮(DLE)、深部红斑狼疮和亚急性皮肤型红斑狼疮(SCLE)。皮肤型红斑狼疮可分为急性、亚急性和慢性3个亚类，每个亚类都有其特征性表现(表20-1)。由于急性皮肤型红斑狼疮通常是SLE的表现，所以将在SLE中讨论。SCLE和慢性红斑狼疮通常只局限于皮肤，所以大多数患者都达不到SLE的诊断标准。

Tab. 20-1 Lesions of cutaneous LE(表20-1 皮肤型红斑狼疮的皮损)

Acute(急性)	Progression in a few days(几天内进展); butterfly rash, alopecia, palmar erythema, aphthus ulcers(蝴蝶斑、脱发、掌红斑、阿弗他溃疡)
Subacute (亚急性)	Progression in a few weeks to several months (几周到几月内进展); papulosquamous lesions and annular to polycyctic erythema (丘疹鳞屑性损害和环状-多环状红斑)
Chronic(慢性)	Progression over long periods of time (进展的时间很长); discoid lupus erythematosus, lupus panniculitis, lupus profundus, nodular cutaneous lupus mucinosis (DLE、狼疮性脂膜炎、深部红斑狼疮、结节性皮肤狼疮黏蛋白病)

1. Systemic lupus erythematosus (SLE)

一、系统性红斑狼疮(SLE)

SLE is an autoimmune disease with an unknown etiology. Young females are most frequently affected by SLE. This is a chronic immunologic inflammatory disease that can affect various

系统性红斑狼疮(systemic lupus erythematosus, SLE)是一种自身免疫性疾病，其确切病因未明。青年女性最为

organs of the body, such as the kidneys, heart, joints, hematologic system and the central nervous system. Multiple organ failure may occur in severe cases.

常见。它能产生慢性免疫性炎症反应，累及肾脏、心脏、关节、血液系统和中枢神经系统，甚至发生多器官功能衰竭。

The typical mucocutaneous manifestations include a malar "butterfly" rash, DLE, oral ulcer, solar photosensitivity and alopecia.

典型的皮肤黏膜损害为颧部蝶形红斑、DLE、口腔溃疡、光敏和脱发。

Laboratory tests reveal positive responses for antinuclear antibody (ANA), anti-dsDNA antibody and anti-Sm antibody, existence of LE cells and a false positive serologic test for syphilis, along with hypocomplementemia and pancytopenia.

实验室检查有抗核抗体阳性、抗双链 DNA 抗体阳性、抗 Sm 抗体阳性、狼疮细胞阳性、血清学梅毒反应假阳性、补体减少和全血细胞减少。

Oral glucocorticoids are still the first choice for SLE treatment.

本病的主要治疗手段是口服糖皮质激素。

【Epidemiology】

The age at onset tends to be from 10 to 30. It is more common (with a ratio of roughly 10 : 1) in females than in males. In other words, the vast majority of patients are women of childbearing age.

【流行病学】

多于 10 到 30 岁之间起病。女性多于男性，男女的发病率为 1 : 10。所以大多数的患者是育龄期的女性。

【Etiology and Pathogenesis】

SLE is an autoimmune disease in which the human immune system mistakenly attacks healthy tissue although the pathogenesis has not been completely clarified. Hereditary predisposition, viral infection, gonadal hormones and other factors are thought to interact in a complex manner to trigger an immune overreaction. As a result, ANA, anti-DNA antibody and anti-Sm antibody are all found in this disease. These autoantibodies are presumably responsible for directly attacking the tissues via type Ⅱ hypersensitivity reaction, or by forming immune complexes via activation of complement cascades (type Ⅲ hypersensitivity reaction). By the end of the progression of the disease, these immune responses lead to inflammation and damage to various body tissues.

【病因及发病机制】

SLE 是一种自身免疫性疾病，其确切病因及发病机制尚未完全阐明。一般认为，遗传素质、病毒感染、性激素和其他因素等通过复杂途径相互作用，触发机体免疫紊乱，最终导致 SLE 的发生。SLE 病程中可产生抗核抗体、抗 DNA 抗体和抗 Sm 抗体，这些抗体通过Ⅱ型变态反应直接破坏组织或通过形成免疫复合物产生补体级联反应来破坏组织(Ⅲ型变态反应)，最终导致全身各器官发生炎症反应。

【Clinical Manifestations】

(1) Cutaneous lesions: 80% or more of all SLE cases present with the typical skin lesions. The four main manifestations of the skin in the diagnostic criteria are erythema on the malar areas, chronic DLE, oral ulcers and photosensitivity.

① Erythema on malar areas: also known as a butterfly rash. This is the most characteristic eruption of SLE, and is seen in about 90% of all cases. Edematous erythema appears symmetrically on the malar areas and the nasal bridge, forming the butterfly pattern. Generally, this erythema spares the nasolabial folds. The margin of the erythema is relatively well-defined, and is slightly elevated (Fig. 20-1). Blistering is rare. The patients are otherwise asymptomatic or have mild subjective symptoms, such as a slight

【临床表现】

(1) 皮肤损害　80%以上的 SLE 患者会有典型的皮肤损害。SLE 的诊断标准中四个主要的皮肤症状为颧部红斑、慢性 DLE、口腔溃疡和光敏。

①颧部红斑：又称为蝶形红斑，这是最典型的皮损，可见于约 90% 的患者。颧部水肿性红斑对称性扩大并在鼻背部连接而形成蝴蝶形，通常不会超过鼻唇沟。红斑边缘相对明显并有轻微隆起(图 20-1)。水疱很少见。患者无症状或有轻微的主观症状，如轻微的灼热感。愈后不留瘢痕。

burning sensation. The rash will heal without scarring.

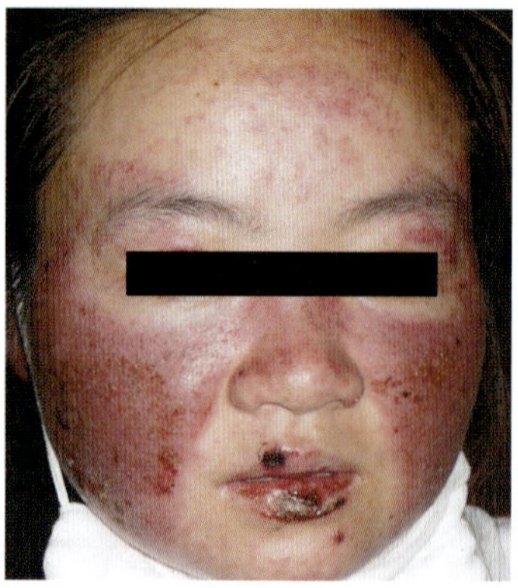

Fig. 20-1 SLE-butterfly rash(图 20-1 系统性红斑狼疮-蝶形红斑)

②Discoid erythema:DLE is a well-defined discoidal erythema. It is seen in 30% of the patients with SLE, and occurs predominantly on sun-exposed sites such as the face, lips and ears. Adherent keratotic scaling and crusts are often seen. The skin lesions gradually evolve into atrophic scarring and cause alopecia when the scalp is involved (described below).

②盘状红斑:DLE 的皮损表现为边界清楚的圆盘状红斑,可见于 30%的 SLE 患者,主要发生在暴露部位如面部、嘴唇和耳廓,常有黏着性角化性鳞屑和痂。盘状红斑逐渐进展为瘢痕萎缩性皮损,累及头皮时会产生脱发(见后面相关章节)。

③Palmar erythema: this is seen in about 50% of SLE cases. Diffuse erythema occurs on the palms particularly on the thenar and hypothenar areas. The lesions are hyperkeratotic and often accompanied by scaling.

③掌红斑:可见于约 50%的 SLE 患者,弥漫性红斑会出现在手掌,尤其是大、小鱼际,皮损过度角化,常覆有鳞屑。

④Alopecia: the occurrence of short, thin, broken hairs at the front margin of the scalp results in uneven hair length (lupus hair). The severity of the alopecia usually correlates with SLE progression.

④脱发:前缘发际会出现细短的断发,形成长短不一的头发(狼疮发)。脱发的严重程度可反映 SLE 的进展。

⑤Enanthema: this occurs in about 40% of SLE cases. Small hemorrhagic lesions with a red halo and small ulcers appear on the lips, oral mucosa, pharynx and pharyngeal mucosa. They may be found in DLE as well when the mucous membranes are involved.

⑤黏膜疹:可见于约 40%的 SLE 患者。在嘴唇、口腔黏膜和咽喉部黏膜上会出现小的出血性皮损,带有红晕和小溃疡。在 DLE 也可见到这种黏膜损害。

⑥Photosensitivity: photosensitive erythema rash is often localized or diffuse in sun-exposed areas of the face, arms, or hands, and generally lasts for more than 1 day.

⑥光敏:光敏性皮损通常为暴露部位如脸部、手臂或者双手处的局限性或弥漫性红斑,持续 1 天以上。

⑦Subcutaneous nodules: often presenting on the face, buttocks and upper arms. This condition is also known as lupus erythematosus profundus (described later).

⑦皮下结节:可发生在面部、臀部和上臂,也称为深部红斑狼疮(见后面相关章节)。

⑧Other cutaneous symptoms: these include palmoplantar keratosis, purpura, Raynaud's phenomenon, erythema multiforme, and ulcers on the extremities.

⑧其他皮肤症状:包括掌跖角皮症、紫癜、Raynaud 现象、多形红斑和四肢溃疡。

(2) Systemic Symptoms: the symptoms of SLE vary greatly from person to person. They may begin suddenly with fever, fatigue, arthralgia and generalized edema accompanied by the cutaneous eruptions described above.

(2) 系统症状 SLE 的症状因人而异,可以突然发热、全身疲乏、关节痛和水肿起病,伴随上述皮肤症状。

①Renal symptoms: lupus nephritis is the most common renal impairment and it can cause considerable damage to SLE patients. Therefore it has often been used as a measure of the prognosis of the condition. The main pathogenic changes for SLE are proteinuria, hematuria, nephrotic syndrome and renal failure.

①肾脏症状：狼疮性肾炎是最常见的肾损害，严重威胁 SLE 患者的健康。因此它常被用来度量 SLE 的预后。SLE 对肾脏造成的损害主要有蛋白尿、血尿、肾病综合征和肾功能衰竭等。

②Arthritis: this occurs in more than 90% of patients. It may affect one joint or several joints at the same time. Usually, the symptom lasts for a short period of time. Proximal interphalangeal and metacarpophalangeal joints, knee, shoulder and elbow joints are most frequently affected presenting as tenderness, swelling and effusions which are symmetric, nonerosive, and usually nondeforming.

②关节炎：可见于 90%以上的 SLE 患者，为单发或多发，多数患者持续时间短暂，近端指(趾)间关节及掌指关节、膝、肩和肘关节最常受累。SLE 的关节炎为对称性、非侵蚀性的，并且通常关节不变形，表现为关节疼痛、肿胀以及渗出。

③Cardiac symptoms: there are a variety of symptoms that can occur due to involvement of the heart in SLE such as Libman-Sacks endocarditis, pericarditis and cardiac tamponade.

③心脏症状：SLE 累及心脏时可产生许多症状，主要有利-赛疣状心内膜炎、心包炎和心包压塞。

④Mental and neurological symptoms: central nervous system (CNS) manifestations such as convulsions, altered consciousness, depression, schizophrenia-like symptoms or cognitive deficit can be observed in about 20% of all cases during the acute active period. However, it may sometimes be difficult to differentiate CNS lupus from similar symptoms caused by the side effects of long-term use of glucocorticoids.

④精神和神经症状：中枢神经系统损害，如惊厥、意识损害、抑郁症、精神分裂症或认知缺陷，可在约 20%的急性活动期患者中出现。有时，中枢性狼疮与长期使用糖皮质激素的副作用难以区分。

⑤Blood abnormalities: hemolytic anemia (autoimmune hemolytic anemia), leukocytopenia and thrombocytopenia are present.

⑤血液异常：可见溶血性贫血(自身免疫性溶血性贫血)、白细胞减少和血小板减少。

【Complications】

The most common complications of SLE are similar to those of other connective tissue diseases such as rheumatoid arthritis, scleroderma, Sjögren syndrome and dermatomyositis or overlap syndrome. As a result of the reduction of cellular immunity in SLE, viral infections (e. g., herpes zoster), bacterial infections and fungal infections may occur in some cases.

【并发症】

SLE 的最常见并发症与其他结缔组织病如类风湿关节炎、硬皮病、Sjögren 综合征和皮肌炎或重叠综合征类似。由于细胞免疫功能的低下，有些 SLE 患者会并发病毒感染(如带状疱疹)、细菌感染和真菌感染。

【Laboratory Findings】

Routine blood counts may reveal anemia, leukocytopenia, lymphocytopenia and thrombocytopenia. The erythrocyte sedimentation rate (ESR) is often elevated as a result of the generalized inflammatory reactions, but C-reactive protein (CRP) is only slightly increased in most cases. Serum protein electrophoresis may show increased human immunoglobulins and IgG and decreased complements (C3, C4, and CH50 specifically). The blood tests commonly used for definite diagnosis of SLE will detect a variety of autoantibodies such as anti-nuclear antibodies, anti-DNA antibodies especially anti-double-stranded DNA (anti-dsDNA) antibodies and

【实验室检查】

可见贫血、白细胞减少、淋巴细胞减少和血小板减少。由于全身性炎症，血沉加快，但 C 反应蛋白(CRP)只略增高。血清蛋白电泳显示人免疫球蛋白和 IgG 增高，补体特别是 C3、C4 和 CH50 降低。SLE 是自身免疫性疾病，血清中可检测到各种抗体，如抗核抗体、抗 DNA 抗体(尤其是抗双链 DNA 抗体)和抗 ENA 抗体。当血清中抗磷脂抗体阳性时，梅毒血清学试验呈假阳性。

anti-ENA antibodies. However, while antiphospholipid antibodies are positive, one should be aware that these antibodies are sometimes correlated with a false positive serologic test for syphilis.

【Histopathology】

Pathological findings of SLE vary depending on the stage of the disease at presentation. The skin biopsy may reveal epidermal atrophy, keratotic plugs, vacuolar degeneration and edema in the superficial dermis, mucin deposition, or perivascular and periadnexal inflammatory infiltration of lymphocytes in the dermis. Under immunofluorescence microscopy, IgG, IgM and C3 may be found to accumulate in the BMZ of the unaffected normal-appearing skin around the margin of a skin lesion (so-called lupus band test, Fig. 20-2).

【组织病理】

病理检查结果也因人而异，这主要与每位患者的病程有关，可见表皮萎缩、角质栓、空泡变性、真皮浅层水肿、黏蛋白沉积和血管周围及附属器周围淋巴细胞的炎症性浸润。在皮损边缘看似正常皮肤处进行活检，行免疫荧光检查后可见基膜带有 IgG、IgM 和 C3 沉积(即狼疮带试验，图 20-2)。

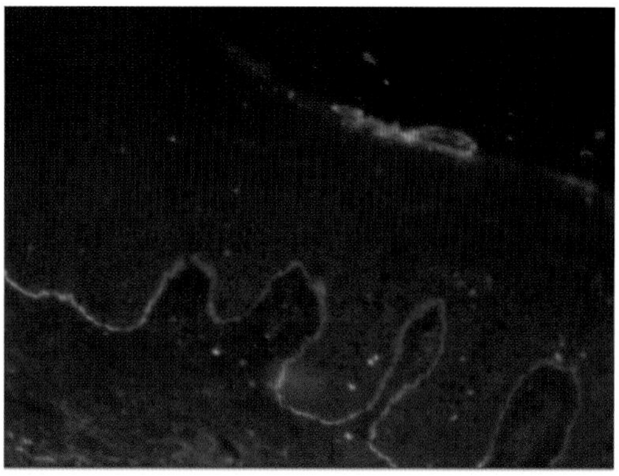

Fig. 20-2　Lupus band test(图 20-2　狼疮带试验)

【Diagnosis】

Tab. 20-2 below lists the 1997 update of the American College of Rheumatology (ACR) criteria for the diagnosis of SLE. As a rule, SLE patients must meet 4 or more of the 11 diagnostic criteria shown in Tab. 20-2 for an SLE confirmation, although the 4 criteria may not all necessarily appear at the same stage of the disease, and some symptoms may appear later. The doctor will therefore need to observe and follow up carefully with the patient.

【诊断】

目前普遍采用美国风湿病学会 1997 年修订的 SLE 分类标准(表 20-2)。通常，满足分类标准 11 项中的 4 项或 4 项以上可诊断为 SLE。有的患者暂不能同时满足 4 项标准，但会在日后陆续出现其他症状，因此需要认真观察和随访。

Tab. 20-2　Updated (1997) American College of Rheumatology Diagnostic Criteria for SLE

(表 20-2　美国风湿病学会 1997 年修订的 SLE 分类标准)

Criterion (标准)	Definition (定义)
SLE can be diagnosed if any 4 or more of the following 11 criteria are present, serially or simultaneously, during any interval of observation(在病程中任何阶段逐渐或者同时出现分类标准 11 项中的 4 项或 4 项以上可诊断为 SLE)	
1. Malar rash (颊部红斑)	Fixed, flat or raised erythema over the malar eminences, tending to avoid the nasolabial folds(固定红斑，扁平或高起，在两颧突出部位，不累及鼻唇沟)
2. Discoid rash (盘状红斑)	Erythematous raised patches with adherent keratotic scaling and follicular plugging (older lesions may demonstrate atrophic scarring)(片状高起于皮肤的红斑，黏附有角化鳞屑和毛囊栓；陈旧病变可发生萎缩性瘢痕)

续表

Criterion（标准）	Definition（定义）
3. Photosensitivity（光敏）	Skin rash as a result of unusual reaction to sunlight, by patient history or physician observation（对日光异常的反应引起的皮疹，从病史中得知或医师观察到）
4. Oral ulcers（口腔溃疡）	Oral or nasopharyngeal ulcers, usually painless, observed by a physician（经医师观察到的口腔或鼻咽部溃疡，一般为无痛性）
5. Arthritis（关节炎）	Nonerosive arthritis involving 2 or more peripheral joints, characterized by tenderness, swelling, or effusion（非侵蚀性关节炎，累及 2 个或更多的外周关节，有压痛、肿胀或积液）
6. Serositis（浆膜炎）	(A) Pleuritis: convincing history of pleuritic pain or friction rub heard by a physician or evidence of pleural effusion（(A)胸膜炎：经医师听到的胸膜摩擦音或者胸膜炎性痛可靠病史，或者胸膜渗出的证据）
	(B) Pericarditis: documented by ECG or rub or evidence of pericardial effusion（(B)心包炎：心电图记录或者心包摩擦音或者心包渗出的证据）
7. Renal disorder（肾脏病变）	(A) Persistent proteinuria ＞0.5 g/24 h or ＞3＋ if quantification not performed（(A)尿蛋白定量(24 h)＞0.5 g 或定性＋＋＋以上）
	(B) Cellular casts: may be red blood cell, hemoglobin, granular, tubular, or mixed（(B)细胞管型：红细胞、血红蛋白、颗粒、管状或混合管型）
8. Neurologic disorder（神经病变）	(A) Seizures: in the absence of offending drugs or known metabolic derangements (e.g., uremia, ketoacidosis, electrolyte imbalance)（(A)癫痫发作：除外药物或已知的代谢紊乱如尿毒症、酮症酸中毒、电解质失衡）
	(B) Psychosis: in the absence of offending drugs or known metabolic derangements, e.g., uremia, ketoacidosis, electrolyte imbalance（(B)精神病：除外药物或已知的代谢紊乱如尿毒症、酮症酸中毒、电解质失衡）
9. Hematologic disorder（血液学异常）	(A) Hemolytic anemia: with reticulocytosis（(A)溶血性贫血：伴网织红细胞增多）
	(B) Leukopenia: ＜4000/mm^3 total on at least 2 occasions（(B)白细胞减少：＜4000/mm^3，2 次或 2 次以上）
	(C) Lymphopenia: ＜1500/mm^3 on at least 2 occasions（(C)淋巴细胞减少：＜1500/mm^3，2 次或 2 次以上）
	(D) Thrombocytopenia: ＜100000/mm^3 in the absence of offending drugs（(D)血小板减少：＜100000/mm^3，除外药物因素）
10. Immunologic disorder（免疫学异常）	(A) Anti-DNA: antibody to native DNA in abnormal titer（(A)抗 DNA 抗体：抗天然 DNA 抗体异常滴度）
	(B) Anti-Sm: presence of antibody to Smith (Sm) nuclear antigen（(B)抗 Sm：存在抗 Sm 核抗原的抗体）
	(C) Positive finding of antiphospholipid antibodies based on ①an abnormal serum level of IgG or IgM anticardiolipin antibodies; ②a positive test result for lupus anticoagulant using a standard method; ③a false-positive serologic test for syphilis known to be positive for at least 6 months and confirmed by *Treponema pallidum* immobilization or fluorescent treponemal antibody absorption tests（(C)抗磷脂抗体阳性，包括：①抗心磷脂抗体的 IgG 或 IgM 血清水平异常；②用标准方法检测狼疮抗凝物结果阳性；③梅毒血清学假阳性至少 6 个月，并经梅毒螺旋体固定试验或荧光梅毒螺旋体抗体吸收试验证实）
11. Antinuclear antibody (ANA)（抗核抗体，ANA）	An abnormal titer of antinuclear antibody by immunofluorescence or an equivalent assay at any point in time and in the absence of drugs known to be associated with drug-induced lupus syndrome（经免疫荧光试验或等同的方法任何时候检测有异常的抗核抗体滴度，并排除药物诱发的红斑狼疮综合征）

【Treatment】

The regimens for SLE are based primarily on immunosuppressants such as glucocorticoids, cyclophosphamide, azathioprine and cyclosporine. In severe intractable cases, a regimen known as glucocorticoids pulse therapy may be performed to suppress the symptoms. Psychiatric treatments may also need to be considered for a patient with CNS involvement. Other supportive measures may be beneficial such as lifestyle guidance, avoidance of exposure to sunlight and cold, avoidance of physical exhaustion, and improved family planning since SLE tends to be aggravated during pregnancy.

【治疗】

主要治疗手段为使用免疫抑制剂，如糖皮质激素、环磷酰胺、硫唑嘌呤和环孢菌素。危重病例可采用糖皮质激素冲击疗法。在中枢性狼疮中尚需要进行心理治疗。其他支持措施同样很重要，如生活方式的指导、避免阳光直接照射和寒冷、避免过度疲劳。应尽量避免怀孕，因为怀孕可使 SLE 加重。

【Prognosis】

SLE is a chronic and relapsing condition, often with long periods of remission. In the past, patients with renal disorders had a poor prognosis; but today, with renal dialysis being widely employed in clinical practice, the mortality rate of such patients has been greatly reduced (the 5-year survival rate now exceeds 90%). But the fatality rate due to CNS damage or cardiac failure is increasing, and infections resulting from long-term glucocorticoid use have also become one of the leading causes of death.

【预后】

SLE 病程进展缓慢，伴有反复加重和缓解。过去认为 SLE 伴有肾脏损害的患者一般预后很差。然而，由于肾脏透析治疗的广泛应用，死亡率已大大下降(5 年生存率已超过 90%)。但是，中枢神经系统和心脏衰竭造成的死亡人数却有所增加。长期应用糖皮质激素导致的感染已成为致命的因素之一。

2. Discoid lupus erythematosus (DLE)

The term discoid lupus erythematosus (DLE) is named according to the morphology of the skin lesions, whereas SLE is the term for the clinical condition with systemic involvement beyond the skin (e.g., fever, arthralgia). Some but not all patients with DLE may therefore also meet the criteria for SLE. In other words, in most cases of DLE, the skin is the only organ involved. Patients with SLE may have DLE rashes.

二、盘状红斑狼疮

盘状红斑狼疮(discoid lupus erythematosus, DLE)是以皮损命名的，而 SLE 是指伴随有系统症状的狼疮的临床状态如发热、关节痛等。有些 DLE 患者可符合 SLE 的诊断标准，但不绝对。对大多数 DLE 患者来说，皮肤是唯一受累器官。SLE 的患者可有 DLE 的皮损。

【Clinical Manifestations】

Single or Multiple round or oval sharply demarcated rose-pink lesions accompanied by adherent scaling and follicular dilation appear on sun-exposed sites. These lesions tend to appear most often on the face, scalp and auricular regions (Fig. 20-3), and rarely on areas below neck level. Scaling and ulcerative lesions may occur on the lips. When DLE develops on the scalp, scarring alopecia may be seen due to the destruction of hair follicles by this disease (Fig. 20-4). These eruptions are often aggravated by sun exposure and leave scars and hyperpigmentation at the center of the lesions after they are healed. When a large number of DLE eruptions occur in areas below the neck level at the same time, the condition is termed widespread DLE (Fig. 20-5), and may progress into SLE with systemic involvement.

【临床表现】

在皮肤暴露部位出现单个或多个圆形或椭圆形的皮损，边界清楚，呈玫瑰红色，上黏附鳞屑，毛囊口扩张，好发于面部、头皮和耳廓(图 20-3)，少数情况下可发生在颈部以下。嘴唇的皮损可覆盖鳞屑和形成溃疡。当 DLE 发生在头部时，可因毛囊被破坏而形成瘢痕性脱发(图 20-4)。皮损可因日晒加重，愈后留下瘢痕，皮损中央会留有色素沉着。当颈部以下区域出现大量皮损时称为播散性 DLE(图 20-5)，这可能进展为伴有系统症状的 SLE。

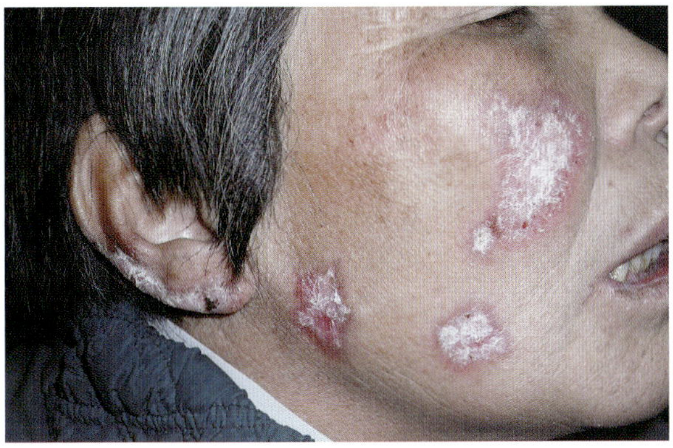

Fig. 20-3　DLE on auricle and face
(图 20-3　盘状红斑狼疮-耳廓和面部)

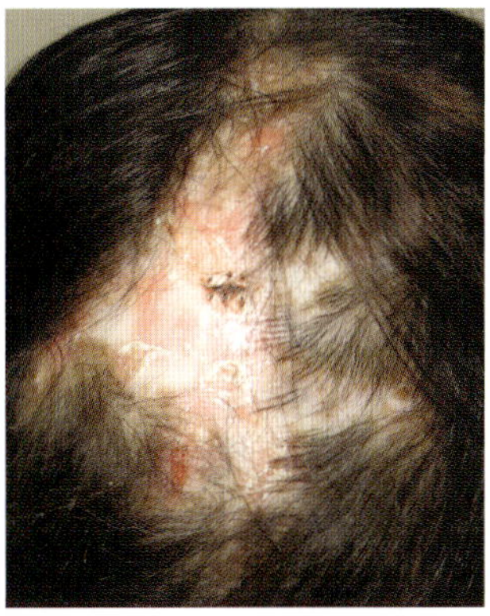

Fig. 20-4　DLE-scarring alopecia
(图 20-4　盘状红斑狼疮-瘢痕性脱发)

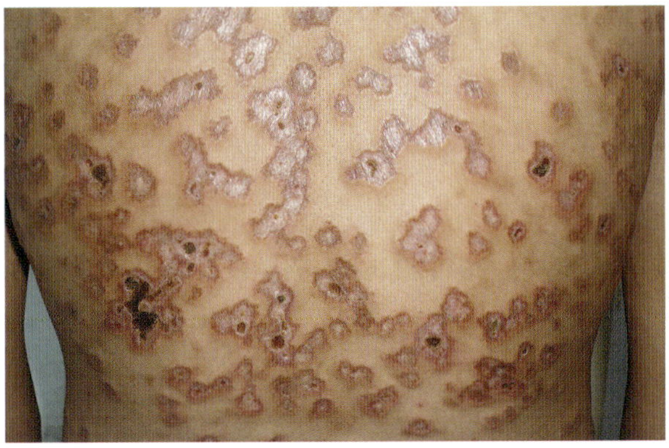

Fig. 20-5　Widespread DLE(图 20-5　播散性盘状红斑狼疮)

【Laboratory Findings】

Since the inflammatory reactions are primarily confined to the skin in this type of LE, laboratory findings are usually normal for most patients except in cases of widespread DLE. However, antinuclear antibodies and anti-DNA antibodies may be positive in some patients. In widespread DLE, hypocomplementemia may accompany SLE progression.

【实验室检查】

损害只发生于皮肤。大多数实验室检查都是正常的(播散性 DLE 除外),但有的患者抗核抗体、抗 DNA 抗体可呈阳性,播散性 DLE 向 SLE 进展时可伴随低补体血症。

【Histopathology】

The typical histopathological findings of DLE include: ①formation of follicular plugging; ②flat atrophy of the epidermis; ③ vacuolar degeneration of the basal cell layer; ④ dense focal infiltration (usually lymphocytic) around the appendages and blood vessels; ⑤ mucin deposits in the dermis. Linear deposition of immunoglobulins can be detected in the basement membranes of the lesions in most cases of DLE (lupus band test (positive), Fig. 20-2).

【组织病理】

DLE 组织病理特征有:①毛囊性角栓;②表皮平坦萎缩;③基底细胞空泡变性;④附属器和血管周围高密度的局灶性浸润(通常为淋巴细胞性);⑤真皮内的黏蛋白沉积。大多数 DLE 患者可检测到皮损基底层免疫球蛋白线状沉积(狼疮带试验阳性,图 20-2)。

【Differential Diagnosis】

Patients with DLE eruptions need to be differentiated from SLE cases with DLE eruptions. Other skin disorders that should be distinguished from DLE are polymorphous light eruptions, lichen

【鉴别诊断】

单纯 DLE 患者应与伴有 DLE 皮损的 SLE 患者鉴别。另需与多形性日光疹、扁平苔藓和结节病相鉴别。

planus and sarcoidosis.

【Treatment】

Patients with DLE should avoid sunlight. Topical application of glucocorticoids and tacrolimus are effective.

【治疗】

DLE 患者需避免日晒。局部应用糖皮质激素和他克莫司有效。

3. Lupus erythematosus profundus

Lupus erythematosus profundus, also known as lupus panniculitis, is a subtype of LE with major skin damage in the subcutaneous tissue. It is a nonspecific inflammation of fatty tissue.

三、深部红斑狼疮

深部红斑狼疮(lupus erythematosus profundus)又称为狼疮性脂膜炎(lupus panniculitis),是指主要损害发生在皮下组织的一种亚型。它的特征是脂肪组织的非特异性炎症。

【Clinical Manifestations】

Lesions occur as subcutaneous indurations, most frequently on the face, shoulders and buttocks, sometimes accompanied with DLE skin lesions. The color of the lesions is either unchanged or rosy pink. Depressed lesions may also appear and leave atrophic scars after healing (Fig. 20-6). Lupus erythematosus profundus may occur independently; however, more than half of all cases are accompanied by SLE and DLE.

【临床表现】

损害多发生在面部、肩部和臀部,表现为皮下硬结,颜色正常或呈玫瑰红色。在深部红斑狼疮发生部位可产生 DLE。在深部红斑狼疮的病程中可形成凹陷性的损害,愈后留下萎缩性瘢痕(图 20-6)。深部红斑狼疮可独立发生,但半数以上的患者伴有 SLE 或 DLE。

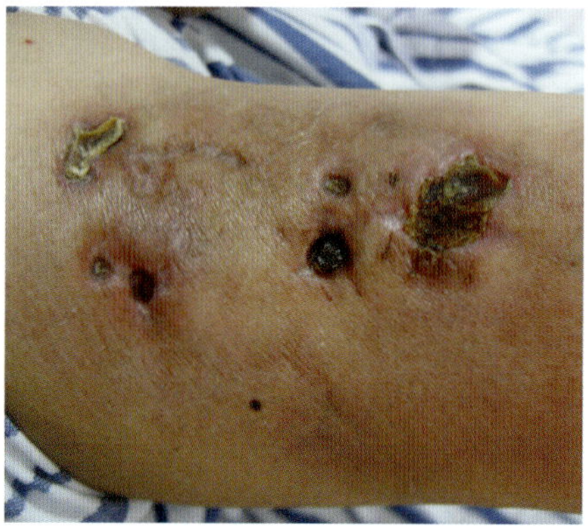

Fig. 20-6　Lupus erythematosus profundus-on upper arm(图 20-6　深部红斑狼疮-上臂)

【Histopathology】

Perivascular lymphocytic infiltration, mucin deposits and dense lymphocytic infiltration are found in subcutaneous tissues. Interlobular inflammation is gradually replaced by fibrosis. Deposits of immunoglobulins and complements may be seen on blood vessel walls and at dermo-epidermal junctions.

【组织病理】

皮下组织内可见血管周围淋巴细胞浸润、黏蛋白沉积和致密的淋巴细胞浸润。小叶间炎症逐渐变为纤维性。血管壁和真皮表皮交界处可见免疫球蛋白和补体沉积。

【Treatment】

Topical or oral glucocorticoids are the main treatments for this disease.

【治疗】

主要治疗手段是局部应用或口服糖皮质激素。

4. Subacute cutaneous lupus erythematosus (SCLE)

Subacute cutaneous lupus erythematosus (SCLE) is an intermediate variant of LE, in which the course and duration of the

四、亚急性皮肤型红斑狼疮

亚急性皮肤型红斑狼疮(subacute cutaneous lupus erythematosus, SCLE)

skin lesions are somewhere between those of chronic DLE and those of the acute LE seen in SLE.

皮损的经过和持续时间介于慢性 DLE 和 SLE 的急性 LE 之间。

【Clinical Manifestations】

Multiple eruptions appear symmetrically on sun-exposed sites on the body. There are two types of SCLE that have been described: annular-polycyclic SCLE, with hypopigmentation patches among the erythema (Fig. 20-7); and papulosquamous (psoriasiform) SCLE, with eruptions resembling psoriasis. Both subtypes of SCLE heal without scarring but tend to recur. About half of the patients with SCLE meet the diagnostic criteria for SLE. The disease may be accompanied by mild systemic symptoms such as arthralgia and fever. Severe renal symptoms and CNS manifestations are rare for this type.

【临床表现】

身体日光暴露部位出现对称性的多发性皮损。SCLE 有两种类型：①环状-多环状 SCLE，红斑中间会有色素减退（图 20-7）；②丘疹鳞屑性（银屑病样）SCLE，其皮损似银屑病。两种类型愈后都不留瘢痕且都会再发。大约半数 SCLE 患者可符合 SLE 的诊断标准。SCLE 可伴随有轻微的系统症状，如关节痛和发热。很少有严重的肾脏和中枢神经系统表现。

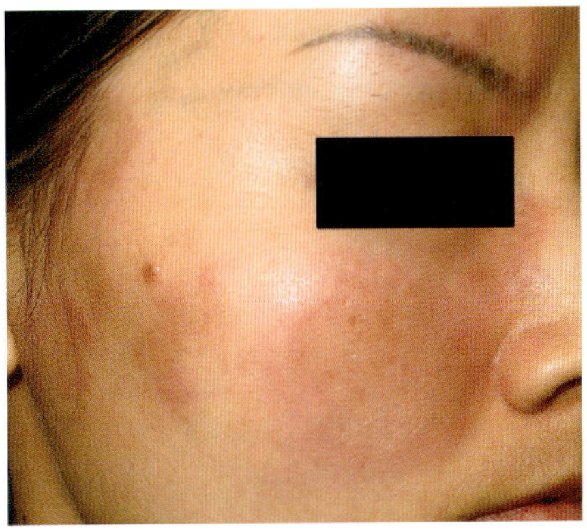

Fig. 20-7 Subacute cutaneous lupus erythematosus(图 20-7 亚急性皮肤型红斑狼疮,SCLE)

【Laboratory Findings】

Antinuclear antibodies (such as anti-SS-A antibodies and anti-SS-B antibodies) are positive in more than half of all cases. A correlation between SCLE and HLA-B8 or HLA-DR3 has also been reported.

【实验室检查】

半数以上的患者抗核抗体（如抗 SS-A 抗体和抗 SS-B 抗体）阳性。据报道 HLA-B8 或 HLA-DR3 与 SCLE 相关。

【Histopathology】

Characteristic histological findings of SCLE include epidermal atrophy, vacuolar degeneration in basal cell layers, as well as perivascular, periadnexal and subepidermal lymphocytic infiltration.

【组织病理】

SCLE 的病理特点有表皮萎缩，基底层细胞空泡变性和血管、附属器周围以及表皮下淋巴细胞浸润。

【Treatment】

The main treatments are glucocorticoids either applied topically or administered orally in small doses. Antimalarials such as hydroxychloroquine or chloroquine are also effective.

【治疗】

主要的治疗方式是局部应用或小剂量口服糖皮质激素以及抗疟药如羟基氯喹或氯喹。

5. Neonatal lupus erythematosus

This is a special type of LE. An annular erythema occurs in newborns whose mothers have SLE or Sjögren's syndrome with positive anti-SS-A and/or SS-B antibodies; however, the mother may sometimes be asymptomatic for both diseases. The skin lesions

五、新生儿红斑狼疮

新生儿红斑狼疮（neonatal lupus erythematosus）是红斑狼疮的一种特殊类型。表现为新生儿的环形红斑，其母亲患有 SLE 或 Sjögren 综合征，且抗 SS-are most commonly seen on the face of the neonate.

A 抗体和抗 SS-B 抗体阳性。有时其母亲无症状。皮损最常累及面部。

【Pathogenesis】

It is believed that anti-SS-A antibodies and anti-SS-B antibodies are passively transported across the placenta to the newborns, resulting in neonatal lupus erythematosus. The presence of an anti-SS-A antibody that can react with a 52 kD antigen indicates that this condition is strongly linked to an autoimmune response. The cutaneous symptoms often subside in 6 months, which is also the time when maternally derived antibodies normally disappear in the newborns, again implying the involvement of those transported antibodies in the pathogenesis of the disease.

【发病机制】

新生儿红斑狼疮的发病机制与通过胎盘传给胎儿的抗 SS-A 抗体和抗 SS-B 抗体有关。能与 52 kD 抗原反应的抗 SS-A 抗体尤其可疑。6 月后新生儿胎传抗体消失后，皮肤症状消退，提示本病的发生有抗体的参与。

【Clinical Manifestations】

The skin lesions often occur in the first month of life, and resemble the annular erythema found in Sjögren's syndrome or in DLE-like annular eruptions (Fig. 20-8). They may heal within 6 months, leaving abnormal hyperpigmentation. In addition to systemic symptoms associated with SLE (fever, hepatosplenomegaly, anemia, thrombocytopenia), congenital cardiac block can be found in some cases. As the cardiac block is irreversible, once it manifests, this condition requires the physician's full attention.

【临床表现】

皮损发生于出生 1 月以内的新生儿，类似于伴随有 Sjögren 综合征的环形红斑或 DLE 样的环形皮损(图 20-8)，6 个月内痊愈留下异常的色素沉着。除了伴随 SLE 的系统症状(发热、肝脾肿大、贫血和血小板减少症)之外，有些患儿还有先天性心脏传导阻滞。心脏传导阻滞是不可逆的，所以应引起医师的高度重视。

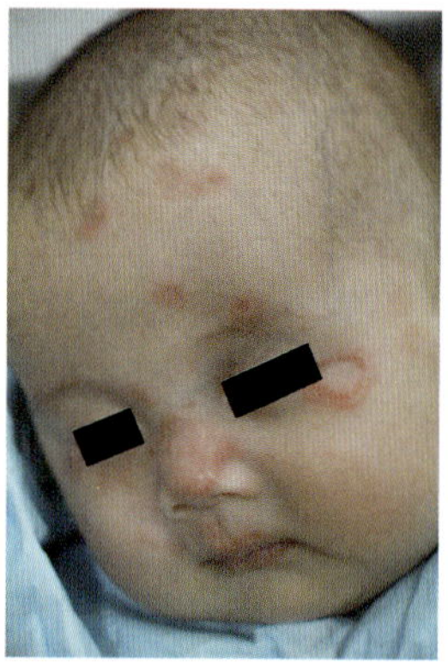

Fig. 20-8　Neonatal lupus erythematosus

(图 20-8　新生儿红斑狼疮)

【Treatment】

Symptomatic relief for the eruptions and systemic symptoms are the main concerns for neonatal LE. A pacemaker may have to be implanted (often permanent for life) in patients with cardiac block.

【治疗】

主要治疗手段是对皮损和系统症状的对症治疗。对有心脏房室传导阻滞的患者可安装心脏起搏器，且常为永久性的。

6. Nodular cutaneous lupus mucinosis

Nodular cutaneous lupus mucinosis is one subtype of cutaneous LE. A number of papules and nodules occur on the back and upper arms. These lesions are caused by abundant mucin

六、结节性皮肤狼疮黏蛋白病

结节性皮肤狼疮黏蛋白病(nodular cutaneous lupus mucinosis)是皮肤红斑狼疮的一个亚型。后背和上臂出现较多

deposits in the dermis, and they are often accompanied by SLE.

丘疹和结节。皮损是真皮内大量黏蛋白的沉积所致,通常伴有 SLE。

7. Bullous systemic lupus erythematosus

Bullous systemic lupus erythematosus is an autoantibody-mediated subepidermal blistering disease that occurs in patients with SLE. Antinuclear antibodies in the serum and autoimmune antibodies against type Ⅶ procollagen in the basement membranes are thought to cause the blistering. Blisters may form on normal skin or on LE lesions.

七、大疱性系统性红斑狼疮

大疱性系统性红斑狼疮(bullous systemic lupus erythematosus)是由自身抗体介导的表皮下大疱病,发生于 SLE 患者。血清中的抗核抗体和基膜中的Ⅶ型前胶原自身免疫性抗体与大疱的形成有关。大疱可出现在正常的皮肤或狼疮性红斑上。

Section Two Dermatomyositis

The common cutaneous findings in dermatomyositis (DM) include heliotrope (also called "lilac") rash, Gottron's sign, poikiloderma, and periungual telangiectasia. The muscle weakness usually starts with the proximal muscles, and laboratory tests will show elevated levels of CPK, aldolase and urinary creatine, which indicate the myositis. Malignant tumors are one of the common complications for DM. In general, patients with interstitial pneumonia may deteriorate rapidly and have a poor prognosis. Therapies for this condition mainly involve glucocorticoids.

第二节 皮 肌 炎

皮肌炎(dermatomyositis, DM)的皮损表现为紫红色斑疹、Gottron 征、皮肤异色症和甲周毛细血管扩张。肌无力症状常由近端肌肉开始。CPK 值、醛缩酶和尿肌酸增加提示有肌炎,常并发恶性肿瘤。伴有间质性肺炎者进展迅速,预后差,主要采用糖皮质激素治疗。

【Epidemiology】

The incidence of DM is apparently lower than for other connective tissue diseases such as SLE or scleroderma. DM most commonly affects adults aged 30-60 years, or children, with a male to female ratio of about 1∶2. When the clinical manifestations are limited to the muscles without cutaneous lesions, the condition is more properly called polymyositis (PM).

【流行病学】

皮肌炎的发病率低于其他结缔组织病(如 SLE 或硬皮病),最常发生于 30～60 岁的成年人和儿童,男女发病率约为 1∶2。多肌炎(PM)是指本病没有皮肤损害的病例。

【Etiology and Pathogenesis】

Although the cause of DM remains unclear, it has been proposed that the disease is caused by autoimmune responses of the muscles and skin tissues to some endogenous or exogenous triggers such as viral infection, allergy, a malignant tumor or chronic infections.

【病因及发病机制】

皮肌炎的发病原因还不清楚,皮肌炎可能与病毒感染、变态反应、恶性肿瘤或慢性感染等内、外因素诱发肌肉和皮肤的自身免疫反应有关,但具体发病机制未明。

【Clinical Manifestations】

Cutaneous symptoms: edematous purplish-red patches (heliotrope rash) on the face, especially the eyelids (Fig. 20-9), and flat elevated violaceous papules with scaling on the extensor surface of the interphalangeal joints, knees and elbows (Gottron's sign) (Fig. 20-10) are diagnostically significant. Seborrheic dermatitis-like erythema on the cheeks and scalp often progresses to butterfly-rash-like skin lesions in children (Fig. 20-11). Dermatitis-like diffuse edematous erythema may appear on the neck and trunk, and

【临床表现】

皮肤症状:面部尤其是眼睑的水肿性紫红色斑疹(图 20-9)及指间关节、膝和肘关节的伸面覆鳞屑性紫红色扁平隆起丘疹即 Gottron 征(Gottron's sign)(图 20-10)具有诊断意义。儿童颊部及头皮脂溢性皮炎样红斑常进展为蝴蝶斑样皮损(图 20-11)。颈部和躯干的泛发性水肿性红斑类似皮炎,有时可在躯干

sometimes shows a linear distribution on the trunk and extremities (linear dermatitis). These eruptions may leave hyperpigmentation or depigmentation patches, skin atrophy, scaling and telangiectasia, and may present as poikiloderma over time. Erythema of perionychia and hair loss are also seen frequently. Panniculitis resembling lupus erythematosus profundus may be seen in some cases as well.

和四肢呈线性分布(线性皮炎)。皮疹导致色素沉着或色素脱失、皮肤萎缩、脱屑和毛细血管扩张,称为皮肤异色症。指甲周围红斑和脱发常见,可见类似深部红斑狼疮的脂膜炎。

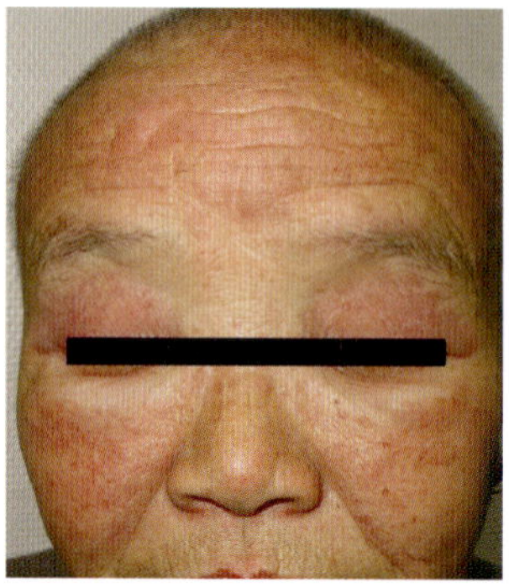

Fig. 20-9　Dermatomyositis
(图 20-9　皮肌炎)

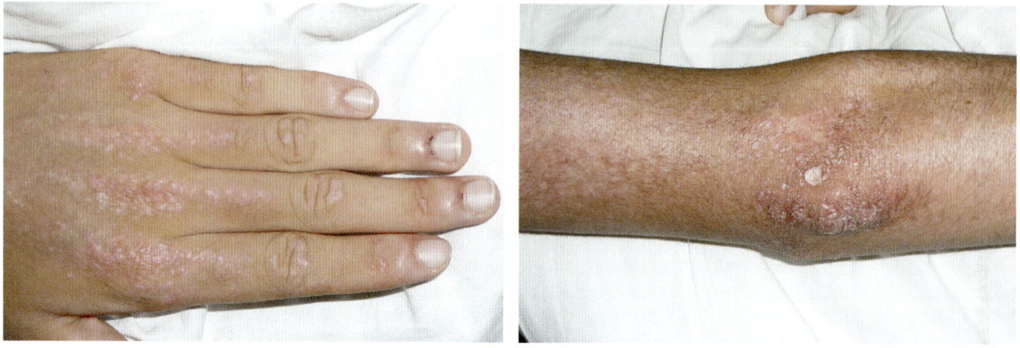

(a)　　(b)

Fig. 20-10　Dermatomyositis-Gottron's sign
(图 20-10　皮肌炎-Gottron 征)

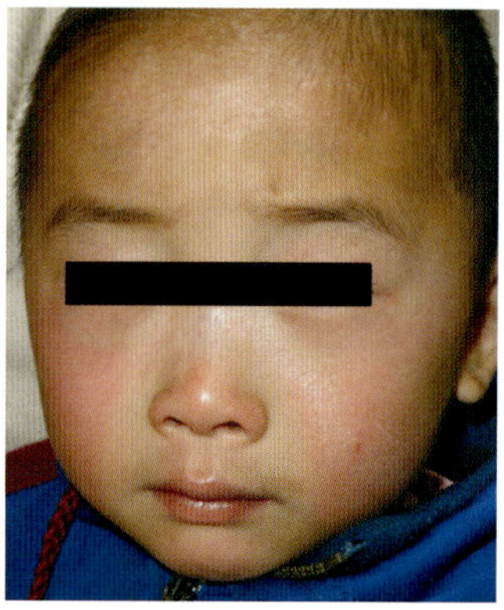

Fig. 20-11　Dermatomyositis in children(图 20-11　儿童皮肌炎)

Muscular symptoms: muscle pain (spontaneous pain, tenderness, "twinges", and gripping pain) and weakness usually occur symmetrically on the trunk, the proximal regions of the extremities, and the neck. The involvement of proximal muscles may cause difficulty in walking, especially when climbing (or descending) stairs. Weakness of the pharyngeal muscle group may lead to dysphagia, dysphonia and dyspnea.

肌肉症状:躯干、四肢近端和颈部可有肌肉痛(自发性疼痛、触痛、刺痛、拧痛)和肌无力,常对称性发生。近端肌肉运动不协调导致上下楼和其他行走困难。咽喉部肌肉无力可导致吞咽困难、发声困难和呼吸障碍。

Other symptoms: Raynaud's syndrome, multiple arthralgia, subcutaneous calcium deposits, diffuse interstitial pulmonary fibrosis, myocarditis and even interstitial pneumonia may occur in some cases.

其他症状:可有 Raynaud 综合征、多发性关节痛、皮下钙沉积、弥漫间质性肺纤维化及心肌炎,有时可发生间质性肺炎。

Dermatomyositis in children: this may develop after a vaccination or after a viral or bacterial infection. Cutaneous

儿童皮肌炎:可继发于疫苗接种及病毒和细菌感染。肌肉症状出现在皮肤

symptoms are typically preceded by muscular symptoms. Subcutaneous and muscular calcium deposits may occur in as many as 10%-20% of child patients, with resultant dyskinesia. The course of dermatomyositis in children is usually quite slow, with myoatrophy, articular contracture, and calcinosis of the skin or muscle as the main consequences. Fever and muscle weakness are common presentations in this subgroup of patients. Patients may die of multiple severe ulcers in the gastrointestinal tract.

症状之前。10%～20%的病例出现皮下和肌肉中钙沉积,这常常导致运动障碍。儿童皮肌炎患者进展相当缓慢。可有肌萎缩、关节挛缩和皮肤或肌肉钙沉积。常常发生发热和肌无力。患者可死于胃肠道多发性溃疡。

【Complications】

Malignant tumors are found in as many as 30%-40% of adult cases. This risk of cancer is even higher when severe edema and intense itching are present. The most common cancers that have been detected in dermatomyositis are stomach cancer, ovarian cancer, breast cancer, lung cancer and malignant lymphoma. However, DM-associated malignancies are rarely seen in children.

【并发症】

成人病例中30%～40%的患者合并恶性肿瘤。当患者有重度水肿和剧烈瘙痒时,恶性肿瘤的发生率更高。胃癌、卵巢癌、乳腺癌、肺癌和恶性淋巴瘤常见。儿童中并发恶性肿瘤的发生率极低。

【Laboratory Findings】

Nonspecific inflammatory reactions such as leukocytosis and elevated erythrocyte sedimentation rates are the positive findings in the early stages of the disease. Rheumatoid factors and antinuclear antibodies are positive in 60%-80% of all cases. During the course of DM, serum myogenic enzymes such as CPK (creatine phosphokinase), aldolase, GOT (glutamic oxaloacetic transaminase) and LDH (lactate dehydrogenase) may elevate significantly, together with increased creatine and myoglobin in the urine. Specific antibodies such as anti-Jo-1 (histidyl tRNA synthetase) and anti-PL-7 (threonyl tRNA synthetase) can be detected to provide further diagnostic clues. Skin and muscle biopsy findings and myogenic changes in electromyography are also valuable for confirming the diagnosis.

【实验室检查】

早期仅有非特异性炎症反应,如白细胞增多和血沉加快。60%～80%的病例类风湿因子和抗核抗体阳性。血清中肌酶(如CPK、醛缩酶、GOT和LDH)增高,由于存在肌炎,尿中的肌酸和肌红蛋白增高,可见特异性抗体,如抗Jo-1(组氨酰tRNA合成酶)抗体和抗PL-7(苏氨酰tRNA合成酶)抗体。皮肤和肌肉活检及肌电图中肌源性改变对诊断都很重要。

【Histopathology】

Edema in the superficial dermis and mild thickening of the basement membranes (PAS positive) are major findings in the early stages of erythematous eruptions. As the lesions progress, epidermal atrophy, vacuolar degeneration of the basal cell layer, mucin deposits, telangiectasia, swelling of collagen fibers, lymphocytic infiltrates and increased macrophages in the tissue are found, similar to the histologic changes in erythema lesions of SLE. Immunoglobulins and complement depositions on the skin are rarely observed. The typical myositic features are best revealed from a muscle sample biopsied from the site where the patient is reporting pain.

【组织病理】

真皮浅层水肿和基膜的轻微增厚(PAS染色阳性)是红斑早期的主要检查所见。随着皮损的进展可看到表皮萎缩、基底层细胞空泡变性、黏蛋白沉积、毛细血管扩张、胶原纤维肿胀、淋巴细胞浸润和组织中巨噬细胞的增加,这些病理改变类似于SLE红斑损害的组织学变化。皮肤中免疫球蛋白和补体的沉积少见。在肌肉痛区取肌肉活检最能显示典型的肌炎性改变的特点。

【Diagnosis】

Several diagnostic criteria for idiopathic inflammatory

【诊断】

虽然迄今为止已有多种不同的特发

myopathies (IIMs) have been proposed, but none of them have been properly validated. The first diagnostic criteria were elaborated in 1975 by Bohan & Peter. One of the major criticisms addressed to Bohan & Peter's criteria was that they cannot clearly distinguish DM and PM from inclusion body myositis (IBM) or other myopathies, particularly dystrophies, leading to misdiagnosis and inappropriate therapy. A new set of muscle-biopsy-based diagnostic criteria were then proposed by Dalakas & Hohlfeld in 2003 (Tab. 20-3). In their classification, MHC-1/CD8 complex is used as a specific marker for differentiating PM and IBM from other muscular diseases, particularly dystrophies. By 2004, the European Neuromuscular Centre (ENMC) had further refined the inclusive and exclusive criteria for idiopathic inflammatory myopathies, and also for some uncommon types of myositis, so that immune-mediated necrotizing myopathy and nonspecific myositis were all included. Tab. 20-4 shows the comparison among three classification criteria.

性炎症性肌病的诊断标准被提出，但均未予以恰当验证。第一个诊断标准由 Bohan 和 Peter 在 1975 年提出。B/P 标准的最大缺陷在于它不能将皮肌炎和多肌炎与包涵体肌炎等其他肌病相鉴别，特别是肌营养不良，因此常常导致误诊及不恰当的治疗。2003 年 Dalakas 和 Hohlfeld 提出了肌肉活检为基础的诊断标准(表 20-3)。该标准将 MHC-1/CD8 分子复合物作为多肌炎和包涵体肌炎区别于其他肌病特别是肌营养不良的特殊标志。接着，在欧洲神经肌肉疾病中心(ENMC)2004 年提出的诊断标准中，特发性炎症性肌病的不同组别，包括免疫介导的坏死性肌病以及非特异性肌炎也被考虑在其中。三种诊断标准的比较见表 20-4。

Tab. 20-3 Dalakas & Hohlfeld's diagnostic criteria for dermatomyositis

(表 20-3 Dalakas 和 Hohlfeld 的皮肌炎诊断标准)

Criterion (诊断标准)	Myopathic DM(肌病性皮肌炎)		Amyopathic DM(无肌病性皮肌炎)
	Definite (确诊)	Probable (可能)	Definite (确诊)
Myopathic muscle weakness (肌病性肌无力)	Yes (有)	Yes (有)	No (无)
Serum skeletal muscle enzymes (血清肌酶)	High or normal(升高或正常)	High (升高)	High or normal(升高或正常)
Electromyographic findings(肌电图)	Myopathic(肌源性)	Myopathic(肌源性)	Myopathic or non-specific (肌源性或非特异性)
Muscle biopsy abnormalities (肌肉活检异常)	Perifascicular, perimysial or perivascular infiltrates (束周、肌束膜周围或血管周围炎症细胞浸润)	Perifascicular atrophy (束周萎缩)	Non-specific or non-diagnostic for DM(非特异性改变)
Rash or calcinosis(皮损或钙化)	Present (有)	Non detected (无)	Present (有)

Tab. 20-4 Comparison among three classification criteria

(表 20-4 三种诊断标准的比较)

Authors/year (作者/年)	Point of strength(优势)	Concerns (缺陷)	Sensitivity (敏感性)	Specificity (特异性)
Bohan & Peter/1975	Useful as a screening tool. Used until now for enrolling patients in clinical trial (作为疾病的筛选工具，至今仍用于临床验证中患者的入组标准)	Unable to differentiate PM from IBM or dystrophies. Imaging and autoantibodies are not considered (不能将 PM 区别于 IBM 或者肌营养不良。影像学及自身抗体不作为诊断标准)	0.943	0.294

续表

Authors/year（作者/年）	Point of strength（优势）	Concerns（缺陷）	Sensitivity（敏感性）	Specificity（特异性）
Dalakas & Hohlfeld/2003	Very high specificity. Patients with ADM are considered. Definition of histological features is precise（特异性很高。无肌病性皮肌炎患者考虑在内。组织学特征的定义非常精确）	Low sensitivity of some items. Imaging and autoantibodies are not considered（对疾病中某些亚型的敏感性较低。影像学及自身抗体不作为诊断标准）	0.771	0.999
ENMC/2004	Imaging and autoantibodies are considered. Definition of histological features is precise（将影像学及自身抗体作为诊断标准。组织学特征的定义非常精确）	Overlap and paraneoplastic DM are not considered. Complex to use in clinical practice（重叠以及副肿瘤性皮肌炎不被考虑在内。临床应用过于复杂）	0.714	0.824

ADM：amyopathic dermatomyositis.（ADM：无肌病性皮肌炎。）

【Treatment and Prognosis】

When malignancy is found in patients with dermatomyositis, the priority is to remove the tumor. The mainstay of therapy for muscle and skin symptoms is to systemically administer glucocorticoids. In severe cases, glucocorticoids pulse therapy or immunosuppressants may also be effective.

If glucocorticoids therapy is given in the early stages, reduced muscular symptoms and decreased serum CPK will be observed in about 80% of cases. However, most DM cases require a prolonged glucocorticoid treatment. Life expectancy for patients with this disease depends primarily on the severity of any malignant tumors and on any heart or lung complications. The mortality rate is particularly high for patients undergoing complications from interstitial pneumonia. However, patients with onset during their youth tend to have a good life expectancy.

【治疗和预后】

如果并发肿瘤，对肿瘤的处理是最主要的。主要的治疗手段是全身应用糖皮质激素。严重病例可用糖皮质激素冲击疗法治疗，也可应用免疫抑制剂。

在病程早期应用糖皮质激素疗法可使约 80%的患者减轻肌肉症状并可降低血清 CPK 值，但许多患者需要长期应用糖皮质激素治疗。预期寿命与恶性肿瘤的严重程度以及心脏或肺脏的并发症有关。并发有间质性肺炎的患者的死亡率尤其高。青年时期起病的患者的预期寿命长。

Section Three　Scleroderma

Scleroderma is characterized by sclerosis of the skin, and it typically follows a course of erythematous edema, sclerosis and finally atrophy. It can be classified into systemic sclerosis (SSc) and localized scleroderma. The former frequently presents a variety of manifestations of the internal organs, whereas the latter has no internal organ involvement.

1. Systemic sclerosis (SSc)

SSc is also known as progressive systemic sclerosis (PSS) or diffuse cutaneous scleroderma, and has an unknown etiology. It typically manifests as generalized cutaneous sclerosis, fibrous degeneration of the synovium and small arteries, and Raynaud's phenomenon. Multiple internal organs can be involved in SSc. Positive anti-Scl-70 antibodies and positive anti-centromere

第三节　硬　皮　病

硬皮病(scleroderma)以皮肤硬化为特征，其典型经过按红斑水肿、硬化、萎缩的过程发展，可分为系统性硬化症(SSc)和局限性硬皮病。在系统性硬化症中，内脏器官可出现各种各样的损害，而在局限性硬皮病中，内脏器官不受累。

一、系统性硬化症

系统性硬化症(systemic sclerosis，SSc)又称进行性系统性硬化症(progressive systemic sclerosis，PSS)、弥漫性皮肤硬皮病，其病因不明。典型表现为全身性皮肤硬化、滑膜和小血管的纤维变性及 Raynaud 现象，可影响多种

antibodies can be observed. The treatment relies mainly on penicillamines and nonsteroidal anti-inflammatory drugs (NSAIDs).

内脏器官,抗Scl-70抗体和抗着丝粒抗体可阳性,主要应用青霉胺和非甾体类抗炎药(NSAIDs)治疗。

【Etiology and Pathogenesis】

【病因及发病机制】

The fundamental etiology for scleroderma remains unknown. It rarely runs in families.

基本病因未明。SSc具有家族史者罕见。

Environmental predisposition: patients with silicosis are prone to developing SSc. Also, SSc-like symptoms have been observed in workers who handle polyvinyl chloride or epoxy resins. Finally, some of the side effects of bleomycin resemble the symptoms of SSc.

环境因素:矽肺患者易得SSc,接触聚氯乙烯或环氧树脂的患者可有SSc样症状,另外博来霉素的副作用也类似SSc。

One type of SSc, called human adjuvant disease, occurs in half of those who have received silicon or paraffin injections or implants for cosmetic purposes. In those cases the condition often appears 10 years or more after the original operation. Due to these and other complications, these cosmetic materials are rarely used today.

有一类SSc称为佐剂病,它发生于一半接受硅或石蜡注射或埋植来达到美容目的的患者身上。疾病发生于手术后10年或10年以上。由于其并发症,这些物质现已不再应用了。

【Classification】

【分类】

There are two classification systems for SSc: Barnett, and LeRoy-Medsger. The classification is based on the degree and affected area of skin hardening, which is also used to describe the severity of SSc (Tab. 20-5).

SSc有两种分类方法:Barnett法和L-M法。以皮肤的硬化程度分类。分类法可用来描述SSc的严重程度(表20-5)。

Tab. 20-5 Classification of systemic sclerosis (SSc)

(表20-5 系统性硬化症的分类)

a. Barnett classification (a. Barnett法)	
Type Ⅰ(类型Ⅰ)	Cutaneous symptoms include Raynaud's phenomenon and hardening of the fingers (皮肤症状为Raynaud现象和手指硬化)
Type Ⅱ(类型Ⅱ)	Hardening of the skin occurs on the extremities and face (肢端和面部皮肤硬化)
Type Ⅲ(类型Ⅲ)	Hardening of the skin spreads to the trunk(皮肤硬化扩展到躯干)
b. LeRoy-Medsger classification (b. L-M法)	
Limited cutaneous type (局限性皮肤型)	The skin hardening only occurs on the extremities below the elbows. Visceral involvement is mild. The prognosis is commonly good. Most cases with positive anti-centromere antibodies (ACA) fall into this type(皮肤硬化仅限于肘部以下肢端,内脏损害轻;预后好;多数抗着丝粒抗体阳性者属于此型)
Diffuse cutaneous type (弥漫性皮肤型)	Hardening of the skin spreads to proximal sites, including the trunk and upper arms. Internal organ involvements including interstitial lung disease, oliguric renal failure, diffuse gastrointestinal disease and myocardial ailment progress quickly. The prognosis is poor in many cases. Cases included in this type are often positive for anti-DNA-topoisomerase Ⅰ (anti-Scl-70) antibody (皮肤硬化累及近端,包括躯干和上肢;内脏损害进展快,如间质性肺病、少尿性肾功能衰竭、弥漫性胃肠道疾病及心肌受累;多数病例预后差;此型患者抗DNA拓扑异构酶Ⅰ(抗Scl-70)抗体常阳性)
c. Other classifications(其他分类法)	
CREST Syndrome (CREST综合征)	A subtype of SSc, it is characterized by five symptoms: calcinosis, Raynaud's phenomenon, esophageal dysfunction, sclerodactylia and telangiectasia. This type is usually positive for ACA, and is a limited form of cutaneous SSc (SSc的一个亚型,特征性表现5个症状,即钙化、Raynaud现象、食管功能障碍、指端硬化和毛细血管扩张。血清抗着丝粒抗体常呈阳性,是一种局限于皮肤的SSc)

【Clinical Manifestations】

SSc frequently occurs in adults aged 30-50 years. The disease is more common in females than in males with a ratio of (3-4) ∶ 1. One of the common signs of SSc is Raynaud's phenomenon or arthralgia, which worsens in winter. The affected skin gradually hardens, often beginning at peripheral sites of the body. The skin lesions may vary in appearance depending on the sites affected and the individual, but edema, induration and atrophy are common skin presentations for most cases.

As SSc progresses, the fingers will show difficulty in flexion and extension. Furthermore, the fingers become pointed, crooked, or swollen like sausages (Fig. 20-12). Small ulcers may also appear on the finger tips as a result of poor circulation, which leave intractable, depressed scars with a worm-eaten appearance. These skin changes tend to extend proximally from the fingers to the upper arms. Telangiectasia, hyperpigmentation, depigmentation and calcium deposits also can appear along with the skin hardening.

(1) SSc of the face (mask-like face): wrinkles on the face disappear as a result of the edematous skin hardening. Characteristically, the nose becomes pointed and radial perioral furrowing can be found (Fig. 20-13).

【临床表现】

SSc好发于30～50岁的成年人。女性的发病率高，男女发病率为1∶(3～4)。冬天Raynaud现象或关节痛加重。受累皮肤由外周皮肤开始逐渐变硬。根据不同患者受累部位的不同，皮损表现出各自特异性的临床特征，通常是肿胀、硬化和萎缩。

随着SSc的进展，手指无法伸屈。病程进一步进展时，手指变尖或呈钩形，如香肠般肿胀（香肠样手指）（图20-12）。由于循环差，手指端形成小溃疡，最终形成顽固性凹陷性虫蚀状瘢痕。这些皮肤损害可从手指向上播散至上臂。伴随皮肤的硬化还可见毛细血管扩张、色素沉着、色素减退和钙沉积。

(1) 面部SSc（假面具样面容）　面部水肿性硬化导致面部皱纹消失，鼻子变尖，口周放射状沟纹，具有特征性（图20-13）。

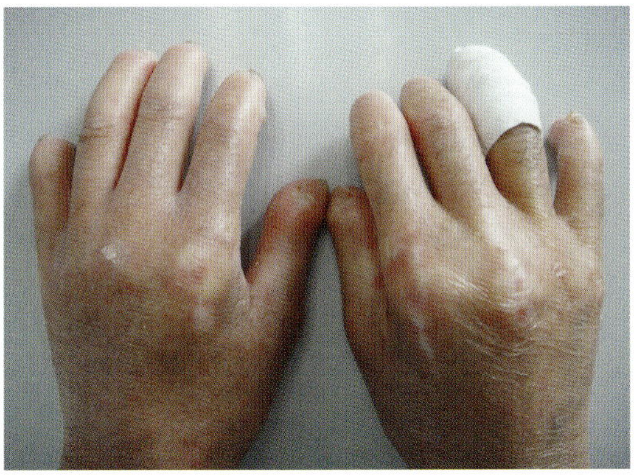

Fig. 20-12　Systemic sclerosis-sausage-like fingers
（图20-12　系统性硬化症-香肠样手指）

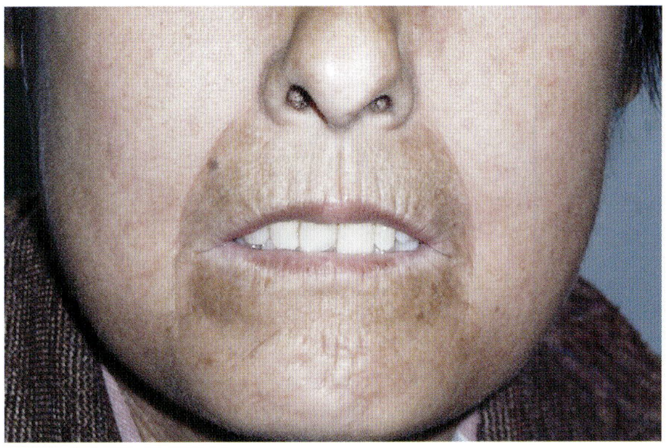

Fig. 20-13　Systemic sclerosis-mask-like face
（图20-13　系统性硬化症-假面具样面容）

Microstomia: patient has difficulty opening the mouth, which makes the mouth appear smaller than normal. Microglossia (i. e., tongue-tied): the patient has difficulty sticking out the tongue.

(2) SSc in other organs: other symptoms beyond skin lesions are arthralgia and joint swelling, decreased esophageal peristalsis, dilation of the lower esophagus, lung fibrosis, cardiac symptoms (arrhythmia, conduction defects), maldigestion, renal involvements (malignant hypertension, and sclerodermatous kidneys in severe cases) and chronic thyroiditis (Hashimoto's thyroiditis).

小口畸形：开口困难，使嘴看上去变小。小舌畸形（如舌系带过短）：舌难伸出。

(2) 其他器官SSc　其他器官的主要症状是关节痛及肿胀、食管蠕动性下降、食管下端扩张、肺部纤维化、心脏症状（心律不齐、传导紊乱）、消化不良症状、肾脏病症状（表现为恶性高血压，严重症状称为硬皮病性肾病）及慢性甲状腺炎（Hashimoto甲状腺炎）。

【Laboratory Findings】

Anti-Scl-70 antibodies are frequently seen in diffuse cutaneous SSc, and anti-centromere antibodies are commonly seen in limited cutaneous SSc and CREST syndrome.

Other laboratory findings in SSc are similar to those in other connective tissue disorders, such as positive rheumatoid factor, false positive serologic test for syphilis, and positive antinuclear antibodies (in a speckled or nucleolar pattern). Nonetheless, unlike SLE, a patient with SSc will show negative LE cell detection and anti-DNA antibodies; also, the serum complements titer will be in the normal range.

【实验室检查】

在弥漫性皮肤型SSc中抗Scl-70抗体常为阳性。在局限性皮肤型SSc和CREST综合征中抗着丝粒抗体常阳性。

SSc的其他检查所见与其他结缔组织病类似：类风湿因子阳性、梅毒血清学假阳性、抗核抗体阳性(呈斑点型或核仁型)。然而，LE细胞和抗DNA抗体阴性且血清补体滴度正常，这与SLE不同。

【Histopathology】

In the early stage of SSc, collagen fibrils are swollen, appearing with interstitial edema, hardening, and lymphocytic infiltrates in the middle and lower layers of the dermis. As the lesions progress, atrophy in the epidermis and appendages, deposition of collagen fibers parallel to the epidermis, and acid mucopolysaccharides (the major component of which is chondroitin sulfate) in the dermis will be observed. Unlike SLE, no deposits of immunoglobulins or complements will be seen in the majority of cases.

【组织病理】

在SSc早期，真皮中层到深层可见胶原纤维肿胀、间质水肿硬化和淋巴细胞浸润。随着损害的进展可见表皮和附件萎缩、胶原纤维平行沉积于真皮和酸性黏多糖(主要成分为硫酸软骨素)沉积。多数病例免疫球蛋白和补体的沉积是阴性的，这与SLE不同。

【Diagnosis and Differential Diagnosis】

Several sets of criteria are available for the diagnosis of SSc. Usually the typical cutaneous symptoms noted above will be sufficient for a conclusive diagnosis. The skin biopsies and tests for specific autoantibodies will be useful in difficult cases. During the edematous stage of SSc, it should be carefully differentiated from mixed connective tissue disease (MCTD) and overlap syndrome.

The current standards for classification of SSc are based on 1980 criteria that were developed by the American College of Rheumatology (ACR). However, patients in the early stages of SSc did not trigger the correct diagnosis due to the insensitivity of those criteria. In 2013, these diagnostic criteria were further reviewed and revised by the ACR and European League Against Rheumatism (EULAR) as shown in Tab. 20-6 below.

【诊断与鉴别诊断】

有多种诊断标准。在典型病例中，皮肤症状就足以得出最后诊断。诊断有困难时，可用皮肤活检和特异性自身抗体辅助诊断。水肿期SSc应与混合结缔组织病(MCTD)和重叠综合征仔细鉴别。

目前临床上常用的标准是1980年美国风湿病学会(ACR)提出的SSc分类标准。但是该标准的敏感性较低，无法对早期的SSc做出诊断。因此2013年ACR及欧洲抗风湿病联盟(European League Against Rheumatism, EULAR)修订了新的诊断标准(表20-6)。

Tab. 20-6 The American College of Rheumatology/European League Against Rheumatism criteria for the classification of systemic sclerosis

(表20-6 美国风湿病学会/欧洲抗风湿病联盟的系统性硬化症分类标准)

Item(s)(主要条件)	Sub-item(s)(次要条件)	Weight/score(权重/分值)
Skin thickening on the fingers of both hands extending proximal to the metacarpophalangeal joints (sufficient criterion)(双手指并延伸至近端掌指关节的皮肤硬化，充分依据)	—	9

续表

Item(s)(主要条件)	Sub-item(s)(次要条件)	Weight/score (权重/分值)
Skin thickening of the fingers (only count the higher score)(指硬化,记得分较高的一项)	Puffy fingers (香肠样手指)	2
	Sclerodactyly of the fingers (distal to the metacarpophalangeal joints but proximal to the proximal interphalangeal joints)(指硬化:远至掌指关节,近至近端指间关节)	4
Fingertip lesions (only count the higher score)(指端损害,记得分较高的一项)	Digital tip ulcers (指尖溃疡)	2
	Fingertip pitting scars (指尖凹陷性瘢痕)	3
Telangiectasia (毛细血管扩张)	—	2
Abnormal nailfold capillaries (甲襞微血管异常)	—	2
Pulmonary arterial hypertension and/or interstitial lung disease(maximum score is 2)(肺动脉高压和/或间质性肺疾病,最大分值为 2 分)	Pulmonary arterial hypertension (肺动脉高压)	2
	Interstitial lung disease (间质性肺病)	2
Raynaud's phenomenon (Raynaud 现象)	—	3
SSc-related autoantibodies (anti-centromere, anti-topoisomerase Ⅰ(anti-Scl-70), anti-RNA polymerase Ⅲ) (maximum score is 3)(SSc 相关自身抗体:抗着丝点型、抗拓扑异构酶Ⅰ(亦称抗 Scl-70)或抗 RNA 聚合酶Ⅲ,最大分值为 3)	Anti-centromere (抗着丝点型); anti-topoisomerase Ⅰ (抗拓扑异构酶Ⅰ); anti-RNA polymerase Ⅲ (抗 RNA 聚合酶Ⅲ)	3

The criteria are not applicable to patients with skin thickening sparing the fingers or to patients who have a SSc-like disorder that can be explained by other diseases such as nephrogenic sclerosing fibrosis, generalized morphea, eosinophilic fasciitis, scleredema diabeticorum, scleromyxedema, erythromyalgia, porphyria, lichen sclerosis, graft-versus-host disease, diabetic cheiroarthropathy. The total score is determined by adding the maximum weight (score) in each category. A total score≥9 will confirm the diagnosis of SSc.

此标准不适用于不累及手指的皮肤增厚患者及类 SSc 样疾病的患者。患者类似 SSc 的临床表现可以用另一疾病诊断更好地进行解释,如肾源性硬化纤维化、泛发型硬斑病、嗜酸性筋膜炎、糖尿病性硬肿病、硬化性黏液水肿、红斑肌痛症、卟啉症、硬化性苔藓、移植物抗宿主病或糖尿病手关节病变等。每一条目中的最大权重(分值)相加即为总分,患者得分≥9 分则可归类为 SSc。

【Treatment】

The patients in the early stage of SSc can be treated with moderate dosages of oral glucocorticoids to reverse the hardening of the skin. Various vasodilators (e. g., calcium antagonists or prostaglandin E1) are effective for Raynaud's phenomenon. Non-steroidal anti-inflammatory drugs (NSAIDs) may be used for relief of arthralgia. For severe patients, immunosuppressants and hematopoietic stem-cell transplantation are possible choices. Bed rest, warmth, and massaging the extremities are effective against cutaneous lesions.

【治疗】

早期口服应用中等剂量的糖皮质激素可用来治疗皮肤硬化。对 Raynaud 现象可用各种各样的血管扩张剂(如钙拮抗剂、前列腺素 E1)治疗。非甾体类抗炎药可用于缓解关节痛。严重病例可用免疫抑制剂和造血干细胞移植来治疗。卧床休息、热敷和按摩四肢对治疗皮损有效。

【Prognosis】

SSc tends to run a chronic course, with the skin hardness progressing gradually. The prognosis depends primarily on the severity of the damage to the kidneys and lungs. Infection may appear at some point during the treatment, and in some cases that may be fatal. Sudden death due to heart failure may also occur.

【预后】

SSc 趋向于慢性过程，皮肤硬化逐渐形成。预后取决于肾脏和肺脏受累的严重程度。治疗过程中可导致感染，这对某些患者来说是致命的。心脏衰竭可导致猝死。

2. Localized scleroderma

Localized scleroderma is sclerosis of the dermis, which only affects the skin. Unlike SSc, there is neither Raynaud's phenomenon nor visceral involvement in this form of scleroderma.

二、局限性硬皮病

局限性硬皮病(localized scleroderma)是真皮的硬化症，只累及皮肤。不像 SSc，局限性硬皮病没有 Raynaud 现象或内脏器官损害。

【Etiology and Pathogenesis】

The pathogenesis is unknown. However, one known trigger for localized scleroderma is external injury. Involvement of *Borrelia* infections has also been reported recently to be related to linear scleroderma.

【病因及发病机制】

发病机制未知，外伤可致病。近来报道，包柔氏螺旋体感染与线状硬皮病有关。

【Clinical Manifestations】

Localized scleroderma occurs most frequently in adults aged 20-40 years and sometimes in children. The ratio of female to male patients is roughly 3 ∶ 1. Raynaud's phenomenon is rarely seen. Systemic symptoms, if present, are mild. However, the specific manifestations of localized scleroderma vary individually.

(1) Morphea (circumscribed plaques): localized round or oval indurated lesions occur on the trunk. The lesions are silvery at the center, and may be surrounded by a purplish-red halo called a lilac ring (Fig. 20-14). Morphea may be further categorized by the size and number of eruptions as localized, guttate or generalized. Generalized morphea is defined by multiple morphea or morphea accompanied by other localized sclerodermatous lesions.

(2) Linear scleroderma (linear morphea): this subtype of localized scleroderma may appear with facial hemiatrophy. Linear or band-like indurated lesions resembling morphea occur on the body. When the forehead is affected, it is called sclérodermie en coup de sabre (sword-cut scleroderma), as it usually spreads to the scalp, leading to alopecia (Fig. 20-15). Linear scleroderma generally tends to penetrate to the deeper layers of the skin. Lilac rings are rarely seen in this group.

【临床表现】

局限性硬皮病好发于 20～40 岁的成人，有时发生于儿童，男女发病率约为 1 ∶ 3，Raynaud 现象罕见，即使有系统性症状也很轻微，局限性硬皮病包括许多表现。

(1) 硬斑病(morphea)(局限性斑块) 本病为发生在躯干部的局限性圆形或椭圆形皮损，中间为银白色，皮损周围的紫红色红晕称为淡紫色环(图 20-14)。根据皮损的大小和数量可将硬斑病分为局限性、点滴状或泛发性硬斑病。泛发性硬斑病是多发性的硬斑病或是伴随有其他局限性硬皮病皮损的硬斑病。

(2) 线状硬皮病(linear scleroderma)(线状硬斑病) 此病可伴有半侧面萎缩。躯干上发生类似于硬斑病的线状或带状的硬结性皮损。当前额受累时，称为刀砍样硬皮病。此病可向头皮蔓延并导致脱发(图 20-15)。线状硬皮病可穿透至皮肤深层。淡紫色环极少见。

【Histopathology and Laboratory Findings】

The histopathological changes of localized scleroderma are similar to that of SSc, but the abnormal laboratory findings that are characteristic of SSc are rarely seen in localized scleroderma.

【组织病理和实验室检查】

局限性硬皮病与 SSc 的病理学检查类似。但 SSc 的特征性实验室检查结果在局限性硬皮病一般很少见到。泛发性

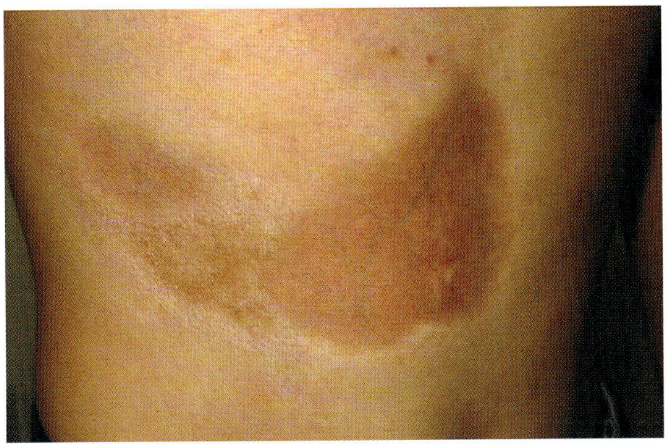

Fig. 20-14　Morphea
（图 20-14　硬斑病）

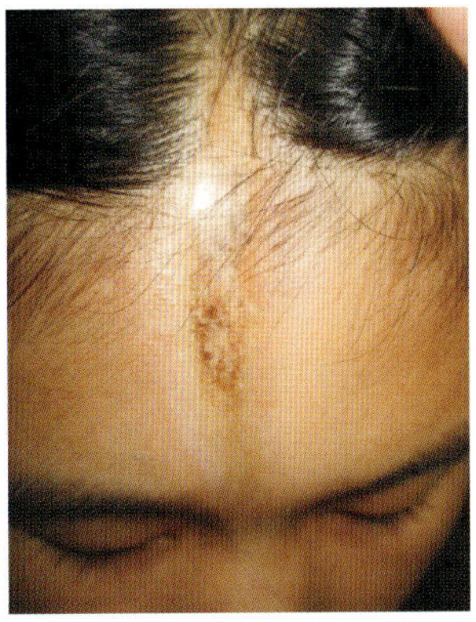

Fig. 20-15　Linear scleroderma(linear morphea)
（图 20-15　线状硬皮病(线状硬斑病)）

Rheumatoid factor and antinuclear antibodies may be positive in patients with generalized morphea.

硬斑病的类风湿因子和抗核抗体可呈阳性。

【Treatment】

Glucocorticoids are topically applied or locally injected. Oral glucocorticoids may be administered for severe cases. If no spreading tendency is observed for a certain period of time, surgery may be considered.

【治疗】

局部外用或注射糖皮质激素。严重病例可口服糖皮质激素治疗。若患者在一段时间内暂无播散趋势，可考虑手术治疗。

【Prognosis】

Patients with localized scleroderma have a good life expectancy; however, the condition is usually chronic. Indurated patches will gradually shrink, leaving hyperpigmentation.

【预后】

局限性硬皮病的患者预期寿命良好，病程通常呈慢性经过。硬斑逐渐萎缩，出现色素沉着。

Section Four　Overlap Syndrome

第四节　重叠综合征

An overlap syndrome is an autoimmune disease in which the patients present with symptoms of two or more connective diseases that meet the individual diagnostic criteria for each condition, such as SLE, SSc and dermatomyositis/polymyositis (DM/PM). Also, even when these conditions overlap, they don't necessarily have to have begun at the same time in order to be categorized as overlap syndrome. The common example of overlap syndrome is a patient with symptoms that fit the diagnostic criteria of both SLE and SSc.

重叠综合征(overlap syndrome)是指患者的症状满足两种或两种以上结缔组织病，如 SLE、SSc 或皮肌炎(DM)/多肌炎(PM)各自的诊断标准的一种自身免疫性疾病。几种结缔组织病不需同时发生。重叠综合征的典型例子为患者同时满足 SLE 和 SSc 的诊断标准。

【Etiology and Pathogenesis】

The pathogenesis of overlap syndrome is unknown. Hereditary factors and environmental factors are thought to be related, even though the responsible hereditary factors have not yet been identified. Usually the specific antibodies for each connective tissue disease (i. e., marker antibodies) are shown independently or simultaneously in overlap syndrome.

【病因及发病机制】

发病机制未明。遗传因素和环境因素与重叠综合征的发病有关。但致病的遗传因素未知。每种结缔组织病都用各自的特异性抗体(标志性抗体)来检测，这些抗体可单独出现或同时出现。

【Clinical Manifestations】

About 92% of the patients with overlap syndrome are females. In patients with SLE and SSc occurring concurrently, symptoms are

【临床表现】

约 92%重叠综合征的患者是女性。当患者同时是 SLE 和 SSc 患者时，常常

more likely to include fever, Raynaud's phenomenon, polyarthritis, ulceration of the fingertips, and pericarditis. Vascular involvement also occurs quite often in such patients, which indicates a poor prognosis.

有发热、Raynaud 现象、多关节炎、指尖溃疡和心包炎，常有血管损害，预后差。

【Laboratory Findings】

An elevated erythrocyte sedimentation rate and polyclonal hypergammaglobulinemia are both commonly seen. The specific antibodies for SLE (anti-dsDNA and anti-Sm antibodies), for SSc (anti-Scl-70 antibodies), and for PM (anti-Jo-1 antibodies), are all positive. Anti-Ku antibodies are also often positive when SSc and PM occur simultaneously (Tab. 20-7).

【实验室检查】

常见血沉加快和多克隆高球蛋白血症。SLE 特异性抗体(抗双链 DNA 抗体、抗 Sm 抗体)、SSc 特异性抗体(抗 Scl-70 抗体)和 PM 特异性抗体(抗 Jo-1 抗体)阳性。当 SSc 和 PM 同时发生时，抗 Ku 抗体阳性(表 20-7)。

Tab. 20-7　Major specific autoantibodies in connective tissue diseases and diseases related to connective tissue disease

(表 20-7　结缔组织病和结缔组织相关疾病的主要特异性自身抗体)

Disease(疾病)	Autoantibody(自身抗体)
SLE (系统性红斑狼疮)	Anti-dsDNA antibody, anti-Sm antibody (抗双链 DNA 抗体、抗 Sm 抗体)
SSc (系统性硬化症)	Anti-Scl-70 antibody, anti-centromere antibody (ACA), anti-Mi-2 antibody (抗 Scl-70 抗体、抗着丝粒抗体(ACA)、抗 Mi-2 抗体)
DM/PM(皮肌炎/多肌炎)	Anti-Jo-1 antibody, anti-PL-7 antibody, anti-Mi-2 antibody (抗 Jo-1 抗体、抗 PL-7 抗体、抗 Mi-2 抗体)
Mixed connective tissue disease(MCTD)(混合性结缔组织病(MCTD))	Anti-RNP antibody(Anti-U1-RNP antibody)(抗 RNP 抗体(抗 U1-RNP 抗体))
Overlap syndrome(重叠综合征)	Anti-dsDNA antibody, anti-Sm antibody, anti-Scl-70 antibody, anti-Jo-1 antibody, anti-Ku antibody (抗双链 DNA 抗体、抗 Sm 抗体、抗 Scl-70 抗体、抗 Jo-1 抗体、抗 Ku 抗体)
Sjögren syndrome (Sjögren 综合征)	Anti-SS-A antibody, anti-SS-B antibody(抗 SS-A 抗体、抗 SS-B 抗体)

【Diagnosis】

The symptoms of overlap syndrome need to meet the diagnostic criteria for each connective tissue diseases separately. When anti-U1-RNP antibodies appear positive and the clinical symptoms meet the diagnostic criteria for MCTD, the diagnosis for MCTD can be established.

【诊断】

重叠综合征必须同时满足几种结缔组织病各自的诊断标准。当抗 U1-RNP 抗体阳性且符合 MCTD 诊断标准时，通常诊断为 MCTD。

【Treatment】

As a general rule, the most significant symptom should be treated according to the treatment guidelines for each connective tissue disease.

【治疗】

根据通常规则，每种结缔组织病中最显著的症状将依据指南进行治疗。

Section Five　Mixed Connective Tissue Disease

第五节　混合性结缔组织病

Mixed connective tissue disease (MCTD) has been characterized as the disease condition with all the overt symptoms of SLE, SSc, and PM/DM, while nevertheless not completely meeting any of the diagnostic criteria of any of these diseases individually. Anti-U1-RNP antibodies and Raynaud's phenomenon are usually positive. Sausage-like fingers may also be found.

混合性结缔组织病(mixed connective tissue disease, MCTD)可见 SLE、SSc 和 PM/DM 的症状，然而却不满足这些疾病的任何诊断标准。抗 U1-RNP 抗体和 Raynaud 现象常阳性，可有香肠样手指。可并发肺动脉高压，并显著影响预后。

Pulmonary hypertension may occasionally develop as a complication, which can significantly affect the patient's prognosis. To date, the question of whether MCTD is an independent entity is controversial.

MCTD 是否是独立发生还存在很多的争议。

【Clinical Manifestations】

MCTD often affects females in their 40s. The typical clinical features are Raynaud's phenomenon, multiple arthralgia (or inflammation), and swelling in the dorsal hands (e.g., sausage-like swelling of the fingers). SLE-like symptoms such as erythema and fever, SSc-like symptoms such as lung fibrosis and esophageal constriction, and PM-and DM-like symptoms such as myositis and muscular weakness may occur in MCTD as well, but renal or CNS disorders are not normally present. These symptoms may give rise to suspicions that the patients have some sort of connective tissue disease; however, most cases cannot meet the diagnostic criteria for SLE, SSc or DM/PM.

【临床表现】

MCTD 的好发人群是 40 岁以上的女性。典型的临床特征有 Raynaud 现象、多发性关节痛(炎症)和手背肿胀(手指香肠样肿胀)。可见 SLE 样症状(如红斑和发热)、SSc 样症状(如肺纤维化和食管缩窄)以及 PM 样、DM 样症状(如肌炎和肌无力)。一般没有肾脏和中枢神经系统症状。如有这些症状可怀疑有结缔组织病,但大多数患者不符合 SLE、SSc 或 DM/PM 的诊断标准。

【Laboratory Findings】

High serum titers of anti-U1-RNP antibodies are of diagnostic significance for MCTD confirmation. Other positive laboratory findings for connective tissue diseases which may be seen in this group of patients include rheumatoid factor, reduction in pulmonary diffusing capacity, and elevation of myogenic enzymes, pancytopenia and hypergammaglobulinemia.

【实验室检查】

MCTD 以血清中抗 U1-RNP 抗体高滴度为特征。其他见于结缔组织病的阳性结果包括类风湿因子阳性、肺弥散功能降低、肌酶升高、全血细胞减少和高丙种球蛋白血症。

【Diagnosis】

Sharps, Kasukawa and Alarcón-Segovia all proposed their diagnostic criteria respectively in 1986 in Tokyo Japan. Kahn raised new criteria in 1991. Previous study revealed that criteria by Alarcón-Segovia (Tab. 20-8) had the highest sensitivity and specificity.

【诊断】

1986 年在日本东京举行的 MCTD 会议上, Sharps, Kasukawa 和 Alarcón-Segovia 宣布了各自的诊断标准,1991 年 Kahn 提出了新的标准。研究表明 Alarcón-Segovia 诊断标准(表 20-8)的敏感性及特异性均最高。

Tab. 20-8　Alarcón-Segovia's criteria for MCTD(表 20-8　Alarcón-Segovia 诊断标准)

Clinical criteria(临床标准)	Serological criterion(血清学标准)
1. Puffy hands(手肿胀)	Anti-U1-RNP-antibodies with a titer of more than 1 : 1600 at the hemagglutinin assay(抗 U1-RNP >1 : 1600 (血凝法))
2. Acrosclerosis with or without proximal SSc(肢端硬化伴或不伴 SSc)	
3. Raynaud's phenomenon(Raynaud 现象)	
4. Myositis: biologically or histologically proven(生物学或组织学证实的肌炎)	
5. Synovitis(滑膜炎)	

Diagnosis of MCTD: the serological criterion is present and more than 3 clinical criteria are present (if 1, 2 and 3 are present, 4 and 5 are also required to distinguish MCTD from SSc).

确诊标准:血清学标准及至少 3 条临床标准(如果 1、2、3 存在,则需要第 4 及第 5 条将 MCTD 区别于 SSc)

【Treatment】

Systemic glucocorticoids are fairly effective for MCTD.

【治疗】

全身应用糖皮质激素相当有效。血

Vasodilators such as calcium antagonists and NSAIDs are the main medications to treat patients with Raynaud's syndrome and arthralgia. Also, systemic glucocorticoids, oxygen inhalation, and vasodilators are helpful for those patients with pulmonary hypertension.

管扩张剂(如钙拮抗剂和非甾体类抗炎药)是治疗 Raynaud 综合征和关节痛的主要手段。全身应用糖皮质激素、吸氧和血管扩张剂可改善肺动脉高压现象。

【Prognosis】

Since the kidneys and CNS are unlikely to be affected, and glucocorticoids are highly effective in MCTD, the condition generally has a good prognosis. However, when complications involving pulmonary hypertension arise, the prognosis may be poor.

【预后】

由于肾脏和中枢神经系统不受累,糖皮质激素高度有效,MCTD 预后好。但一旦并发肺动脉高压则预后差。

Section Six Sjögren's Syndrome

第六节 Sjögren 综合征

Sjögren's syndrome (SS) is an autoimmune disease in which the main targets of the immune response are the exocrine glands, such as the salivary and lacrimal glands. The typical skin lesions often present as annular erythema or purpura due to vasculitis. The hallmark symptoms of SS usually occur as well, and these include xerostomia (dry mouth), keratoconjunctivitis sicca (dry eye) and distal renal tubular acidosis. An increased incidence of dental caries is somewhat common due to the dryness of the mouth. Anti-SS-A antibodies and anti-SS-B antibodies are usually positive for this condition. Hashimoto's disease (chronic thyroiditis) and B-cell lymphoma may also occur as complications. The treatment is generally symptomatic and supportive, and glucocorticoids may be administered in patients with severe complications.

Sjögren 综合征(Sjögren's syndrome, SS)是主要攻击外分泌腺的一种自身免疫性疾病,如唾液腺和泪腺。皮肤特征性损害是由血管炎造成的环形红斑和紫癜,可出现口干燥症、干燥性角结膜炎和远端肾小管酸中毒,口干可导致牙齿被腐蚀的发生率增加。本病抗 SS-A 和抗 SS-B 抗体呈阳性,常并发 Hashimoto 病(慢性甲状腺炎)和 B 细胞淋巴瘤,主要治疗手段是对症支持治疗,有严重并发症者可用糖皮质激素。

【Pathogenesis】

The pathogenesis of SS is still unclear.

【发病机制】

本病的发病机制尚未明确。

【Classification】

SS can be classified into primary SS and secondary SS. The former is defined as the condition presenting with typical SS symptoms without any other connective tissue disease (this is also known as sicca syndrome), the latter is applied to cases associated with other connective tissue diseases such as SLE.

【分类】

Sjögren 综合征可分为原发性和继发性,当只有 Sjögren 综合征的特征性症状而不伴有其他结缔组织病时称为原发性 Sjögren 综合征(干燥综合征)。伴有其他结缔组织病(如 SLE)的患者诊断为继发性 Sjögren 综合征。

【Clinical Manifestations】

SS most commonly occurs in adults aged 30-50 years. Male to female ratio is 1 : 9. The characteristic cutaneous symptoms include annular erythema and purpura with vasculitis, recurrent punctate hypergammaglobulinemic purpura on the lower extremities, and diffuse macular purpura. In addition, edematous or urticarial, well-demarcated annular erythema may be seen, 1-5 cm in diameter. There seems to be a close relationship between anti-SS-B antibodies

【临床表现】

Sjögren 综合征的好发人群是 30～50 岁的成年人,男女发病率是 1 : 9。皮肤的特征性损害是环形红斑和紫癜,伴随有血管炎。下肢可见复发性小斑点的高丙种球蛋白血症性紫癜,也可见弥散的斑点状紫癜。另可见水肿性或荨麻疹性环形红斑,境界清楚,直径为 1～5 cm。

and edematous annular erythema. This annular erythema often occurs on the face, healing spontaneously in about 2 weeks but sometimes persisting longer. Other cutaneous manifestations are dry skin, telangiectasia, hair loss, butterfly rash, chilblain erythema and nodular erythema.

抗 SS-B 抗体阳性与水肿性环形红斑的发生有密切联系。环形红斑好发于面部，可在 2 周或更长时间内自愈，另有皮肤干燥、毛细血管扩张、脱发、蝶形皮疹、冻疮样红斑和结节性红斑。

Eye symptoms: these commonly appear as keratoconjunctivitis sicca, photophobia, pain, itching and lacrimal disorders.

眼部症状：有干性角膜结膜炎、畏光、疼痛、瘙痒和流泪障碍。

Oral symptoms: dryness of the mouth, dysphagia, and sharp pain in the mouth are the results of salivary gland involvement. Tooth caries, angular cheilitis and oral candidiasis may occur in some cases.

口腔症状：因唾液腺受累引起口腔干燥、吞咽困难和口腔刺痛，并继发牙齿腐蚀、口角炎和口腔念珠菌病。

Other mucosal symptoms: lesions may be found in the nasal cavity, pharynx, larynx, bronchial tubes, external genitalia and alimentary mucosa.

其他黏膜症状：损害累及鼻腔、咽喉部、细支气管、外生殖器和消化道黏膜。

Miscellaneous symptoms: Raynaud's phenomenon, arthralgia, fever, fatigue, myalgia, lymphadenopathy and interstitial pneumonia can occur. Once B-cell lymphoma appears as a complication in such patients, the prognosis is poor.

其他症状：有 Raynaud 现象、关节痛、发热、疲乏、肌肉痛、淋巴结肿大和间质性肺炎，一旦并发 B 细胞淋巴瘤，则预后不良。

【Complications】

SS tends to appear in conjunction with SLE or rheumatoid arthritis. However, SSc, polyarteritis nodosa, polymyositis, idiopathic thrombocytopenic purpura, Hashimoto's disease, autoimmune hemolytic anemia, primary biliary cirrhosis, renal tubular acidosis and malignant lymphoma may also appear in association with this condition.

【并发症】

Sjögren 综合征常与 SLE 和类风湿关节炎同时发生。可并发 SSc、结节性多动脉炎、多肌炎、特发性血小板减少性紫癜、Hashimoto 病、自身免疫性溶血性贫血、原发性胆汁性肝硬化、肾小管性酸中毒和恶性淋巴瘤。

【Laboratory Findings】

Schirmer's test, Rose-Bengal test and fluorescent dye tests are performed by ophthalmologists to identify lacrimal gland abnormalities. Parotid gland radiography and parotid gland scintigram can be used to evaluate the morphology and function of the parotid glands. Antinuclear antibodies, anti-SS-A antibodies, anti-SS-B antibodies and anti-RNP antibodies are also usually positive for this condition. Elevated levels of immunoglobulins, salivary amylase and rheumatoid factor may be present as well. In general, anti-SS-A antibodies have high sensitivity and anti-SS-B antibodies have high specificity for SS.

【实验室检查】

眼科医师应用席尔默试验、孟加拉玫瑰试验和荧光染料试验来确定泪腺是否异常。耳科医师应用腮腺放射线摄影来确定形态，而腮腺功能可用腮腺闪烁曲线来确定。血清抗核抗体、抗 SS-A 抗体、抗 SS-B 抗体和抗 RNP 抗体阳性。可有免疫球蛋白增多，唾液淀粉酶和类风湿因子阳性。Sjögren 综合征抗 SS-A 抗体是高敏感性的，而抗 SS-B 抗体是高度特异性的。

【Histopathology】

The annular erythema shows pathological features similar to those of SLE and SCLE. Typically, the secretory glands are densely infiltrated by lymphocytes and plasma cells. A labial biopsy of the minor salivary glands will have some prognostic value. A skin biopsy of the purpura lesions will show vasculitis in the small blood vessels. Immunoglobulin deposition may also be found in the blood

【组织病理】

环形红斑的病理特征与 SLE 及 SCLE 类似。具有代表性的是分泌腺被大量淋巴细胞和浆细胞浸润。唇部的小唾液腺活检对疾病预后有指导价值。皮肤紫癜部位活检可见小血管的血管炎。血管可见免疫球蛋白沉积。

vessels.

【Diagnosis】

Currently, the diagnosis is made when the clinical features meet the European diagnostic criteria (Tab. 20-9).

【诊断】

近来，Sjögren 综合征需对照欧洲诊断标准进行诊断(表 20-9)。

Tab. 20-9 Revised version of the European classification criteria for SS (2002)

(表 20-9 Sjögren 综合征的分类标准欧洲修订版，2002 年)

Ⅰ. Ocular symptoms: a positive response to at least 1 of the following questions (Ⅰ. 眼部症状:对相应问题至少有 1 条是肯定的)	(1) Have you had daily, persistent, troublesome dry eyes for more than 3 months? (是否有 3 个月以上的每天持续性的令人烦恼的眼干燥?) (2) Do you have a recurrent sensation of sand or gravel in the eyes? (是否眼内有反复的沙子或沙砾的感觉?) (3) Do you use tear substitutes more than 3 times a day? (是否每天使用人工眼泪 3 次以上?)
Ⅱ. Oral symptoms: a positive response to at least 1 of the following questions (Ⅱ. 口腔症状:对相应问题至少有 1 条是肯定的)	(1) Have you had a daily feeling of dry mouth for more than 3 months? (是否有 3 个月以上每天感到口干燥?) (2) Have you had recurrently or persistently swollen salivary glands as an adult? (作为成人是否有反复和持续的唾液腺肿胀?) (3) Do you frequently drink liquids to aid in swallowing dry food? (是否经常饮用液体以便于吞干的食物?)
Ⅲ. Ocular signs: objective evidence of ocular involvement defined as a positive result for at least 1 of the following 2 tests (Ⅲ. 眼部体征:至少有相应 2 个试验中的 1 个阳性的眼部受累的客观证据)	(1) Shirmer's test, performed without anaesthesia (≤5 mm in 5 minutes) (不采用麻醉的情况下做席尔默试验，5 min 内≤5 mm) (2) Rose bengal score or other ocular dye score (≥4 according to van Bijsterveld's scoring system) (根据 van Bijsterveld 积分系统，孟加拉玫瑰试验积分或其他眼部染料积分≥4)
Ⅳ. Histopathology (Ⅳ. 组织病理)	In minor salivary glands (obtained through normal-appearing mucosa) focal lymphocytic sialoadenitis, evaluated by an expert histopathologist, with a focus score≥1, defined as a number of lymphocytic foci (which are adjacent to normal-appearing mucous acini and contain more than 50 lymphocytes) per 4 mm^2 of glandular tissue (从小的唾液腺(外观正常的黏膜)取材有局部淋巴细胞浸润，由一位组织病理专家判定局部积分≥1，即腺体组织每 4 mm^2 有许多淋巴细胞区域(临近外观正常的黏膜腺泡，含有 50 个以上的淋巴细胞))
Ⅴ. Salivary gland involvement: objective evidence of salivary gland involvement defined by a positive result for at least 1 of the following diagnostic tests (Ⅴ. 唾液腺受累:有相应表示唾液腺受累的诊断试验之一阳性的客观证据)	(1) Unstimulated whole salivary flow (≤1.5 mL in 15 minutes) (非刺激性全唾液流量，15 min 内≤1.5 mL) (2) Parotid sialography showing the presence of diffuse sialectasias (punctate, cavitary, or destructive pattern), without evidence of obstruction in the major ducts (腮腺造影显示弥漫性腮腺末梢导管扩张呈点状、腔洞样或破坏性模式，而主导管无阻塞的证据) (3) Salivary scintigraphy showing delayed uptake, reduced concentration and/or delayed excretion of tracer (腮腺闪烁曲线测定显示示踪剂的摄入延迟、浓度降低和/或分泌延迟)
Ⅵ. Autoantibodies: presence in the serum of the following autoantibodies (Ⅵ. 血清中有相应自身抗体)	Antibodies to Ro(SSA) or La (SSB), or both (抗 Ro(SSA) 或 La(SSB) 抗体，或二者)

Vitali C, *et al*. Classification criteria for Sjögren's syndrome: a revised version of the European criteria proposed by the American-European Consensus Group. Ann Rheum Dis 2002; 61: 554-558.

【Treatment】

Specific treatment is not yet available for SS. The main strategy is to use symptomatic therapies and supportive treatments. Oral hygiene should be maintained by mouthwash to prevent periodontal disease. Artificial saliva and artificial tears for protection of the cornea have been shown to be effective for patients with dry mouth and dry eyes. Large dosage of glucocorticoids and immunosuppressants are administered in severe cases (e. g., ones with generalized angiopathy or malignant lymphoma).

【治疗】

主要的治疗手段是对症支持治疗，因为尚无有效的药物治疗手段。用漱口剂保持口腔卫生以预防牙周病，对口干和眼干者应用人工唾液和人工泪液来有效保护角膜。并发全身血管性损害或恶性淋巴瘤的严重病例可用大剂量的内服糖皮质激素和免疫抑制剂治疗。

Section Seven Undifferentiated Connective Tissue Disease

第七节 未分化结缔组织病

The term undifferentiated connective tissue disease (UCTD) refers to unclassifiable systemic autoimmune diseases which share clinical and serological manifestations with definite connective tissue diseases (CTDs) but which do not adequately satisfy any of the existing classification criteria. Evolution is the most common characteristic of UCTD: about 30% of patients with undifferentiated onset will evolve to some definite CTD, and about 70% will remain as such over time. CTDs evolved from UCTDs are characterized by a simplified clinical profile and the absence of severe organ involvement.

未分化结缔组织病(undifferentiated connective tissue diseases, UCTD)的临床特征为具有结缔组织病的症状和体征，但是不符合任何结缔组织病的诊断标准。演变是未分化结缔组织病疾病过程中最为突出的特点，约 30%可演变为结缔组织病，约 70%维持未分化结缔组织病的状态。经未分化结缔组织病演变而来的结缔组织病，病情相对轻微，重要器官损害较少。

【Etiology and Pathogenesis】

UCTD and fully developed systemic autoimmune diseases are typically multi-etiological entities, where genetic and environmental abnormalities along with derailed immunoregulatory processes contribute to the development of the disease. Immunoregulatory disturbances are an important etiology of UCTD according to the clinical characteristics and the autoantibody profiles of UCTD. Decrease of thymus natural T-regulatory cell populations and overproduction of IFN-γ are the basic pathogenesis of UCTD, and are also the typical cause for the evolution of UCTD.

【病因及发病机制】

UCTD 与完全分化的系统性自身免疫性疾病的发病机制类似，都是复杂的多因素导致的疾病，病因包括遗传、环境因素以及免疫紊乱。根据 UCTD 的临床特点和自身抗体，提示免疫紊乱是 UCTD 重要的发病机制。其中胸腺天然调节 T 细胞下降和 IFN-γ 生成水平的异常亢进是 UCTD 基本的发病机制，也是 UCTD 发生演变的基本病因。

【Clinical Manifestations】

Most of the patients are females in the age of 30-50 years. As mentioned, about 70% of patients will remain as undifferentiated over time. These patients with stable UCTD appear to have a mild clinical profile characterized by the presence of articular manifestations (non-erosive arthritis), mild Raynaud's phenomenon and hematological manifestations (mild leucopenia or thrombocytopenia). In other words, these patients do not develop erosive or deforming arthritis, severe cutaneous manifestations,

【临床表现】

女性多见，发病年龄 30～50 岁。约 70%的 UCTD 患者将一直维持未分化的状态。这些稳定型的 UCTD 临床表现轻微，常见的症状、体征有关节症状(非侵蚀性关节炎)，轻微的 Raynaud 现象以及血液学表现(轻度白细胞减少或者血小板减少)。这些患者一般不会有侵蚀性或者致畸性关节炎、严重的皮损表现、严

severe Raynaud's phenomenon, or capillaroscopic alterations (suggestive of SSc) and do not have renal or neurological involvement.

With respect to the autoantibody profile, ANA positivity is high, ranging from 58% up to 90%; anti-Ro/SSA and anti-RNP antibodies appearing to be the most frequent specificities, followed by anti-dsDNA antibodies. Nevertheless, it should be kept in mind that other autoantibodies are observed with lower frequencies.

重的 Raynaud 现象或者毛细血管镜下表现(提示 SSc),并且不伴有肾脏或者神经系统累及。

自身抗体中 ANA 阳性率达 58%到 90%;抗 Ro/SSA 抗体和抗 RNP 抗体阳性最为常见,其次为抗双链 DNA 抗体,其余自身抗体的阳性率较低。

【Evolution of UCTD】

Data from the literature show clearly that 30% of patients with an undifferentiated onset will later develop a defined CTD. In addition, the evolution to defined CTD occurs in the majority of cases within 3-5 years of the diagnosis of UCTD, and the likelihood of developing CTD decreases over that time. Patients who develop a defined CTD late tend to have a milder form of the disease, with a lower incidence of serious adverse events and a better prognosis. Among the UCTD patients who evolved to CTDs, SLE is the most frequent final form of the disease (20%-60%).

【UCTD 的演变】

文献报道 30%的 UCTD 患者会演变成 CTD,并且在起病后 3~5 年 UCTD 演变为 CTD 发生率较高,随着病程的延长,演变发生率逐渐降低。愈晚发生演变的患者其疾病的严重程度更加轻微,严重不良事件的发生率更低,且预后更好。其中,UCTD 患者最常演变为 SLE(20%~60%)。

【Diagnosis】

The history of UCTD dates back to 1980, when LeRoy proposed the concept of undifferentiated connective tissue syndromes (UCTS) to define early phases of CTD. Classification criteria are still a matter of debate. The preliminary criteria to identify patients with stable UCTD by Mosca *et al* were the following: (i) signs and symptoms suggestive of a CTD, but not fulfilling any of the criteria for defined CTDs; (ii) positive antinuclear antibodies; (iii) disease duration of at least 3 years. However these criteria do not distinguish stable UCTD from incomplete forms of defined CTD or some overlap syndromes (i. e., mixed connective tissue disease). A possible solution to this problem would be to add exclusion criteria at disease onset.

【诊断】

UCTD 是 1980 年 LeRoy 等在提出未分化结缔组织综合征的基础上发展而来,目前尚无公认的诊断分类标准。1999 年 Mosca 等人初步提出了稳定型 UCTD 的标准是:①具有 CTD 的症状和体征,但不符合任何 CTD 诊断;②抗核抗体阳性;③自身免疫性疾病病程至少 3 年。但是该标准亦不能将稳定型 UCTD 与特定 CTD 的不完全形式或者一些重叠综合征(比如混合性结缔组织病)区分开来,可能的解决方法是在发病时增加一些排除标准。

【Treatment】

In accordance with this simplified clinical profile, these patients are generally treated with short courses of low dose corticosteroids, non-steroidal anti-inflammatory drugs (NSAIDs) and antimalarial drugs to control arthralgia, dysfunction, myalgia and fever, although they may also be left completely untreated. Immunosuppressive drugs are generally reserved for treating specific clinical manifestations, or when there is major organ involvement. Patient education should focus on symptomatic treatment.

【治疗】

由于 UCTD 的临床症状和体征轻微,治疗以控制关节痛、功能局限、肌痛和发热为目的,治疗的基本药物为短疗程的小剂量糖皮质激素,非甾体类抗炎药和羟氯喹,或不做任何治疗。某些特定的临床表现或者重要器官受累时需要免疫抑制剂治疗。故患者教育应以对症治疗为主。

Min ZHENG(郑敏), Hua-li CAO(曹华莉), Sui-qing CAI (蔡绥勍)

Chapter Twenty-one Autoimmune Bullous Dermatoses

第二十一章 自身免疫性大疱性皮肤病

Blisters are accumulations of fluid within or beneath the epidermis. However, diseases presenting with blisters and pustules induced by physical injuries (e. g., frostbite and burns), infections (e. g., those by bacteria or by viruses such as herpes), and ischemia (e. g., vasculitis) are not included in this autoimmune bullous dermatoses group.

水疱的形成是由于液体在表皮内或表皮下储积。由物理损伤(如冻伤或灼伤)、感染(如由细菌或病毒引起的疾病如疱疹等)或缺血(如血管炎)引起的水疱和脓疱性疾病则不列于自身免疫性大疱性皮肤病。

Bullous dermatoses can be divided into inherited (congenital) and acquired types. Congenital blistering diseases such as epidermolysis bullosa are caused by the mutations in the genes which encode for epidermal basement membrane structural proteins. Acquired blistering diseases such as pemphigus and bullous pemphigoid are autoimmune diseases. Autoantibodies against epidermal structural proteins are induced, immunopathological effects of which result in an increased fragility of the epidermis and blister formation.

大疱性皮肤病分为先天遗传性和获得性两类。前者如大疱表皮松解症是由于编码表皮基膜结构蛋白基因突变引起。后者如天疱疮和大疱性类天疱疮均为自身免疫性疾病,是由于体内产生针对表皮结构蛋白的自身抗体,从而导致表皮脆性增加、产生水疱。

The acquired bullous dermatoses can be further categorized into intraepidermal and subepidermal blistering dermatoses. The intraepidermal immunobullous disorders comprise all subtypes of pemphigus. The subepidermal immunobullous disorders comprise bullous pemphigoid, epidermolysis bullosa acquisita, linear IgA bullous dermatosis, and dermatitis herpetiformis. All of these immunobullous diseases will be discussed below. However, one must be aware that an intraepidermal split may be the only pathological finding due to blister re-epithelialization when a biopsy sampling is from an older subepidermal blister.

获得性的大疱性皮肤病通常分为表皮内水疱和表皮下水疱性皮肤病。表皮内免疫大疱性疾病包括各种亚型天疱疮,而大疱性类天疱疮、获得性大疱性表皮松解症、线状 IgA 大疱性皮病、疱疹样皮炎则均属于表皮下免疫大疱性疾病。本章主要介绍以上这些免疫大疱性疾病。尽管分类如此,但我们必须要认识到由于大疱表皮的再生化,陈旧性的表皮下水疱活检有时候可以表现为表皮内裂隙。

Section One Pemphigus

第一节 天疱疮

Pemphigus is derived from the Greek "pemphix", meaning blister or bubble. Pemphigus is a severe and potentially life-threatening condition. The two major subtypes, pemphigus vulgaris and pemphigus foliaceus, are distinguished by the site of cleavage within the epidermis. Splitting is suprabasal in pemphigus vulgaris and its rare vegetating form, pemphigus vegetans. Blistering is more superficial in the foliaceus and its variant erythematosus types.

天疱疮(pemphigus)源于希腊语"pemphix",意思为大疱或水疱。天疱疮病情重,有潜在致命危险。天疱疮两个主要亚型,即寻常型天疱疮和落叶型天疱疮,二者的区别在于其在表皮裂隙的位置深浅。寻常型天疱疮及其变异型增殖型天疱疮水疱裂隙位置在基底层上。落叶型天疱疮及其变异型红斑型天疱疮水疱裂隙位置则更加表浅。

【Etiology and Pathogenesis】

【病因及发病机制】

Predisposition to pemphigus is linked to genetic factors. First-degree relatives of patients with pemphigus vulgaris are more likely to develop autoimmune diseases than controls. Certain major

天疱疮易感性与遗传因素关联。寻常型天疱疮一级亲属较对照组更易罹患自身免疫性疾病。一些主要组织相容性

histocompatibility complex (MHC) class Ⅱ molecules, in particular an allele of human leukocyte antigen (HLA)-DR4 (DRB1 * 0402), are commonly found in patients with pemphigus vulgaris.

复合物Ⅱ类分子,特别是一些特殊的位点的表达,如 HLA-DR4 (DRB1 * 0402) 位点,在寻常型天疱疮患者中较常见。

All types of pemphigus are autoimmune diseases in which pathogenic IgG antibodies bind to antigens within the epidermis. The antigen-antibody mediated reaction disrupts the adhesion between epidermal cells, causing the keratinocytes to fall apart. The main antigens are desmoglein 3 in pemphigus vulgaris and desmoglein 1 in pemphigus foliaceus. Both of them are cell-adhesion molecules of the cadherin family, which are found mainly in desmosomes. Patients with active disease have antibodies for both IgG1 and subclasses of IgG4, but the latter is pathogenic. Most of the studies have concluded that there is a correlation between disease activity and antibody titers.

各型天疱疮的发生是由于致病性的 IgG 抗体与表皮内的相应抗原结合而引起的自身免疫性疾病。正是由于抗原-抗体反应干预了细胞间黏附,从而导致角质形成细胞松解脱落。寻常型天疱疮主要抗原是桥粒芯糖蛋白 3,而落叶型天疱疮的主要抗原是桥粒芯糖蛋白 1。桥粒芯糖蛋白 3 和桥粒芯糖蛋白 1 均为在桥粒中存在的钙黏素家族细胞黏附分子。活动期患者的抗体有 IgG1 和 IgG4 亚型,后者为致病性抗体。大部分研究表明抗体滴度与病情活动程度平行。

【Clinical Manifestations】

【临床表现】

The common forms of pemphigus include pemphigus vulgaris and its variants, pemphigus foliaceus and its variants, drug-induced pemphigus, IgA pemphigus, paraneoplastic pemphigus, and neonatal pemphigus.

天疱疮临床常见的类型有:寻常型天疱疮及变异型、落叶型天疱疮及变异型、药物诱导的天疱疮、IgA 天疱疮、副肿瘤天疱疮、新生儿天疱疮。

(1) Pemphigus vulgaris and variants:

(1) 寻常型天疱疮及变异型

Pemphigus vulgaris most frequently affects middle-aged and elderly people. It is characterized by flaccid blisters of the skin and mouth, although most patients develop the mouth lesions first. After the blisters rupture, widespread painful erosions appear (Fig. 21-1). Erosions form in the oral cavity and esophageal mucosa, causing dysphagia. When the eruptions become widespread, electrolyte abnormalities resulting from body fluid loss or hypoproteinemia can be found; this can be fatal once secondary infections arise. Blistering can also be artificially produced in patients with this disease by rubbing the normal-appearing skin (Nikolsky's sign). When the blisters are pressed without breaking, the fluid contents extend to the peripheral normal skin around the blisters (blister diffusion phenomena, also known as Nikolsky's sign) (Fig. 21-2).

寻常型天疱疮(pemphigus vulgaris)好发于中年人及老年人。特征性表现为皮肤及口腔松弛性大疱,大疱破裂后可出现广泛的疼痛性糜烂面(图 21-1)。大部分患者在口腔先出现皮损,当糜烂出现在口腔和食管黏膜时则导致吞咽困难。当出现大面积皮损时,可因为体液的丢失出现电解质紊乱和低蛋白血症,并发感染时则危及生命。当轻轻摩擦看似正常的皮肤时可人工产生大疱(尼氏征),或者是从疱顶按压大疱,疱液可向疱的周围扩散,此为水疱扩展征,也为尼氏征阳性(图 21-2)。

Pemphigus vegetans is a benign subtype of pemphigus vulgaris whose onset is marked by the formation of vesicles and erosions which have a tendency to develop excessive granulomatous tissues and crusting. At the periphery of the lesions, new vesicles and pustules are commonly seen (Fig. 21-3). There is usually a bad odor accompanying these pustules, and the disorder frequently occurs on areas exposed to friction, such as the axillary fossa, umbilical fossa, and the periphery of the oculonasal and perioral regions. Pemphigus vegetans can be of the Neumann type or Hallopeau type. The onset

增殖型天疱疮(pemphigus vegetans)是寻常型天疱疮的良性型,其特点为水疱和糜烂,并易形成过多的肉芽组织和结痂,边缘常出现新生水疱和脓疱(图 21-3),常有臭味。皮损好发于腋窝、脐周、眶周、鼻周及口周等易受摩擦的部位。增殖型天疱疮有两型:Neumann 型和 Hallopeau 型。Neumann 型大疱糜烂更明显,可出现寻常型天疱疮样的糜烂

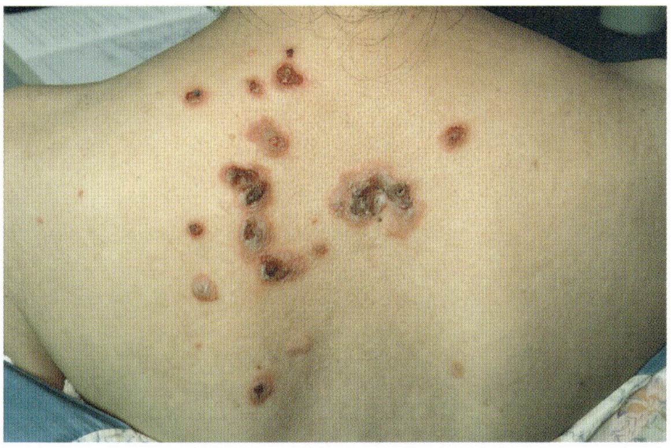

Fig. 21-1　Pemphigus vulgaris(图 21-1　寻常型天疱疮)

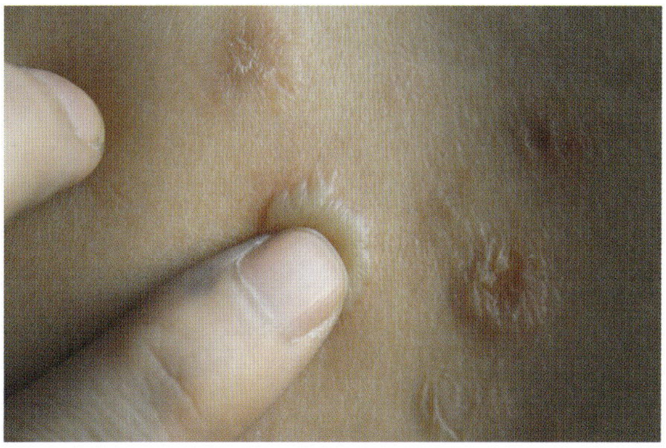

Fig. 21-2　Nikolsky's sign positive(图 21-2　尼氏征阳性)

of the Neumann type is marked by blistering, and the formation of pemphigus vulgaris-like blistered erosions. Pustules mainly occur in the Hallopeau type, which has a better prognosis.

(2) Pemphigus foliaceus and variants:

Pemphigus foliaceus also commonly affects the middle-aged and elderly people. Extremely fragile flaccid vesicles are ruptured easily, followed by the formation of loose flaky exfoliations. The scalp, face, chest, and back are the most commonly affected areas. When the disorder progresses and spreads over the whole body, it resembles exfoliative erythroderma. Nikolsky's sign is positive. Unlike pemphigus vulgaris, pemphigus foliaceus does not involve the mucosa.

Pemphigus erythematosus (also known as Senear-Usher syndrome) is a variant of pemphigus foliaceus. Its sufferers have the same age range as pemphigus foliaceus. It frequently affects the seborrheic zones on the scalp, face, chest, and back (Fig. 21-4). Systemic lupus erythematosus (SLE)-like erythema or seborrheic dermatitis-like eruptions occur on the face, and pemphigus foliaceus-like intraepidermal blisters may be found on the trunk. Mucosae are not often involved.

面；而 Hallopeau 型，则主要是出现小脓疱，愈后相对较好。

（2）落叶型天疱疮及变异型

落叶型天疱疮（pemphigus foliaceus）好发于中年人及老年人。表浅松弛的小水疱易破裂，形成疏松的叶片状表皮剥脱。皮损好发于头、面及胸背部。当皮损进展波及全身时则出现剥脱性红皮病样外观。尼氏征为阳性。本型不同于寻常型天疱疮，不侵犯黏膜部位。

红斑型天疱疮（pemphigus erythematosus）（又名 Senear-Usher 综合征）为落叶型天疱疮变异型，也好发于中年及老年人。主要累及头皮、面部及胸背部这些脂溢区（图 21-4）。通常可在面部出现系统性红斑狼疮样红斑或脂溢性皮炎样皮疹，在躯干可出现落叶型天疱疮样表皮内水疱样皮损。黏膜通常不受侵犯。

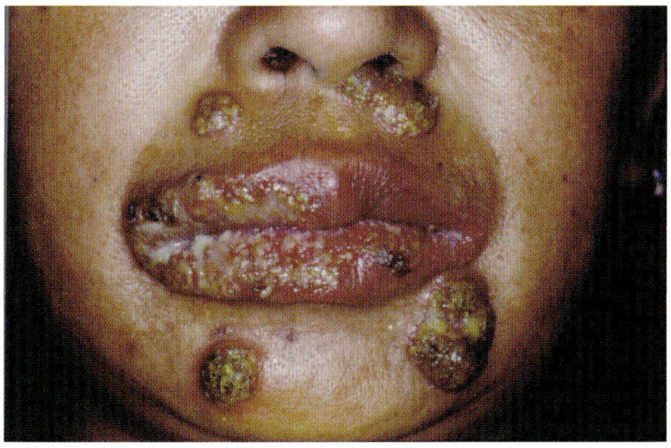

Fig. 21-3　Pemphigus vegetans(图 21-3　增殖型天疱疮)

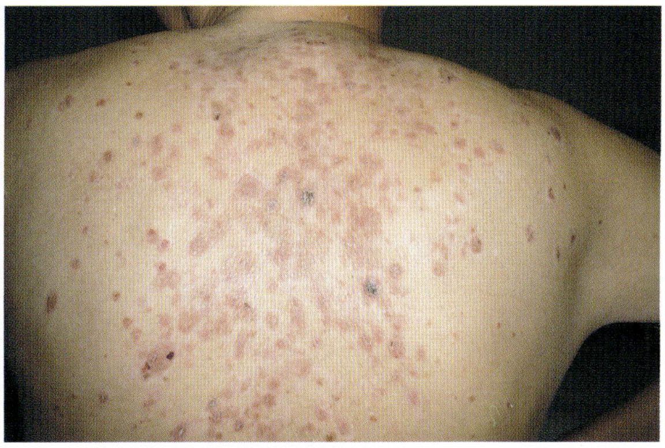

Fig. 21-4　Pemphigus erythematosus(图 21-4　红斑型天疱疮)

(3) Drug-induced pemphigus:

Drug-induced pemphigus is a catchall term for various diseases that cause lesions that resemble pemphigoid clinically and immunologically, which manifest with various clinical symptoms, along with histological and immunohistological findings. Acantholysis (separation of prickle cells) is one common finding at affected skin lesions. However, IgA deposits may sometimes be evident in the lesional epidermis. Drug-induced pemphigus is most frequently induced by drugs that contain residues of sulfhydryl groups, such as penicillamine and captopril.

(3) 药物诱发的天疱疮

药物诱发的天疱疮(drug-induced pemphigus)准确的界定较困难，如同类天疱疮一样，其临床表现、组织学及免疫组织学特征可多样。通常皮损表皮可出现棘层松解。有时还可发现 IgA 在病变的表皮沉积。引起药物诱发的天疱疮的最常见的是含有巯基结构的药物，如青霉胺和卡托普利。

(4) IgA Pemphigus:

IgA pemphigus is a rare variant of pemphigus characterized by epidermal intercellular IgA deposits, primarily affecting middle-aged and elderly people. Vesicles and pustules appear, usually on the trunk and extremities, and can be arranged in an annular pattern when the axilla and groin are involved. The disease may have a prolonged course. Some cases are not clinically differentiable from subcorneal pustulosis. IgA pemphigus manifest into two main subtypes: subcorneal pustular dermatosis (SPD) and intraepidermal neutrophilic dermatosis (IEN).

(4) IgA 天疱疮

IgA 天疱疮(IgA pemphigus)是罕见的天疱疮亚型，主要是由于表皮的细胞间 IgA 沉积引起。主要累及中老年患者，表现为在躯干和肢端特别是腹股沟和腋窝的水疱和脓疱，可呈环形排列，有时可演变成慢性。有些病例在临床上与角层下脓疱病鉴别较困难。IgA 天疱疮主要表现为两种亚型：角层下脓疱性皮病(SPD)型和表皮内嗜中性皮病(IEN)型。

(5) Paraneoplastic pemphigus:

As its name suggests, this disease accompanies malignant or benign neoplasms, especially lymphoproliferative disorders. Typically, it presents with severe mucosal erosions along with various cutaneous lesions on the other parts of the body. In severe cases, erosions, ulceration, and bloody crusts are all seen on mucous membranes of the oral cavity, pharynx, and lips (Fig. 21-5). Pseudomembranous conjunctivitis may lead to blepharosynechia. Autoantibodies against several epidermal proteins such as desmogleins and plakin family molecules can be positive. The two keys to diagnose this disease are the detection of IgG autoantibodies and evidence of tumors.

(5) 副肿瘤性天疱疮

副肿瘤性天疱疮(paraneoplastic pemphigus)可与各类良恶性肿瘤伴发，特别是淋巴增生性疾病。副肿瘤性天疱疮可出现严重的黏膜糜烂，身体其他部位皮肤的皮疹表现可多样。严重时口腔、咽喉及嘴唇黏膜可出现糜烂、溃疡和血痂(图 21-5)。假膜性的结膜炎可导致睑球粘连。自身抗体可针对表皮蛋白，如桥粒芯和桥斑蛋白分子家族。本病最重要的是检测 IgG 自身抗体同时寻找伴发的肿瘤。

(6) Neonatal pemphigus:

Neonatal pemphigus is seen in newborns whose mother usually has pemphigus. The maternal IgG autoantibodies cross the placenta and attack the skin of the newborn infant. The clinical symptoms, histopathological and immunohistopathological findings of pemphigus are transiently present in neonatal pemphigus.

(6) 新生儿天疱疮

新生儿天疱疮(neonatal pemphigus)患儿一般其母亲患有天疱疮。主要原因是患儿母亲自身 IgG 抗体通过胎盘导致胎儿的皮肤患病。新生儿天疱疮的临床特征、组织病理及免疫组织病理学表现均为暂时的。

【Histopathology and Immunopathology】

Acantholysis causes intraepidermal blistering. In pemphigus vulgaris, blisters occur suprabasally. The basal cells remain attached to the basement membrane but shrink from one another

【组织病理和免疫病理】

棘层松解导致表皮内水疱，寻常型天疱疮的大疱出现在基底层上，疱底由于基底细胞黏附于基底膜，但彼此分离，

and appear to be isolated and free-standing appearing like a set of tombstones (Fig. 21-6). A smear taken from the base of a blister or oral erosion (Tzank preparation) will contain acantholytic cells (round keratinocytes floating freely within the blister cavity). The vegetating lesions in pemphigus vegetans are hyperkeratotic, acanthotic, and papillomatous. Some suprabasal clefts may contain eosinophils, but acantholytic cells are rarely present.

形似“墓碑”(图 21-6)。从水疱的基底或口腔的糜烂面刮片检查(Tzank 试验),可见在水疱中漂浮的圆形角质形成细胞(即棘层松解细胞)。增殖型天疱疮病理表现为角化过度、棘层肥厚和乳头瘤样增生。基底层上的裂隙中可见嗜酸性粒细胞,而棘层松解细胞则少见。

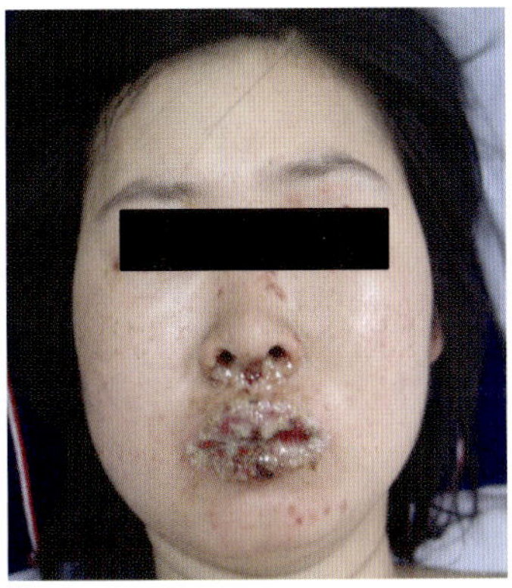

Fig. 21-5 Paraneoplastic pemphigus
(图 21-5 副肿瘤性天疱疮)

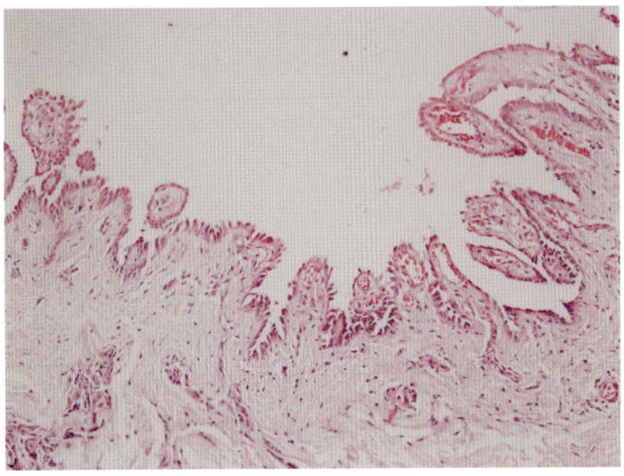

Fig. 21-6 Histopathology of pemphigus vulgaris
(图 21-6 寻常型天疱疮组织病理)

In early lesions of pemphigus foliaceus, vacuoles form in the intercellular spaces in the upper levels of the epidermis. These coalesce to form clefts or superficial bullae in the upper granular layer or immediately below the *stratum corneum*. Dyskeratotic cells in the granular layer of older lesions will distinguish pemphigus foliaceus from pemphigus vulgaris. The presence of a subcorneal blister, with acantholytic cells and scattered eosinophils, is highly suggestive of pemphigus foliaceus.

落叶型天疱疮的早期皮损可见表皮上部细胞间空泡形成,以后在颗粒层上部或角质层下形成裂隙或水疱,陈旧性皮损中颗粒层可见角化不良细胞,此有别于寻常型天疱疮。一般出现角质层下水疱,伴有棘层松解细胞及散在的嗜酸性粒细胞,高度提示落叶型天疱疮。

Pemphigus erythematosus blends the immunohistological findings of pemphigus foliaceus and lupus erythematosus. Patients often have a positive serum antinuclear antibody. Immunofluorescence yields both an intercellular deposition of immunoreactants and a “lupus band” of immunoreactants along the BMZ.

红斑型天疱疮兼具落叶型天疱疮和红斑狼疮的免疫组织学特征,患者通常血清抗核抗体阳性,免疫荧光可以出现棘细胞间免疫反应物的沉积,可以出现沿基膜带的“狼疮带”反应。

In the SPD type, subcorneal vesicopustules or pustules can be observed, usually with minimal acantholysis. However, in the IEN type, intraepidermal vesicopustules or pustules with variable numbers of neutrophils are present.

在 SPD 型中,可见角层下脓性水疱或脓疱,常仅有少许棘层松解,而在 IEN 型中,可见表皮内脓性水疱或脓疱伴有不等数量的中性粒细胞。

Biopsies from paraneoplastic pemphigus patients show necrosis of keratinocytes or vacuolar interface dermatitis in addition to suprabasal clefting. In one single study, 27% of cases had only suprabasilar acantholysis alone. Therefore, the specificity of these histological findings has come into question.

副肿瘤型天疱疮的病理显示除了基底层上的裂隙改变,还可出现角质形成细胞的坏死或基底细胞空泡化的界面皮炎改变。有研究显示,27%的副肿瘤型天疱疮病理仅表现为基底层上的棘层松解,因此病理是否具有特异性仍有待考证。

The diagnosis of pemphigus is confirmed by direct

直接免疫荧光(DIF)可确诊天疱疮,

immunofluorescence (DIF), which shows IgG and C3 deposits in the intercellular spaces in a reticular pattern when viewing biopsies from the lesions or the surrounding skin (Fig. 21-7). In rare cases, intercellular IgA can be detected by direct immunofluorescence in IgA pemphigus. Circulating intercellular antibodies are detected in 80%-90% of patients by indirect immunofluorescence (IIF), but the sensitivity of this test depends upon the substrates. The titer of these antibodies correlates closely with clinical activity of the disease and may guide changes in the dosage of systemic glucocorticoids.

皮损或皮损周围皮肤取材可见棘细胞间有 IgG 和 C3 呈网状沉积(图 21-7)。在罕见的 IgA 型天疱疮中,抗体的沉积主要为 IgA。80%～90%患者通过间接免疫荧光试验可检测到抗棘细胞间的循环抗体,其敏感性依赖于底物。抗体的滴度与病情活动度密切相关,并可指导糖皮质激素用量。

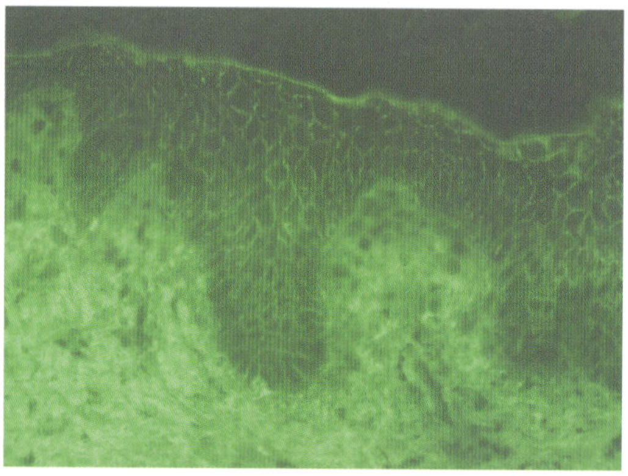

Fig. 21-7 DIF of pemphigus vulgaris

(图 21-7 寻常型天疱疮直接免疫荧光)

In paraneoplastic pemphigus, DIF reveals a "net-like" epidermal deposition of IgG and complement C3 on the surfaces of keratinocytes and a linear deposition at the BMZ. Indirect immunofluorescence assay is positive in both stratifying and non-stratifying epithelia. The pathogenicity of these antigens has been established by passive transfer studies. The autoantibodies recognize a number of heterogeneous intracellular and extracellular antigens including desmoplakin Ⅰ (250 kD), desmoplakin Ⅱ (210 kD), the bullous pemphigoid antigen (230 kD), periplakin (190 kD), and a 170 kD antigen that is unnamed yet.

在副肿瘤天疱疮中,直接免疫荧光揭示免疫球蛋白 IgG 和/或补体 C3 除了于角质形成细胞表面形成"网状"沉积,同时也线状沉积于基膜带。间接免疫荧光揭示循环抗体既可与鳞状上皮结合,也可与非鳞状上皮结合。抗原的致病性可通过被动转移试验建立。自身抗体识别的抗原包括一系列异质性的胞内和胞外抗原,这些抗原有桥斑蛋白Ⅰ(250 kD)、桥斑蛋白Ⅱ(210 kD)、大疱性类天疱疮抗原(230 kD)、斑周蛋白(190 kD)以及一个尚未命名的 170 kD 的抗原。

【Diagnosis and Differential Diagnosis】

The diagnosis of pemphigus can be confirmed by histology combined with immunofluorescence. The quantity of antibodies in the serum indicates the severity of the pemphigus. When desmoglein 3 is detected alone, the disease is often limited to the membrane-dominant pemphigus vulgaris, in which minor blistering of the skin is expected. However, when desmoglein 1 and 3 are detected at the same time, blisters often appear at both the oral mucosa and the skin of the rest of the body. It is necessary to differentiate the disease from dermatitis herpetiformis, bullous

【诊断与鉴别诊断】

皮肤病理结合免疫荧光可以对天疱疮进行确诊。患者血清中抗体的量反映着天疱疮的严重程度。当血清中仅能检测到桥粒芯蛋白 3,则反映为膜结合型的寻常型天疱疮,患者皮肤出现轻度的小水疱。当血清中同时能检测到桥粒芯蛋白 1 和 3,患者口腔黏膜和全身均出现水疱。本病需要与疱疹样皮炎、大疱性类天疱疮、脓疱疮、烧伤、大疱性药疹、多形

pemphigoid, impetigo, burns, bullous drug eruptions, erythema multiforme, and Stevens-Johnson syndrome.

红斑以及 Stevens-Johnson 综合征相鉴别。

【Treatment】

Therapeutic means are chosen according to the patient's age, the affected area, the subtype of pemphigus, and the progression of the condition. Nevertheless, systemic glucocorticoids are the mainstay of any of these therapies. In order to reduce side effects for any systemic glucocorticoids, adjuvant glucocorticoid sparing drugs can be initiated along with or after glucocorticoid treatment. Although there is a lack of controlled studies on this subject, most experts believe that immunosuppressive agents possess a glucocorticoid sparing effect, and therefore it can decrease the side effects of glucocorticoids by allowing the use of lower glucocorticoids dosages and increase remission rates.

The most commonly used agents are cyclophosphamide (1.5-2.5 mg/(kg · d)) and azathioprine (1.5-2.5 mg/(kg · d)). In patients who do not respond well to conventional immunosuppressants, intravenous immunoglobulin (IVIG) appears to be an effective alternative treatment, and its early use is of significant benefit in patients who may experience life-threatening complications from immunosuppression. IVIG is effective even when used alone. However, several courses of treatment may be required to obtain a durable remission, and follow-up is needed to determine if prolonged treatment is required.

Antibiotics, fluid replacement, nutrition management, and the use of topical glucocorticoids may help. Treatment is withdrawn when patients are clinically free of symptoms and when they have a negative finding on direct immunofluorescence. The titer of circulating antibody has a rough correlation with disease activity, but it is not accurate enough by itself to determine when to stop therapy.

【治疗】

应根据患者的年龄、皮损累及范围以及病变进展的程度、临床亚型综合考虑来制订一个合适的治疗方案。系统使用糖皮质激素仍然是天疱疮的主要治疗方法。由于系统使用糖皮质激素具有许多潜在的不良反应，所以同时应给予辅助治疗，一般在使用激素的同时或使用激素后应用辅助治疗。尽管没有进行过对照研究，但大多数的学者认为免疫抑制剂具有延长激素间隔作用，可以通过减少激素的用量以减少激素的副作用，并可提高病情的缓解率。

临床上最常应用的免疫抑制剂是环磷酰胺(1.5～2.5 mg/(kg · d))和硫唑嘌呤(1.5～2.5 mg/(kg · d))。当常规免疫抑制剂治疗疗效欠佳时，静脉注射免疫球蛋白(IVIG)是一个良好的选择。在免疫抑制剂可能威胁患者生命时，应及早使用 IVIG。IVIG 单独使用有效。通常需要使用几个疗程才能获得病情持久缓解。延长治疗时有必要进行规则随访。

抗生素的使用、电解质和营养的补充以及局部外用糖皮质激素对治疗均很有帮助。当患者临床症状消失，并且直接免疫荧光为阴性时可考虑停药。循环抗体的滴度测定可以大致了解疾病的活动情况，但不能作为是否停药的依据。

Section Two　Bullous Pemphigoid

Bullous pemphigoid (BP) is a group of rare, relatively benign autoimmune subepidermal bullous diseases of the elderly. Bullous pemphigoid often starts with pruritic urticarial erythematous lesions. Later, large, tense blisters develop both on erythematous and normal skin. Mucosa can also be involved with blisters and erosions.

第二节　大疱性类天疱疮

大疱性类天疱疮(bullous pemphigoid, BP)是一组少见的、相对良性的自身免疫性表皮下大疱性疾病，好发于老年人。通常大疱性类天疱疮首发皮损为瘙痒性荨麻疹性红斑，继而可以在红斑以及正常皮肤上出现紧张性大疱，黏膜部位也可累犯，出现紧张性大疱和糜烂。

【Etiology and Pathogenesis】

Bullous pemphigoid is mediated by autoantibodies that bind to the bullous pemphigoid antigens 230 (BP230, a cytoplasmic component) and 180 (BP180, a transmembrane glycoprotein component of hemidesmosomes in epidermal basal cells). Skin-fixed and circulating IgG autoantibodies target one or both BP antigens. These IgG autoantibodies are found both circulating and bound in the lamina lucida region of the BMZ of the epidermis. The BMZ-bound autoantibodies result in activation of complement and chemotaxis, degranulation of mast cells and release of inflammatory mediators. The activated inflammatory cells release proteolytic enzymes that cleave the target antigens and disrupt the hemidesmosomes, resulting in subepidermal blisters.

【病因及发病机制】

大疱性类天疱疮由针对类天疱疮抗原230(BP230,一种胞质成分)和180(BP180,一种表皮基底细胞半桥粒的跨膜糖蛋白)的自身抗体介导。皮肤和循环中的自身抗体IgG可以结合一种或两种BP抗原。这些自身抗体出现在外周血并沉积在表皮基膜带透明层。沉积在表皮基膜带的自身抗体导致补体和趋化因子的激活、肥大细胞脱颗粒以及炎性介质的释放。活化的炎症细胞释放蛋白水解酶,蛋白水解酶裂解靶抗原、破坏半桥粒,导致表皮下大疱的形成。

【Clinical Manifestations】

The eruption is usually generalized, sites of predilection being the lower part of abdomen, the groin, and the flexor surfaces of the arms and legs. The palms and soles can also be affected in some cases. Oral blisters (24%), if present, are mild and transient. Involvement of genital mucous membranes occurs in 7% of patients. Mucosal involvement is sometimes present, but, unlike pemphigus, it is rarely the first site of involvement. Bullous pemphigoid begins with a localized area of edematous erythema or with wide-spread pruritic urticarial plaques that gradually become more edematous and extensive. The condition is usually misdiagnosed as urticaria before the appearance of blisters. The degree of itching varies but is usually moderate to severe. The typical lesions are tense bullae (Fig. 21-8). Most bullae rupture within a week, leaving an eroded base that, unlike the situation with pemphigus, does not spread and heals rapidly. Nikolsky's sign is negative.

【临床表现】

皮损通常泛发全身,最常见的发病部位是下腹部、腹股沟、四肢屈侧,掌跖部位亦可受累。24%的患者出现口腔大疱,通常轻微短暂,7%的患者发生生殖器黏膜受累。有别于天疱疮的是大疱性类天疱疮首发罹患部位罕见于黏膜。大疱性类天疱疮发病初期皮损表现为局限性水肿性红斑和广泛的荨麻疹样瘙痒性斑块,皮损逐渐水肿明显、泛发。在水疱出现前,该病经常误诊为荨麻疹。瘙痒程度不一,通常为中重度。典型皮损为张力性大疱(图21-8),大多数大疱在一周内破溃,形成糜烂面。但是与寻常型天疱疮不同的是,其糜烂面不扩大,愈合快。尼氏征阴性。

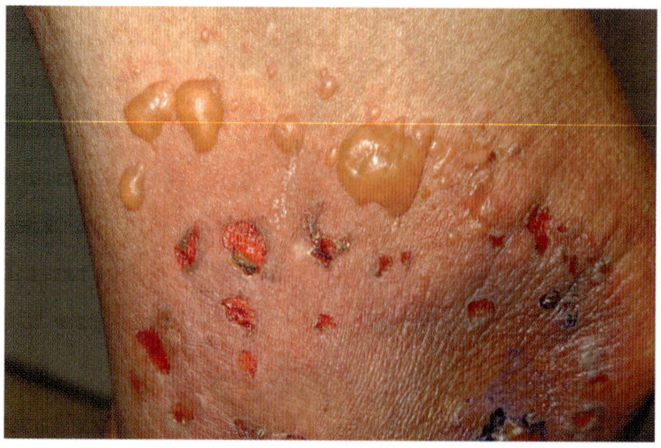

Fig. 21-8　Bullous pemphigoid(图21-8　大疱性类天疱疮)

Cicatricial pemphigoid refers to a heterogeneous group of scarring, subepidermal blistering disorders caused by a variety of

瘢痕性类天疱疮是一组异质性瘢痕性表皮下水疱性疾病,由多种自身抗体

autoantibodies. Tense bullae that heal with scarring are a common theme. Most subtypes involve oral or ocular mucosa. Pemphigoid gestationis (also known as herpes gestationis) relates to a vesiculobullous condition occurring in gravid women; it has essentially the same histopathologic and immunohistologic findings as typical bullous pemphigoid. Paraneoplastic variants have been described in the literature as well. Other localized variants of bullous pemphigoid are also reported clinically, including vesicular, nodular, vegetating, hyperkeratotic, and erythrodermic types, all having the same histologic and immunologic characteristics as generalized bullous pemphigoid. The diagnosis is usually confirmed by histologic studies and direct and/or indirect immunofluorescence assays.

引起，常表现为紧张性水疱，继而以瘢痕愈合，大部分亚型均可累及口腔或眼部黏膜。妊娠类天疱疮（又称妊娠疱疹）是发生于妊娠期妇女的水疱大疱性疾病，其免疫组织学及病理组织学与一般的大疱性类天疱疮表现相同。另外，有文献报道存在副肿瘤型类天疱疮的亚型。大疱性类天疱疮存在许多局限型的临床亚型，如水疱型、结节型、增殖型、角化过度型和红皮病型，它们的组织病理学和免疫学特征与泛发性类天疱疮相同。确诊需要组织病理学和直接或间接免疫荧光检查。

【Histopathology and Immunopathology】

The histopathology shows subepidermal blisters, often filled with eosinophils (Fig. 21-9). Cicatricial pemphigoid usually demonstrates fewer eosinophils than bullous pemphigoid. Neutrophilic microabscesses in the dermis may appear in new lesions. Direct immunofluorescence (DIF) shows a linear band of IgG and C3 along the BMZ (Fig. 21-10). Elston *et al*. have also reported that linear deposition of C3 and IgG along the dermoepidermal junction in samples adjacent to the skin lesion forms an N-serrated pattern by direct immunofluorescence assay. Indirect immunofluorescence, using serum from the patient, can detect IgG antibodies that react with the BMZ in 70% of patients. Biopsy specimens treated with 1 mol/L sodium chloride will split the lamina lucida (this is so-called "salt-split skin"). By direct immunofluorescence, the IgG will appear predominantly or exclusively on the epidermal side in bullous pemphigoid. One needs to bear in mind that immunoreactivity for a certain antigen is not always restricted to one disease entity. For instance, BP180 (BPAG2) is the target antigen for several autoimmune bullous disorders, including bullous pemphigoid, cicatricial pemphigoid, pemphigoid gestationis, and linear IgA bullous dermatosis.

【组织病理和免疫病理】

组织病理学检查显示，类天疱疮的大疱位于表皮下，疱腔内有嗜酸性粒细胞浸润（图 21-9）。瘢痕性类天疱疮病理上通常较大疱性类天疱疮出现更少的嗜酸性粒细胞浸润，在新发性皮损中真皮有时候可以发现中性粒细胞微脓肿。直接免疫荧光检查显示 IgG 和 C3 在基膜带处呈线状沉积（图 21-10），并且 Elston 等人发现皮损周边皮肤直接免疫荧光检查显示 C3 和 IgG 在基膜带处呈"N"形锯齿状线状沉积。用患者血清进行间接免疫荧光检查发现 70%的患者可出现 IgG 抗体与基膜带进行反应。用 1 mol/L NaCl 处理后的活检标本可在表皮透明层处产生裂隙（盐裂皮肤直接免疫荧光试验），并可见 IgG 主要在或只在大疱的表皮侧沉积。需要强调的是免疫荧光特定抗原反应并非严格指向特定的疾病。例如针对 BP180 (BPAG2)靶抗原的免疫荧光反应除了大疱性类天疱疮以外，还有瘢痕型类天疱疮、妊娠类天疱疮、线状 IgA 大疱性皮病。

【Treatment】

The treatment depends on the affected area and the disease's rate of progression. Systemic glucocorticoids combined with immunosuppressive agents such as azathioprine, cyclophosphamide, methotrexate, and chlorambucil have been therapies of choice for this disease. The general dosage of systemic glucocorticoids is 0.5 mg/(kg · d) and it should be reduced gradually. Antibiotics,

【治疗】

根据病变的程度及病情进展的速度确定治疗方案。系统使用糖皮质激素联合免疫抑制剂如硫唑嘌呤、环磷酰胺、甲氨蝶呤、苯丁酸氮芥是主要的治疗方法。系统使用糖皮质激素量一般为 0.5 mg/(kg · d)，然后逐渐减量。抗生素、氨苯

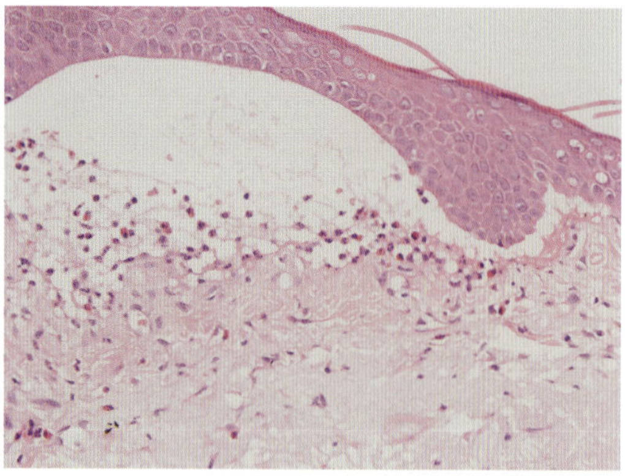

Fig. 21-9 Histopathology of bullous pemphigoid
(图 21-9 大疱性类天疱疮组织病理)

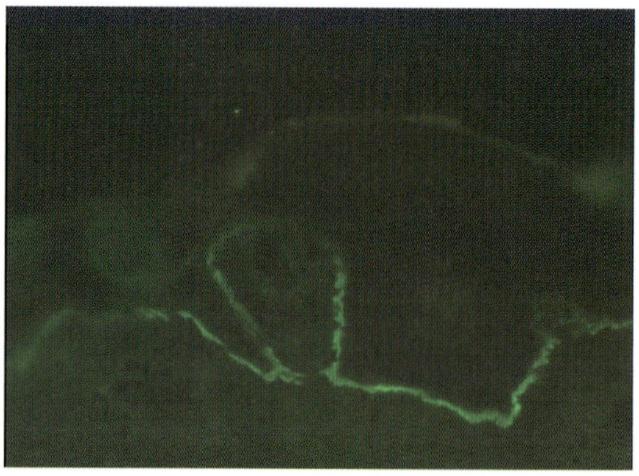

Fig. 21-10 DIF of bullous pemphigoid
(图 21-10 大疱性类天疱疮直接免疫荧光)

dapsone, and topical glucocorticoids may be a safe and effective alternative for some patients. Topical glucocorticoid therapy is effective for limited, moderate, and severe bullous pemphigoid.

砜、局部糖皮质激素外用可以作为一些患者安全、有效的替代疗法。外用糖皮质激素对于局限性、中度、重度大疱性类天疱疮均有效。

Studies have also demonstrated an excellent clinical response when a localized or generalized bullous pemphigoid was treated with tetracycline, minocycline, or erythromycin, with or without niacinamide. These drugs may suppress the inflammatory response at the BMZ, inhibit neutrophil chemotaxis, and increase cohesion of the dermoepidermal junction. The effect may be enhanced by the synergetic effect of niacinamide. Dehydration and secondary infections should be carefully avoided, and nutrition management is important for elderly patients. Plasma exchange therapy may also be performed in severe cases.

研究表明,单独应用四环素、米诺环素或红霉素,或联合应用烟酰胺对于局限型或泛发型大疱性类天疱疮具有良好的临床疗效。这些药物可以抑制皮肤基膜带的炎症反应,抑制中性粒细胞的趋化,增强真皮表皮的黏附。烟酰胺可能起协同作用。同时要注意脱水和继发感染,老年患者要注意补充营养。对危重患者,可考虑血浆置换。

Section Three Dermatitis Herpetiformis

第三节 疱疹样皮炎

Dermatitis herpetiformis is a rare, chronic, intensely burning, pruritic vesicular skin disease associated commonly with a subclinical gluten-sensitive enteropathy and IgA deposits in the upper dermal papillae.

疱疹样皮炎(dermatitis herpetiformis)是一种罕见的慢性水疱性皮肤病,损害有剧烈烧灼感和瘙痒,通常伴有临床症状不明显的谷胶敏感性肠病和真皮乳头上部 IgA 沉积。

【Etiology and Pathogenesis】

【病因及发病机制】

All patients with this disease have an underlying gluten-sensitive enteropathy, although this may be asymptomatic. The IgA deposits in the dermal papillae are gluten dependent. These deposits clear slowly after the introduction of a gluten-free diet. Recent study indicates that epidermal transglutaminase-3 is the autoantigen for dermatitis herpetiformis. HLA typing in dermatitis herpetiformis patients showed a tight correlation between this disease and DR3 or DQW2. Granular deposits of IgA and C3 in the superficial dermis under the BMZ induce an inflammatory reaction, which then separates the epidermis from the dermis to

尽管有时不出现症状,但疱疹样皮炎患者都伴发谷胶过敏性肠病,IgA 真皮乳头沉积是谷胶依赖性的,在采用严格的无谷胶饮食后,这些沉积的抗体可以逐渐清除。最近有研究表明转谷氨酰胺酶-3 是疱疹样皮炎的自身抗原。HLA 的研究表明,疱疹样皮炎患者大多与 HLA-DR3 及 HLA-DQW2 基因的表型具有强相关性,在基膜带下真皮浅层的 IgA 和 C3 颗粒状沉积可诱导炎症反应,导

form subepidermalblister.

致表皮和真皮的分离产生表皮下水疱。

【Clinical Manifestations】

Dermatitis herpetiformis usually begins in the age of 20-60, but many cases have been reported in children. Dermatitis herpetiformis presents initially with a few mild itchy papules or vesicles, but with time the disease evolves into its classic presentation of intensely burning urticarial papules, vesicles, and rarely bullae, either isolated or in groups such as in herpes simplex or zoster (hence the term herpetiformis). Blisters are usually distributed symmetrically on the elbows, knees, scalp, neck, shoulder, and buttock. Mucosal involvement occurs rarely.

【临床表现】

疱疹样皮炎发病年龄通常在 20～60 岁，但儿童亦好发。疱疹样皮炎最初表现为少数瘙痒性丘疹或水疱，症状轻微，此后病情逐渐发展为典型的临床表现，出现风团样丘疹、水疱，少数可见大疱，损害呈散在或群集分布，有的类似单纯疱疹或带状疱疹样皮疹(因此称为疱疹样)，伴有剧烈烧灼感。水疱对称分布，发生于肘、膝、头皮、颈、肩和臀部。黏膜受累少见。

【Histopathology and Immunopathology】

Microabscesses composed mainly of neutrophils and a few eosinophils are found in the subepidermal vesicles and dermal papillae. Direct immunofluorescence of uninvolved skin shows granular IgA, usually accompanied by C3 deposits in the dermal papillae and superficial dermis. The IgA and C3 deposits can be found not only in the samples from the peripheral skin of the lesions but also in samples from normal-appearing areas of skin. The granular deposition of IgA distinguishes dermatitis herpetiformis from linear IgA bullous dermatosis. Granules have a vertical "picket fence" appearance. Other immunoglobulins can be present in dermatitis herpetiformis; for example, IgM is found concurrently in more than 30% of cases.

【组织病理和免疫病理】

表皮下疱及真皮乳头内可见由中性粒细胞及少量嗜酸性粒细胞形成的微脓肿。取未受累的皮肤直接免疫荧光检查示 IgA 呈颗粒状沉积在真皮乳头及真皮浅层，并常伴有 C3 的沉积。此 IgA 和 C3 的沉积不仅见于皮损周围，亦见于外观正常的皮肤。疱疹样皮炎的 IgA 颗粒状沉积区别于线状 IgA 大疱性皮病的线状 IgA 沉积，颗粒状沉积在真皮乳头呈垂直的尖桩篱栅样外观。其他的免疫球蛋白也可以在疱疹样皮炎沉积，30%以上的疱疹样皮炎病例免疫荧光检查发现有 IgM 的沉积。

【Diagnosis and Differential Diagnosis】

Dermatitis herpetiformis is diagnosed by the clinical features (such as rashes, intense itching), subepidermal blistering, and granular IgA deposits in the papillae. The symptoms are improved remarkably by dapsone, and this fact also has diagnostic significance. Dermatitis herpetiformis is relatively rare in the Chinese population, and should be distinguished from other subepidermal blistering disorders such as linear IgA bullous dermatosis, bullous pemphigoid, herpes gestationis, and erythema multiforme.

【诊断与鉴别诊断】

依据临床特点(如皮疹、伴剧烈瘙痒)、表皮下水疱、真皮乳头颗粒状 IgA 沉积可做出诊断。口服氨苯砜症状能明显缓解，对帮助诊断有显著意义。疱疹样皮炎在中国人发病较罕见。本病需与其他表皮下大疱病如线状 IgA 大疱性皮病、大疱性类天疱疮、妊娠疱疹及多形红斑相鉴别。

【Treatment】

Dapsone has been found to be more effective than the somewhat safer alternative sulfapyridine and is the first choice for the treatment of the disease. For adults, the typical initial dosage of dapsone is 100-150 mg given orally once daily. Itching and burning can be controlled in 12-48 hours with this dose, and new lesions gradually stop appearing.

【治疗】

本病的治疗氨苯砜较磺胺吡啶更加有效。首选氨苯砜(dapsone, DDS)，成人常用剂量为 100～150 mg/d，一般在服药 12～48 h 后症状即可缓解，水疱消退，无新发水疱，瘙痒和灼烧感减轻。

Attention needs to be paid when dapsone is prescribed due to its severe side reactions. This compound can induce dose-related hemolysis, anemia, methemoglobinemia, and dapsone hypersensitivity syndrome in some severe cases. Therefore, a leukocyte count and hemoglobin level should be monitored weekly when possible during the first month, then monthly for 6 months, and semiannually thereafter. Sulfapyridine, a short-acting sulfonamide (starting dosage 500-1500 mg/d), can be converted to dapsone metabolically in the body and does not cause neuropathy. Strict adherence to a gluten-free diet (avoid foods containing wheat, rye, oats, triticale or barley) for at least 6 months allows most patients to begin a decreased dosage or possibly a discontinuation of dapsone therapy. The diet has to be followed for a long period (often 2 years) after medication is discontinued.

值得注意的是，氨苯砜可引起溶血性贫血、高铁血红蛋白血症，这些与剂量有关，严重时可出现氨苯砜超敏反应综合征。在用药的第一个月内应该每周检查血常规，以后 6 个月内每月检查一次，此后每半年检查一次。磺胺吡啶是一种短效的氨苯磺胺类药物(初始剂量为 500～1500 mg/d)，体内可代谢为氨苯砜，但不会导致神经病变。同时应该严格进行无谷胶饮食(避免含有谷胶的食物，如小麦、黑麦、燕麦、黑小麦和大麦)，至少 6 个月后大多数患者方可减少或停用氨苯砜，并且通常在停药后 2 年内均应维持无谷胶饮食。

Section Four　Linear IgA Bullous Dermatosis

第四节　线状 IgA 大疱性皮病

Linear IgA bullous dermatosis (LABD) is a chronic acquired subepidermal bullous disease that affects both children and adults, with cutaneous and mucosal involvement, and is characterized by linear IgA deposits on the BMZ of the lesions detected with immunofluorescence. It has clinical features similar to those of dermatitis herpetiformis, but the histologic and immunofluorescence patterns are different and there is no association with diseases of the small intestine. Drug-induced linear IgA bullous dermatosis is rare but increasing in frequency.

线状 IgA 大疱性皮病(linear IgA bullous dermatosis, LABD)系成人和儿童慢性获得性的表皮下大疱性疾病，累及皮肤和黏膜，皮损的免疫荧光检查示皮肤基膜带有线状 IgA 的沉积。线状 IgA 大疱性皮病与疱疹样皮炎临床表现非常相似，但组织病理和免疫荧光表达模式有所不同，并且与肠病无关。药物诱导的线状 IgA 大疱性皮病尽管罕见，但发病率正在增加。

【Etiology and Pathogenesis】

There is a strong association between linear IgA bullous dermatosis and the extended autoimmune haplotypes HLA-B8, HLA-CW7, and HLA-DR3, and possession of one of these haplotypes is associated with an early onset of disease. Drugs are also inducers of linear IgA bullous dermatosis, among which vancomycin is the most common causative agent and diclofenac less commonly. Vancomycin alone accounts for approximately half of the drug-induced cases. However, a large range of drugs have been reported as causative agents beyond these two. The incidence of lymphoproliferative disorders is higher among adult patients with linear IgA bullous dermatosis, which may occur even after the skin disease is in remission.

The autoantibodies in linear IgA bullous dermatosis are IgA molecules, which is unusual for an autoimmune disease; hence the presence of these autoantibodies has diagnostic significance. The IgA antibodies are directed to a number of different target antigens within the adhesion complex, including two that may be unique to

【病因及发病机制】

线状 IgA 大疱性皮病发病与自身免疫单倍型 HLA-B8、HLA-CW7、HLA-DR3 强相关，并且这些单倍型与早年起病相关。药物诱导的线状 IgA 大疱性皮病确实存在，万古霉素引起的最常见，有报道约半数药物诱导的线状 IgA 大疱性皮病与万古霉素相关。双氯芬酸引起的也不少见，同时还有很多其他药物引起的报道。在成人型线状 IgA 大疱性皮病中，患有淋巴增生性疾病的发病率增高，并且很多出现在线状 IgA 大疱性皮病缓解过程中。

线状 IgA 大疱性皮病的自身抗体是 IgA，这在自身免疫性疾病中不多见，因此，这些自身抗体的存在具有诊断价值。IgA 抗体针对的是黏附复合物中众多的不同的靶抗原，这些抗原包括分子量为

linear IgA bullous dermatosis, with molecular weights of 285 kD and 97/120 kD. Other targets include the BP230 and BP180 antigens, and collagen Ⅶ, the anchoring fibril component, as well as some still uncharacterized antigens. In *in vitro* studies, indirect evidence has shown that these antibodies are pathogenic and can cause splitting of the skin and infiltration of neutrophils along the BMZ.

285 kD 和 97/120 kD 的线状 IgA 大疱性皮病的特异性抗原、BP230 和 BP180、胶原蛋白Ⅶ、锚丝组分以及其他尚未鉴定出来的未知抗原。有间接证据表明这些抗体都存在致病性，可以引起体外培养的皮肤裂解以及导致中性粒细胞在基膜带的浸润。

【Clinical Manifestations】

Linear IgA bullous dermatosis is divided into childhood LABD, whose symptoms appear in children under age 10, and adult LABD, which occurs in adults aged 40 or older. The two conditions are more frequently seen in China than elsewhere, where it is about one-third as common as bullous pemphigoid. Moreover, one-third of Chinese patients are children. Erythema multiforme-like lesions and tense blisters occur over the entire body accompanied by intense itching which is similar to the manifestations of dermatitis herpetiformis. The lesions comprise urticarial plaques and papules, and annular, polycyclic lesions, often with blistering around the edges, forming the so-called "string of pearls sign" (Fig. 21-11). Lesions may also occur in the mucous membranes. The lesions tend to aggregate on the genitalia and inner regions of the thighs in children. In some cases, it may heal spontaneously.

【临床表现】

本病分为儿童型和成人型。儿童型一般在 10 岁以下发病，成人型在 40 岁以上发病。线状 IgA 大疱性皮病在中国发病率较高，约为大疱性类天疱疮发病率的 1/3，其中 1/3 的患者为儿童型。皮肤损害与疱疹样皮炎相似，主要表现为全身的多形红斑样皮损、紧张性的大疱以及剧烈的瘙痒。皮损包括荨麻疹性的斑块和丘疹，以及环形和多环形损害，特征性表现为环形红斑边缘的大疱，此谓"串珠征"(图 21-11)。黏膜损害并不少见。儿童型的皮疹多见于外阴等腔口周围、腹股沟部位。一些患者能自行缓解。

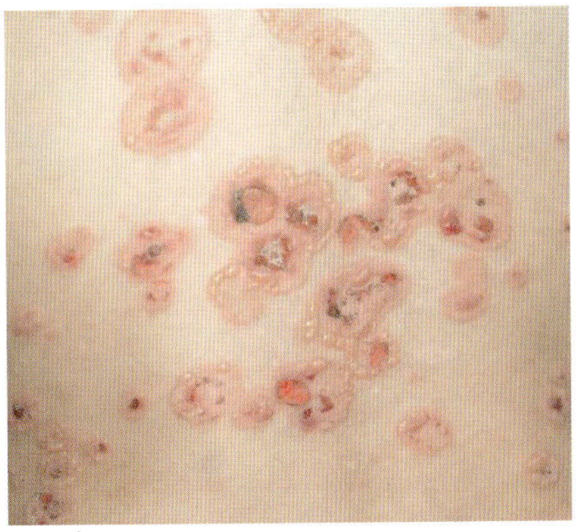

Fig. 21-11 Linear IgA bullous dermatosis

(图 21-11 线状 IgA 大疱性皮病)

【Histopathology and Immunopathology】

Subepidermal blistering is evident. Neutrophils are seen both at the tips of papillae and along the tips of rete ridges, a diagnostic feature for LABD. By direct immunofluorescence, linear IgA and C3 (in some cases) can be found along the epidermal basement membrane zone in samples taken from normal-appearing skin around the lesions. Anti-epidermal basement membrane zone IgA autoantibodies may be detected in the patient's serum by indirect immunofluorescence. Indirect immunofluorescence for basement

【组织病理和免疫病理】

组织病理示表皮下水疱。真皮乳头顶部及沿棘突处有中性粒细胞浸润(此点对 LABD 有诊断价值)。皮损周围皮肤直接免疫荧光检查示基膜带线状 IgA 沉积，部分病例可发现补体 C3 的沉积。以患者血清做间接免疫荧光检查，可以检测出抗表皮基膜带 IgA 的自身抗体。儿童型的自身抗体阳性率(约 80%)明显

membrane zone IgA autoantibodies is more often positive in children (about 80%) than in adults (about 30%), but the titers are usually low. However, the use of normal human skin split through the lamina lucida with 1 mol/L salt will increase sensitivity and give additional information to the site of the target antigen.

较成人型自身抗体(约 30%)高,但抗体滴度通常较低,若以 1 mol/L NaCl 的盐裂皮肤做底物,则可提高敏感性,并能获得靶抗原的位置等相关信息。

【Diagnosis and Differential Diagnosis】

The diagnosis of LABD is confirmed by ①the disease has an onset within 5-6 years of birth for children, or in the ages between 60-80 for adults; ② there is no gluten-sensitive enteropathy; ③annular erythematous patches with tense blisters at edges, the "string of pearls sign"; ④subepidermal blisters and neutrophils at the tips of papillae and linearly aligned along the dermal-epidermal junction; ⑤linear IgA and C3 along the dermal-epidermal junction (immune deposits localized to the roof of the blister in most cases). LABD should be distinguished from dermatitis herpetiformis, bullous pemphigoid, herpes gestationis, and bullous lupus erythematosus.

【诊断与鉴别诊断】

诊断依据:① 儿童一般 5～6 岁起病,成人为 60～80 岁起病;② 无谷胶敏感性肠病;③ 表现为环形红斑边缘的大疱,出现"串珠征";④ 表皮下水疱,真皮乳头顶部及真皮表皮交界处有中性粒细胞聚集;⑤ 皮损直接免疫荧光示真皮表皮交界处线状 IgA 和 C3 沉积,免疫复合物一般沉积在疱顶。鉴别诊断:本病主要应与疱疹样皮炎、大疱性类天疱疮、妊娠疱疹以及大疱性红斑狼疮相鉴别。

【Treatment】

Mild cases can be controlled with topical glucocorticoids alone. In severe cases, dapsone can be given in the early stage of the disease at a dose of 0.5 mg/(kg · d) (for children) and 25-50 mg/d (for adult). The dosage may be slowly increased to 1 mg/(kg · d) in children and 100-150 mg/d in adults. Most patients can be treated at this dosage with no obvious side effects.

Sulphapyridine (250 mg to 3 g daily) is an alternative that usually suppresses the eruptions rapidly, but the dose may need frequent adjustments. Dapsone and sulphapyridine can also be used together. When patients do not respond to either of these, glucocorticoids may need to be added. Azathioprine or cyclosporine may also be effective for recalcitrant cases. Tetracycline and nicotinamide are also suggested as alternative treatments.

The cutaneous lesions are always much more responsive than the mucosal lesions, which can be treated with topical glucocorticoids. Because of the good prognosis in the majority of patients, attempts should be made to avoid over-treatment and the risks of severe side effects of glucocorticoids.

【治疗】

某些患者症状较轻,局部外用糖皮质激素即可。严重患者,儿童早期给氨苯砜 0.5 mg/(kg · d)、成人 25～50 mg/d,然后逐渐加到儿童 1 mg/(kg · d)、成人 100～150 mg/d,此剂量大部分患者反应良好,无明显副作用。

磺胺吡啶作为一个替代药品,每天 250 mg 至 3 g 通常能很快控制症状,但剂量需要频繁地调整。有时可以联合应用氨苯砜和磺胺吡啶。对上述治疗无反应者可加用糖皮质激素。对于特别顽固治疗的患者可以考虑选用硫唑嘌呤或环孢菌素。也可选用四环素和烟酰胺。

皮肤损害对治疗的反应较黏膜损害好,后者可以局部加用糖皮质激素。由于大部分患者预后较好,应避免过度治疗,以免产生糖皮质激素的严重副反应。

Section Five Epidermolysis Bullosa Acquisita

Epidermolysis bullosa acquisita (EBA) is a rare, chronic, subepidermal, mucocutaneous blistering disease characterized by skin fragility and spontaneous or trauma-induced blisters that heal with scarring and milia formation. The causative antigen of the disease is collagen Ⅶ. The disease has a distinctive immunopathology.

第五节 获得性大疱性表皮松解症

获得性大疱性表皮松解症(epidermolysis bullosa acquisita, EBA)是一种罕见的慢性皮肤黏膜表皮下大疱性疾病。临床特征是皮肤脆性增加,自发或外伤诱发,大疱愈后遗留有瘢痕和粟丘疹。该病的靶抗原为Ⅶ型胶原，具有明显的免疫病理学特征。

【Etiology and Pathogenesis】

The pathogenesis of EBA is not clearly understood, but a number of conditions have been proven to be associated with EBA, namely amyloidosis, inflammatory bowel disease, carcinoma of the lung, multiple myeloma, systemic lupus erythematosus, and lymphoma. Collagen type Ⅶ, the major component of the anchoring fibrils, is the target antigen recognized by autoantibodies from patients with EBA. Collagen type Ⅶ is made up of a globular amino non-collagenous domain (NC1) and a collagenous triple helix domain. The autoantibodies in EBA react to the epitopes within the fibronectin-like region at the globular amino non-collagenous NC1 domain. Evidence shows that the autoantibodies are pathogenic. Complement-binding autoantibodies from patients with EBA bind to skin and attract neutrophils to the BMZ, resulting in subepidermal blisters.

【病因及发病机制】

尽管EBA发病机制尚不清楚，但已证实淀粉样变、炎症性肠病、肺癌、多发性骨髓瘤、系统性红斑狼疮以及淋巴瘤等诸多因素与其发病相关。Ⅶ型胶原是锚纤维的主要组分，为EBA的靶抗原，患者血液中自身抗体能识别。Ⅶ型胶原包含一个球形氨基非胶原结构域(NC1)和一个胶原三螺旋结构域。EBA自身抗体结合的抗原表位是NC1中一个类似于纤连蛋白(fibronectin)的区域。有证据表明EBA自身抗体是致病性的，其结合补体并结合于皮肤，吸引中性粒细胞至表皮基膜带，导致表皮下水疱形成。

【Clinical Manifestations】

EBA can be divided into three subtypes: the classical variant, the cicatricial pemphigoid-like variant, and the bullous pemphigoid-like variant.

(1) Classical variant of EBA: the classical or mechanobullous form of EBA is characterized by skin fragility, trauma-induced blisters, and erosions with mild mucous membrane involvement and healing with scarring. It resembles the dystrophic forms of inherited epidermolysis bullosa. Classical EBA presents with tense blisters on a non-inflammatory base. They appear in trauma-prone areas of the palms, soles, elbows, and knees. The lesions heal with scarring and milia formation that resemble porphyria cutanea tarda (Fig. 21-12). Some of these patients may have some scarring alopecia at specific sites or nail dystrophy.

【临床表现】

EBA主要有三个临床亚型：经典型EBA、瘢痕性类天疱疮样EBA及大疱性类天疱疮样EBA。

(1) 经典型EBA　又称为机械性EBA，临床特征为皮肤脆性增加，外伤后起疱、糜烂，伴黏膜轻度受累，愈后遗留瘢痕，类似于营养不良型遗传性大疱性表皮松解症。经典型EBA的临床表现为正常皮肤上张力性大疱，好发于易受外伤的部位，包括掌跖、肘、膝。皮损愈后遗留有瘢痕和粟丘疹，与迟发性皮肤卟啉病相似(图21-12)。一些患者可出现瘢痕性脱发和指(趾)甲营养不良。

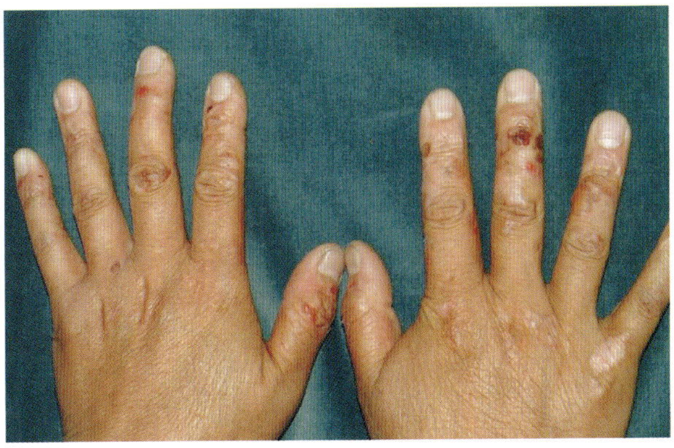

Fig. 21-12　Epidermolysis bullosa acquisita
(图21-12　获得性大疱性表皮松解症)

(2) Cicatricial pemphigoid-like variant of EBA: this type of EBA may extensively (or even predominantly) affect mucosal epithelia in a manner resembling cicatricial pemphigoid. Ocular involvement is common, but visual loss is rare.

(3) Bullous pemphigoid-like variant of EBA: approximately 50% of patients with EBA present this type of clinical picture in the early course of the disease. Tense blisters on an erythematous base are widely distributed on the trunk and flexural surfaces. The lesions present with itching and fragile skin, and may heal without scarring or milia formation.

(2) 瘢痕性类天疱疮样 EBA　此型 EBA 也可像瘢痕性类天疱疮一样广泛(或者大部分)累及黏膜上皮。眼部受累常见,但很少引起失明。

(3) 大疱性类天疱疮样 EBA　大约 50%的患者在疾病的早期表现为此种类型。红斑基础上发生张力性大疱,广泛分布于躯干和身体的屈侧。皮损瘙痒,皮肤脆性小,一些皮损愈后无瘢痕和粟丘疹。

【Histopathology and Immunopathology】

The blistering is subepidermal, but the precise histological findings depend on the stage of the disease. In the inflammatory stage of the disease, a heavy infiltrate can be seen, in which neutrophils predominate. By contrast, little or no infiltrate is found during the mechanobullous, non-inflammatory phase. With DIF assay, linear IgG deposits at the BMZ are found in the normal-appearing skin in all patients, but linear IgA and IgM, and even C3 may also be seen. Typically, linear depositions of IgG and C3 at the dermoepidermal junction form a U-serrated pattern, which is different from the n-serrated pattern of bullous pemphigoid. The skin split test with 1 mol/L salt showed that skin split occurs at the lamina lucida and the IgG antibodies are bound to the dermal aspect of the blister. Positive indirect immunofluorescence can be obtained in approximately half of the patients when tested with circulating autoantibodies specific to the BMZ. Immunoelectron microscopic studies have shown that the IgG were deposited in the upper dermis beneath the basal lamina and within the sublamina densa zone.

【组织病理和免疫病理】

组织病理检查示表皮下水疱,但准确的病理表现取决于疾病的阶段。在炎症期,可见疱内有以大量的中性粒细胞为主的浸润。在机械性大疱及非炎症阶段,通常只有稀疏或很少的细胞浸润。外观正常皮肤 DIF 示所有患者的基膜带均有 IgG 线状沉积,同时也可见 IgA、IgM 甚至 C3,IgG 和 C3 通常表现为"U"形锯齿形线状沉积,有别于大疱性类天疱疮的"n"形锯齿形线状沉积。患者的皮肤用 1 mol/L 的 NaCl 做盐裂试验,显示裂隙位于透明板及 IgG 沉积在大疱的真皮侧。约半数患者做间接免疫荧光可以显示循环自身抗体结合于基膜带。免疫电镜示 IgG 的沉积发生在致密板下的真皮上部及致密板下带。

【Diagnosis and Differential Diagnosis】

The absence of a hereditary history of blistering formation is an important clue for diagnosis. The most reliable methods for EBA diagnosis are indirect immunofluorescence and immunoblot assay following testing for skin splitting with 1 mol/L NaCl. Certain blistering diseases need to be differentiated from EBA including bullous pemphigoid, pemphigus, porphyria, drug-induced eruptions, or amyloidosis. In severe cases, cutaneous symptoms may be similar to a dystrophic form of inherited epidermolysis bullosa, presenting as nail deformity and coalescence of fingers and toes.

【诊断与鉴别诊断】

大疱的形成无遗传病史对诊断有重要帮助。诊断 EBA 的最可靠的方法为通过盐裂皮肤做间接免疫荧光检查和免疫印迹试验。本病需要与大疱性类天疱疮、天疱疮、卟啉病、药疹以及淀粉样变进行鉴别。在严重患者,可以出现营养不良型遗传性大疱性表皮松解症的症状(指(趾)甲畸形以及指(趾)的融合),需要予以鉴别。

【Treatment】

Glucocorticoids in combination with dapsone or sulfapyridine may be the preferred first-line treatment, but EBA in general is resistant to this treatment. Some patients are refractory to high-

【治疗】

糖皮质激素联合氨苯砜或者磺胺吡啶可能是最好的一线治疗方法,但大部分患者对治疗的反应差。一些患者即使

dose prednisone therapy. Then, colchicine (0.6-1.5 mg/d for up to 4 years) or cyclosporine (6 mg/(kg · d)), administered in conjunction with intravenous immunoglobulins may be effective alternatives.

用大剂量的泼尼松也疗效不佳。秋水仙碱(0.6～1.5 mg/d，持续 4 年)、环孢素(6 mg/(kg · d))和静脉注射免疫球蛋白可能有效。

Ye-qiang LIU (刘业强)

Chapter Twenty-two Disorders of the Mucous Membrane

第二十二章 黏膜疾病

The mucous membranes are linings of mostly endodermal origin, covered in epithelial layers, which are involved in absorption and secretions. They are coterminous with the skin at the nostrils, lips, ears, genitalia and anus. As with the structure of the skin next to them, the epithelial layers of mucosa are also thin in those sites, but lack the thickened protective cornified layer. Many mucous membranes have glands that secrete the sticky, thick fluid known as mucus which protects against pathogens.

黏膜起源于内胚层内面，表面覆盖具有吸收和分泌功能的上皮层。鼻、唇、耳、生殖器和肛门部位的黏膜与皮肤相互移行。黏膜的结构与皮肤类似，但其上皮层稍薄，缺乏具有保护作用的厚角质层。多数黏膜有分泌黏液的腺体，其分泌的黏液可抵御病原体侵袭。

Abnormalities of the mucous membranes may be associated with the following conditions: developmental disorders, infections, inflammatory cutaneous diseases, heritable dermatoses, and benign or malignant tumors. The chronic inflammation of the mucosa can result from dryness or chapping of the mucous membranes, sustained lip licking or some chronic inflammatory reaction arising from a specific chronic irritation. The differences in the clinical features between the mucous membranes and skin lesions exist, for example, bullae are not likely to appear in mucous membrane disorders. Such characteristics will be necessary in making decisive conclusion regarding treatment in a clinical setting when dealing with mucous membrane disorders.

黏膜异常可能与以下状态相关：发育异常、感染、炎症性皮肤病、遗传性皮肤病、良恶性肿瘤。黏膜的慢性炎症可由黏膜干燥、皲裂、长期舔唇或其他特定慢性刺激导致的慢性炎症反应所引起。黏膜与皮肤损害的临床特征是不同的，比如黏膜疾病不表现为大疱，而皮肤可以。这些特征对于临床黏膜疾病的诊断和治疗是必要的。

Section One Recurrent Aphthous Stomatitis

第一节 复发性阿弗他口腔炎

Recurrent aphthous stomatitis, also known as recurrent aphthous ulcer, is the most common oral mucosal disease, and the causes remain poorly understood. The most common presentation is single or multiple recurrent painful ulcers which appear in the mouth and sometimes in the genital area.

复发性阿弗他口腔炎（recurrent aphthous stomatitis）又称为复发性口疮，是最常见的口腔黏膜疾病，病因不明，多表现为单个或多发的、复发性、疼痛性口腔溃疡，也可发生于生殖器部位。

【Etiology and Pathogenesis】

【病因及发病机制】

Many local and systemic factors have been proven to be associated with this condition. Some studies showed that genetic factors and/or immunopathogenic mechanisms may contribute to the development of recurrent aphthous stomatitis. There is also a definite genetic component to the factors that govern susceptibility to this disorder. More than 42% of patients who report first-degree relatives with a history of the disease will develop this disease at some point of their lives. When both parents of the patient have or have had the disease, then the likelihood rises to 90%. By contrast, the likelihood is less than 20% among patients who report neither parent having recurrent aphthous stomatitis.

许多局部因素和系统因素已被证实与复发性阿弗他口腔炎相关，有研究提示遗传因素和/或免疫机制与本病发生有关。遗传因素在复发性阿弗他口腔炎的易感性中起主导地位，一级亲属患病的患者中有超过42%在其生命过程中可发生本病，双亲患病（既往或现患病）的患者发生本病的风险高达90%，而双亲不患病的患者发病风险不到20%。

A cell-mediated immune response has been linked to this

本病的发病机制与细胞免疫有关，T

disease's pathogenesis. Here TNF-α induced by T-cells and other leukocytes affects endothelial cells and stimulates neutrophil chemotaxis to produce an inflammatory response at the site. Other cytokines (such as IL-2) can activate NK cells and will also play important roles in this condition.

细胞及其他白细胞产生的 TNF-α 通过影响内皮细胞、活化中性粒细胞的趋化作用从而在局部引起炎症反应。其他细胞因子(如白介素 2)通过活化 NK 细胞参与本病的发生。

Some foods such as chocolate, coffee, nuts, strawberries, cheese, tomatoes and wheat gluten all are implicated in this disease; therefore, about 50% of patients may improve clinically when these suspected foods are precluded from the diet. Patch tests to benzoic acid or cinnamaldehyde are positive in some patients. Deficiencies of vitamins B1/B2/B6/B12, folic acid and iron may also be associated with this condition.

某些食物与本病有关,如可可、咖啡、坚果、草莓、奶酪、土豆、含谷胶面粉。约 50%的患者避免食用这些食物后症状可缓解。部分患者苯甲酸、肉桂醛斑贴试验可为阳性。维生素 B1、维生素 B2、维生素 B6、维生素 B12、叶酸、铁缺乏可能也与本病相关。

Exposure to certain drugs, such as nicorandil, or to non-steroidal anti-inflammatory drugs may induce aphthae-like ulcers in older people (but rarely in younger patients). Trauma, depression, tobacco smoking, hormonal imbalance, and gastrointestinal diseases may also provoke the formation of these ulcers.

老年人使用尼可地尔和非甾体类抗炎药可能诱发阿弗他样溃疡,年轻人少见。创伤、抑郁、吸烟、内分泌失调、胃肠疾病可诱发溃疡形成。

【Clinical Manifestations】

【临床表现】

Recurrent aphthous stomatitis is possibly the most common oral mucosal disease, and can be classified into three variants based on the clinical features. The genital area and/or anus may also be involved occasionally in addition to the oral sores. Females are more likely to be affected than males.

复发性阿弗他口腔炎是最常见的口腔黏膜疾病,根据其临床特征可分为 3 种临床变异型。除了常见的口腔损害,偶尔也会累及外阴和/或肛门,其中女性发病率较高。

Recurrent aphthous stomatitis minor is the most common variant. It is characterized by recurrent, round, discrete, small and painful well-defined ulcers that are usually covered by a grayish-yellow pseudomembrane (fibrinous exudate) with an erythematous halo. The ulcers heal without scarring within 10-14 days.

轻型复发性阿弗他口腔炎最常见,表现为散在分布、小的、圆形、边界清楚的疼痛性复发性溃疡,表面覆盖灰黄色假膜(纤维素性渗出),周围有红晕,10～14 天溃疡愈合,不留瘢痕。

Recurrent aphthous stomatitis major is less common and exhibits larger ulcers (greater than 5 mm in diameter) than the minor type. Also, the ulcers may coalesce and often have an irregular border. This variety usually lasts for 6 weeks or longer, and the lesions frequently leave scars after healing.

重型复发性阿弗他口腔炎相对少见,溃疡较轻型复发性阿弗他口腔炎大,直径超过 5 mm,可融合,边缘不规则,愈合时间常超过 6 周,有瘢痕形成。

The third variant of recurrent aphthous stomatitis is herpetiform ulcers, which presents as multiple small clusters of pinpoint vesicles and ulcers that may coalesce to form a single large irregular ulcer which takes 7-10 days to heal.

第 3 种类型为疱疹样溃疡,损害初发为群集性针尖大小的水疱、溃疡,相互融合形成大的不规则溃疡,7～10 天愈合。

Despite the clinical forms of recurrent aphthous stomatitis, the ulcers are mostly confined to the nonkeratinized mucosa of the mouth, sparing the dorsum of the tongue, the gingiva, and the hard palate. In general, patients have no symptoms other than submandibular lymphadenopathy and rarely fever.

不管哪种临床类型,溃疡多发生在口腔黏膜角化不显著的地方,而舌背、牙龈、硬腭等部位黏膜不累及。除了下颌下淋巴结肿大,偶有发热,一般不出现其他症状。

【Histopathology】

Non-specific chronic inflammation may be found under microscopy. In the early stage, a predominantly lymphocytic infiltrate in the epithelium, edema and vacuolation of the epithelial cells are present. In the later stages of the condition, vasculitis in the dermis can be seen and the infiltrate is mainly composed of neutrophils, lymphocytes and plasma cells. Scarring by connective tissue regeneration may be evident in old lesions.

【组织病理】

镜下表现为非特异性慢性炎症。早期表皮以淋巴细胞浸润为主，并出现上皮细胞水肿、空泡形成。晚期表现为真皮血管炎，以中性粒细胞、淋巴细胞、浆细胞浸润为主。陈旧性皮损由于结缔组织再生，故有明显瘢痕形成。

【Diagnosis】

The diagnosis of recurrent aphthous stomatitis is made on the basis of its recurrent history and the clinical features. There are no specific laboratory tests available, so each type of recurrent aphthous stomatitis needs to be differentiated from the following diseases:

(1) Behçet syndrome: a form of vasculitis that can lead to ulceration in oral mucous membranes but is often accompanied by other symptoms such as genital ulcers, eye inflammation, or skin lesions (papulopustules, folliculitis, and erythema nodosum and acneiform lesions).

(2) Herpes simplex: a viral disease caused by herpes simplex virus type Ⅰ. Intraoral herpes appearing inside the mouth is sometimes mistaken for recurrent aphthous stomatitis, but aphthous ulcers usually lack the characteristic vesicular stage of herpes.

【诊断】

复发性阿弗他口腔炎的诊断主要依靠反复发作的病史和临床特点，缺乏特异性实验室检查，因此不同类型的复发性阿弗他口腔炎需与下列疾病鉴别。

(1) 白塞氏综合征　白塞氏综合征是一种可引起口腔溃疡的血管炎，但常伴有其他表现，如生殖器溃疡、眼部炎症、皮肤损害(丘脓疱疹、毛囊炎、结节性红斑、痤疮样皮损)。

(2) 单纯疱疹　由单纯疱疹病毒Ⅰ型感染引起的病毒性皮肤病，发生在口腔内的单纯疱疹容易与复发性阿弗他口腔炎混淆，阿弗他口腔炎缺乏单纯疱疹特征性的水疱期。

【Treatment】

Management of this condition depends on the clinical presentation and symptoms. The available therapeutic list below is intended to alleviate the symptoms and shorten the healing time.

(1) Topical therapy: topical glucocorticoids, when used for a short period, have a very safe profile and should be the first line of treatment for recurrent aphthous stomatitis. Since early intervention is the key to optimum resolution, high-potency topical glucocorticoids may be prescribed at the beginning. Antibiotic ointments may be used to prevent bacterial infection. Topical use of anesthetics may be recommended for pain relief. Some growth factors may also be of benefit for ulcer recovery.

(2) Systemic therapy: vitamin B group and vitamin C are useful for recurrent aphthous stomatitis patients. Systemic anti-inflammatory drugs, particularly glucocorticoids can be used for severe cases to reduce inflammation and pain. Antimicrobial and analgesic drugs may be given in some patients.

【治疗】

复发性阿弗他口腔炎的治疗主要根据患者的临床表现及症状，以减轻症状和缩短愈合时间为目的。

(1) 局部治疗　首选短期局部应用糖皮质激素，安全性好，建议选用强效外用糖皮质激素进行早期干预，效果良好。抗生素软膏可预防细菌感染。疼痛明显可以局部使用麻醉剂。某些生长因子可以促进溃疡愈合。

(2) 系统治疗　服用 B 族维生素和维生素 C 有一定效果。还可系统性应用抗炎药物，如糖皮质激素可明显减轻重症患者的炎症和疼痛。抗生素和镇痛药也可使用。

【Prevention】

It is essential to educate the patient regarding the nature of

【预防】

健康教育，告知患者疾病的特点。

this condition. Avoidance of suspected foods should accelerate the improvement in the patient's condition.

避免某些食物可以改善临床症状。

Section Two Lichen Sclerosus

Lichen sclerosus is a chronic disease of the skin and mucosa. The terms lichen sclerosus *et* atrophicus, kraurosis vulvae, and balanitis xerotica obliterans are synonymous but lately have all been replaced by the single term lichen sclerosus (LS). LS can present from childhood to old age and occurs in all races.

【Etiology and Pathogenesis】

The pathogenesis of LS is poorly understood. Autoimmune diseases (thyroid disease, vitiligo, alopecia areata, and pernicious anemia) occur in between one-fifth and one-third of women with LS, but are much less common in men. Psoriasis is increased in women with LS, accounting for 7.5%-17% of patients according to the literature. Autoantibodies to extracellular matrix protein (ECM1) are found in 80% of LS patients (as compared to 4% of controls and 7%-10% of patients with other autoimmune diseases). The titer of the ECM1 autoantibody is correlated to the severity of the disease. However, the implication of humoral autoimmunity in the pathogenesis of LS is still unclear.

【Clinical Manifestations】

The initial lesions of LS are white, polygonal, flat-topped papules, plaques, or atrophic patches. Lesions may be surrounded by an erythematous to violaceous halo. Within atrophic lesions, the skin is smooth, slightly wrinkled, soft, and white (Fig. 22-1). Bullae, often hemorrhagic, telangiectasias, and purpura may occur on the surface of the patches.

About 40% of women with LS are asymptomatic. However, when men are referred to specialists for diagnosis, virtually 100% are symptomatic. Itching is frequently severe, especially when the lesion affects the anogenital area. In the genital area, fissuring and erosion may occur. This may result in dysuria, urethral and vaginal discharge, dyspareunia, and burning pain. Normal anatomic structures may be obliterated, with loss of the labia minora, clitoral hood, and urethral meatus. In women, this perineal involvement typically affects the vulvar and perianal areas, giving a "figure-eight" or "hourglass" appearance (Fig. 22-1). Introital stenosis or fusion may occur. However, the vaginal and cervical mucosae are not involved in LS in contrast to lichen planus. In males, lesions are atrophic and may be markedly hypopigmented or depigmented, resembling vitiligo. Lesions usually involve only the glans penis, but may extend on to the shaft of the penis and scrotum.

第二节 硬化性苔藓

硬化性苔藓(lichen sclerosus)是一种慢性皮肤黏膜疾病。硬化萎缩性苔藓、女阴干枯症、闭塞性干燥性龟头炎均属同一疾病,现统称为硬化性苔藓(LS)。儿童和老人均可发病,可见于所有人种。

【病因及发病机制】

LS的发病机制尚不明确。有五分之一到三分之一患有LS的女性患者罹患自身免疫性疾病(甲状腺疾病、白癜风、斑秃和恶性贫血),而男性患者较少见。LS女性患者银屑病的发病率有所上升,占7.5%~17%。与对照组的4%及其他自身免疫性疾病的7%~10%相比,LS患者中存在针对ECM1的抗体的比例为80%。ECM1抗体滴度与病情严重程度相关。体液免疫在LS的发病机制中的作用尚不清楚。

【临床表现】

LS的原发损害为白色的、多角形平顶丘疹、斑块或萎缩性斑片。皮损周边有红晕,有时可为紫色。萎缩性皮损表现为白色、柔软、表面光滑、稍带皱纹的皮肤(图22-1),还可出现出血性大疱、毛细血管扩张和紫癜。

40%的LS女性患者无自觉症状,而几乎100%的LS男性患者均有自觉症状。表现为严重的瘙痒,特别是在肛门、生殖器部位。在生殖器区域常可能表现为裂隙和糜烂。这可导致排尿困难、尿道阴道瘘、性交困难和烧灼痛。小阴唇、阴蒂冠和尿道口的正常解剖结构可消失。女性患者会阴部的典型病变是累及外阴和肛周部位,形成"8"字形或"沙漏"样表现(图22-1),可发生阴唇狭窄或融合。与扁平苔藓相反,阴道及子宫颈黏膜不受累。男性患者表现为萎缩性皮损,同时可伴明显色素减退或脱色,类似于白癜风。皮损常仅累及龟头,也可累及阴茎和阴囊。

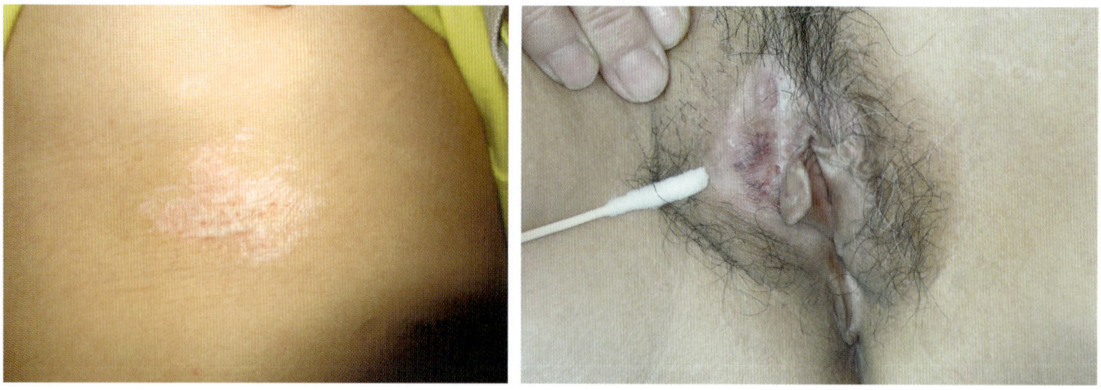

(a)　　(b)

Fig. 22-1　Lichen sclerosus(图 22-1　硬化性苔藓)

Extragenital lesions are most frequent on the upper back, chest, and breasts, and are usually asymptomatic otherwise. The tongue and oral mucosa may also be involved. Patients having only extragenital lesions with histologic features of both LS and morphea have been reported.

生殖器以外的损害最常见于上背、胸部和乳房,通常无症状。舌和口腔黏膜亦可受累。有报道称仅有生殖器外损害的 LS 患者,其病理学表现同时具有 LS 和硬斑病的组织学特征。

【Histopathology】

【组织病理】

Early lesions are characterized by interface dermatitis with vacuolar alteration of keratinocytes. As the disease progresses, the epidermis becomes thinner and the rete ridges are flattened and accompanied by compact hyperkeratosis and follicular and eccrine plugging. The upper dermis is edematous, with collagen in this layer being homogenized. Immediately beneath the altered papillary dermis, a sparse band-like and perivascular lymphoid infiltrate are seen (Fig. 22-2). In pruritic lesions, coexistent changes of lichen simplex chronicus may be seen, with acanthosis rather than atrophy of the epidermis.

早期损害以伴有角质形成细胞空泡变性的界面皮炎为特征。随疾病进展,表皮逐渐变薄,表皮突变平,伴有致密的角化过度及毛囊与小汗腺角质栓。真皮浅层水肿,真皮上部胶原组织均质化。病变的真皮乳头层下方可见稀疏的带状和血管周围淋巴样浸润(图 22-2)。瘙痒性皮损中可同时伴有慢性单纯性苔藓的棘层增厚改变,而不是皮肤萎缩改变。

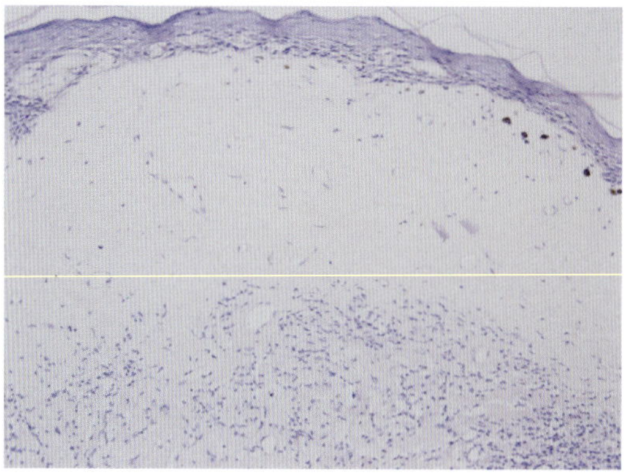

Fig. 22-2　Lichen sclerosus-histopathology(图 22-2　硬化性苔藓-组织病理)

【Differential Diagnosis】

【鉴别诊断】

Extragenital LS must be differentiated from guttate morphea and lichen planus, especially from the atrophic type of lichen planus. Anogenital LS must be distinguished from genital lichen planus, lichen simplex chronicus, vulvar intraepithelial neoplasia

生殖器外 LS 必须与点滴状硬斑病和扁平苔藓鉴别,特别是与萎缩性扁平苔藓鉴别。肛门生殖器 LS 必须与生殖器扁平苔藓、慢性单纯性苔藓、女阴上皮

(SCC *in situ*), and extramammary Paget's disease. The white color and atrophic surface are characteristic, and a biopsy from the affected site can make a confirmative diagnosis.

内肿瘤(原位 SCC)和乳房外 Paget's 病相鉴别。皮损具有特征性的白色、萎缩性表面,对该部位组织进行活检可明确诊断。

【Treatment】

The use of superpotent topical glucocorticoids has remarkable potential for the management of anogenital LS. They are accepted universally as one of the best choices for all forms of genital LS. Most patients will respond to once daily application of these agents and can subsequently be tapered to less frequent applications (once or twice a week) or to lower-strength steroids. Penile, vulvar, and prepubertal LS in girls have all been documented to respond to this form of treatment. Coexistent candidiasis may be present or appear after this treatment, and can be managed with topical or oral antifungal agents.

Topical 0.1% tacrolimus ointments have also been demonstrated to be effective in genital LS. Topical retinoic acid can be used for patients in whom superpotent topical glucocorticoids are ineffective or not tolerated. Topical calcipotriol may also be of benefit. Topical testosterone was found to be no more effective than a simple emollient. As extragenital LS is very difficult to treat, in cases where superpotent topical glucocorticoids and alternative means mentioned above are ineffective, potassium p-aminobenzoic acid, PUVA, UVA1, narrow-band UVB, calcipotriol, or antimalarials may be considered for use.

【治疗】

局部使用超强效糖皮质激素可明显改善肛周外生殖器的 LS。所有类型的生殖器部位 LS 均可采用此种治疗方式。一般来说,大部分患者对每天 1 次应用这些制剂有效,然后可逐渐减少使用次数(1～2 次/周)或使用相对弱效的类固醇激素制剂。阴茎、女阴和女性青春期前 LS 用此方法治疗均有效。念珠菌感染可同时存在或在激素治疗后出现,可局部外用和口服抗真菌药物来治疗。

已证实局部使用 0.1%他克莫司软膏对生殖器部位 LS 有效。对局部应用超强效糖皮质激素无效或不能耐受的患者,可选用外用维 A 酸类药物。外用卡泊三醇也有一定疗效。局部使用睾酮不会比润滑剂有效。生殖器外 LS 治疗困难。如果超强效局部糖皮质激素和上面提及的其他方法无效,可试用对氨基苯甲酸钾、PUVA、长波紫外线 1(UVA1)、窄谱 UVB、卡泊三醇或抗疟药。

Section Three　Contact Cheilitis

Contact cheilitis is a medical condition involving inflammation of the lips when they come into direct contact with particular allergens.

第三节　接触性唇炎

接触性唇炎(contact cheilitis)是唇部接触特定变应原后发生的唇部炎症。

【Etiology】

A variety of allergens have been associated with contact cheilitis. These include cosmetics and other materials that normally come into contact with the lips (e.g., lipsticks, sunscreens, lip fragrances, skin care agents, nail polish, cigarette holders, rubber, metals, and toothpaste); foods (e.g., oranges, lemons, artichokes, mangoes, sugar cane) and even reeds for music instruments such as saxophones or clarinets. Some medications may also act as the allergens for this condition.

【病因】

接触性皮炎与多种变应原有关,包括化妆品和唇部接触用品(唇膏、防晒产品、唇香油、护肤品、亮甲剂、烟嘴、橡皮、金属、牙膏)、食物(橘子、柠檬、洋蓟、芒果、甘蔗),甚至是萨克斯管或单簧管的簧片。某些药物也会引起变应性接触性唇炎。

【Clinical Manifestations】

Lesions in vermillion border are the most common, with dryness, scaling and an uncomfortable sensation. In severe cases, edema, vesicles, crusting, and fissuring may occur, with a burning

【临床表现】

本病通常表现为唇红干燥、脱屑和不适,严重者局部红肿、水疱、结痂、皲裂,伴有烧灼感,瘙痒也是常见的症状。

sensation on the lips. Pruritus is also a common complaint with allergic contact cheilitis.

【Diagnosis】

The diagnosis can usually be made from the history of contact with the specific allergen, coupled with the clinical features of the lips.

【诊断】

根据变应原接触史和唇部临床表现可以诊断。

【Treatment】

Avoidance of suspected antigens and reduction of any irritation are both usually of benefit for patients with allergic contact cheilitis, since it is not hard to eliminate virtually all possible sources of irritation. Topical glucocorticoids and systemic anti-histamines may also be used to relieve the symptoms.

【治疗】

避免接触可疑过敏原,减少局部刺激,这是简单易行的方法。局部使用糖皮质激素和系统抗组胺药都有效。

Section Four Actinic Cheilitis

第四节 光线性唇炎

Actinic cheilitis, also known as solar cheilitis, is a diffuse inflammation of the vermilion border of the lips which results from excessive exposure to UV light (usually but not always from sunlight). It primarily affects persons with light complexions, especially those with a tendency to sunburn easily.

光线性唇炎(actinic cheilitis),又称为日光性唇炎,是日光(也有可能是其他的紫外光)过度照射引起的唇红部弥漫性炎症改变,常发生于肤色浅易晒伤的人群。

【Etiology】

Actinic cheilitis is caused by chronic and excessive exposure to ultraviolet radiation. Other etiologic factors include tobacco, lip irritation, poor oral hygiene, and ill-fitting dentures.

【病因】

光线性唇炎的发生与长期或过度紫外线照射有关。吸烟、唇刺激、口腔卫生差、不适当的牙套等也可导致该病发生。

【Clinical Manifestations】

Actinic cheilitis is more common in older males and in individuals with a light complexion who have history of chronic sun exposure. Farmers, fishers and sportsmen are easily affected. Almost every case begins at the vermilion of the lower lip due to this area's more direct exposure to sunlight. There are two forms of actinic cheilitis that have been described in clinical terms.

(1) Acute actinic cheilitis: patient has a history of excessive exposure to sunlight before onset. The typical clinical features are redness, erosion, exudation and crusts with burning or pain on sun exposed lips. Scar formation is rare.

(2) Chronic actinic cheilitis: the labial changes progress so slowly that the patient is frequently unaware of them; they begin with mild swelling, dryness, scaling and vermilion zone atrophy, and are often combined with pallor and erythema spots. The normal demarcation line between the vermilion zone and the skin of the lip becomes blurred or may even disappear. As the lesion progresses, rough, scaly areas develop on the drier portions of the vermilion, and the appearance is somewhat like leukoplakia. Painful ulceration may develop in one or more sites, and these may remain unhealed

【临床表现】

光线性唇炎多见于老年男性,浅肤色且有长期日晒史的个体如农民、渔民、运动员易患本病。皮损好发于下唇唇红部,与该部位易直接暴露于日光中有关。临床上,光线性唇炎有两种类型。

(1) 急性光线性唇炎 发病前有强烈阳光照射史,急性发作,表现为局部红肿、糜烂、渗出、结痂,伴有烧灼感或疼痛。很少有瘢痕形成。

(2) 慢性光线性唇炎 缓慢发病,病情轻微,以致被忽视。早期表现为轻微肿胀、干燥、脱屑,以及伴有红斑或苍白斑点的唇红部位萎缩。唇红与皮肤的分界线模糊或消失。随着病情进展,唇红更干燥的部位表面变得粗糙、脱屑严重,有时表现为类似黏膜白斑样的损害。可出现单发或多发的疼痛性溃疡,长期愈合不良,约10%的患者在此基础上可发

for a long period of time and will then lead to squamous cell carcinoma (SCC) in about 10% of patients.

【Histopathology】

Hyperkeratosis, parakeratosis, acanthosis, edema and elongation of the rete ridges may be seen in the epidermis. In the upper dermis, telangiectasis, degeneration of elastic tissue (solar elastosis) and chronic inflammatory infiltration are usually seen. Epithelial dysplasia of the basal and suprabasal layers may also present in actinic mucosal leukoplakia.

【Diagnosis】

Diagnosis is based on the onset of the disease in association with known or suspected previous exposure to UV radiation and typical clinical manifestations.

【Prevention and Treatment】

Prevention of any further exposure to sunlight is important. Also, immediate cooling of the affected areas, if possible, can greatly reduce the severity of the condition. Application of topical glucocorticoid creams or oral hydroxylchloroquine 0.1-0.2 g, two times a day may be effective for patients in the early stages. Topical 5-fluorouracil (5-FU) has been shown as an effective therapy for diffuse proliferative actinic cheilitis. Localized lesions respond well to cryotherapy. Surgical excision may be considered in patients with actinic mucosal leukoplakia or precancerous lesions.

展为鳞状细胞癌。

【组织病理】

表皮表现为角化过度和角化不全、棘层肥厚、水肿，表皮突延长；真皮浅层常见毛细血管扩张，弹性组织变性（日光性弹力纤维变性）及慢性炎症细胞浸润。光线性黏膜白斑患者在基底层和基底层上部可有上皮间变。

【诊断】

根据发病情况与已知或可疑的紫外线暴露史以及典型的临床表现即可诊断。

【预防与治疗】

避免日晒是相当重要的，及时对受累处进行冷疗能显著改善病情。早期患者可外用糖皮质激素霜或口服羟氯喹，0.1～0.2 g，每日 2 次；外用 5-氟尿嘧啶对于弥漫性增殖性光线性唇炎有效。局限性皮损冷冻治疗效果良好。光线性黏膜白斑或癌前病变应考虑手术切除。

Section Five　Exfoliative Cheilitis

Exfoliative cheilitis is a recurrent chronic superficial desquamative inflammation of the lips.

【Etiology】

The etiology is unknown, although some cases may be factitious. Exfoliative cheilitis in the upper lip is often a primary disorder, but lesions in the lower lip are more likely to be indications of some other disease, such as seborrheic dermatitis, atopic dermatitis or may even be a side reaction to retinoid therapy.

A wide variety of irritants have been linked to cheilitis, including lipsticks, toothpaste, mouthwashes, shaving materials, nail polish, excessive lip licking and ultraviolet radiation.

【Clinical Manifestations】

The lower lip is more often involved in young females and inflammation is likely to be confined to the vermilion zone. Exfoliative cheilitis is a desquamative, mild inflammatory recurrent condition of the lips that is characterized by dryness and scaling in the vermilion zone. Fissures, crusts and pain will present only in

第五节　剥脱性唇炎

剥脱性唇炎（exfoliative cheilitis）是唇部反复脱屑的慢性浅表性炎症。

【病因】

病因不明，有的病例可能是人为引起的。发生在上唇的剥脱性唇炎常常是原发的，下唇损害可以是其他疾病的表现，如脂溢性皮炎、特应性皮炎，甚至可能是维 A 酸药物治疗的副反应。

唇炎相关刺激因素有：唇膏、牙膏、含漱液、剃须用制剂、亮甲剂、过度舔唇、紫外线辐射。

【临床表现】

下唇受累多见于青年女性，损害可能局限于唇红部位。剥脱性唇炎炎症轻，反复发作，主要表现为唇红处干燥、脱屑，严重者有皲裂、结痂和疼痛（图 22-3）。慢性病程，可持续数月或数年。

severe cases (Fig. 22-3). The condition may persist for months or years.

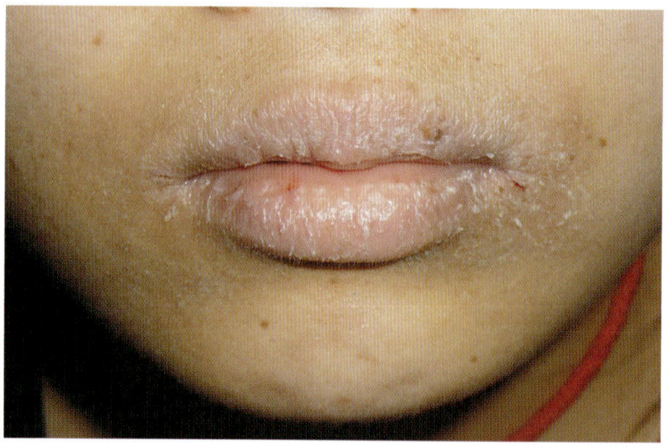

Fig. 22-3 Exfoliative cheilitis(图 22-3 剥脱性唇炎)

【Diagnosis】

The diagnosis is based on desquamative chronic inflammation in the vermilion zone with no clear causative factor. Cheilitis from other causes will need to be ruled out.

【诊断】

根据唇红部位慢性脱屑性炎症、诱因不明即可诊断。必须排除其他原因引起的唇炎。

【Treatment】

It is important to avoid all presumed irritants in order to reduce any further damage. The lesions may improve with topical glucocorticoid ointments.

【治疗】

避免所有可疑刺激因素,减少进一步损害,局部外用糖皮质激素软膏可改善皮损。

Section Six Fordyce Disease

第六节 Fordyce 病

Fordyce disease (also known as Fordyce's spots) presents as enlarged sebaceous glands in the mucosae of the mouth and genitals. The spots are a form of ectopic sebaceous gland.

Fordyce 病(Fordyce disease)又称为 Fordyce's 斑,表现为口腔和外阴黏膜皮脂腺肥大,是一种皮脂腺异位。

【Etiology and Pathogenesis】

While there seems to be a genetic component, the cause for this condition is idiopathic. Local irritation or trauma may affect the natural course of the disease.

【病因及发病机制】

本病是一种特发性疾病,可能与遗传有关。局部刺激和创伤也可能在发病中起作用。

【Clinical Manifestations】

Fordyce's spots are common in adult males. At birth the papules are present but may not become evident until a child reaches puberty. The condition can appear either as a single lesion or in a symmetrical group of up to one hundred. The typical lesions are small, white or yellow, 1-2 mm in diameter, painless, raised papules. They usually occur on the shaft of the penis or on the labia, as well as on the inner surface and vermilion border of the lips (Fig. 22-4).

【临床表现】

本病成年男性常见。丘疹出生即有,直到青春期才变得明显。皮损可以单发,或近百颗对称分布。典型皮损表现为高出皮面的白色或黄色小丘疹,直径为 1～2 mm,无疼痛感。皮损发生于阴茎和阴唇,也可见于唇红缘及其内侧(图 22-4)。

【Diagnosis】

Diagnosis is based on patient history and the clinical appearance of the rashes.

【诊断】

依靠病史及皮损的临床特点即可确诊。

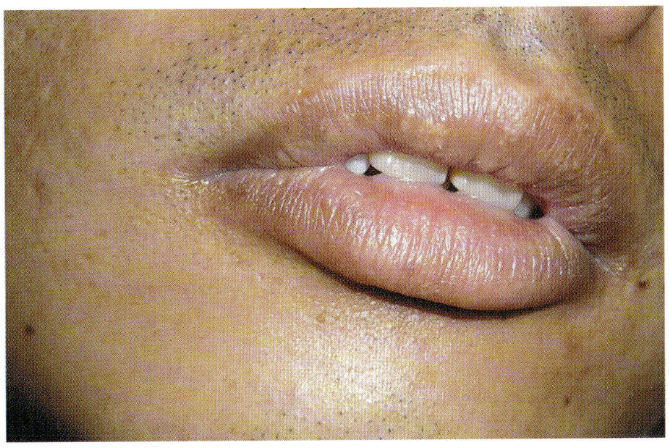

Fig. 22-4 Fordyce disease(图 22-4 Fordyce 病)

【Treatment】

Treatment is not necessary in many cases. Tretinoin gels or creams can reverse the effects of the condition and prevent it from getting worse. CO_2 laser or electrodesiccation has also been used with some success to ameliorate the appearance of this condition.

【治疗】

一般不需治疗。维 A 酸凝胶或霜剂可以改善皮损，并防止其进一步恶化。CO_2 激光和电离子治疗可以改善外观。

Section Seven Pearly Penile Papules

第七节 珍珠状阴茎丘疹

Pearly penile papules are also known as hirsutoid papillomas of the penis. Pearly white papules appear circumferentially around the coronal margin of the glans penis.

珍珠状阴茎丘疹（pearly penile papules）又称为阴茎多毛状乳头瘤，主要表现为在龟头的冠状沟缘环绕排列的白色珍珠样丘疹。

【Etiology and Pathogenesis】

The cause of pearly penile papules is unknown. It has been considered to be a physical ectopic condition.

【病因及发病机制】

珍珠状阴茎丘疹病因不明，目前认为属于一种生理性变异。

【Clinical Manifestations】

Pearly penile papules most commonly develop in uncircumcised males between the ages of 20 and 30. They tend to be less visible with age. Lesions typically appear as small, smooth, skin-colored papules on the penis, often in one or more rows encircling the sulcus or corona (Fig. 22-5). It is often otherwise asymptomatic, asymmetrically distributed and may persist for many years.

【临床表现】

本病好发于未行包皮环切的 20～30 岁男性，随着年龄增长皮损数目减少甚至不明显。典型皮损表现为阴茎龟头边缘及冠状沟处环绕的一行或数行小的皮色丘疹，表面光滑（图 22-5），分布不对称，无自觉症状，常持续数年。

【Histopathology】

These lesions show a rich vascular network surrounded by dense connective tissue.

【组织病理】

皮损病理表现为致密结缔组织包绕的丰富的血管网。

【Diagnosis and Differential Diagnosis】

The diagnosis is based mainly on clinical features. Clinically, these lesions can be easily confused with condyloma acuminatum and ectopic sebaceous glands, but they should be differentiated by medical history, clinical features, response to treatment, and their histopathological appearance.

【诊断与鉴别诊断】

诊断主要依靠临床特征。临床上容易与尖锐湿疣和皮脂腺异位症相混淆，但通过病史、临床特点、治疗反应和组织病理学表现则容易鉴别。

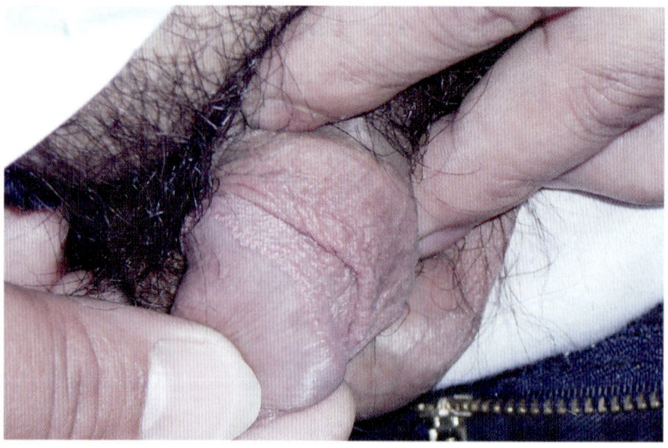

Fig. 22-5　Pearly penile papules(图 22-5　珍珠状阴茎丘疹)

【Treatment】

The condition is considered as a normal variation, and therefore no treatment is required. Patients with pearly penile papules usually seek dermatologic consultation because of concerns about sexually transmitted disease or cancer. The only effective treatment is removal, either through CO_2 laser or electrodesiccation.

【治疗】

珍珠状阴茎丘疹属于正常变异，不需治疗。某些患者可能因担心为性传播疾病或癌症而就诊。CO_2 激光和电切除治疗有效。

Section Eight　Balanoposthitis

第八节　包皮龟头炎

Balanoposthitis is used to describe acute or chronic forms of inflammation occurring on the glans penis and prepuce.

包皮龟头炎(balanoposthitis)是指包皮和龟头的急性或慢性炎症。

【Etiology and Pathogenesis】

The condition tends to be more common among uncircumcised males. The etiology of the disease is complicated. A wide variety of causes or predisposing factors have been associated with balanoposthitis as follows.

(1) Irritants: long prepuce, phimosis, poor hygiene, detergents, retained smegma or inadequate drying may cause an irritant dermatitis.

(2) Trauma: frictional trauma and accidental wounds may cause fissures, erosions or erythema and edema in this localized area.

(3) Infections: this is the most common cause of balanoposthitis. Candidal, bacterial, trichomonal, amoebic, mycoplasmal or chlamydial infections may be involved in this condition.

【病因及发病机制】

本病在未行包皮环切的男性中更为常见，病因复杂，下列因素与包皮龟头炎的发生有关。

(1) 刺激　包皮过长、包茎、个人卫生差、洗涤剂、包皮垢和不恰当干燥均会引起刺激性皮炎。

(2) 创伤　裂伤或意外伤可造成局部皲裂、糜烂或红斑水肿。

(3) 感染　最常见的病因，念珠菌、细菌、滴虫、阿米巴、支原体和衣原体感染都与之相关。

【Clinical Manifestations】

Balanoposthitis can be classified into a number of clinical variants according to the different etiological causes and clinical features.

(1) Acute superficial balanoposthitis: here the main causes are mechanical or chemical factors. It presents as an acute inflammation. Redness, vesicles, erosion and exudates can be seen

【临床表现】

包皮龟头炎根据病因和临床特点可分为多种临床型。

(1) 急性浅表性包皮龟头炎(acute superficial balanoposthitis)　物理化学刺激是主要原因，表现为急性炎症，包皮

on the glans penis and prepuce area (Fig. 22-6). Ulceration is usually followed by secondary infections. Pain, tenderness or burning sensations may be present.

和龟头出现潮红、水疱、糜烂和渗出(图22-6),继发感染可形成溃疡,可自觉疼痛、感觉敏感、触痛或烧灼感。

(2) Circinate erosive balanoposthitis: there are two subtypes of this form of balanoposthitis. One type is a condition associated with Reiter's disease. The other is a persistent recurrent balanoposthitis. Red macules are the early manifestation, and they gradually become circular. Erosions, exudates and ulcers can sometimes be seen.

(2) 环状糜烂性包皮龟头炎(circinate erosive balanoposthitis) 包括两种亚型,一种是 Reiter's 病的表现之一,另一种情况是持久性复发性包皮龟头炎。早期表现为红斑,逐渐变成环状,局部可发生糜烂、渗出,有时形成溃疡。

(3) Candidal balanoposthitis: candidal infection appears to be the most common cause of this disease. It most frequently follows intercourse with an infected sexual partner. The pathogenicity of the candidal specifies yeast depends on the host conditions and may be further influenced by chronic diseases such as diabetes. The clinical features include a non-purulent redness with a slightly scaly surface. Satellite vesicles, erosions and pustules at the edges of the lesions can be revealed (Fig. 22-7). The entire groin area may also be affected in some cases. Microscopic examination and cultures should confirm the diagnosis.

(3) 念珠菌性包皮龟头炎(candidal balanoposthitis) 念珠菌感染是本病最常见的原因,多由患者的性伴侣通过性交传播。感染发病与宿主因素以及某些慢性疾病有关,如糖尿病。临床表现为非化脓性的红斑,表面有细小鳞屑;皮损周边有散在卫星状分布的水疱、糜烂和脓疱(图 22-7)。腹股沟也可以受累。真菌镜检和培养可确诊。

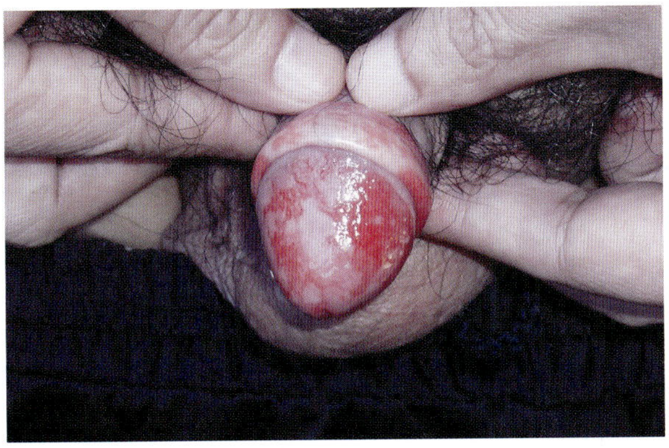

Fig. 22-6　Acute superficial balanoposthitis

(图 22-6　急性浅表性包皮龟头炎)

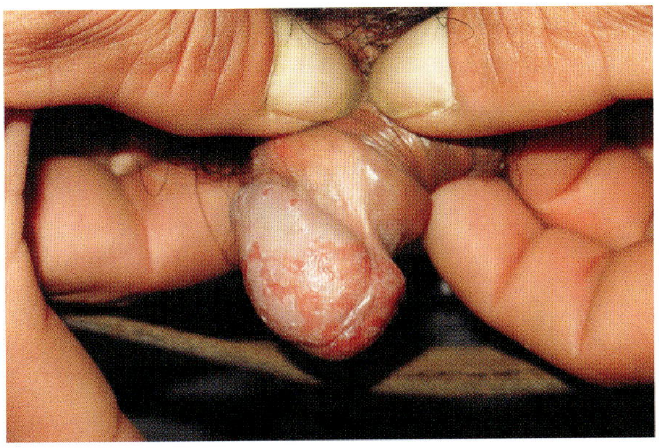

Fig. 22-7　Candidal balanoposthitis

(图 22-7　念珠菌性包皮龟头炎)

(4) Trichomonal balanoposthitis: trichomonas can cause a sexually acquired superficial erosive balanoposthitis. In severe cases, penile abscesses or lesions of chancriform type are occasionally seen. Trichomonal balanoposthitis is often mixed with other infections. Histology of the lesions shows dense lymphocytic infiltration in the upper dermis. This condition responds well to metronidazole.

(4) 滴虫性包皮龟头炎(trichomonal balanoposthitis) 滴虫可以通过性接触引起浅表糜烂性包皮龟头炎。严重者可见硬下疳性损害或脓肿形成。往往存在混合感染。病理学表现为真皮浅层致密淋巴细胞浸润。甲硝唑治疗效果好。

(5) Amoebic balanoposthitis: *Entamoeba histolytica* is the main pathogen. Cutaneous amoebiasis of genitalia extended from balanoposthitis may occasionally occur. It presents as a redness and edema of the prepuce. Erosion and ulcers are also often seen.

(5) 阿米巴性包皮龟头炎(amoebic balanoposthitis) 主要由溶组织内阿米巴引起,偶尔也会波及生殖器区的皮肤引起皮肤阿米巴病。临床表现为包皮红斑水肿,常形成糜烂和溃疡。

(6) Plasma cell balanitis: also known as Zoon's balanitis. This

(6) 浆细胞性龟头炎(plasma cell

is an idiopathic benign penile dermatosis. The lesion is usually a solitary, glistening, red plaque of the glans or prepuce. The lesion may exhibit pinpoint purpuric spotting. Erosive and vegetative variants have been seen (Fig. 22-8).

balanitis) 又称为Zoon's龟头炎(Zoon's balanitis),是一种特发性的良性的龟头疾病。临床表现为包皮或龟头单发的红色斑块,质硬、表面发亮,可见针尖大紫癜样损害,有糜烂或不同程度增生(图22-8)。

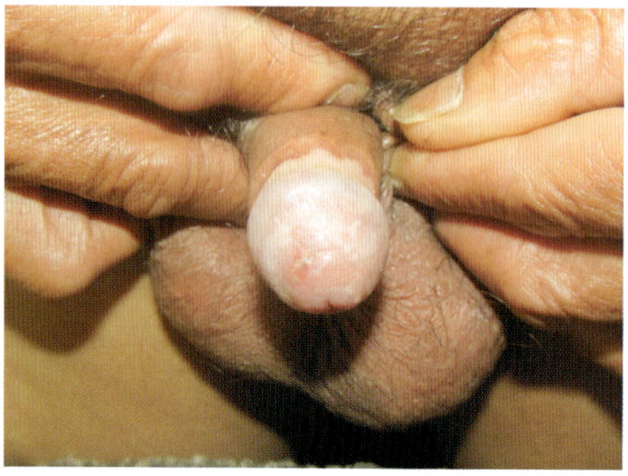

Fig. 22-8 Plasma cell balanitis(图 22-8 浆细胞性龟头炎)

【Diagnosis】

Diagnosis is based on medical history and clinical features. Histopathologically, dense plasma cells infiltration can be seen in the dermis from the lesions of plasma cell balanitis. In chronic unresolving balanoposthitis, the following conditions should be excluded: Bowen's disease, extramammary Paget's disease, lichen sclerosus *et* atrophicus, lichen planus and psoriasis.

【诊断】

根据病史和临床表现可以诊断。浆细胞性龟头炎组织病理上在真皮内有致密的浆细胞浸润。诊断慢性顽固性包皮龟头炎应排除以下疾病:鲍温病、乳房外Paget's 病、硬化性苔藓、扁平苔藓、银屑病。

【Treatment】

Treatment focuses on controlling the acute infection and preventing recurrent inflammations by improvement of local hygiene.

Pathogenic organisms must be eliminated in infectious balanoposthitis, and sexual partners should be treated concurrently. There is a large variety of effective antibiotics and antifungal agents available. Most patients will respond well to topical antibiotics and antifungals. Itraconazole and fluconazole are oral alternatives for severe cases. Mycoplasma balanoposthitis responds to high doses of tetracycline.

Non-specific forms of balanoposthitis respond to repeated topical cool bathing with potassium permanganate (1 : 5000) and the application of a compound of mild antibacterial creams with weak potency glucocorticoids may also be beneficial.

Zoon's balanitis has been successfully treated with CO_2 lasers, but about 40 percent of those treated by this method undergo some relapse. Circumcision may be indicated in recurrent and recalcitrant cases.

【治疗】

治疗原则是保持局部清洁,控制急性炎症,预防复发和感染。

感染性包皮龟头炎患者必须消灭病原体,性伴侣必须同时治疗。可供选择的抗生素和抗真菌药物很多,多数患者局部外用抗生素或抗真菌药物有效,严重病例可口服伊曲康唑或氟康唑。大剂量四环素治疗支原体包皮龟头炎有效。

非特异性包皮龟头炎可用 1 : 5000 高锰酸钾溶液反复冷湿敷,并外用弱效糖皮质激素与抗生素的复方制剂。

CO_2激光治疗 Zoon's 龟头炎有效,但复发率约高达 40%。复发或顽固病例可考虑包皮环切。

【Prevention】

Proper hygiene with frequent washing and drying of the prepuce is an essential preventive measure. Circumcision will prevent balanoposthitis.

【预防】

适当保持包皮清洁、干燥是预防的主要措施。包皮环切能预防包皮龟头炎。

Chao JI(纪超),Bo CHENG(程波)

Chapter Twenty-three Diseases of the Appendages

第二十三章 附属器疾病

Section One Seborrheic Dermatitis

第一节 脂溢性皮炎

Seborrheic dermatitis is a chronic inflammatory dermatosis generally confined to areas where sebaceous (oil) glands are most prominent (known as "seborrheic areas"). Typically, it presents as light erythematous patches covered with greasy scales or crusts.

脂溢性皮炎(seborrheic dermatitis)是发生在皮脂溢出部位的一种慢性炎症性皮肤病,表现为淡红斑片上覆有油腻性鳞屑或痂,常发生于皮脂分泌活跃的部位。

【Etiology and Pathogenesis】

The etiology of seborrheic dermatitis is not yet determined. Multiple factors seem to be involved in its pathogenesis, including immunity, heredity, vitamin B group deficiency or inefficiency, hormones, and neurologic or environmental factors. New data have shown that there existed vast propagation of yeast *Malassezia* in a seborrheic predisposed individual, which have changed the original micro-ecological environment of the skin.

【病因及发病机制】

尚未清楚。可能与免疫、遗传、B族维生素缺乏或不足、激素、神经和环境因素有关。目前研究发现,患者可能在遗传性油脂分泌过多的基础上发生马拉色菌大量繁殖,致使皮肤原有的微生态环境发生了变化。

【Clinical Manifestations】

Seborrheic dermatitis commonly involves areas rich in sebaceous glands, such as the scalp, face, presternal and interscapular regions, and the flexures. The lesions tend to be brown, pale yellow to red in color and covered with greasy scales (Fig. 23-1). Pruritus is common and clinical presentation varies with the locations affected.

【临床表现】

脂溢性皮炎常见于皮脂腺分布较丰富的部位,如头皮、面部、胸部、肩胛间及皱褶部位。皮损多为褐色或淡黄红色斑片,表面覆以油腻性鳞屑(图23-1),常伴瘙痒。根据皮损部位不同,临床表现亦有所不同。

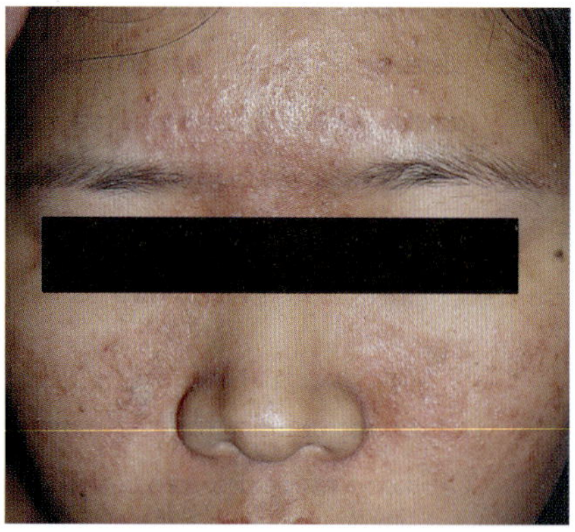

Fig. 23-1 Seborrheic dermatitis(图 23-1 脂溢性皮炎)

In the scalp, mild seborrheic dermatitis may present as diffused erythema and papules with flaky greasy scaling. Pruritus is common. The hair may become sparse in affected scalp areas. Large amounts of greasy scales, crust and even exudation may appear in addition to red papules or erythema in severe cases.

Seborrheic dermatitis is usually accompanied by acne when it appears on the face. Once it involves the trunk, different sized,

头皮脂溢性皮炎轻者表现为弥漫性红斑和丘疹,覆有油腻的糠秕状鳞屑,自觉瘙痒,毛发可稀疏脱落。重者头皮潮红,在丘疹和红斑的基础上出现大量的油腻性鳞屑及痂,可有渗出。

颜面受累时常与痤疮伴发;躯干部位皮损常为大小不等的圆形或椭圆形红

round or oval shaped erythema, papules or plaques with greasy scales are typically displayed. In the axillae, groin, submammary regions, umbilicus and anogenital regions, the lesions may sometimes be confused with tinea corporis, and in fact patients with this condition are often infected secondarily with *Candida*. When the onset of the disease occurs shortly after birth, it is called infantile seborrheic dermatitis

斑、丘疹和斑块，表面有油腻性鳞屑。在腋部、腹股沟、乳房下、脐部、外阴和肛门等皱褶部位的皮损类似体癣，易继发念珠菌感染。于出生不久发病者，称为婴儿脂溢性皮炎（infantile seborrheic dermatitis）。

【Histopathology】

Histopathological slides have no diagnostic value, generally just manifesting the characteristics of chronic dermatitis.

【组织病理】

无诊断价值，一般显示慢性皮炎特征。

【Diagnosis and Differential Diagnosis】

Based on the areas involved and the features of the lesions, the diagnosis is not difficult to make conclusively. However, the condition may be confused with scalp psoriasis, pityriasis rosea, eczema and tinea corporis in some circumstances.

In scalp psoriasis, the lesions usually present as red papules or plaques with silvery scales, also Auspitz's sign is positive and bunched hair can be seen. For pityriasis rosea, the lesions are more likely to be found on the neck, trunk and proximal extremities. The typical lesions of pityriasis rosea are oval macules whose long axis runs parallel to the dermatoglyphic lines with a precursor 'herald patch' prior to eruption. In eczema, the eruptions tend to be pleomorphic, symmetrically distributed, and accompanied by exudation and severe pruritus. Although tinea corporis usually presents with less rash, the clear margin of the eruption where the mycelia reside, and/or positive findings of spores under microscopic examination will indicate tinea corporis.

【诊断与鉴别诊断】

根据好发于皮脂溢出的部位、皮损特点，诊断一般不困难，但需与头皮银屑病、玫瑰糠疹、湿疹及体癣等进行鉴别。

头皮银屑病为表面覆着银白色鳞屑的红色丘疹、斑块，Auspitz 征阳性，可见束状发。玫瑰糠疹的皮疹为好发于颈、躯干、四肢近端的椭圆形斑疹，典型的皮疹其长轴与皮纹一致，常先有母斑。湿疹皮损呈多形性，对称分布，表面常有渗出，瘙痒剧烈。体癣皮损数目少，边界清楚，直接镜检可见菌丝或孢子。

【Treatment】

A low risk lifestyle may be recommended. Alcohol and spicy food should be avoided, and the diet should include a proper amount of vegetables and fruits but less refined sugar and cholesterol. All kinds of mechanical stimulus of the skin (e. g., use of exfoliants) should be avoided.

(1) Systemic therapy: oral vitamins B2, B6 or a B-complex vitamin, lipid and carbohydrate restricted diet may be beneficial for this condition. Oral antihistamines and tranquilizers can be applied in cases with severe pruritus. Oral tetracycline, erythromycin or metronidazole can be prescribed in the cases with exudation or secondary infections.

(2) Topical therapy: the principles of topical regimens are to restrict lipid secretions, suppress inflammation, treat infection and stop pruritus. Sulphur, resorcin (meta-dihydroxybenzene), coal tar, salicylic acid, selenium sulphide and imidazole are commonly

【治疗】

应保持生活规律，忌饮酒及刺激性食物，多食蔬菜及水果，少食多糖及多脂食物，避免各种机械性刺激（如使用去角质剂）。

(1) 系统治疗　口服维生素 B2、维生素 B6 或复合维生素 B，控制脂质和糖类饮食。瘙痒剧烈时可服抗组胺药及镇静剂。渗出明显或继发感染者，可口服四环素、红霉素或甲硝唑。

(2) 局部治疗　原则为去脂、消炎、杀菌、止痒。常用的药物有：硫黄、雷锁辛（间苯二酚）、煤焦油、水杨酸、硫化硒、咪唑类等，按不同部位、不同皮损选用不

prescribed for those purposes. The formulas of topical agents should be chosen according to the features and the locations of the lesions. Medicated shampoos including selenium sulphide, ketoconazole and coal tar have been proven effective for lesions on the scalp.

同的剂型。如头部皮损可用含硫化硒、酮康唑或各类焦油的洗发剂洗头。

Section Two Acne

第二节 痤 疮

Acne is a chronic inflammatory disease of the pilosebaceous units, which mainly occurs on the face and the upper parts of the trunk, areas rich with sebaceous glands. It is commonly seen in adolescents, with males slightly more commonly affected than females. Acne vulgaris is the most common type, manifesting primarily as comedones (whiteheads or blackheads), erythematous papules, pustules and nodules.

痤疮(acne)是一种累及毛囊皮脂腺的慢性炎症性皮肤病,常见于皮脂腺丰富的面部和胸背部,好发于青春期,男性略多于女性,其中寻常痤疮最常见。主要表现为粉刺(白头和黑头)、红斑性丘疹、脓疱、结节等损害。

【Etiology and Pathogenesis】

Acne is a condition with complex causes. Androgen levels, seborrhoea, abnormal keratinization of the pilosebaceous duct and infection by *Propionibacterium acnes* are all contributory factors to its pathogenesis. Hereditary, immune, and endocrine disorders may also be accompanied by this disease in some cases.

(1) Endocrinological factors: acne development is closely related to the body's androgen production and metabolism. As the sebaceous glands are controlled mainly by androgen, their activity and size therefore increase dramatically during puberty.

(2) Abnormal hypercornification: hypercornification of the pilosebaceous duct will cause a narrowing of the discharge passageway that often leads to a blockage of the opening for the hair follicles; as a result, sebum and epithelial debris accumulate locally to form comedones.

(3) Infective factors: *Propionibacterium acnes* (*P. acnes*) is the main infective agent of acne, although *Pityrosporum ovale* and *Staphylococcus albus* have also been associated with the disease. When *P. acnes* replicates inside the hair follicle, it hydrolyzes triglycerides into free fatty acids and low molecular peptides. Once released, these molecules can provoke an inflammation of the hair follicle wall and its surrounding tissues to present as papules, pustules, nodules and cysts in the patient.

(4) Others factors: genetics, food (such as excessive consumption of dairy products), emotional stress, drugs, cosmetics and some occupational factors are also thought to play important roles in the pathogenesis of acne.

【病因及发病机制】

痤疮是一种多因素的疾病,主要与雄激素水平、皮脂分泌增多、毛囊皮脂腺导管异常角化、痤疮丙酸杆菌感染等因素有关。部分病例尚与遗传、免疫、内分泌障碍有关。

(1) 内分泌因素 痤疮的发生与体内雄激素水平及其代谢密切相关,皮脂腺主要受雄激素调控,青春期后雄激素使皮脂腺增大,皮脂分泌活动增加。

(2) 角化异常 毛囊皮脂腺导管角化过度,导管口径变小,毛囊口阻塞,使皮脂排出不畅,上皮细胞和皮脂积聚于毛囊口而形成粉刺。

(3) 感染因素 以痤疮丙酸杆菌为主,其次为卵圆形糠秕孢子菌和白色葡萄球菌。毛囊内的痤疮丙酸杆菌可水解皮脂中甘油三酯产生游离脂肪酸,并可产生一些低分子多肽,刺激毛囊壁及其周围组织而产生丘疹、脓疱、结节和囊肿等皮肤损害。

(4) 其他 遗传、饮食(如过多进食牛奶)、情绪、药物、化妆品及某些职业等亦与痤疮的发病有关。

【Clinical Manifestations】

(1) Acne vulgaris: acne vulgaris often runs a chronic course in

【临床表现】

(1) 寻常痤疮(acne vulgaris) 本病

males or females aged 15-30 years. Most patients’ skin is greasy. The severity of the disease is correlated with the quantity of the sebum secretion. The lesions are predominantly seen on the face, forehead, followed by the chest and back. At the early stage, the lesions appear as cone-shaped papules, either whiteheads (closed comedones) or blackheads (open comedones). A curd-like substance can be squeezed out of the whiteheads. Lipid plugs formed from oxidized sebum constitute the blackheads. The lesions can manifest as follicular papules, pustules, nodules and cysts, leaving atrophic scars after the condition subsides (Fig. 23-2). The lesions tend to be symmetrical and are usually accompanied by seborrhoea. Red follicular papules and pustules are often observed. Usually, more than one kind of lesions can be found in one patient. Patients may have mild pruritus and pain. In addition, deep papules, nodules, cysts, or even abscesses can occur in severe or inadequately treated cases, resulting in scarring once healed.

多发于 15～30 岁的男女，慢性病程，多数痤疮患者为油性皮肤，而且痤疮的严重程度与皮脂分泌量有一定的相关性。皮损好发于面颊、额部，其次为胸部及背部。皮损初起为与毛囊一致的圆锥形丘疹，如白头粉刺（闭合性粉刺）及黑头粉刺（开放性粉刺），白头粉刺可挑挤出白色豆渣样物质，而黑头粉刺内含脂栓，由皮脂氧化所致。皮损可发展成毛囊性丘疹、脓疱、结节和囊肿，消退后可遗留萎缩性瘢痕（图 23-2）。皮损多对称性分布，常伴有皮脂溢出。毛囊性红色丘疹和脓疱常见，也常有多种皮损共存，自觉轻微痒痛，病情严重或治疗不彻底者，继续发展可形成深在性丘疹、结节或囊肿，甚至脓肿，愈合后形成瘢痕。

(2) Acne conglobata: this is a rare variant of acne. It is more severe than acne vulgaris, and is usually seen in young males. The lesions tend to appear at the chest, shoulder, back and retrocollic area. The buttock, thighs, forearms and face are sometimes also affected. There are several types of eruptions in acne conglobata, in which papulopustules, abscesses, nodules and cysts are seen. It usually follows a protracted course and heals with scars (Fig. 23-3). If the patient happens to be female, it is necessary to determine whether the disease is caused by a polycystic ovary syndrome, which results in an increased level of androgen.

（2）聚合性痤疮（acne conglobata）本病少见，病情较寻常痤疮重得多，常见于青年男性。皮损常位于胸、肩、背及后颈部。同时也可在臀部、大腿、前臂及面部发生。皮疹包括多种损害，以丘脓疱疹、脓肿、结节和囊肿为主，病程慢性，愈合后留下明显瘢痕（图 23-3）。若发生于女性，则应检查是否存在多囊卵巢综合征导致体内雄激素水平增高。

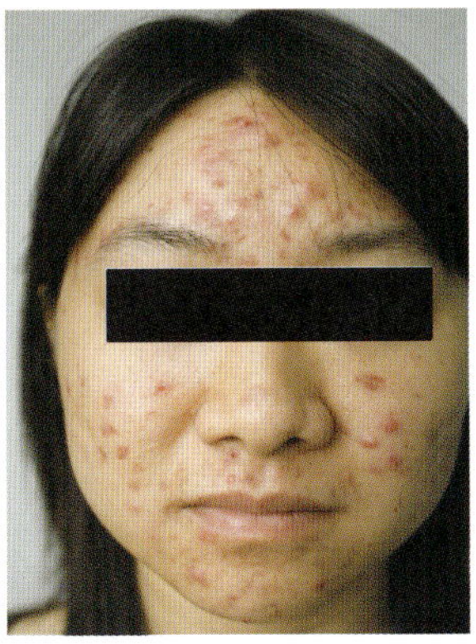

Fig. 23-2　Acne vulgaris(图 23-2　寻常痤疮)

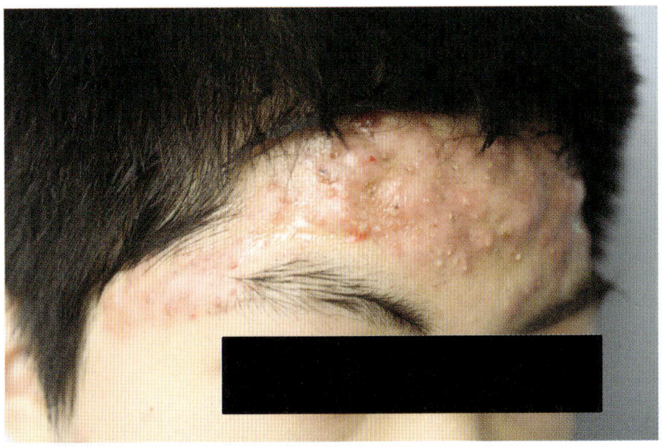

Fig. 23-3　Acne conglobata(图 23-3　聚合性痤疮)

(3) Neonatal acne: this mainly happens within 3 months after birth. The affected infant usually has a family history of seborrhoea. The incidence rate in male infants is higher than in female infants. Some believe that maternal estrogen in the fetus is the cause of this condition. The skin lesions usually occur on the forehead and face, and mainly present as comedones, papules and pustules. The lesions tend to heal spontaneously within 6 months.

（3）新生儿痤疮（neonatal acne）本病主要发生于出生后 3 个月内，男性多于女性，有皮脂溢的家族史。也有学者认为是由于母体雌激素在胎儿阶段进入体内引起。皮疹发生在额部、面颊，主要为粉刺、丘疹和脓疱。一般在半岁之内可自行消退。不留后遗症，患者青春

This particular condition does not leave sequelae; however, the patient is more prone to severe acne in adolescence.

期更易发生严重痤疮。

【Diagnosis and Differential Diagnosis】

As most of the patients are teenage males or females, and since the skin lesions usually occur in the seborrheic areas and present as comedones, papules, pustules, nodules or cysts, the diagnosis of acne is usually straightforward. However, it may need to be differentiated from rosacea and lupus miliaris disseminatus faciei. Rosacea commonly affects middle-aged people, and the lesions mainly present as telangiectatic erythema, papules or pustules in the middle part of the face. Lupus miliaris disseminatus faciei mostly affects adults, with the eruptions appearing on the face, mainly in the periorbital and perioral areas. The skin lesions present as soft red papules or nodules, which show an apple-jelly-like color on diascopic examination.

【诊断与鉴别诊断】

根据患者多为青年男女，皮疹好发于脂溢部位，有粉刺、丘疹、脓疱、结节、囊肿等，一般不难诊断，但需与酒渣鼻、颜面播散性粟粒性狼疮相鉴别。酒渣鼻好发于中年人，皮损为以面中部为主的毛细血管扩张性红斑、丘疹或脓疱。颜面播散性粟粒性狼疮好发于成年人，发生于颜面，主要在眼周和口周。皮疹为红色的丘疹、结节，触之较软，玻片压之出现苹果酱色。

【Treatment】

The principle for the selection of medications for the treatment of acne is according to the pathogenesis of acne. It is generally believed that patients with acne should adjust their diet, avoid spicy foods, restrict intake of fats and refined sugar, and consume more vegetables and fruits. The skin should be kept clean and dry (oily or powdery cosmetics should be avoided in particular), and squeezing or scratching of the comedones and blackheads should be avoided as well. Patients may also have to change their living habits in order to reduce stress due to lack of sleep or other general ailments such as constipation.

【治疗】

原则是针对多个痤疮致病环节选择药物，根据病情注意调节饮食，避免辛辣刺激食物，控制脂肪和糖类食品，多吃蔬菜、水果。保持皮肤清洁，避免使用油性及粉质化妆品，忌用手挤压、搔抓粉刺和黑头。此外劳逸适度，纠正便秘。

(1) Systemic therapy:

①Antiandrogens: the purpose of antiandrogens is to regulate or inhibit sebum secretion. Diane-35 (Cyproterone acetate 2 mg + ethinyl estradiol 0.035 mg), used for female patients only, one pill daily, may be started on the first day of menstruation and continued for 21 days, and be repeated in this way in the next menstruation. Spironolactone, 40-60 mg/d for 1 month is an alternative which does not need to be synchronized with the patient's menstrual cycle.

(1) 系统治疗

①抗雄激素药物：通过调节或抑制体内雄激素水平，从而减少皮肤油脂分泌。达英-35(醋酸环丙孕酮 2 mg＋乙炔基雌二醇 0.035 mg)，仅适用于女性，月经第一天开始连服 21 天，每天一粒，下一月经周期再服。螺内酯，每日 40～60 mg，连服 1 个月，不需与月经同步服用。

②Antibiotics: oral tetracycline, minocycline or doxycycline can inhibit *P. acnes* replication and suppress the chemotaxis of neutrophils, which effectively decreases the concentration of free fatty acids in the sebum. The recommended dosage for tetracycline is 1.0 g once daily for 4 weeks; then 0.5 g each morning for 8 weeks. Minocycline or doxycycline can also be prescribed with a dosage of 100 mg once or twice daily for 6-8 weeks.

②抗生素：口服四环素或米诺环素或多西环素能抑制痤疮丙酸杆菌和抑制中性粒细胞趋化，使面部皮脂中游离脂肪酸浓度下降。四环素的用法为 1.0 g/d，连服 4 周后改为每晨服 0.5 g，连服 8 周。米诺环素或多西环素 100 mg，每日 1 次或 2 次，连用 6～8 周。

③ Isotretinoin: isotretinoin can inhibit the activity of the

③异维 A 酸：此药物抑制皮脂腺功

sebaceous gland, and thereby decrease the secretion of sebum, and can also reverse abnormal keratinization and the formation of blackheads. Isotretinoin can prevent the spread of *P. acnes* directly. This medicine is particularly effective for patients with nodular, cystic, and conglobata acne types.

能，可减少皮脂分泌，控制异常角化和黑头粉刺的形成，并抑制痤疮丙酸杆菌，对结节性、囊肿性和聚合性痤疮效果好。

④ Glucocorticoids: anti-inflammatory effects have been demonstrated when small doses of prednisone or dexamethasone have been applied in severe cases of nodular acne, acne conglobata, and during the inflammatory stages of cystic acne and acne fulminans. Here the recommended therapy is simply prednisone 15-30 mg/d. However, long term use of this drug should be discouraged due to systemic side effects such as diabetes, obesity, hypertension, osteoporosis and a vascular necrosis of the long bones.

④糖皮质激素：小剂量的泼尼松或地塞米松具有抗炎作用，适用于严重结节性痤疮、聚合性痤疮、囊肿性痤疮的炎症期和暴发性痤疮。常用泼尼松 15～30 mg/d，但应避免长期使用，以免引起糖尿病、肥胖、高血压、骨质疏松和长骨的缺血性坏死等系统性副作用。

(2) Topical therapy: the principle in choosing topical medications is to eliminate grease, dissolve keratin plugs, and fight bacterial growth.

（2）局部治疗　选择含有去脂、溶解角质、杀菌性能的外用药。

① Tretinoin: the anti-keratinization effects of tretinoin can be used to dissolve the comedones, inhibit secretion of the sebaceous glands and reduce inflammation. All-trans retinoic acid compound (of which tretinoin is one example) may be used as a topical cream or gel with a concentration of 0.05%-0.1%. Side effects of tretinoin include local irritation, erythema, desquamation and burning sensations; therefore the dosage may need to be reduced in order to reduce irritation.

①维 A 酸类：抗角化的作用可溶解粉刺，也有抑制皮脂分泌和抗炎的作用。可用 0.05%～0.1%维 A 酸（全反式）霜或凝胶。不良反应有局部刺激、皮肤发红、脱屑及烧灼感等。注意维 A 酸类外用药需少量点涂，以减少刺激症状。

② Benzoyl peroxide: being a peroxide, benzoyl peroxide can slowly release oxygen and benzoic acid that will kill *P. acnes* on the skin. This compound also has an anti-keratinization effect and inhibits the hyperactivity of the sebaceous glands.

②过氧化苯甲酰：过氧化苯甲酰为过氧化物，可缓慢释放新生态氧和苯甲酸，杀灭痤疮丙酸杆菌，还有抗角化及抑制皮脂腺功能的作用。

③ Antibiotics: tetracycline, erythromycin and clindamycin can be used in concentrations of 1%-4%, usually in ointment or lotion form.

③抗生素：四环素、红霉素或克林霉素，可配制成 1%～4%软膏或洗剂。

(3) Physical therapy: this is the alternative option for patients who cannot tolerate or are not willing to receive medical treatment. Currently, the commonly used effective therapy is red-blue light therapy, photodynamic therapy, laser therapy and alpha hydroxy acids peeling therapy, etc. Photodynamic therapy is a combination of red and blue light irradiation, which can destroy the *P. acnes* by photodynamic effect and reduce the inflammatory reaction. The main adverse reactions are pain and pigmentation.

（3）物理疗法　对于不能耐受药物治疗或是不愿接受药物治疗的痤疮患者，物理治疗是最好的选择。目前，常用的有效疗法有红-蓝光、光动力疗法、激光治疗和果酸疗法等。光动力疗法是联合应用红-蓝光照射，可通过光动力学效应破坏痤疮丙酸杆菌，减轻炎症反应。主要不良反应是疼痛、色素沉着。

Section Three　Rosacea

第三节　酒　渣　鼻

Rosacea is a chronic inflammatory disorder seen mainly in middle-aged people, characterized by erythema, papules, pustules

酒渣鼻(rosacea)是一种主要发生于中年人面部中央的红斑、丘疹、脓疱和毛

and telangiectasia in the central area of the face. Lesions have a progressive course and rhinophyma can form at the late stage.

细血管扩张的慢性炎症性疾病。病变呈进行性发展,晚期可形成鼻赘。

【Etiology and Pathogenesis】

The causes of rosacea remain unclear. It may be connected to psychological, gastrointestinal or endocrinological disorders, alcohol, spicy foods, temperature extremes, and parasitism by *Demodex folliculorum*. Rosacea often develops from seborrhea; therefore, the stimuli from the local infection, diet, environment factors all contribute to the dysfunction of the facial neurovasomotor response, which eventually results in a local chronic inflammation presenting as capillary dilation, pustules and pus formation, and tissue hyperplasia.

【病因及发病机制】

本病的病因不明,可能与精神因素、胃肠功能紊乱、内分泌功能失调、嗜酒、辛辣食物、冷热刺激、气候影响和毛囊蠕形螨的寄生等有关。酒渣鼻往往在皮脂溢出的基础上发生,由于感染、饮食、环境的因素的刺激,造成调节颜面部血管运动的神经功能障碍,毛细血管持续扩张,脓疱和脓液及组织增生,形成了局部的慢性炎症。

【Clinical Manifestations】

Rosacea mostly affects middle-aged adults. Women are more commonly affected than men, but the disease usually follows a much more severe course in male patients. The eruptions are most likely to appear in the central convex areas of the face (nose, cheeks, chin and forehead). Rosacea is classified into three stages: erythematotelangiectatic, papulopustular, and rhinophymatous stage respectively. The three stages may overlap in a single individual.

【临床表现】

本病好发于中年人,女性较多,但男性患者病情常较严重。皮疹较集中分布在面中部的鼻、面颊、颏及额部。酒渣鼻分为三期:红斑毛细血管扩张期、丘疹脓疱期、鼻赘期。同一患者可有不同期的重叠。

(1) Erythematotelangiectatic stage (stage Ⅰ): rosacea may be triggered by specific stimuli such as food, a sudden change in environmental temperature, or emotional agitation. The eruption presents as a symmetrical persistent erythema, accompanied by mild telangiectasia, especially in the central convex areas of the face (Fig. 23-4).

(1)红斑毛细血管扩张期(Ⅰ期)　起初为进食刺激性食物、外界温度突然改变及情绪激动后,发生对称性红斑,久之红斑持久不退,并出现浅表毛细血管扩张,以面中部明显(图 23-4)。

(2) Papulopustular stage (stage Ⅱ): as the course of rosacea progresses, pinhead to bean-sized papules, pustules and nodules can develop in addition to erythema and telangiectasia, and the telangiectasia becomes more extensive (Fig. 23-5).

(2) 丘疹脓疱期(Ⅱ期)　病情继续发展时,除红斑和毛细血管扩张外,在红斑的基础上出现针头至绿豆大小丘疹、脓疱、结节,毛细血管扩张更加广泛(图 23-5)。

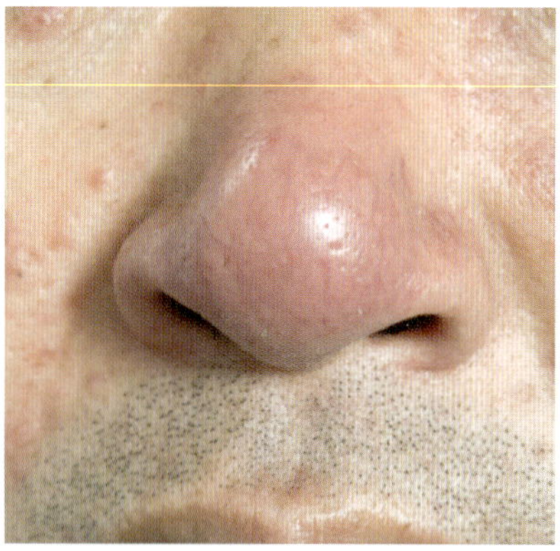

Fig. 23-4　Erythematotelangiectatic stage-stage Ⅰ
(图 23-4　红斑毛细血管扩张期-Ⅰ期)

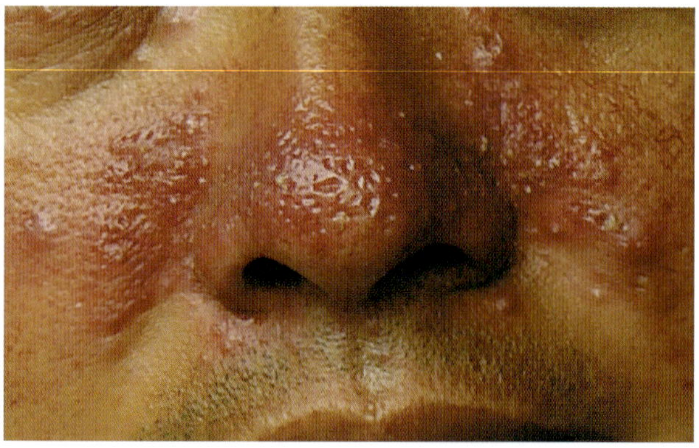

Fig. 23-5　Papulopustular stage-stage Ⅱ
(图 23-5　丘疹脓疱期-Ⅱ期)

(3) Rhinophymatous stage (stage Ⅲ): usually this is seen in male patients. The telangiectasia becomes more extensive, there is sebaceous hyperplasia and proliferation of the connective tissues forming various-sized and shaped nodular indurations. This is called granulomatous rosacea, which most commonly affects the nose (and is then called rhinophyma), although other areas can be affected, such as the chin, forehead, and the eyebrows. Rhinophyma is usually accompanied by enlargement of the pilosebaceous orifices and an increased secretion of sebum.

(3) 鼻赘期(Ⅲ期) 常见于男性患者，毛细血管扩张更广泛，局部皮脂腺及结缔组织增生，形成不同大小和形状的结节状隆起，称为肉芽肿性酒渣鼻。因常发生在鼻部，又称为鼻赘。这些损害也可见于其他部位，如颏部、前额和眉弓。鼻赘常伴有毛囊皮脂腺口的扩大和皮脂的分泌增加。

Rosacea also can involve the eyes and surrounding areas, manifesting as blepharitis, keratitis, iritis and conjunctivitis, and is known as ocular rosacea (Fig. 23-6).

酒渣鼻还可累及眼及其周围，表现为眼睑炎、角膜炎、虹膜炎、结膜炎等，称为眼型酒渣鼻(图 23-6)。

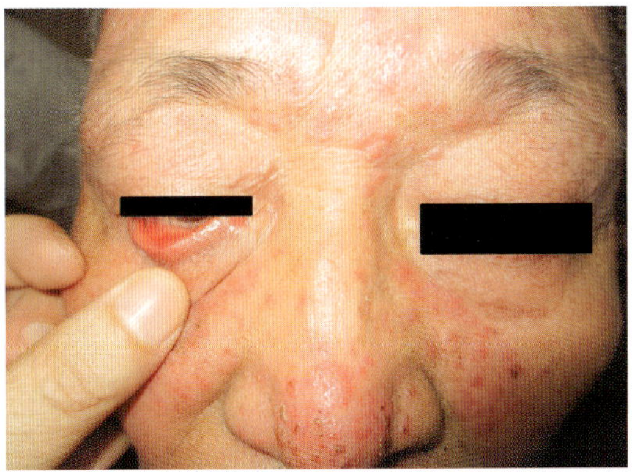

Fig. 23-6 Ocular rosacea(图 23-6 眼型酒糟鼻)

【Diagnosis and Differential Diagnosis】

Generally rosacea can be diagnosed in a middle-aged adult presenting with typical skin lesions. It should be differentiated from acne vulgaris, seborrheic dermatitis and steroid dependent dermatitis (steroid-induced rosacea-like eruption). Acne vulgaris mostly affects a younger age group, and presents with more extensively distributed whiteheads or blackheads, but lacks facial erythema. Seborrheic dermatitis is more extensively distributed than rosacea, and has greasy scales covering the lesions and exhibits no telangiectasia. Steroid dependent dermatitis often has a long-term history of topical use of fluorinated corticosteroid preparations. The skin lesions are steadier than rosacea, without flush or bleeding, and paroxysmal worsening is rare.

【诊断与鉴别诊断】

根据好发于中年人面中部的典型皮损可以诊断。本病需与寻常痤疮、脂溢性皮炎和激素依赖性皮炎(激素诱导的酒糟鼻样皮疹)进行鉴别。痤疮好发于年轻人，常有白头或黑头粉刺，分布广泛，不伴面部红斑。脂溢性皮炎比酒渣鼻的分布可更广泛，有油腻状鳞屑，不发生毛细血管扩张。激素依赖性皮炎有长期局部外用含氟糖皮质激素制剂的病史，皮损较酒渣鼻稳定，无潮红出血，无阵发性加重表现。

【Treatment】

Symptomatic treatments are normally given since the causes of rosacea are unclear. Any functional disorders of the gastrointestinal and endocrine systems should be corrected. The efforts also should be made to avoid known trigger factors such as strong sunlight, extreme temperature fluctuations, alcohol, and spicy foods. Finally, maintaining a healthy lifestyle and keeping regular bowel

【治疗】

由于病因不明，治疗常为对症性，纠正肠胃功能，调整内分泌。避免各种已知的或加重的因素，如烈日暴晒及温度骤变，忌饮酒及辛辣食物。保持大便通畅，生活规律，尽量避免使用含氟糖皮质激素制剂。

movements, and avoiding fluorinated corticosteroids are all necessary for deferring this condition.

(1) Systemic therapy: the systemic treatments for rosacea include tetracycline and tetracycline derivatives such as doxycycline or minocycline. In patients who do not tolerate or are allergic to tetracyclines, erythromycin and related medications can be used. In refractory cases, isotretinoin is indicated. Patients with excess facial oil secretion or a high density of hair follicles, metronidazole is available. Vitamin B group have adjuvant therapeutic roles for this disease. Hydroxychloroquine can be used for patients who have an aggravated history after sun exposure.

(1) 系统治疗　酒渣鼻的全身治疗主要是采用四环素类及四环素衍生物，如多西环素或米诺环素。对不能耐受或对四环素类过敏者可用红霉素及其相关药物。对难治病例可以系统应用异维A酸。面部油性分泌物多或毛囊密度大者，可用甲硝唑。B族维生素有辅助治疗作用，对日晒后加重者可服用羟氯喹。

(2) Topical therapy: the use of glucocorticoids should be avoided. Application of 10% sulphur cream, 1%-3% metronidazole cream, or washing with a soap containing 2.5% selenium sulphide can be effective.

(2) 局部治疗　避免使用糖皮质激素制剂。可以使用10%硫黄霜、1%～3%甲硝唑霜、2.5%硫化硒洗剂。

(3) Others: in spite of systemic and local medicines, other regimens as follows are also available for this disease. An adjustable long pulse variable multiple 532 nm laser or intense pulse light therapy can be used in patients with obvious telangiectasia. For patients at the rhinophymatous stage, ultra-pulsed CO_2 laser, dermabrasion, and surgical treatment can be effective alternatives.

(3) 其他　毛细血管扩张明显者，可用可调长脉冲变倍数532 nm激光或强光治疗，皮赘期可用超脉冲CO_2激光、皮肤磨削术以及外科手术等治疗。

Section Four　Alopecia Areata

第四节　斑　秃

Alopecia areata is one type of hair loss that typically causes baldness in patches. Any hairy parts of the body can be involved. It usually appears suddenly without subjective symptoms and tends to heal spontaneously.

斑秃(alopecia areata)是一种突然发生的局限性斑片状脱发，任何有毛部位均可受累，无自觉症状，可自行缓解。

【Etiology and Pathogenesis】

The causes of alopecia areata are still not clear, although psychological factors, genetic factors, endocrinological disorders and autoimmune disorders have all been postulated to be important for pathogenesis at present. It is notable that about 25% of patients have a family history, which may imply a genetic predisposition. Also, alopecia areata is often complicated by autoimmune diseases, suggesting that this disease may also be ascribed to polygenic factors.

【病因及发病机制】

发病原因尚不完全清楚。目前认为与精神因素、遗传、内分泌失调、自身免疫等因素有关。遗传易感性是斑秃发病的一个重要因素，约25%的患者有家族史。该病可能属于多基因病，自身免疫性疾病常合并斑秃。

【Clinical Manifestations】

Alopecia areata can be seen at any age, but appears mostly in young adults. It is often noticed unconsciously by the patient or by close associates, and the onset is often sudden. Lesions often appear as single or multiple round or oval well-defined bald patches, ranging from 1-10 cm in diameter (Fig. 23-7). The skin in the bald area appears normal, and is usually otherwise asymptomatic.

【临床表现】

本病可发生于任何年龄，但以青壮年多见，患者常于无意中发现或为他人发现。皮损为突然出现的单个或多个圆形或椭圆形、直径为1～10 cm、边界清楚的脱发区(图23-7)，局部皮肤正常，常无自觉症状。按病期可分为进展期、静止

According to the normal progression of the disease, alopecia areata can be divided into active, stationary and regrowth phases.

期及恢复期。

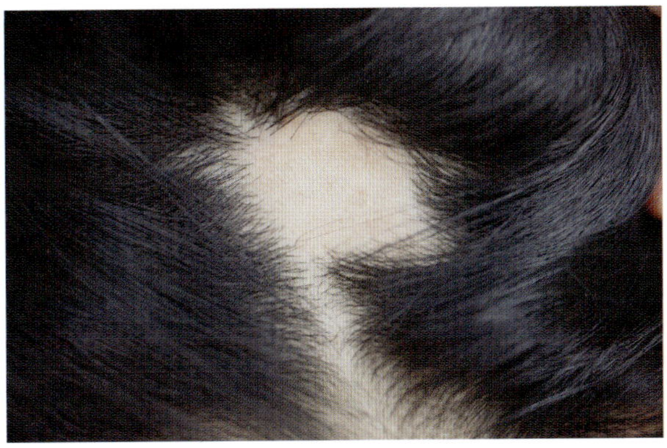

Fig. 23-7　Alopecia areata(图 23-7 斑秃)

In the active phase, easily extractable short broken hairs are often seen at the margins of the bald patches, and microscopic examination shows hair atrophy (atrophia pilorum propria) at the skin entry points in the hair proximal areas that may give an "exclamation mark" appearance, since the proximal ends are narrower than the distal ends of the hair shaft. The term alopecia totalis refers to cases with total or nearly total loss of scalp hair, while alopecia universalis means loss of hair over the entire body. In the stationary phase, the hair is no longer easily extracted at the margins of the bald patches; most patients with bald patches may enter the regrowth phase after 3-4 months. In the regrowth phase, new hair growth is soft and woolly hair, and may be nonpigmented initially, subsequently becoming coarser and darker, and ultimately becoming indistinguishable from normal hair.

进展期脱发区边缘有短的毛发，松动易拔出，显微镜下可见毛发萎缩，表现为进入头皮处的近端的发干萎缩变细，远端发干粗黑，也称为"惊叹号发"。如头发全部脱落者称为全秃，全身各处长毛、短毛均有脱落者为普秃。静止期脱发斑边缘的头发不再松动，大多数患者在脱发静止 3～4 个月后进入恢复期。恢复期有新毛发长出，开始多为柔软的细毛，色淡，逐渐毛发变黑、变粗乃至恢复正常。

【Diagnosis and Differential Diagnosis】

The diagnosis of alopecia areata can be based on typical clinical manifestations. In the active phase, the hair on the edge of the advanced lesions are loose and easily pulled out and the "exclamation mark" shape of the hair root has diagnostic significance. However, alopecia areata should be differentiated from tinea capitis, pseudopelade and syphilitic alopecia. The diagnosis of tinea capitis is made according to a fungal microscopic examination. The bald patches of pseudopelade are usually irregularly shaped and are accompanied by atrophy of the follicular orifices and permanent hair loss. Finally, a moth-eaten bald pattern may imply syphilitic alopecia.

【诊断与鉴别诊断】

根据典型临床表现本病一般容易诊断。进展期病灶周边有毛发松动，易拔出，发根部呈"惊叹号"有诊断意义。本病应与头癣、假性斑秃及梅毒性脱发相鉴别。头癣根据真菌镜检可确诊，假性斑秃秃发区常不规则，且患处毛囊口萎缩，毛发永久性脱落。梅毒为虫蚀样脱发。

【Treatment】

The onset of alopecia areata is usually related to psychological factors. Most patients with alopecia areata will experience hair loss, and recover spontaneously, within 6-12 months. Doctors should be

【治疗】

本病发生常与精神因素有关，且大多数患者会经历脱发，并可在 6～12 个月内自然痊愈，故应耐心向患者解释病

patient in explaining the course and prognosis of alopecia areata in order to help relieve the psychological burden on the patients. Therefore, removing possible promoting factors and counseling the adoption of a healthier lifestyle should greatly help this group of patients. For those afflicted with alopecia totalis or alopecia universalis, wearing a wig may be recommended in order to reduce psychological stress, but this is not absolutely necessary.

程及预后,解除患者精神负担。祛除可能的诱因因素,生活保持规律。对秃发范围广或全秃和普秃患者,宜带假发以减轻心理负担。

(1) Systemic therapy: patients with alopecia totalis or alopecia universalis may benefit from prednisone 15-30 mg/d for a few weeks, then tapering off within 2-3 months. Relapses are common after discontinuation of the therapy, and given the psychological factors involved it is generally good that the patient be warned of this in advance. Also, the side effects of long term use of glucocorticoids should always be taken into consideration, since this disease is generally self-limiting.

(1) 系统治疗　对全秃及普秃者,可口服泼尼松,15～30 mg/d,数周后逐渐减量。维持 2～3 个月可见效,但停药后可能复发,由于心理因素在该病中的作用,预先告知患者这种可能性对患者是有益的。由于该病为自限性,还应注意长期应用会发生糖皮质激素的不良反应。

(2) Topical therapy: intralesional injection or topical application of glucocorticoids is generally useful. Topical use of 1%-3% minoxidil tincture or cream and 10% capsicum tincture can improve blood flow to the affected area in order to promote hair growth. If applied twice daily, effects are generally noticed after 2-3 months. By the same token, ultraviolet irradiation or PUVA therapy can also be used for the acceleration of hair growth. In the end, hair transplantation can be performed on patients with intractable hair growth.

(2) 局部治疗　可局部皮损部位注射或外用糖皮质激素制剂。外用 1%～3%米诺地尔(敏乐啶)酊剂或霜剂、10%辣椒酊等,可改善局部血液循环,促进毛发生长,一般每日外用 2 次,2～3 个月可见效果。紫外线照射或 PUVA 治疗也有促进毛发生长作用。对毛发不能生长者可施行毛发移植术。

Section Five　Androgenetic Alopecia

第五节　雄激素源性脱发

Androgenetic alopecia (AGA) is also known as male pattern alopecia or premature alopecia. It is characterized by the typical progression of baldness noted in men, and is caused by the involvement of genetic factors and the actions of androgenic hormones.

雄激素源性脱发(androgenetic alopecia, AGA)又称为男性型脱发(male pattern alopecia),也称为早秃(premature alopecia),是有遗传因素参与的,且依赖雄激素作用的以进行性脱发为特征的秃发。

【Etiology and Pathogenesis】

【病因及发病机制】

AGA often shows a family history, demonstrates autosomal dominant inheritance, and is androgen-dependent. The activity of 5α-reductase, which can transform testosterone into dihydrotestosterone, is higher in the bald areas than in non-bald areas of the scalp. This observation implies that AGA is related to some genetic abnormalities of 5α-reductase. Scientists believe that inhibition of the activities of abnormal 5α-reductase is the key to preventing AGA.

AGA 常有家族史,表现为常染色体显性遗传,但其遗传特性需在雄激素作用下才表现出来。5α-还原酶能使睾酮转变为二氢睾酮,在头皮秃发区,5α-还原酶的活性比非脱发区明显增高,因此 AGA 可能与遗传性质的 5α-还原酶异常有关。科学家相信抑制异常的 5α-还原酶活性可能是防治本病的主要途径。

【Clinical Manifestations】

【临床表现】

AGA mostly affects male patients, and the symptoms are more

本病多见于男性,男性症状比女性

severe than in female patients. The age of onset is 20-30. The typical pattern of male baldness begins at the frontal hairline, where existing hair often becomes finer and shorter. Similar changes also occur at the scalp vertex. The hairs at the margins of the occipital and temporal areas are not affected (Fig. 23-8). As the disease progresses, the hairs on top of the scalp eventually are lost completely, leaving smooth skin. In females, the symptoms are much less severe, usually presenting simply as thinning of hair density at the scalp vertex. The course of hair loss in AGA patients is slow and takes place over a long period of time (years to decades). It is usually an asymptomatic condition but may be slightly itchy. However, the growth of eyebrows, beard, eyelashes, armpit hair, pubic hair and other short body hair is not affected.

重，常在20～30岁发病，常从前额角发际开始，毛发变为纤细而稀疏，逐渐伸延至头顶，但枕部及两颞部发缘毛发不受影响（图23-8）。随着病情进展，头顶部头发可脱光，皮肤光滑。女性症状较轻，多为头顶部的毛发稀疏。AGA患者脱发的过程一般很慢（几年到几十年），一般无自觉症状或有微痒。眉毛、胡须、睫毛、腋毛、阴毛和身体其他短毛等的生长不受影响。

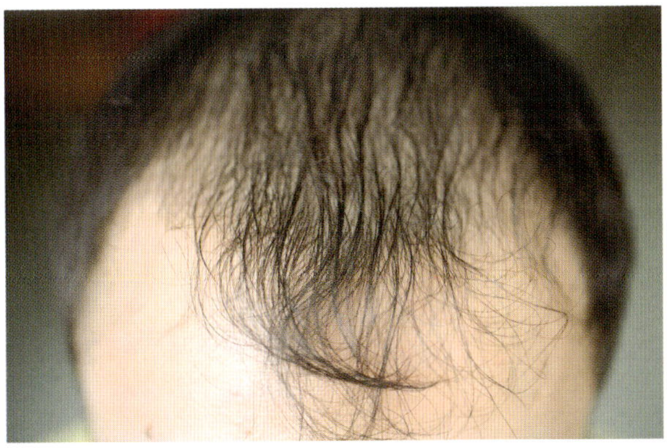

Fig. 23-8 Androgenetic alopecia（图 23-8 雄激素源性脱发）

【Diagnosis and Differential Diagnosis】

The diagnosis is straightforward when patients present with a typical patterned hair loss with a family history of similar condition. However, it should be differentiated from other causes of long-term hair loss, such as malnutrition, drugs, endocrine diseases (hyper/hypothyroidism) and iron deficiency anemia.

【诊断及鉴别诊断】

根据家族史、秃发模式等临床表现，本病的诊断不难。应与其他原因导致的脱发进行鉴别，如营养不良、药物、内分泌疾病（甲状腺功能亢进症或减退症）以及缺铁性贫血等。

【Treatment】

The disease lacks any effective treatment. However, avoidance of local irritation and psychological stress is beneficial. Most drugs show their clinical efficacy by affecting androgen metabolism and androgen receptors. Finasteride (a new type 5α-reductase inhibitor) 1 mg/d for 6-12 months can reduce hair loss, and even promote hair regrowth, although its effects are only manifest after about 6 months. Topical use of 2%-5% minoxidil solutions or gels, twice daily, can also stimulate the hair development, but again the effects begin to appear after several months. If the systemic and topical treatments show no results, hair transplantation may be considered. A wig can often obtain satisfactory cosmetic results.

【治疗】

本病缺乏有效的治疗方法，应减少局部刺激，解除思想负担，药物多通过雄激素代谢作用与雄激素受体而发挥作用。非那雄胺为一种新型5α-还原酶抑制剂，1 mg/d，连续服药6～12个月，可减少毛发脱落，促进头发生长，一般服药6个月可有一定效果。2%～5%米诺地尔溶液或凝胶外用，每日2次，可刺激头发的生长，使用数月后有疗效。药物治疗效果不佳者可选择毛发移植术。假发可以获得较满意的美容效果。

Section Six Hyperhidrosis

Hyperhidrosis is the local or systemic production of excessive amounts of sweat, beyond what would be expected under the environmental or physiological circumstances. Under strenuous exercise or work, under hot weather or drugs, people can often sweat to excess, and this is not considered evidence of hyperhidrosis.

【Etiology and Pathogenesis】

The causes of hyperhidrosis can be broken down into organic diseases and functional disturbances. The term organic diseases here include endocrine disorders such as hyperthyroidism and diabetes mellitus, neurological disorders such as cerebral concussion and hemiplegia, and infectious diseases such as tuberculosis. In functional hyperhidrosis, most patients suffer from some sort of psychiatric distress due to strong emotional stimuli, such as nervousness or fear. All the factors listed above may cause sympathetic nerve disturbances resulting in hyperhidrosis in some patients.

【Clinical Manifestations】

Clinically, hyperhidrosis can be divided into two types.

(1) Localized hyperhidrosis: this type affects both genders, with an onset in childhood or puberty. It can persist for many years and can alleviate after age 25. Localized hyperhidrosis occurs predominantly in the palmoplantar, axillary, groin and pubic areas; followed by the forehead, nose apex and chest areas. Palmoplantar hyperhidrosis may be persistent or episodic, being caused typically by emotional fluctuations, and does not change with the seasons. Palmoplantar hyperhidrosis usually presents with wet and cold extremities, and may be accompanied by hyperkeratinization (Fig. 23-9). In addition, any part of the sympathetic nerve projection can cause localized hyperhidrosis, where hyperhidrosis recurs asymmetrically, or is restricted to only a certain small part of the body.

(2) Generalized hyperhidrosis: this type of hyperhidrosis is typically caused by organic diseases such as febrile infection, which arises from the regulatory effects of the nervous system or the effects of oral antipyretics. Other possible causes include central nervous system disorders, such as cortical and basal ganglion disorders. Spinal cord or peripheral nervous system disorders can result in hyperhidrosis as well.

【Treatment】

(1) Topical therapy: special care must be taken with skin

第六节 多汗症

多汗症(hyperhidrosis)是指正常生活环境和条件下患者局部或全身皮肤异常多汗。正常人在剧烈运动或高强度工作、天气炎热及药物作用下,可以大量出汗,这些都是正常的生活现象,不属于多汗症。

【病因及发病机制】

多汗症的原因一般可分为器质性疾病和功能性失调两种。前者主要见于内分泌失调,如甲状腺功能亢进症、糖尿病;神经系统病患,如脑震荡和偏瘫;亦见于感染过程中及感染后,如结核病。功能性多汗症一般以精神性出汗较多,由于高度情绪刺激(如紧张、痛苦、害怕等)造成,为交感神经失调而致多汗。

【临床表现】

多汗症一般分为两型。

(1) 局限性多汗症　此型男女均可发生,常始于儿童或青春期,可以持续多年,至25岁以后常自然减轻。局限性多汗症多见于掌跖、腋下、腹股沟、会阴部,其次为前额、鼻尖和胸部。掌跖多汗症可为持续性或周期性的,由情绪波动造成,没有季节区别。常出现手足湿冷,可伴手足角化过度表现(图23-9)。此外交感神经任何支配部位均可引起局限性多汗症,此种多汗症反复出现于一侧或局限于某一小片部位。

(2) 全身性多汗症　此型主要由器质性疾病引起,如感染性高热,由于神经系统的调节或口服退热剂以出汗来散发热量,中枢神经系统(如皮质及基底神经节)、脊椎或周围神经系统的损害可以造成全身多汗。

【治疗】

(1) 局部治疗　首先应注意皮肤清

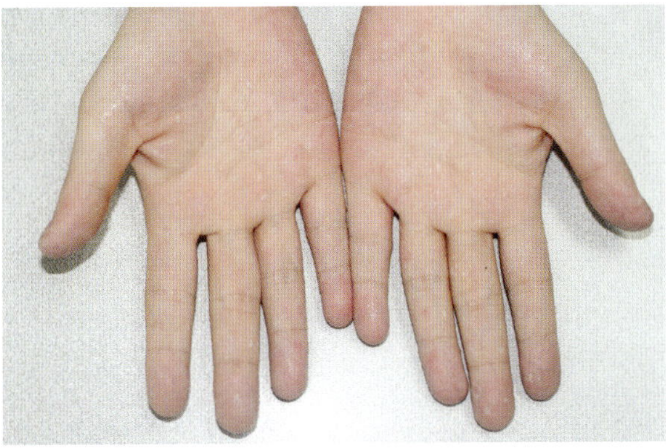

Fig. 23-9 Palmoplantar hyperhidrosis(图 23-9 掌跖多汗症)

hygiene, such as applying an absorbent powder such as talcum after cleansing the axillary area to keep it dry. Application of 5% formaldehyde solution, 1% formaldehyde solution, 0.5% aluminum acetate solution, or 5% alum solution (hydrated aluminum sulfate) in the palmoplantar area is usually helpful.

洁，腋部可于清洁后扑粉以保持干燥。掌跖多汗症可用5%甲醛溶液外搽，1%甲醛溶液、0.5%醋酸铝溶液、5%明矾溶液浸泡或涂搽掌跖部。

(2) Systemic therapy: anticholinergic drugs such as atropine and belladonna have temporary effects, but dry mouth, flushing and palpitations may develop as side effects of these drugs. The application of sedatives, such as bromine agents, phenobarbital or chlorpromazine, is effective against psychiatric hyperhidrosis.

(2) 系统治疗 抗胆碱能药物，如阿托品、颠茄等，具有暂时性效果，但有口干、皮肤潮红、心悸等不良反应。镇定药，如溴剂、苯巴比妥、氯丙嗪等，对精神性多汗症有效。

(3) Physical therapy: superficial X-ray irradiation inhibits the secretion of sweat glands, and can have a certain effect on severe hyperhidrosis.

(3) 物理治疗 严重多汗症可用浅层X线照射抑制汗腺分泌，有一定疗效。

(4) Surgical treatment: is the best method for treating axillary hyperhidrosis.

(4) 手术治疗 治疗腋窝多汗症的最佳方法。

Section Seven Bromhidrosis

第七节 臭 汗 症

Bromhidrosis refers to a particular offensive odor arising from the sweat.

臭汗症(bromhidrosis)是指所出汗液带有特殊的臭味。

【Etiology and Pathogenesis】

Bromidrosis, when caused by the eccrine glands, is due to the decomposition of some substances on the skin surface facilitated by epidermal bacteria, usually accompanied by hyperhidrosis. Bromidrosis, when caused by the apocrine glands, is a result of the production of free fatty acids and ammonia by the interactions of some bacteria with the organic substances in the secretions from the apocrine glands. Since the apocrine glands are affected by sex hormones, bromidrosis usually presents during adolescence and may disappear as the patients grow older. Mental or nervous system diseases (such as paranoia, schizophrenia, etc.) can also occur along with bromidrosis. The cause of bromidrosis may be related to genetic factors.

【病因及发病机制】

外泌汗腺引起的臭汗症多由表皮细菌分解皮肤表面物质引起，常与多汗症伴发；顶泌汗腺引起的臭汗症多由该部位各种细菌与顶泌汗腺分泌物中所含的有机物质互相作用后产生的游离脂肪酸和氨所致。由于顶泌汗腺的分泌受性激素影响，故多在青春期开始，至老年后逐渐消失。精神或神经系统疾病(如偏执狂、精神分裂等)也可产生臭汗症，臭汗症的发生可能与遗传因素有关。

【Clinical Manifestations】

The offensive smell produced by bromidrosis arises predominantly in the following areas: axillary, plantar, pubic areas and toe webs and the perianal and groin areas. The fovea umbilicalis and submammary areas are less frequently involved. The unpleasant smell is primarily related to perspiration and is aggravated in the summer, especially during puberty. Bromidrosis usually subsides once the patient has grown older. The intensity of the odor differ in individuals and races; in severe cases it may present as a pungent odor, while in mild cases, it may not present at all when there is no perspiration.

【临床表现】

臭汗气味主要发生在腋下、足底、会阴部、趾缝、肛周和腹股沟，其次为脐窝和乳房下，大多与汗液有关，因此夏季加重，以青春发育期臭味最浓，随年龄增长而减轻。臭汗气味轻重随个体、种族差异显著不同。重的为一种刺鼻的特殊气味，轻的在不出汗时几乎无气味发生。

【Treatment】

The skin must be kept clean and dry. The patient should shower and change clothes frequently, keep the skin dry, and concurrently treat any accompanying hyperhidrosis in order to control perspiration and reduce the population of epidermal bacteria. Topical application of 3%-5% formaldehyde solution or 5% alum solution twice daily can reduce perspiration. In cases of podobromidrosis (smelly feet), feet may be soaked in a potassium permanganate solution (1 : 8000) once a day for 10 minutes. In severe cases surgery can be taken into consideration, including total or partial gland excisions.

【治疗】

应注意清洁卫生，经常洗澡，勤换衣服，保持皮肤干燥。同时治疗多汗症，因汗液减少可使皮肤表面的细菌大大减少，局部外用3%～5%甲醛溶液或5%明矾溶液，每日两次，可减少出汗。足臭可用1∶8000高锰酸钾溶液浸泡，每次10 min，每日1次。如臭汗症病情严重者可行腺体全切术、部分切除术。

Lie-hua DENG(邓列华)

Chapter Twenty-four Diseases of Subcutaneous Fat

Section One Erythema Nodosum

Panniculitis is a group of diseases involving inflammations of subcutaneous adipose tissue, among which erythema nodosum is the most common form.

【Etiology and Pathogenesis】

Erythema nodosum is presumed to be a reactive inflammation in the deep dermis and subcutaneous adipose tissue to a variety of etiologic factors. It has been associated with systemic conditions such as infections, rheumatic diseases, sarcoidosis, pregnancy, inflammatory bowel diseases, medications, autoimmune disorders, or malignancies. It is well known that upper respiratory infections by group A β-hemolytic *Streptococcus* are closely correlated with erythema nodosum, especially in children and young adults. However, the exact etiology of erythema nodosum is never made certain in a significant percentage of cases.

【Clinical Manifestations】

Erythema nodosum may present clinically in an acute or chronic form. The acute form of erythema nodosum is more common, and may occur at any age and in both sexes but is most common in young women. The typical eruption of erythema nodosum consists of a sudden onset of multiple, bilateral, symmetrical, tender, erythematous, warm and slightly raised nodules or plaques varying from 1-10 cm in diameter. These nodules are usually located on the anterior aspects of the lower extremities, especially on the shins, ankles and knees (Fig. 24-1), also on the upper legs, extensor arms, neck, but rarely on the face. The abrupt onset is always accompanied by malaise, leg swelling, and arthritis or arthralgia of the ankles, knees, or wrists. Fever, headache and some gastrointestinal complaints may also be present in severe cases. The individual lesion lasts from a few days to several weeks, before the inflammation slowly fades and finally resolves without atrophy or scarring. Ulceration is never seen in erythema nodosum.

Chronic erythema nodosum has been described under different names, including erythema nodosum migrans or subacute nodular migratory panniculitis. The lesions tend to develop in old women, and are not often associated with any underlying systemic diseases. In contrast to acute erythema nodosum, lesions of chronic erythema nodosum are usually unilateral, or asymmetrical if bilateral, and usually manifest without pain or even mild tenderness. A single

第二十四章 皮下脂肪组织疾病

第一节 结节性红斑

脂膜炎(panniculitis)是发生于皮下脂肪组织的炎症。结节性红斑是最常见的脂膜炎。

【病因及发病机制】

结节性红斑(erythema nodosum)被视为是发生于真皮深层和皮下脂肪组织、由不同病因引起的反应性炎症,与感染、风湿性疾病、肉样瘤病、妊娠、炎性肠病、药物、自身免疫性疾病和肿瘤等多种系统性因素有关。特别是在儿童和青年人中,A 组乙型溶血性链球菌的上呼吸道感染与结节性红斑的关系已广为人知。然而,结节性红斑的大多数病例的病因仍不能确定。

【临床表现】

结节性红斑可表现为急性型或慢性型。急性型结节性红斑更常见,可在任何年龄及两性中均可发生,但多数病例见于年轻成年女性。结节性红斑的典型皮疹由突然发生的多个、双侧对称、有触痛的、红色、皮温高的、轻度隆起的结节或斑块构成,其直径为 1～10 cm,通常位于下肢伸侧,尤其常见于胫部、踝部和膝部(图 24-1),皮损也可见于大腿、上肢伸侧、颈部,罕见于面部。结节性红斑的急性起病常伴有全身不适、下肢水肿,踝、膝或腕的关节炎或关节痛。重者还可有发热、头痛和某些胃肠道症状。其自然病程持续数天至数周,然后缓慢退化,最终痊愈而无萎缩或瘢痕形成,但从不会发生溃疡。

慢性结节性红斑也以不同的名称被描述,包括游走性结节性红斑或亚急性结节性游走性脂膜炎。其皮损倾向于发生在老年女性,且不伴有潜在疾病。与急性结节性红斑不同,慢性结节性红斑的皮损常单侧发生,即使是两侧均有但并不对称,无痛或有比急性结节性红斑

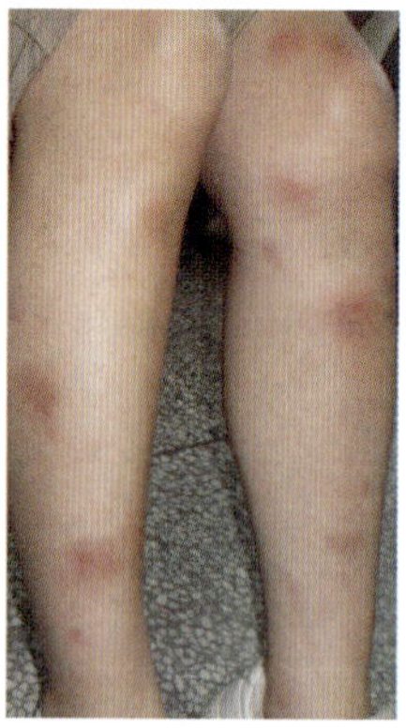

Fig. 24-1 Erythema nodosum(图 24-1 结节性红斑)

primary lesion tends to resolve spontaneously, but tends to migrate centrifugally, and will form an annular subcutaneous induration with central clearing. Chronic erythema nodosum is more persistent and usually lasts from a few months to years.

皮损为轻的触痛。起病时的单个皮损倾向于缓解,但离心性地向外扩展,形成中央消退的环状皮下斑块。慢性结节性红斑具有数月至数年的持续较长的病程。

【Laboratory Findings】

The initial laboratory workup for erythema nodosum should include complete blood count, urinalysis, erythrocyte sedimentation rates (ESR), antistreptolysin-O (ASO) titers and C-reactive protein (CRP) detection, throat culture, intradermal tuberculin (also known as purified protein derivative, PPD) test and a chest X-ray. Normal or slightly raised white blood cell counts, elevated ESR, and increased CRP levels are all typically found in patients with erythema nodosum.

【实验室检查】

结节性红斑的初步实验室检查应包括血常规、尿液分析、血沉、抗链球菌溶血素 O(ASO)、C-反应蛋白(CRP)、咽部培养、结核菌素皮试(也称 PPD 试验)和胸部 X 片。在结节性红斑患者中可发现白细胞计数正常或轻度升高、血沉快和C-反应蛋白水平升高。

【Histopathology】

Histopathologically, erythema nodosum is a septal panniculitis. The inflammatory infiltrate principally involves the septa of connective tissue lying between fat lobules throughout the entire affected area. The infiltrate is mainly composed of either neutrophils (at early stages of erythema nodosum) or a mixture of lymphocytes, histiocytes and/or multinucleated giant cells (during the late stages of the disease), depending on the stage of the disease when the biopsy is taken. It is characteristic that leukocytoclastic vasculitis is not a histologic feature of erythema nodosum.

【组织病理】

在组织病理学上,结节性红斑为间隔性脂膜炎。在整个受累区域,炎性浸润主要累及脂肪小叶之间的结缔组织间隔。炎性浸润在早期由中性粒细胞组成,在晚期则由淋巴细胞、组织细胞和/或多核巨细胞等混合组成,这取决于活检取材皮损所处的病期。应注意的是,白细胞碎裂性血管炎不是结节性红斑的组织学特征。

【Diagnosis】

Most of cases of erythema nodosum can be diagnosed based on history and clinical appearance, but biopsy is recommended for confirmation. A deep skin incisional biopsy is needed in order to properly sample the subcutaneous tissue.

【诊断】

大多数结节性红斑患者可根据其病史、临床表现做出诊断。皮损活检的组织病理学有助于明确诊断,活检时应取材较深,以获取足够的皮下组织。

【Differential Diagnosis】

Erythema nodosum needs to be distinguished from erythema induratum of Bazin, nodular vasculitis, superficial thrombophlebitis,

【鉴别诊断】

结节性红斑需要与 Bazin 硬红斑或结节性血管炎、浅表血栓性静脉炎、皮肤

cutaneous polyarteritis nodosa, subcutaneous sarcoidosis, and subcutaneous panniculitis-like T-cell lymphoma. Histopathological examination will provide the necessary clues for the differential diagnosis.

结节性多动脉炎、皮下肉样瘤病和皮下脂膜炎样 T 细胞淋巴瘤等进行鉴别诊断。组织病理学检查对结节性红斑的鉴别诊断很有帮助。

【Treatment】

Treatment of erythema nodosum should be directed towards eliminating the underlying associated conditions once it is diagnosed. Non-steroidal anti-inflammatory drugs (NSAIDs) such as indomethacin may be helpful to relieve the lesional inflammation and arthralgia. Potassium iodide can be chosen for patients with persistent lesions. Systemic glucocorticoids are not often prescribed for erythema nodosum, but if used, the possible side effects on the underlying infection should be considered and ruled out before treatment. Rapid resolution of lesions and symptoms after using systemic glucocorticoids or intralesional injections of triamcinolone acetonide has been demonstrated as well.

【治疗】

结节性红斑的治疗应注意针对潜在的相关情况。非甾体类抗炎药(如吲哚美辛)有助于缓解皮损炎症及关节痛。碘化钾可用于持久性皮损的治疗。结节性红斑很少系统使用糖皮质激素，如需使用，应排除潜在感染。系统使用糖皮质激素将导致皮损的迅速消退。曲安奈德皮损内注射也可使皮损消退。

【Prognosis】

Prognosis of erythema nodosum is self-limiting and benign. Most cases of erythema nodosum regress spontaneously within a few weeks or months without atrophy or scarring. Ulceration is never seen during the course of erythema nodosum. Recurrences of erythema nodosum are not uncommon, especially when the underlying conditions or infection still exists.

【预后】

结节性红斑呈自限性，预后良好。多数结节性红斑的病例可在几周或数月内自发消退，而无萎缩或瘢痕。病程中不发生溃疡。结节性红斑复发并非少见，尤其是在某些潜在情况或感染存在时。

Section Two　Cold Panniculitis

第二节　寒冷性脂膜炎

Cold panniculitis is an inflammation of the subcutaneous adipose tissue resulting from a localized cold injury, usually limited to the body areas exposed to the cold.

寒冷性脂膜炎(cold panniculitis)是由局部寒冷损伤所致的皮下脂肪组织的炎症，通常限于暴露于寒冷的部位。

【Etiology and Pathogenesis】

Cold panniculitis has been documented in the cheeks of children who suck ice or popsicles or in the upper lateral thighs of women during the winter months because of exposure to the cold environment. It is believed that localized cold injury induces an inflammation of the subcutaneous adipose tissue.

【病因及发病机制】

寒冷性脂膜炎已有报道发生在吮吸冰棒的儿童颊部和冬月中因寒冷加剧而发生于女性的大腿外上方。局部的寒冷损伤导致了皮下脂肪组织的炎症。

【Clinical Manifestations】

Cold panniculitis particularly affects infants and young children, and is also common in obese adult women. Usually the skin lesions occur a few days after exposure to the cold environment. The distribution of the lesions is characteristically on the face (cheeks and forehead) in children, and on the buttocks, thighs, arms and under the chin, which are areas often poorly protected from the cold in obese women. Lesions present as slightly erythematous or violaceous, with poorly-defined margins, painless,

【临床表现】

婴儿和儿童尤其易发生寒冷性脂膜炎，肥胖的成年女性也易患寒冷性脂膜炎。皮损常在接触寒冷后几天内发生。皮损在儿童特征性地分布于面部(颊部及额部)，在肥胖女性则特征性地分布于臀部、股部、上臂和颌下等易受寒冷的区域。皮损表现为淡红色或紫色、非触痛性、质硬的皮下结节，局部皮温低，边界

indurated subcutaneous nodules with a low skin temperature. Nodules may be raised slightly above the skin and can sometimes be painful (Fig. 24-2).

欠清晰。结节可轻微隆起于皮面，可有疼痛感(图 24-2)。

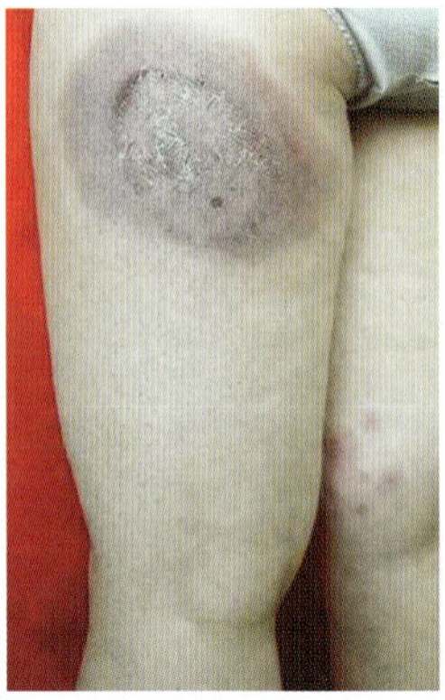

Fig. 24-2　Cold panniculitis(图 24-2　寒冷性脂膜炎)

【Histopathology】

The classic histopathological features of cold panniculitis are lobular panniculitis with necrosis of adipocytes and a mixed inflammatory infiltration that is composed of lymphocytes, histiocytes, foam cells, and/or neutrophils.

【组织病理】

寒冷性脂膜炎在组织病理学上的典型特征主要是小叶性脂膜炎，具有脂肪细胞坏死和由淋巴细胞、组织细胞、泡沫细胞和/或中性粒细胞组成的混合性炎性浸润。

【Diagnosis and Differential Diagnosis】

For cold panniculitis, the diagnosis usually can be made by confirming a history of skin exposure to cold and on the basis of classic presentation with nodular red swellings over the areas so exposed. Cold panniculitis needs to be distinguished from subcutaneous fat necrosis of the newborn, sclerema neonatorum, poststeroid panniculitis, chilblains and frostbite.

【诊断与鉴别诊断】

寒冷性脂膜炎的诊断常根据皮肤暴露于寒冷的病史和发生于遇冷区域的结节性红肿的典型表现而确定。寒冷性脂膜炎需要与新生儿皮下脂肪坏死、新生儿硬肿症、皮质类固醇激素后脂膜炎、冻疮和冻伤等进行鉴别诊断。

【Treatment】

In most instances, cold panniculitis is a self-limiting disorder and requires only supportive treatment for symptomatic relief. Most patients are able to recover in a few days or weeks after the skin lesions are slowly warmed up.

【治疗】

多数情况下，寒冷性脂膜炎是具有自限性的疾病，仅需对症支持处理。许多患者在缓慢复温后经数天至数周可痊愈。

【Prognosis】

The prognosis of cold panniculitis is excellent due to its self-limiting natural course. No complications are known.

【预后】

由于多数病例可在几周内自然缓解而无不良反应发生，故寒冷性脂膜炎的预后极佳。

Wei HE(何威)

Chapter Twenty-five Non-infectious Granulomas

Section One Sarcoidosis

Sarcoidosis is a systemic, non-caseous granulomatous disease of unknown etiology. While numerous organs may be involved, the lungs, lymph nodes and skin are the most commonly affected. The first case of cutaneous sarcoidosis was documented in the late 1800s, in which it was described as "multiple benign sarcoid of the skin", because the lesions resembled sarcomas but were benign.

【Etiology and Pathogenesis】

Sarcoidosis is a multisystem granulomatous disease characterized by hyperactivity of the cell-mediated immune system. Although the immunopathogenesis of sarcoidosis remains unknown, the interplay between extrinsic antigens and immunogenetic response of individuals is believed to be responsible for the development and progression of the disease. Presumably, antigen-presenting cells such as macrophages and dendritic cells recognize, process, and present the processed antigen to $CD4^+$ T-cells via HLA class Ⅱ molecules. These activated macrophages produce interleukin (IL)-12, which induces lymphocytes to polarize towards a Th1 profile, and in turn prompts these activated T-cells to release IL-2、IFN-γ and chemotactic factors that further recruit and activate monocytes and macrophages. The end result is the occurrence of multinucleated giant cells and the formation of granulomas. Although the identity of the putative antigen(s) of sarcoidosis is unknown, infectious organisms might be among the leading causes, including mycobacteria, HHV-8, EBV, etc. In addition, genetic susceptibility to sarcoidosis has been associated with HLA-1, HLA-B8, and HLA-DR3 alleles.

【Clinical Manifestations】

(1) Clinical course: sarcoidosis is a chronic disease and multiple organs can be involved. As the symptoms might be subtle and nonspecific, the diagnosis of sarcoidosis is often delayed or missed entirely. For example, 30%-60% of patients with pulmonary sarcoidosis are asymptomatic. Other than the lungs, the skin, eye, liver, and peripheral lymph nodes are often affected as well.

(2) Cutaneous symptoms: skin lesions are seen in 20% to 35% of cases of systemic sarcoidosis. Some cases exhibit skin lesions only. Cutaneous lesions of sarcoidosis are divided into two categories: specific and nonspecific. The specific type has clear granulomas in histology, while the nonspecific type is caused by

第二十五章 非感染性肉芽肿

第一节 结 节 病

结节病(sarcoidosis)是一种系统性、非干酪肉芽肿性、病因不明的疾病。多数器官均可受累,而肺、淋巴结及皮肤是最常见的受累部位。结节病的皮肤表现最早于19世纪晚期被报道,当时被描述为一种"良性的类似肉瘤样的皮损"。

【病因及发病机制】

结节病是多系统肉芽肿性疾病,以细胞免疫活性升高为特点。尽管其免疫发病机制不明,但外源性抗原及其诱发的个体免疫应答与该病的发生发展密切相关。目前,关于结节病的免疫发病机制的理论为:在潜在抗原的存在下,抗原递呈细胞,如巨噬细胞或树突状细胞通过HLA-Ⅱ型分子识别、处理抗原并将处理后的抗原呈递给$CD4^+$ T细胞,同时产生IL-12,激活$CD4^+$ T细胞向Th1细胞的分化,促进Th1型反应。Th1细胞释放IL-2、IFN-γ及其他趋化因子,趋化并活化单核细胞和巨噬细胞,最终引起多核巨细胞的产生以及肉芽肿的形成。结节病的潜在致病抗原尚不清楚,可能来源于感染性微生物,包括分枝杆菌、人类疱疹病毒-8及EB病毒等。另外,结节病的遗传易感性与HLA-1, HLA-B8及HLA-DR3等位基因有关。

【临床表现】

(1)病程 结节病常表现为慢性病程,可累及多个器官,症状轻微非特异,因此常常被误诊和漏诊。30%～60%的肺部结节病患者没有任何症状。除了肺部以外,皮肤、眼、肝脏及外周淋巴结是结节病最常累及的器官。

(2)皮肤症状 20%至35%的系统性结节病出现皮肤表现,有些甚至只有皮肤表现。结节病的皮肤表现可分为特异性皮肤表现及非特异性皮肤表现。特异性的表现在皮肤病理中可见清晰的肉

reactive response but lacks sarcoidal granulomas in histological findings.

Specific sarcoidal lesions favor the face, lips, neck, upper trunk, and extremities, and are fairly symmetric in distribution. Papules and plaques are commonly present, and are often red-brown in color (Fig. 25-1). Less common presentations include hypopigmentation, subcutaneous nodules, ichthyosiform lesions, alopecia and ulcerations. However, erythroderma and erythema multiforme-like lesions manifest only rarely.

芽肿形成,而非特异性的皮肤表现往往是反应性的,不出现结节病性肉芽肿。

结节病的特异性皮肤表现好发于面部、唇部、颈部、躯干上部及四肢,对称分布。通常表现为丘疹、斑块,红棕色(图25-1)。少见表现为色素减退、皮下结节、鱼鳞病样损害、脱发及溃疡。红皮病及多形红斑样损害则较为罕见。

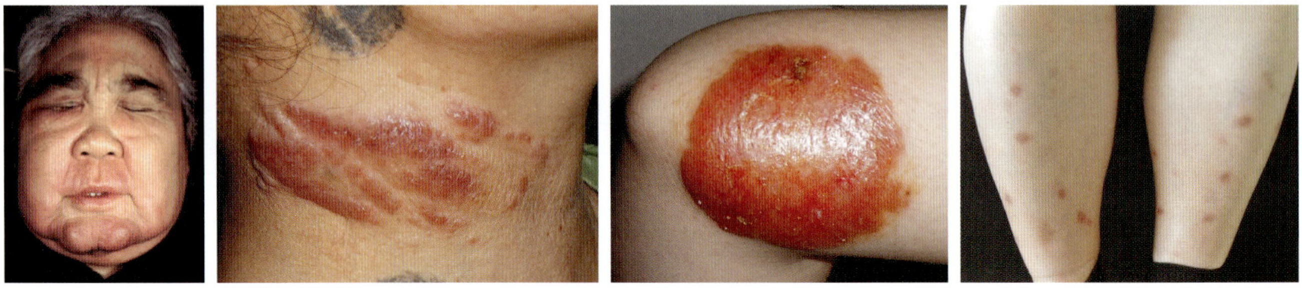

(a)　(b)　(c)　(d)

Fig. 25-1　Sarcoidosis(图 25-1　结节病)

Variants of sarcoidosis include Darier-Roussy disease and lupus pernio. In the Darier-Roussy form of sarcoidosis, deep-seated 0.5-2.0 cm nodules are usually found on the extremities. Lupus pernio is characterized by papules, nodules and plaques arranged in a beaded pattern, primarily affecting exposed areas such as the nose, ears, and cheeks. These two forms of sarcoidosis indicate that systemic organs may be involved.

Erythema nodosum is non-specific cutaneous manifestation of sarcoidosis, which usually resolves spontaneously and generally does not require systemic corticosteroid therapy. Sarcoidosis that manifests as erythema nodosum with hilaradenopathy, fever, migrating polyarthritis, and acute iritis is termed Löfgren's syndrome.

Furthermore, the oral cavity, anogenital area, and nails can also be affected. Nail involvement often implicates a chronic course of the disease, presenting as subungual hyperkeratosis, clubbing, onycholysis, etc.

(3) Systemic symptoms: although various organs may be involved, lungs and eyes are most frequently affected, and pulmonary sarcoidosis is the most common. At the final stage, pulmonary fibrosis is formed in affected lung tissue with bronchiolectasis and the lung parenchyma takes on a "honeycombing" appearance. Hilar and/or paratracheal lymphadenopathy, which is usually asymptomatic unless associated with parenchymal lung disease, occurs in 90% of patients. Ocular sarcoidosis may present

结节病的变异型包括 Darier-Roussy 型及冻疮样狼疮型。Darier-Roussy 型中,通常可见四肢深在的 0.5～2.0 cm 结节。冻疮样狼疮型以串珠状排列的丘疹、结节和斑块为特点,好发于鼻、耳、面颊等暴露部位。这两型结节病是系统受累的征兆。

结节性红斑是结节病的非特异性皮肤表现,通常自发消退,无须系统激素治疗。结节病表现为结节性红斑、肺门淋巴结肿大、发热、游走性多关节炎及急性虹膜炎时,称 Löfgren 综合征(Löfgren's syndrome)。

此外,口腔及肛门生殖器区域、指甲均可受累。指甲病变通常是慢性病变的标志,可表现为甲下角化过度、杵状指、甲松解等。

(3) 系统症状　尽管多器官均可受累,但是肺部及眼部最常受累。肺部结节病是最常见表现,肺部结节病终末期表现为肺部纤维化伴细支气管扩张,及肺实质"蜂窝样变"。90%患者出现肺门和/或气管旁淋巴结肿大,除伴发肺实质病变外,通常无症状。眼结节病可能表现为葡萄膜炎及虹膜睫状体炎。

as uveitis and iridocyclitis.

【Histopathology】

Non-caseous epithelioid cell granuloma is typically observed in sarcoidosis with few lymphocytic infiltration around granuloma (the so-called naked tubercles)(Fig. 25-2). Inclusion bodies such as Schaumann bodies (rounded laminated basophilic inclusions) and asteroid bodies (eosinophilic stellate inclusions) may be seen in the giant cells of granuloma, but these are not specific for sarcoidosis and may occur in other granulomatous reactions.

【组织病理】

结节病的典型病理表现为非干酪性上皮样细胞肉芽肿，外周少量淋巴细胞浸润（裸结节）（图 25-2）。在肉芽肿的巨细胞内，可见包涵体，如 Schaumann 小体（圆形层状的嗜碱性包涵体）及星状体（嗜酸性星状包涵体），这些包涵体对于结节病的诊断并不特异，也可见于其他肉芽肿反应中。

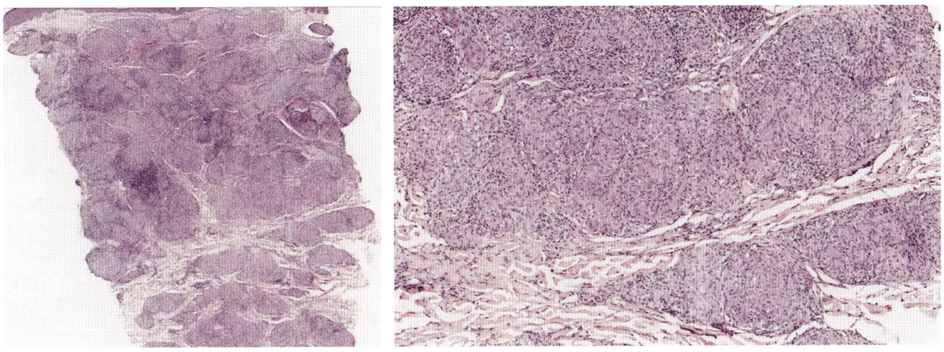

(a) (b)

Fig. 25-2　Sarcoidosis-histopathology（图 25-2　结节病-组织病理）

【Diagnosis and Differential Diagnosis】

Diagnosis of sarcoidosis is a matter of exclusion, at both a clinical and histological level. In order to establish the diagnosis, a supportive clinical history must be accompanied by the histological presence of non-caseous granulomas in at least one organ. A negative result of tuberculin test and elevated levels of angiotensin-converting enzyme (ACE) and calcium further support the diagnosis. In addition, bilateral hilar lymphadenopathy revealed by CT scan is of diagnostic value. Sarcoidosis should be differentiated from tuberculosis cutis, leprosy, granuloma annulare, foreign body granuloma, etc.

【诊断及鉴别诊断】

结节病的临床及组织学诊断均是排除性诊断。除支持性临床病史外，至少存在一个器官系统的非干酪性肉芽肿的组织学表现方可诊断。结核菌素试验结果阴性及血管紧张素转换酶和钙离子的水平升高均有助于诊断。此外，CT 发现双侧肺门淋巴结肿大同样具有诊断价值。结节病应与皮肤结核、麻风、环状肉芽肿及异物肉芽肿等疾病相鉴别。

【Treatment】

Topical or intralesional corticosteroids are the first-line therapy for localized and mild cases that are limited to the skin. Oral corticosteroids are the drug of choice for rapidly progressive lesions or for lesions unresponsive to topical therapies. Anti-inflammatory and immunosuppressive agents are administered as monotherapy or as adjuvants for corticosteroid tapering. Tumor necrosis factor inhibitors have been demonstrated to be beneficial in recalcitrant skin lesions.

【治疗】

局部及皮损内注射糖皮质激素是局限性、较轻的皮肤结节病的一线治疗方案。口服糖皮质激素是快速进展或局部治疗无效的结节病治疗方案。抗炎药和免疫抑制剂可单独用于治疗或作为糖皮质激素减量时的辅助治疗。肿瘤坏死因子抑制剂对于顽固性皮损有一定疗效。

Section Two　Granuloma Annulare

第二节　环状肉芽肿

Granuloma annulare (GA) is a common cutaneous disorder classically presenting with multiple morphologies. The etiology of GA remains unknown and several systemic conditions have been proposed but not yet proven, including diabetes mellitus, malignancy, thyroid disease, etc.

环状肉芽肿(granuloma annulare, GA)是一种常见皮肤病，表现多样，其病因未明，但与许多系统性疾病相关，如糖尿病、恶性肿瘤、甲状腺疾病等，尚未得到明确证实。

【Etiology and Pathogenesis】

GA is a cell-mediated immune response to an unknown antigen. IFN-γ secreting Th1 cells cause a delayed type of hypersensitivity reaction whereby macrophages are differentiated to aggressive effector cells. The end result of this process is the degradation of the connective tissue matrix, which is a typical feature of GA. Generalized GA was found in association with HLA-Bw35. Several systemic diseases have been associated with generalized GA, including diabetes mellitus (DM), malignancy, thyroid disease, lipid abnormalities, infections caused by human immunodeficiency virus (HIV), hepatitis B and hepatitis C, and rheumatoid arthritis.

【病因及发病机制】

环状肉芽肿是对未知抗原的细胞免疫反应。分泌 γ 干扰素的 Th1 细胞引起迟发型过敏反应，导致巨噬细胞分化为侵袭性效应细胞。该过程最终导致结缔组织基质降解(环状肉芽肿的典型表现)。泛发型环状肉芽肿与 HLA-Bw35 相关。与泛发型环状肉芽肿相关的系统性疾病包括糖尿病、恶性肿瘤、甲状腺疾病、脂代谢紊乱、艾滋病、乙型肝炎、丙型肝炎及类风湿关节炎。

【Clinical Manifestations】

The presentation of GA is variable, including localized, generalized, subcutaneous, and perforating forms. Other rare subtypes of GA were reported such as macular or patch type, papular, palmar, photo-distributed, and pustular GA (Fig. 25-3). The lesions of GA are usually asymptomatic but can sometimes be pruritic or painful.

【临床表现】

环状肉芽肿表现多样，包括局限型、泛发型、皮下型及穿通型。少见亚型包括斑疹/斑片型、丘疹型、手掌型、曝光部位型及脓疱型(图 25-3)。环状肉芽肿通常无症状，有时瘙痒或疼痛。

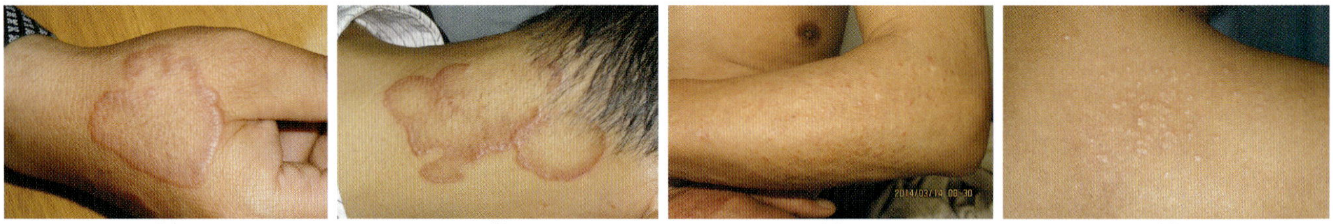

(a)　(b)　(c)　(d)

Fig. 25-3　Granuloma annulare(图 25-3　环状肉芽肿)

(1) Localized GA: it is most frequently found on the lateral or dorsal surfaces of the hands and feet, and is most common in young females. The disease begins with a few asymptomatic, flesh-colored papules that undergo central involution. Over months, a ring of papules slowly increases in diameter to 0.5-5 cm. The duration of the disease is highly variable. Many lesions undergo spontaneous resolution without scarring, whereas others last for years.

(2) Generalized GA: myriad small skin-colored to pink-violet papules arising in a symmetric distribution occur on the trunk and

(1) 局限型环状肉芽肿　好发于年轻女性，常见于手、足的侧面及背面，疾病初期，数个无症状、皮色丘疹向中聚集，数月后增大为直径 0.5～5 cm 的环形皮损。疾病病程各异，多数皮损可自然消退，不留瘢痕，而有些皮损则持续数年。

(2) 泛发型环状肉芽肿　大量皮色至粉紫色的小丘疹对称分布于躯干及四

extremities. Some of these papules may coalesce to form small annular plaques. In about half the cases, the disease is associated with diabetes mellitus.

（3）Subcutaneous GA: a palpable, subcutaneous nodule of normal skin color, it commonly occurs in early childhood. Typical locations are the palms, hands, pretibial areas, feet, as well as the buttocks, scalp and, rarely, the eyelids.

（4）Perforating GA: it is a papule with a centralized concavity that may ulcerate and crust on the dorsal hands and fingers. Dermal excretion of degenerated collagen fibers may occur in some cases. It often arises secondarily after localized GA.

肢，有些丘疹融合成小的环状斑块。约半数病例中，此病与糖尿病密切相关。

（3）皮下型环状肉芽肿　可触及的皮下皮色结节，好发于儿童期。常累及掌、手部、胫前、足、臀部及头皮，眼睑受累罕见。

（4）穿通型环状肉芽肿　临床表现为发生于手背及手指的中央有凹陷的丘疹，可能破溃或结痂。有时排出变性胶原。通常继发于局限型环状肉芽肿。

【Histopathology】

GA is classically characterized by dermal palisading granulomas with central degeneration of collagen, the presence of mucin, and a lymphohistiocytic infiltrate (Fig. 25-4). The presence of mucin is the key feature of histology to distinguish GA from other non-infectious granulomatous diseases.

【组织病理】

环状肉芽肿的经典病理表现为真皮栅栏状肉芽肿伴中间变性的胶原，可见黏蛋白及淋巴组织细胞浸润（图 25-4）。黏蛋白是区别环状肉芽肿与其他非感染性肉芽肿疾病的特征。

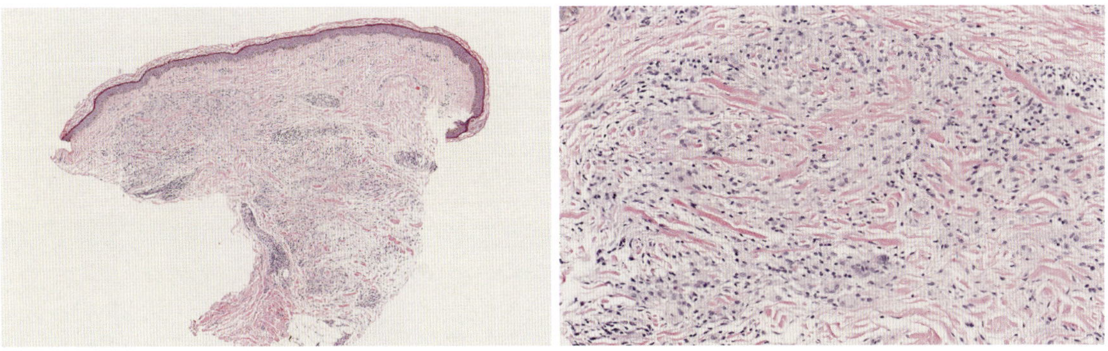

(a)　(b)

Fig. 25-4　Granuloma annulare-histopathology（图 25-4　环状肉芽肿-组织病理）

【Diagnosis and Differential Diagnosis】

The diagnosis can be made upon characteristic clinical presentation and biopsy. Furthermore, a thorough review of systems, risk factors assessment, physical examination, and laboratory and imaging evaluations for underlying conditions such as diabetes mellitus, malignancy, thyroid disease, and dyslipidemia may be useful. The differential diagnosis of GA is broad, including sarcoidosis, necrobiosis lipoidica, tinea, nummular eczema, psoriasis, lupus, leprosy, etc.

【诊断及鉴别诊断】

可根据临床表现及病理活检进行诊断。对潜在的系统性疾病，如糖尿病、恶性肿瘤、甲状腺病、脂代谢紊乱等需要进行系统回顾、危险因素评估、体格检查、进一步的实验室及影像学检查。鉴别诊断需要考虑结节病、类脂质渐进性坏死、癣、钱币样湿疹、银屑病、狼疮、麻风等。

【Treatment】

GA tends to heal spontaneously. Localized GA is most commonly treated with topical high potency corticosteroids or intralesional corticosteroids. Generalized GA has been reported to respond to dapsone, isotretinoin, etretinate, hydroxychloroquine, niacinamide, hydroxyurea, narrow-band ultraviolet B therapy,

【治疗】

环状肉芽肿可以自愈。局限型环状肉芽肿通常可外用强效糖皮质激素或局部注射糖皮质激素治疗。据报道，氨苯砜、异维 A 酸、阿维 A 酯、羟氯喹、烟酰胺、羟基脲、窄谱 UVB 照射及 PUVA 照

psoralen and ultraviolet A therapy (PUVA). If systemic diseases are involved, they should be treated simultaneously.

射治疗对泛发型环状肉芽肿治疗有效。如果发现系统性疾病，应同时治疗。

Section Three Necrobiosis Lipoidica

第三节 类脂质渐进性坏死

Necrobiosis lipoidica (NL) is an inflammatory skin disorder characterized by irregularly shaped, firm, callous lesions with reddish brown pigmentation and atrophy in the centers of the lesions. It was named dermatitis atrophicans lipoidica diabetica by Oppenheim in 1929, and later renamed as necrobiosis lipoidica diabetica by Urbach in 1932.

类脂质渐进性坏死(necrobiosis lipoidica，NL)是一种炎症性皮肤病，特征性皮损为形状不规则、质硬、胼胝样损害，伴褐红色的色素沉着及中央性萎缩。Oppenheim 于 1929 年首先命名本病为糖尿病性类脂质萎缩性皮炎；1932 年，Urbach 再命名为糖尿病性类脂质渐进性坏死。

【Etiology and Pathogenesis】

Necrobiosis lipoidica was thought to be related to diabetes mellitus, and was initially regarded as one of the complications of diabetes mellitus. However, later studies showed that patients with necrobiosis lipoidica did not necessarily suffer from diabetes. A widely accepted theory of its origin is microangiopathy, a consequence of glycoprotein deposition in the vasculature that causes the thickening of blood vessels. Recently, hypoxia has been associated with its pathogenesis as well.

【病因及发病机制】

类脂质渐进性坏死与糖尿病有一定关系，最初有学者认为此病是糖尿病并发症之一，但后来发现某些有类脂质渐进性坏死的患者并没有糖尿病。目前主流理论认为该病涉及微血管病变，由糖蛋白在血管沉积导致血管壁增厚所致。近期研究表明局部低氧也是其发病原因之一。

【Clinical Manifestations】

Necrobiosis lipoidica most commonly appears in people at their 30s and 40s. Most of the patients are females. The lesions are confined to the anterior surfaces of the lower legs, but may also occur on the forearms, hands, feet, and trunk (Fig. 25-5). Three-quarters of cases present bilateral distribution at onset and most of the remaining cases become bilateral later. Lesions may be single but are more often multiple. A wide range of lesions over the body is generally rare. The typical lesion begins as a firm, dull-red papule or plaque, which rapidly enlarges to become a yellowish atrophic plaque with an erythematous edge. The surface is often smooth and telangiectasias become prominent. The disease is often asymptomatic. About 1/3 of the lesions will develop ulcerations over time.

【临床表现】

类脂质渐进性坏死好发于 30～50 岁，大部分为女性。损害主要位于小腿伸面，也多见于前臂、手、足以及躯干部(图 25-5)。3/4 的病例初起即为双侧对称的皮损，大部分病例会进展到双侧累及。皮损可为单个，但多发者更为常见，全身广泛累及者罕见。初起为坚硬、暗红色的丘疹或斑块，辐射状扩大，后形成浅黄色萎缩性斑块，边缘红色，表面光滑，并有明显毛细血管扩张，皮损常无症状，约 1/3 损害可发生溃疡。

【Histopathology】

Histopathological study shows a diffuse palisaded and interstitial granulomatous dermatitis, with "layered" tiers of granulomatous inflammation aligned parallel to the skin surface. The pathological changes involve the entire dermis and extend into the subcutaneous fat septae. The epidermis is normal or atrophic. There is a superficial and deep lymphocytes predominant infiltration with plasma cells and occasionally eosinophils. The

【组织病理】

病理示弥漫性栅栏状和间质肉芽肿性皮炎，肉芽肿浸润呈“层状”分布，与表皮平行排列，累及整个真皮并延伸至皮下脂肪组织间隔，表皮正常或萎缩，真皮浅、深层可见淋巴细胞为主的伴浆细胞及嗜酸性粒细胞的浸润，肉芽肿性炎症可见多核巨细胞，但无星状体(图 25-6)。

granulomatous inflammation includes multinucleated histiocytes but no asteroid bodies (Fig. 25-6).

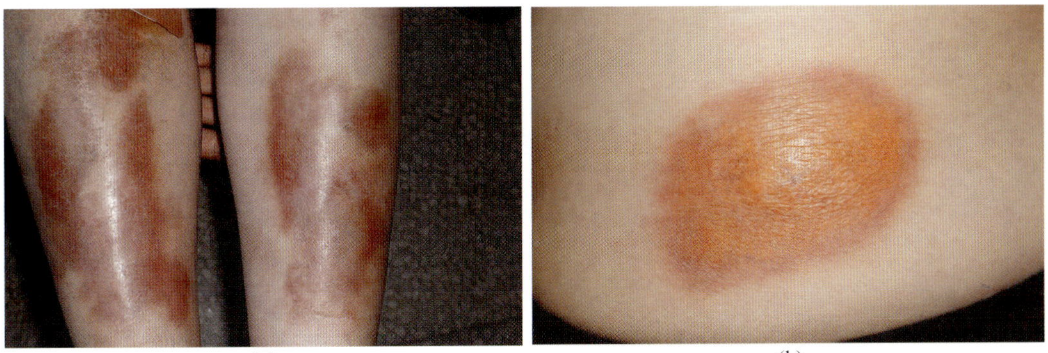

(a)　(b)

Fig. 25-5　Necrobiosis lipoidica(图 25-5　类脂质渐进性坏死)

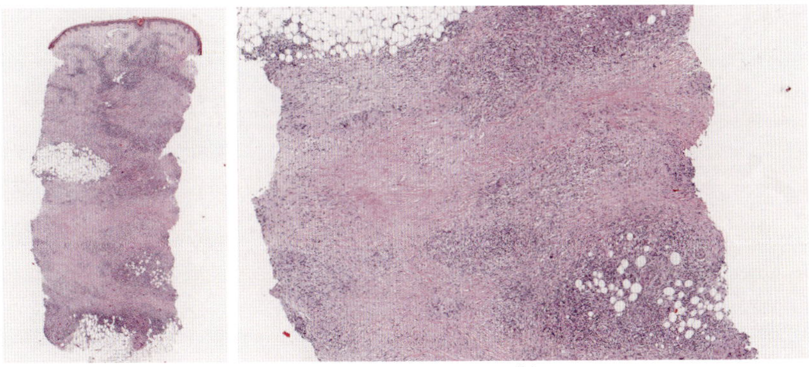

(a)　(b)

Fig. 25-6　Necrobiosis lipoidica-histopathology(图 25-6　类脂质渐进性坏死-组织病理)

【Diagnosis and Differential Diagnosis】

Given the typical clinical features with the histopathological changes, necrobiosis lipoidica can be diagnosed. Necrobiosis lipoidica should be differentiated from xanthomatosis, cutaneous amyloidosis, localized scleroderma and granuloma annulare.

【Treatment】

There are no evidence-based guidelines for the treatment of necrobiosis lipoidica. Topical or intralesional steroids alleviate inflammation but might promote further atrophy. Systemic corticosteroids may alleviate the disease, but they may elevate serum glucose. Other treatments such as cyclosporine, tacrolimus ointment 0.1%, etanercept, pentoxifylline, topical PUVA, infliximab, hydroxychloroquine, and thalidomide are reported to be effective.

【诊断及鉴别诊断】

根据典型的临床表现及组织病理学改变，即可诊断类脂质渐进性坏死。需要鉴别黄瘤病、皮肤淀粉样变、局限型硬皮病和环状肉芽肿。

【治疗】

类脂质渐进性坏死的治疗尚无循证医学证据。局部使用或皮损内注射激素可以减轻炎症，但可能加重萎缩。系统性使用糖皮质激素可以缓解病情，但可能会升高血糖。其余有效治疗包括环孢素、0.1%他克莫司软膏、依那西普、己酮可可碱、局部 PUVA 照射、英夫利昔单抗、羟氯喹、沙利度胺。

Yang WANG(汪旸)

Chapter Twenty-six　Neoplasms of the Skin

第二十六章　皮肤肿瘤

Section One　Epidermal Nevi

第一节　表皮痣

An epidermal nevus (plural: nevi) is a congenital, noncancerous (benign) skin disorder caused by an overgrowth of epidermal cells. Epidermal nevus is typically seen at birth or within the first year of life, but may appear occasionally throughout childhood or even adulthood. The incidence of epidermal nevi is estimated to be 1 in 1000 infants. The majority of epidermal nevi present sporadically, although familial cases have been reported. Males and females are equally affected.

表皮痣(epidermal nevus)是由于表皮细胞增生而引起的非肿瘤性的先天性皮肤疾病，通常出生时即有或在一岁以内出现，极少可以在童年或成年时发生。发生率约为新生儿的千分之一，男女比例相当，在人群中散在分布，但也有家系发病的报道。

【Clinical Manifestations】

Epidermal nevi most commonly present as skin-colored, brown, or grayish papules or raised, velvety patches or plaques. The lesions are soft and sharply demarcated. They may take a linear or atypical zosteriform shape aligning with skin Blaschko lines. As the affected individual ages, the nevus can become thicker and darker and develop a wart-like (verrucous) appearance (Fig. 26-1). The common affected areas are the truck, extremities, or neck. The majority of affected individuals have epidermal nevus only without other abnormalities, but neoplasms such as basal cell carcinoma and squamous cell carcinoma arising from epidermal nevus have been reported. Other systemic defects that may accompany epidermal nevus are in the brain, eyes, bones, central nerve system, cardiovascular system, and urinary system. In these cases, the condition is referred to as epidermal nevus syndrome, in which an epidermal nevus syndrome may be named differently according to the affected organs and systems.

【临床表现】

典型表现为线状排列或不规则长条形排列的皮肤色、黄褐色或浅灰色柔软的天鹅绒样的丘疹或斑片、斑块，边界锐利，有时表皮痣沿着 Blaschko 线分布。表皮痣通常随着年龄而发展，逐渐变厚，颜色变深，呈现疣状外观(图 26-1)。最常见的分布部位为躯干、四肢及颈部。大部分表皮痣患者仅有皮损而无其他异常，但也有伴发基底细胞癌和鳞状细胞癌的报道。有时表皮痣有合并系统受累的可能，包括脑、眼、骨骼、中枢神经系统、心血管系统、泌尿系统等。这时称之为表皮痣综合征，累及器官及系统的不同有多种不同表皮痣综合征的命名。

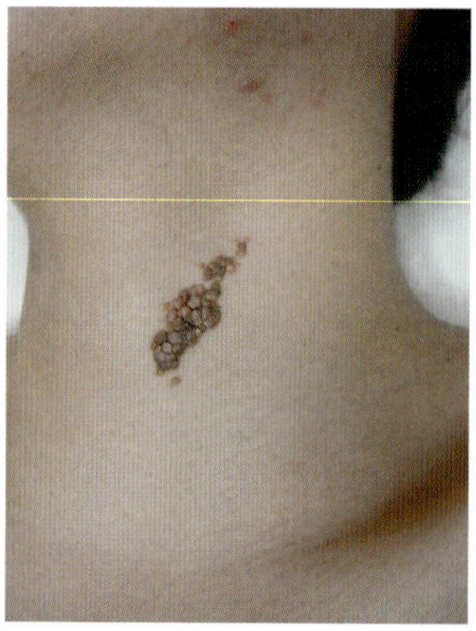

Fig. 26-1　Epidermal nevus(图 26-1　表皮痣)

【Histopathology】

Most epidermal nevi exhibit an epidermal proliferative process

【组织病理】

大部分表皮痣的病理改变局限于表

only; variable degrees of hyperkeratosis, focal parakeratosis, acanthosis, and papillomatosis are commonly seen. Other findings, including epidermolytic hyperkeratosis and focal acantholytic dyskeratosis may also be present. Inflammatory linear verrucous epidermal nevus may have clinical and histologic changes resembling psoriasis. When epidermal proliferation occurs at follicular and sebaceous areas, epidermal nevus is known as organoid nevus.

皮，表现为不同程度的角化过度伴有不同程度的角化不全、棘层肥厚和乳头瘤样增生，也可表现为表皮松解性角化过度或局灶性棘层松解性角化不良。炎性线状疣状表皮痣在临床及组织病理学特征上均与银屑病相似。少数表皮痣可见真皮毛囊及皮脂腺的增生，此时称为器官样痣。

【Treatment】

The treatment of choice for small epidermal nevi is surgical excision. Dermabrasion, electrofulguration, laser, and cryosurgery have each been used to treat epidermal nevi as well. However, superficial means of removal frequently result in recurrence. Aggressive approaches may be more successful, but can be complicated by hypertrophic scars or keloid formation. For example, dermabrasion, if superficial, is associated with a high rate of recurrence, and deep dermabrasion inevitably result in superficial scars. Cryosurgery has similar limitations, along with other disadvantages such as slow healing, swelling, infection, and, not uncommonly, abnormal coloration of the skin. Recent advances in laser technology have increased the reliability, precision, and safety of such treatments; however, recurrences and scar formation are still problematic. Corticosteroids applied under occlusion or by injection, as well as tretinoin ointment applied topically, may be partially effective in some cases. Oral retinoids may be beneficial for the treatment of widespread epidermal nevi, but may require life-long therapy.

【治疗】

小的表皮痣建议手术切除。磨削术、电灼术、激光或冷冻治疗都有报道。需要注意的是，浅表的去除术常易复发而切得太深会不可避免地留下增生性瘢痕或瘢痕疙瘩。比如，磨削太浅会复发而太深会引起浅表瘢痕；冷冻治疗伤口恢复缓慢、易局部肿胀、易引起感染、有愈合后引起皮肤颜色改变的可能；激光治疗具有简单易行、定位准确和安全的特点，但也有引起瘢痕和复发的可能。糖皮质激素局部封包或局部注射、局部外用维 A 酸类软膏可能部分有效。口服维 A 酸药物对于泛发性表皮痣有效，但需要终身治疗。

Wei SHI(施为), Jiang-lin ZHANG (张江林)

Section Two Seborrheic Keratosis

第二节 脂溢性角化病

Seborrheic keratosis (SK), also known as senile warts, is a benign skin mass that derives from keratinocytes. The frequency increases with age.

脂溢性角化病（seborrheic keratosis, SK）又称为老年疣（senile warts），是由于角质细胞过度增生所致的良性增生性皮肤病，随着年龄增长而多见。

【Etiology and Pathogenesis】

No specific etiologic factors have been identified in the pathogenesis of SK. As SK appear commonly on sun exposed areas such as the face, neck, dorsa of the hands, ultraviolet light may play a role. A familial tendency has also been noted in some cases.

【病因及发病机制】

确切病因不明，阳光暴露部位如面部、颈部、手背部等常见，紫外线可能是诱因之一。部分与遗传有关。

【Clinical Manifestations】

The age of onset is typically between 40-50 years. The color of the lesions varies from light tan to black, which may change even within a single lesion. The lesions are round or oval shaped, flat or slightly elevated, and become wart-like with a very rough surface or a velvety surface sometimes (Fig. 26-2). Seborrheic keratoses arise singly or in clusters (1-100) that range in size from very small to 3 cm in diameter, may or may not itch. Because in some cases the lesions are restricted to the top layers of the epidermis, SK often give a 'sticky' appearance. The inflamed lesions may become painful. Conditions associated with an abrupt 'flare' of lesions followed by a regression include pregnancy, coexisting inflammatory dermatoses (in particular erythroderma), and malignancy.

【临床表现】

发病年龄主要在40～50岁，皮损颜色可以为浅褐色至深褐色甚至黑色，甚至同一皮损颜色也会深浅不一。圆形或椭圆形，可以是扁平的或者轻度隆起的，疣状，表面粗糙或似天鹅绒样(图26-2)。大小不一，可以非常小也可以大至直径为3 cm，数量一个至数十个。部分皮损由于只有表皮上部受累，所以经常被描述为黏着性的外观。可有或无痒感，伴发感染时或有疼痛感。在有恶性肿瘤或者妊娠或炎症(如红皮病)时，皮疹可能会突然大批出现之后消退。

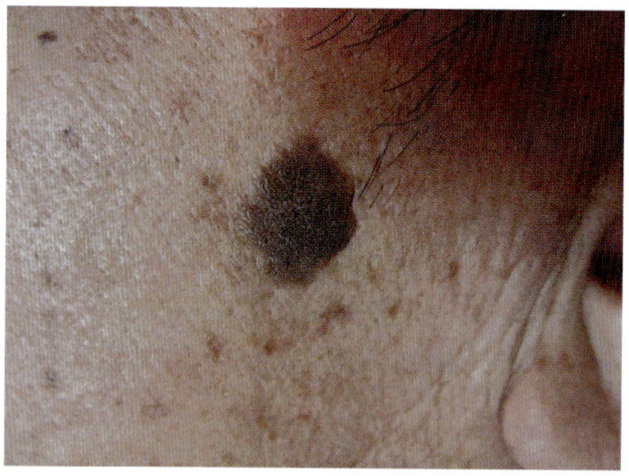

Fig. 26-2　Seborrheic keratosis(图 26-2　脂溢性角化病)

The variants of SK include stucco keratosis, dermatosis papulosa nigra and inverted follicular keratosis. Stucco keratosis typically involves the lower extremities, while dermatosis papulosa nigra is commonly seen in individuals with dark skin, presenting with multiple hyperpigmented papules on the face. Inverted follicular keratosis is typically an asymptomatic, firm, white-tan to pink colored papule on the face of older adults. Some malignant neoplasms may arise within or adjacent to SKs, such as basal cell carcinoma, squamous cell carcinoma, keratoacanthoma, and melanoma. A biopsy should be taken when malignancy is suspected. If SK increases in number and/or size abruptly, the Leser-Trélat sign should be considered. This is a paraneoplastic syndrome and is often associated with visceral neoplasms especially gastrointestinal adenocarcinomas, breast cancer, and lymphoid tissue neoplasms.

特殊类型的脂溢性角化病还包括：①灰泥角化病(stucco keratosis)：通常发生于双下肢。②黑色丘疹性皮病(dermatosis papulosa nigra)：通常发生于深色人种的面部，表现为数个黑色丘疹。③倒置性毛囊角化病(inverted follicular keratosis)：多见于老年人面部，无症状、浅褐色至粉红色的坚实丘疹。脂溢性角化病皮损内或周边可以出现恶性肿瘤，基底细胞癌、皮肤鳞癌、角化棘皮瘤、黑素瘤都有报道。临床疑似恶性肿瘤时必须活检。当脂溢性角化病皮损数目/体积迅速增加时要考虑Leser-Trélat征(Leser-Trélat sign)，这是一种皮肤副肿瘤综合征，常伴发内脏肿瘤特别是胃肠道腺癌、乳腺癌或淋巴瘤。

【Histopathology】

Certain degrees of hyperkeratosis, acanthosis and papillomatosis are easily revealed histologically. These epidermal excrescences tend to

【组织病理】

表现为不同程度的角化过度、棘层肥厚及乳头瘤样增生，不规则地向上、向

expand outward and upward irregularly and may form a 'church steeple' when combined with remnant cornified material on the top. The base of the SK is usually symmetric at the level of the adjacent epidermis. Horn pseudocysts, full of keratinized material due to epidermal invaginations, are highly characteristic. Nine distinct histological types-hyperkeratotic, acanthotic, reticulated (adenoid), clonal (nested), irritated, inflamed, desmoplastic, melanoacanthma, and plane-have been described.

外生长，有时与皮损顶部保留的角质物一起形成"塔尖样"外观。基底面一般与正常表皮平齐，反向的表皮凹陷形成的充满角质的假性角囊肿具有高度特征性。本病至少有九种组织类型，即角化过度型、棘层肥厚型、腺样型或网状型、克隆型或成巢型、刺激型、炎症型、结缔组织增生型、黑色素棘皮瘤型和扁平型。

【Diagnosis and Differential Diagnosis】

SK is easily diagnosed clinically. The differential diagnosis includes verruca vulgaris, solar lentigo, actinic keratosis, Bowen's disease, soft fibroma, melanocytic nevus, and melanoma, etc.

【诊断与鉴别诊断】

大多数脂溢性角化病易于诊断，需要鉴别的疾病包括寻常疣、日光性黑子、日光性角化病、鲍温病、软纤维瘤、黑色素细胞痣和黑素瘤等。

【Treatment】

No treatment is necessary for most cases. However, removal may be considered when SK enlarge suddenly or itch excessively or are easy to be irritated. Small lesions can be removed with electrocautery and larger lesions can be excised by shaving, excision, cryosurgery or CO_2 laser.

【治疗】

脂溢性角化病一般不需要治疗，如果伴有突然长大或者有过度瘙痒等症状或者皮损易受刺激可以考虑去除。小的皮损可以采用电灼，大的皮损可以采用削除术、手术切除术、冷冻或者 CO_2 激光。

Wei SHI(施为), Jiang-lin ZHANG (张江林)

Section Three　Actinic Keratosis

第三节　光化性角化病

Actinic keratosis (AK), also known as solar keratosis, is a precancerous disease. The cases are most common in individuals with light skin at ages of 30-40. The likelihood of AK increases with age.

光化性角化病(actinic keratosis, AK)又称日光性角化病(solar keratosis)。一般被认为是癌前病变，好发于浅肤色人种，一般出现于30～40岁，发病率随年龄增长而升高。

【Etiology and Pathogenesis】

Repeated and prolonged sun exposure is the main contributing factor for AK development.

【病因及发病机制】

反复慢性的日光照射是主要的发病原因。

【Clinical Manifestations】

AK presents clinically as persistent erythematous patches or plaques on sun exposed areas, which persist rather than fade away. The lesions start as erythema or papules of red, brown or ordinary skin color with a rough surface, or covered with white to yellow scales. Hyperkeratosis is common. Lesions become thicker as the condition progresses, with accompanying evidence of solar damage such as depigmentation, telangiectasia, and wrinkling. AKs range from a few millimeters to several centimeters that may coalesce when multiple lesions occur. Affected areas are commonly located on sun exposed parts, such as the face (Fig. 26-3), ear, dorsa of the

【临床表现】

光化性角化病通常表现为光暴露部位持续存在、不消退的红斑性斑片或斑块。早期可以是红色、棕色或皮肤色，表面粗糙，常有白色或者黄色鳞屑的红斑或丘疹。可有角化过度，后期损害表现为典型的肥厚。常伴有日光损伤的背景，如色素脱失、毛细血管扩张和皱纹，直径从数毫米至数厘米不等，多发时可以相互融合。常好发于曝光部位如面部(图26-3)、耳部、手背及前臂伸侧、头顶

hands, extensor side of the forearms, and scalp of bald individuals. However, any region of the body can be affected if enough actinic damage has accumulated at the site. Patients may feel an itchy, stinging, or burning pain.

脱发处。如果光损害足够严重，身体任何其他部位均可以发生。自觉症状包括瘙痒、刺痛、灼痛等。

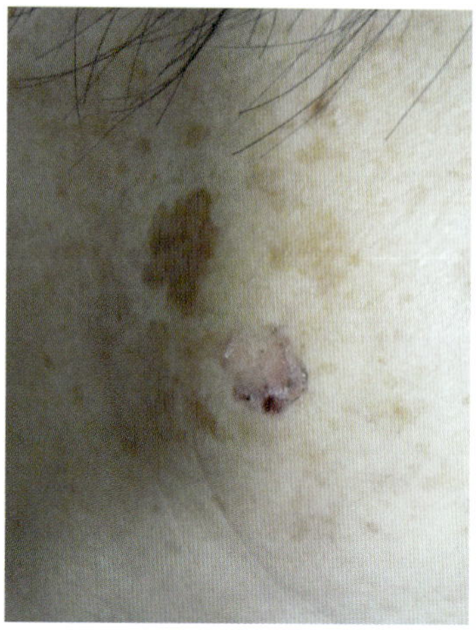

Fig. 26-3　Actinic keratosis(图 26-3　光化性角化病)

Clinical subtypes of AKs include hypertrophic (or hyperkeratotic), pigmented AK, lichenoid, atrophic, Bowenoid AK, AK with cutaneous horn and actinic cheilitis. Caution should be exercised in the event of sudden lesion enlargement, ulceration, bleeding, inflammation, or changes in pain sensation to rule out squamous cell carcinoma.

临床亚型包括：肥厚型(角化过度型)、色素沉着型、苔藓样型、萎缩型、鲍温样型、皮角和光化性唇炎。如果发现突然长大、溃疡、出血、伴发感染、皮损疼痛，需要警惕鳞状细胞癌的发生。

【Histopathology】

Histopathologically, AK is characterized by a focal, atypical keratinocytic proliferation at the epidermal layer. Acrosyringia and acrotrichia are often uninvolved by atypical keratinocytes but highly keratinized at the ostia of these structures, with adjacent parakeratosis, and a characteristic "checkerboard" pattern (often referred to the "flag" sign) may be seen due to alternation of hyper- and para-keratosis changes. Atypical keratinocytes at the basal layer may be clustered and disoriented during their outward maturation path, and may be trapped at the middle and upper parts of the epidermis. Therefore, these atypical keratinocytes are often found in partially-thickened epidermal areas, as opposed to full-thickness atypia occurring in squamous cell carcinoma *in situ*. The dermal changes usually include actinic elastosis.

【组织病理】

特征性的改变为局限性表皮不典型角质形成细胞增生，由于不典型的角质形成细胞常不累及汗管顶端及毛囊顶端，此处的开口处为角化过度，导致角化过度与角化不全交替出现的特征性模式，称为"棋子征"。不典型的角质细胞在基底层聚集，逐渐无序成熟至表皮中上层，常局限于肥厚的表皮处，与原位鳞状细胞癌的全层表皮侵犯不同。真皮层往往伴有日光性弹力纤维变性。

【Diagnosis and Differential Diagnosis】

The palpable hyperkeratotic lesion on sun-exposed regions is meaningful for diagnosis. Hyperkeratotic type AK may develop to cutaneous horns that require biopsy to exclude the possibility of squamous cell carcinoma (SCC). The distinction of AK from SCC can sometimes be difficult; most often a biopsy is warranted.

【诊断与鉴别诊断】

位于曝光部位的可触及的角化过度性皮损是临床诊断的线索。角化过度型光化性角化病可发展为皮角，应做病理切片排除潜在鳞状细胞癌(鳞癌)的可能。有时光化性角化病与鳞癌鉴别困

Further caution should be taken with lesions located on the ears and lips due to their relatively high risk for progression into SCC. Other differential diagnosis include DLE, seborrheic keratosis, lentigo maligna, etc.

难，需要病理检查确诊。警惕发生于唇部及耳廓的光化性角化病，因为其更加容易进展为鳞癌。需要鉴别的疾病还包括盘状红斑狼疮、脂溢性角化病、恶性雀斑样痣等。

【Treatment】

Early treatment is recommended for AK in order to avoid SCC development. Treatments include cryosurgery, electrocautery, shave excision, CO_2 laser, photodynamic therapy, and surgical excision, etc. Topical 5-fluorouracil (5-FU), or imiquimod cream can be used. Topical tretinoin may be useful for long-term management.

【治疗】

推荐早期治疗以防止进展为皮肤鳞癌。方法包括冷冻、电干燥术、削除术、CO_2 激光、光动力治疗或手术切除等。也可以外用 5-氟尿嘧啶或者咪喹莫特，长期局部外用维 A 酸也有效。

Wei SHI(施为), Xiang CHEN(陈翔)

Section Four Epidermal Cysts

Epidermal cyst, also known as epidermoid cyst, keratin cyst, infundibular cyst, or epidermal inclusion cyst, is the most common type of skin cyst. It is characterized by an intradermal or subcutaneous benign tumor that usually grows slowly.

第四节 表皮囊肿

表皮囊肿(epidermal cyst)也称为表皮样囊肿(epidermoid cyst)、角质囊肿、漏斗部囊肿、表皮包涵囊肿，是最常见的皮肤囊肿，是一种缓慢生长的真皮内或皮下良性肿瘤。

【Clinical Manifestations】

Epidermal cyst most often occurs on the face, neck, and trunk, but it can be found anywhere on the body. The epidermal cyst is a commonly fluctuant, tense swelling varying from a half to several centimeters in diameter. The surface of the overlying skin is usually smooth and shiny due to the fact that the skin has been stretched by the upward pressure (Fig. 26-4). Epidermal cysts derive from the follicular infundibulum, hence they are alternatively known as infundibular cysts. These nodules can be moved freely over the underlying tissue along with the surrounding normal skin. The expanded gland duct of the cyst tends to form an opening frequently at its central point, resembling a comedone. The pasty contents of the cysts are primarily a mixture composed of macerated keratin and a cheese-like, lipid material. The lesions can be primary, or may arise from previously disrupted follicular structures. Multiple epidermal cysts may occur in individuals with a significant history of acne vulgaris. Rupture of the cyst can result in an intensely painful inflammatory reaction.

【临床表现】

表皮囊肿常发生于面、颈和躯干，亦可见于任何部位。表皮囊肿通常呈现具有波动性的张力性肿胀区，直径从半厘米到几厘米。由于向上的压力，覆盖表面的皮肤光滑而有光泽(图 26-4)。表皮囊肿起源于毛囊漏斗部，因此又叫漏斗部囊肿，这些结节可移动，与下面的组织不粘连，其表面皮肤通常正常，延伸的腺体导管常开口于皮损中央，类似粉刺。囊肿的糊状内容物主要由浸软的角质和乳酪状脂性物质组成。囊肿可以是原发的，也可以起源于破坏的毛囊结构，多发性表皮囊肿可以见于具有明显寻常痤疮病史的个体。囊肿破裂可以导致炎症反应，伴有剧痛。

【Histopathology】

The cyst sits in the dermis, but the wall of the cyst is composed of a stratified squamous epithelium including granular layer and its cavity is filled with lamellar keratinous materials. A

【组织病理】

囊肿位于真皮内，囊壁由复层鳞状上皮细胞构成，含有颗粒层，囊腔内有层状角化物质。也可以见到囊肿周围的肉

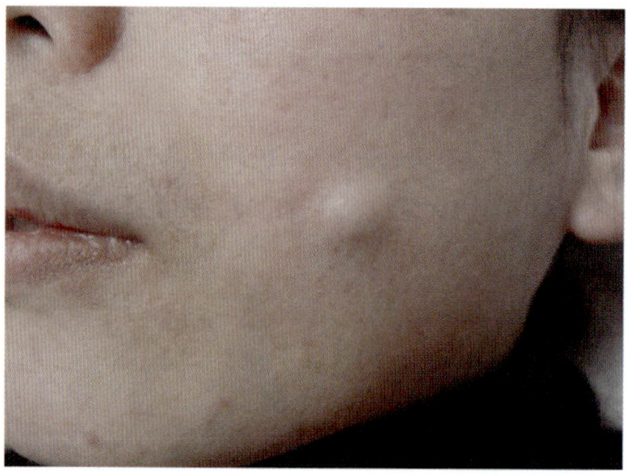

Fig. 26-4 Epidermal cyst(图 26-4 表皮囊肿)

granulomatous response may be seen sometimes around the cyst.

【Diagnosis and Differential Diagnosis】

The diagnosis of an epidermal cyst is based on the clinical features and histological changes. Epidermal cysts are differentiated from pilar cysts (trichilemmal cysts)primarily by their location and the keratinizing fashion of the contents in the cyst. In particular, pilar cysts appear most frequently on the scalp. The keratinization of the contents is trichilemmal in pilar cysts, but epidermoid in epidermal cysts. The epidermal cyst may also sometimes resemble lipoma, especially when it is difficult to demonstrate its freely movable feature. A differentiation from steatocystoma multiplex and neurofibroma may also be considered.

【Treatment】

Excision is curative. Removal may be accomplished by simple excision or extrusion of the cyst contents and wall through a surgical incision. Antibiotic therapy and intralesional triamcinolone may be helpful in resolution of any inflammation. Incision and drainage is the preferred course of action for an inflamed cyst lesion.

芽肿样反应。

【诊断与鉴别诊断】

根据临床特点和病理容易诊断。与毛发囊肿(毛鞘囊肿)的鉴别在于发病部位和囊内容物的角化方式,毛发囊肿最常发生于头皮,病理上其囊内容物表现为外毛根鞘式角化,而表皮囊肿为表皮样角化。脂肪瘤与表皮囊肿非常相似,有时囊肿的自由活动度难以确定,以致与脂肪瘤不易区别。此外,还需与多发性脂囊瘤及神经纤维瘤相鉴别。

【治疗】

手术切除可以治愈。可以单纯切除或者通过手术切口挤出囊内容物或者囊壁。发炎时可以切开引流或者皮损内注射曲安西龙加速炎症消退,有时需要抗生素治疗。

Wei SHI(施为),Jiang-lin ZHANG (张江林)

Section Five Bowen's Disease

Bowen's disease is an intraepidermal squamous cell carcinoma, also called squamous cell carcinoma *in situ* or SCC *in situ*, which may ultimately turn into invasive squamous cell carcinoma.

【Etiology and Pathogenesis】

Lesions occur primarily on sun-exposed surfaces, and are closely correlated to the degree of chronic sun damage on the skin. Lesions induced by chronic arsenicism may present in non-sun-

第五节 鲍 温 病

鲍温病(Bowen's disease)也称为原位鳞状细胞癌(squamous cell carcinoma *in situ*)或原位鳞癌(SCC *in situ*)。本病为表皮内鳞状细胞癌,最终可转变为侵袭性生长的鳞状细胞癌。

【病因及发病机制】

本病皮损主要见于日光暴露部位,并与慢性日光性损伤的程度直接相关。慢性砷中毒引起的鲍温病发生于接触化

exposed sites where the chemical has come in contact with the skin. Bowen's disease may also develop over the lesions of epidermodysplasia verruciformis that are caused by HPV infection.

学物质的非日光暴露部位。本病也可发生于由 HPV 感染引起的疣状表皮发育不良的基础上。

【Clinical Manifestations】

Bowen's disease can be found on any part of the body as an erythematous, slightly scaly, crusted, non-infiltrated patch or slightly elevated plaques. The lesions range from a few millimeters to several centimeters in diameter. The lesions are well demarcated with overlying scales; once removed, the exposed dull undersurface may be papillary and moist (Fig. 26-5). The lesions often arise *de novo* on sun-exposed skin of elderly individuals, or they may arise from a pre-existing AK. The head and neck are the most common sites, followed by the extremities and trunk. The lesions can be multifocal. Any mucosal membranes may be involved, such as the vulva, vagina, nasal mucosa, conjunctiva, and larynx.

【临床表现】

可发生于全身任何部位。表现为红色、轻度鳞屑和结痂、非浸润性的斑片或者轻度隆起的斑块，直径几毫米至几厘米，大小不等。边界清楚，鳞屑较明显，去除鳞屑后露出乳头状、潮湿的表面(图 26-5)。最常见于老年人的曝光部位，可以原发，也可以继发于光化性角化病。累及部位依次为头和颈部、四肢、躯干，可为群集性。可累及黏膜，女阴、阴道、鼻黏膜、眼结膜和喉是最常见的受累部位。

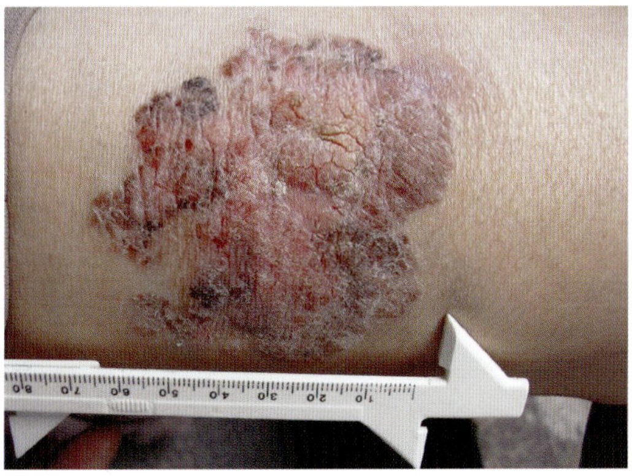

Fig. 26-5 Bowen's disease(图 26-5 鲍温病)

【Histopathology】

The epidermis shows hyperkeratosis, parakeratosis, acanthosis, and widening of the rete ridges. The cellular architecture of the epidermis is completely disorganized, and atypical cells are seen at all layers of the epidermis. These atypical cells have irregular hyperchromatic nuclei and conspicuous nucleoli. Mitoses are commonly seen. Pathologic mitoses and individually keratinizing cells can also be found. However, a sharp delineation between the dermis and epidermis exists, and the basement membrane is intact. The epidermis may become atrophic or hyperplastic. The neoplasm more commonly extends down the adnexa. The Pagetoid variant demonstrates large keratinocytes with abundant pale staining cytoplasm scattered throughout the epidermis, resembling melanoma *in situ* or Paget's disease.

【组织病理】

表皮显示角化过度、角化不全、棘层增厚和表皮突增宽。表皮细胞排列完全紊乱，表皮全层均可见不典型细胞，这些不典型细胞具有不规则、深染的核，核仁明显，核分裂常见，病理性核分裂及单个角化的细胞也可见到，但表皮与真皮的界限清楚，基膜完整。表皮可以萎缩也可以增生，肿瘤常向下延伸至附属器。如果表皮内出现散在分布、大的、苍白的、胞质丰富的角质细胞，类似于原位黑素瘤或者 Paget 病，称为 Paget 样鲍温病。

【Diagnosis and Differential Diagnosis】

The diagnosis of Bowen's disease can be based on the clinical lesions and the histopathology. Bowen's disease is frequently

【诊断与鉴别诊断】

主要根据临床皮损的特点和组织病理进行诊断。本病常易被误诊为钱币状

misdiagnosed as nummular eczema, psoriasis, seborrheic keratosis, superficial basal cell carcinoma, and actinic or arsenical keratoses. Paget's disease may also mimic Bowen's disease, not only clinically but also histopathologically. However, there is no dyskeratosis in Paget's disease, and the intervening nonvacuolated epidermal cells do not appear atypical in Paget's disease. Finally, mucin stains are positive in Paget's disease and negative in Bowen's disease. Bowenoid papulosis may be histopathologically confused with Bowen's disease; however, the presence of multiple lesions clinically and positive markers for HPV are usually helpful.

湿疹、银屑病、脂溢性角化病、浅表性基底细胞癌、日光性或砷角化病。Paget 病的临床表现和组织病理表现均可与鲍温病相似，但 Paget 病无角化不良，其间的非空泡变表皮细胞不是异形变细胞，Paget 病黏蛋白染色为阳性，而鲍温病为阴性。鲍温样丘疹病在组织病理学上与鲍温病相似，但其临床为多发损害及 HPV 标志阳性常对诊断有帮助。

【Treatment】

Simple elliptic excision of small lesions is the best treatment option. Alternatives such as curettage and fulguration, electrocautery, cryotherapy, laser ablation, 5-fluorouracil treatments, photodynamic therapy, and shave excision have all been used at times, with variable success.

【治疗】

手术切除是治疗小块皮损的最佳选择。刮除、电灼、电烙术、冷冻、激光、5-氟尿嘧啶、光动力疗法和削除术均有效。

Wei SHI(施为), Xiang CHEN(陈翔)

Section Six Squamous Cell Carcinoma

第六节 鳞状细胞癌

Squamous cell carcinoma (SCC) is also known as prickle cell carcinoma or epidermoid carcinoma. This carcinoma occurs not only on the skin but on the mucous membranes as well.

鳞状细胞癌(squamous cell carcinoma, SCC)(鳞癌)又名棘细胞癌、表皮样癌。不仅发生于皮肤，还可发生于黏膜。

【Etiology and Pathogenesis】

Ultraviolet light is definitely a major causative factor in light-complexioned individuals and in individuals with significant exposure to sunlight during childhood and adolescence. UVB has long been known to be of prime importance, but UVA is also thought to play a role today. Chronic trauma, scares, inflammation, radiation or chemical exposure have also been known to be pathogenic for developing SCC.

【病因及发病机制】

紫外线对浅肤色者以及在儿童和青少年时期受到强烈日晒者是肯定的致病因素。虽然长期以来认为最主要的致病因素是 UVB，但 UVA 同样也很重要。慢性创伤、瘢痕、炎症、放射和化学暴露均可致病。

【Clinical Manifestations】

The lesions typically occur as superficial, discrete, firm nodules with indurated, rounded and elevated bases. They are mostly dull red with telangiectasias on the surface. In other instances, the tumors may be in the form of small, erythematous, infiltrated, hard, scaly plaques at the beginning, turning into deep nodules or ulcers after a few months. Tumors grow either in an exophytic or endophytic (invasive) manner. In the early phases, tumors are localized, elevated, and freely movable over the underlying structures in the skin; but later they become diffuse, more or less

【临床表现】

本病表现为浅表性、散在性、质硬的损害，基底为圆的隆起性硬结。病损呈暗红色，有毛细血管扩张，或开始为小的红斑性、浸润性质硬的鳞屑性斑块，数个月内损害变大，成为深在性结节和溃疡。肿瘤可以呈现外生性或内生性(侵袭性)混合生长。早期肿瘤呈局限性隆起，基底可活动。继之逐渐扩大，出现程度不同的凹陷，且固定。晚期损害的表面呈

depressed, and fixed. The surface of the advanced lesions may be cauliflower-like, composed of densely packed, filamentous projections, inside of which are clefts filled with viscid, purulent, malodorous exudates(Fig. 26-6).

菜花状，质硬、团块状、纤细突出，裂隙间有恶臭脓性分泌物(图 26-6)。

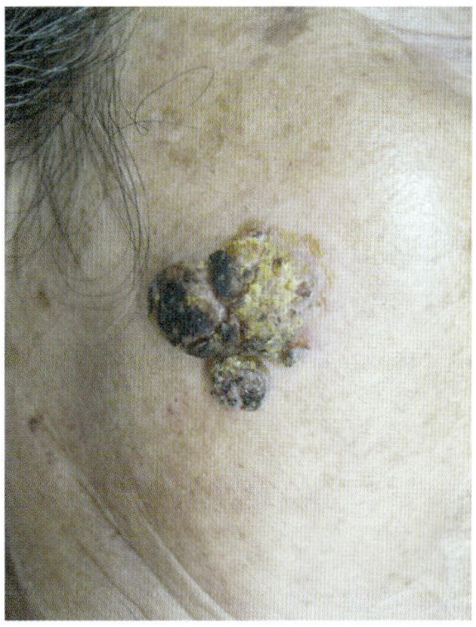

Fig. 26-6 Squamous cell carcinoma(图 26-6 鳞状细胞癌)

【Histopathology】

Invasive SCC is characterized by irregular nests of epidermal cells invading the dermis to a variety of depths. The grade of SCC is classified histologically by the degree of cell differentiation. Well-differentiated SCC generally presents as a downward proliferation of lobules and detached islands composed of glassy, brightly eosinophilic keratinocytes with variant degrees of pleomorphous nuclei and mitosis, sometimes accompanied by keratin pearls and apoptotic cells. The pink color of the cytoplasm arises from an abundance of high-molecular-weight keratin. Invasion is seen as detached tumor islands lying free within the dermis at varying levels. A polymorphous inflammatory infiltrate may be present. Poorly differentiated SCCs should be distinguished from spindle cell melanoma, atypical fibroxanthoma and leiomyosarcoma.

【组织病理】

侵袭性鳞癌的特征是不规则的表皮癌细胞巢侵入真皮中，深度不一，依据癌细胞分化程度进行分级。分化良好的鳞癌表现为小叶状或岛屿状向下增生，由呈玻璃状、强嗜酸性的角质形成细胞构成，可以出现不同程度的核异型性及有丝分裂，同时出现角珠和凋亡细胞，因为丰富的高分子量角蛋白而出现粉红色胞质。在真皮的不同深度可以见到孤立的肿瘤岛。可以伴有炎症细胞浸润。分化较差的鳞癌需要与梭形细胞黑素瘤、不典型黄瘤和平滑肌肉瘤相鉴别。

【Diagnosis and Differential Diagnosis】

The diagnosis of SCC depends on the clinical features of the lesions and histopathology. SCC may be difficult to distinguish from keratoacanthoma. The rapid growth and the presence of a rolled border with a keratotic central plug are typical indicators of keratoacanthoma. A keratoacanthoma typically has a volcano-like architecture and is comprised of well-differentiated keratinocytes with a brightly eosinophilic glassy cytoplasm surrounding a core filled with cornified material. An inflammatory infiltrate around the tumor includes lymphocytes, eosinophils and neutrophils. Other skin conditions that are commonly mistaken for SCC are inverted follicular keratosis, hypertrophic lichen planus, chronic stasis ulcers, and ulcerations developing from burns, some atypical

【诊断与鉴别诊断】

根据临床损害特征及组织病理改变进行诊断。鳞癌有时难以与角化棘皮瘤鉴别，生长迅速和中央有角质栓及卷状边缘明显提示角化棘皮瘤。典型的角化棘皮瘤有火山口样结构，肿瘤由分化良好、胞质呈明亮嗜酸性玻璃状的角质形成细胞组成，中央充满角化的物质，炎性浸润细胞为淋巴细胞、嗜酸性粒细胞及中性粒细胞。倒置性毛囊角化病、肥厚型扁平苔藓、慢性淤积性溃疡、烧伤性溃疡、某些非典型分枝杆菌感染、深部真菌感染常被误诊为鳞癌。可依据临床表现

mycobacterial or deep fungal infections. The clinical features may supply certain information for the differential diagnosis. However, the architectural pattern, recognition of the features of the different cells, and the presence of nuclear atypia are critical in establishing a diagnosis.

相鉴别，但结构模式、细胞识别和核异型性表现对于诊断具有决定意义。

【Treatment】

Tumors should be thoroughly removed because of the possibility of metastasis. Ideally, an excisional surgical specimen with margin control should be performed. The Mohs surgical technique (also known as chemosurgery) is a preferred choice because of its precise margin control. For metastatic or advanced cases, chemotherapy with cisplatin and doxorubicin or bleomycin is frequently used. Electrochemo-therapy and photodynamic therapy are two treatment alternatives currently under development. Radiation therapy is also effective in some cases.

【治疗】

鳞癌的治疗必须彻底切除肿瘤，因为有转移的可能性。理想的外科手术切除必须掌握好切除边缘，Mohs 外科手术(也称为化学外科)因其能准确确定边缘尤其适用。转移性鳞癌或晚期鳞癌常用顺铂、多柔比星或博来霉素等来进行化疗。电化学疗法、光动力疗法也是正在研究的替代治疗方法。放疗对部分患者有效。

Wei SHI(施为), Xiang CHEN(陈翔)

Section Seven Basal Cell Carcinoma

第七节 基底细胞癌

Basal cell carcinoma (BCC) is also known as basal cell epithelioma or basalioma.

基底细胞癌(basal cell carcinoma, BCC)又称为基底细胞上皮瘤(basal cell epithelioma)、基底细胞瘤。

【Etiology and Pathogenesis】

It appears that BCC arises from immature pluripotential cells. Gene mutations contribute to the pathogenesis and the malignant characteristics of BCC. Also, some undetermined factors from stromal cells are known to be important for tumor cell growth and spread, but the exact mechanism is yet to be defined.

【病因及发病机制】

本病起源于未成熟的多潜能细胞。基因突变与本病的发生和恶性特点有关。来源于基质细胞的一些未定因子对于基底细胞癌的生长和扩散也具有重要作用，但其确切机制尚不十分清楚。

【Clinical Manifestations】

BCC can be divided clinically into the following types.

(1) Nodular & ulcerative BCC: nodular & ulcerative BCC are also known as classic BCC. This often occurs as one or several small, waxy, semi translucent nodules formed around a central depression with telangiectasias. As the lesion enlarges, it may or may not be ulcerated, crusted, or even bleeding. The rolled border is characteristic for this type of BCC (Fig. 26-7). Lesions are most frequently found on the face and especially on the nose. Nodular BCCs may grow broadly and extend deeply, producing severe damage on eyelids, nose or ears.

(2) Superficial BCC: this type of BCC frequently presents as

【临床表现】

基底细胞癌临床上可以分为以下几种类型。

(1) 结节溃疡型基底细胞癌　结节溃疡型基底细胞癌也称为经典型基底细胞癌，表现为一个或几个小的具有蜡样光泽、半透明的结节，中央有凹陷，常伴有毛细血管扩张，随着皮损的增大可有溃疡、结痂和出血，也可没有上述表现，卷曲的边缘具有特征性(图 26-7)，皮损最常见于面部，尤其是鼻部。肿瘤体积较大且浸润较深时组织破坏和溃疡是主要表现，可以毁损眼睑、鼻或耳。

(2) 表浅型基底细胞癌　此型多发

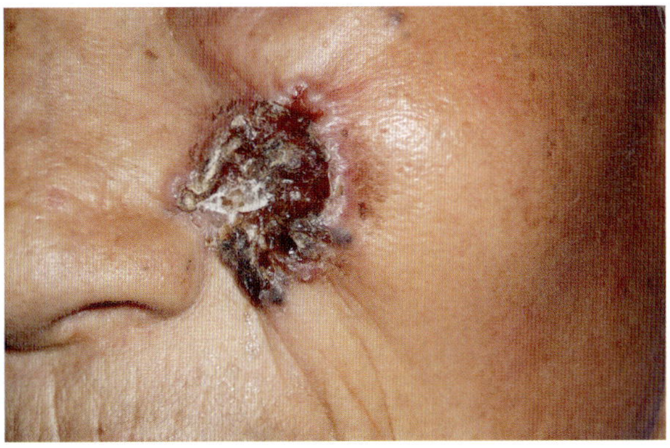

Fig. 26-7　Basal cell carcinoma(图 26-7　基底细胞癌)

one or several erythematous macules or thin plaques. The lesions are more often found on the trunk or limbs, but the head and neck may be affected as well. They are usually superficial and flat, remaining primarily in horizontal growth manner. The growth often exhibits little tendency to invade or ulcerate and enlarges only very slowly. However, the tumor has the potential to invade deeply to form induration, ulceration, and nodule.

(3) Morpheaform BCC: as the name suggests, this type of BCC demonstrates waxy white sclerotic plaques occurring predominantly on the scalp and neck, with the conspicuous absence of a rolled edge. Ulceration and crusting are also absent, whereas telangiectasia is prominent. The tumor presents as a flat, slightly atrophic lesion without well-demarcated border. It is often difficult to differentiate from a scar. The actual spread of the cancer is often significantly beyond the clinical boundaries of the tumor.

(4) Pigmented BCC: this variant of BCC shares all the features of the nodular type, and furthermore, brown or black pigmentation is present. This type of BCC usually evolves extremely slowly.

(5) Fibroepithelioma of Pinkus: the tumor is usually an elevated, skin-colored, sessile lesion on the lower trunk, or on the lumbosacral area, groin, or thigh. The lesion is superficial and sometimes resembles a fibroma.

【Histopathology】

Histopathologically, BCC can be divided into several subtypes such as nodulocystic, adenoid, keratotic, morpheaform, pigmented, superficial, infiltrative, micronodular, fibroepithelioma of Pinkus, etc. Some common features may be shared by the different subtypes of BCC: the tumor nests are composed of basophilic basaloid cells with large, relatively uniform nuclei and hyperchromatins, but scant cytoplasm. Cellular borders are indistinct and desmosomes are not apparent. Some of the tumor nests may connect with the overlying epidermis at the periphery of the cell mass; the columnar cells may

生于躯干或四肢，但头部及颈部也可受累。表现为一个或数个红色斑疹或者薄的斑块。常呈浅表性扁平生长，很少发生浸润和溃疡，生长非常缓慢。多为水平式生长，但也可向下侵袭形成硬结、溃疡和结节。

(3) 硬斑病样型基底细胞癌　此型为发生于头皮、颈部的有蜡样光泽的白色硬化性斑块，没有卷起的边缘，无结痂和溃疡，但有明显的毛细血管扩张，扁平，轻度萎缩，境界不清，常与瘢痕鉴别困难，癌的实际大小常比肿瘤临床表现的宽度大很多。

(4) 色素型基底细胞癌　此型具有结节型所有表现，不同的是有棕色或黑色色素沉着，肿瘤通常进展很慢。

(5) Pinkus 纤维上皮瘤型基底细胞癌　通常为肤色、高起、无蒂的损害，好发于躯干下部、腰骶部、腹股沟或大腿，损害为浅表性，类似于纤维瘤。

【组织病理】

组织病理上，基底细胞癌可分为结节囊肿型、腺样型、角化型、硬斑病样型、色素型、浅表型、浸润型、微结节型、Pinkus 纤维上皮瘤等。不同类型的基底细胞癌具有共同的特点：肿瘤团块由嗜碱性基底样细胞构成，有的与表皮相连，瘤细胞核大、相对一致、浓染、缺乏胞质，细胞边沿不清，桥粒不明显。在细胞团块的周围，柱状细胞特征性排列成栅栏状，有时

be characteristically arranged like a fence (so-called palisading arrangement) with mitoses sometimes appearing in a few cells. A variable degree of fibromyxoid stroma may present within the lesion that is intimately associated with the tumor islands, giving an impression of increased cellular contents. The artifact clefts surrounding the tumor nests as a result of tissue contraction are important indicators for the diagnosis.

可见到少数的有丝分裂现象。伴有数量不等的纤维黏液间质，纤维黏液间质与肿瘤岛紧密结合，表现为细胞结构增加。肿瘤细胞巢周边的人工收缩间隙是重要的诊断线索。

【Diagnosis and Differential Diagnosis】

The histopathology can confirm the diagnosis. It is necessary to distinguish between BCC and SCC. Also, Bowen's disease, Paget's disease, actinic and seborrheic keratosis may mimic BCC. Pigmented BCC is frequently misdiagnosed as melanoma or as a pigmented nevus. Finally, the morpheaform BCC is easily misdiagnosed as scar.

【诊断与鉴别诊断】

组织病理可以明确诊断。基底细胞癌需与鳞状细胞癌相鉴别。Bowen病、Paget病、日光性角化病和脂溢性角化病也可类似于基底细胞癌。色素型基底细胞癌常误诊为黑素瘤或色素痣。硬斑病型基底细胞癌易被误诊为瘢痕。

【Treatment】

As the most frequent site of BCC is on the face, the goal of treatment for BCC is not only a permanent cure but also cosmetic resolution. The treatment varies according to the type of lesion and its location since there is no ideal method of treatment that is effective for every individual. Common therapies include excision, Mohs' microsurgery, ionizing radiation, cryosurgery, curettage, and electrocautery.

【治疗】

因为大部分基底细胞癌位于面部，故治疗目的是永久治愈并获得最佳的美容效果。治疗方法依皮损的类型和发生部位而异，包括切除术、Mohs显微外科术、离子放疗、冷冻、刮除或电灼，没有单一的方法适合于所有损害，需视情况而定。

Wei SHI(施为)

Section Eight　Paget's Disease

Paget's disease is a chronic disease that is characterized by an eczematous rash on the breast or extramammary areas.

第八节　Paget病

Paget病(Paget's disease)是一种发生于乳房或乳房外，表现为湿疹样损害的慢性疾病。

【Etiology and Pathogenesis】

The pathogenesis is not known. Some genes and viral infections, and even genetic tendencies have been associated with this condition.

【病因及发病机制】

确切发病机制尚未明确，与某些基因、病毒感染及遗传倾向性有关。

【Clinical Manifestations】

(1) Mammary Paget's disease: the disease begins as an erythematous crusted or keratotic, circumscribed pruritic patch on the nipple and adjacent areas, and may be confused with eczema or unilateral eczematous neurodermatitis. After months or years, the lesion may evolve into an infiltrated, ulcerated plaque (Fig. 26-8). The disease is less common in males, but carries a worse prognosis in men than in women.

(2) Extramammary Paget's disease: the lesions of extramammary

【临床表现】

(1) 乳房Paget病(mammary Paget's disease)　开始为乳头及周围皮肤的局限性红斑性斑片，表面结痂或角化、瘙痒，类似湿疹或单侧湿疹样神经性皮炎。经数月至数年发生浸润和溃疡性斑块(图26-8)。男性患者少见，但较女性患者预后差　。

(2) 乳房外Paget病(extramammary

Paget's disease are similar to those of mammary Paget's disease. An intractable eczematous patch may persist in the anogenital or axillary region for several years. Pruritus is common, and sometimes pain may be present as well. Extramammary Paget's disease is frequently associated with an underlying adnexal adenocarcinoma or a regional internal carcinoma with or without metastasis. The most common affected site is the vulva (Fig. 26-9), followed (in decreasing frequency) by the perianal area, penis, scrotum, and groin.

Paget's disease）类似乳房 Paget 病的损害，表现为肛门生殖器或腋部难治性湿疹样斑片，皮损持续数年。瘙痒常见，有时可有疼痛。本病常合并皮下附属器腺癌，或局部内在性癌症，可有转移或没有转移。最常发生的部位是女阴(图26-9)，其次为肛周、阴茎、阴囊和腹股沟。

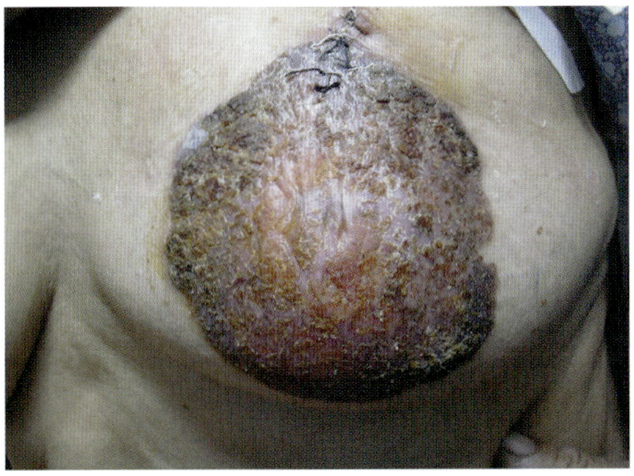

Fig. 26-8　Mammary Paget's disease
(图 26-8　乳房 Paget 病)

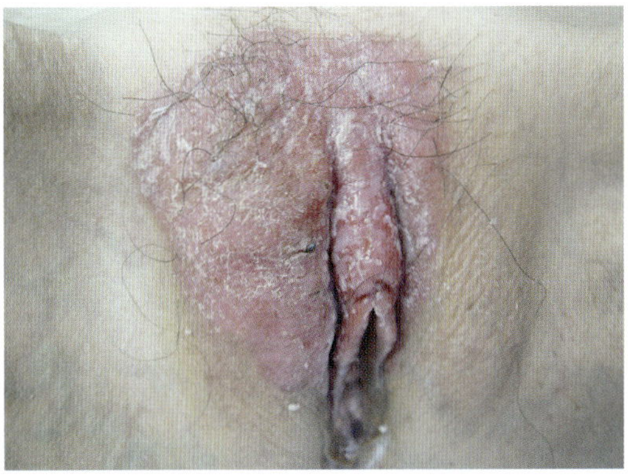

Fig. 26-9　Extramammary Paget's disease
(图 26-9　乳房外 Paget 病)

【Histopathology】

Paget's disease is characterized by the presence of Paget cells; these are large, round, clear-stained cells with large nuclei and absence of intercellular bridges. Furthermore, these Paget cells can be recognized by a positive Periodic Acid-Schiff (PAS) stain even after diastase treatment. A layer of basal cells that separates the Paget cells from the dermis is frequently shown, which is rarely seen in melanoma. An inflammatory reaction is often present in the dermis.

【组织病理】

本病有特征性的 Paget 细胞，为大而圆的淡染细胞，核大，无细胞间桥。Paget 细胞 PAS 染色阳性且耐淀粉酶。在 Paget 细胞与真皮之间常有一层基底细胞分隔，而黑素瘤则无。真皮内常有炎症反应。

【Diagnosis and Differential Diagnosis】

The presence of unilateral eczematous changes of the nipple recalcitrant to conventional treatment is indicative for Paget's disease, and then a biopsy and histological examination should confirm the diagnosis. Usually, the presence of bilateral lesions suggests atopic dermatitis or nummular eczema. Extramammary Paget's disease on the anal, perianal, and perineal areas should be differentiated from other premalignancies and malignancies, such as SCC, BCC, perianal Bowen's disease, and anorectal melanoma.

【诊断与鉴别诊断】

单侧乳头湿疹样损害一般治疗无效时提示此病，此时必须进行活检，确诊有赖于病理。双侧性皮损提示为特应性皮炎或钱币状湿疹。肛门、肛周和会阴区域的乳房外 Paget 病必须与其他的癌前病变和恶性病变区别，如鳞状细胞癌、基底细胞癌、肛周鲍温病和肛门直肠黑素瘤。

【Treatment】

Surgical excision and radiotherapy have been shown to be efficacious in treating Paget's disease. Mastectomy may be necessary in some cases of mammary Paget's disease.

【治疗】

外科切除和放疗对本病有效，乳房 Paget 病可行乳房次全切除术。

Wei SHI(施为)

Section Nine　Sebaceous Nevus

Sebaceous nevus, which is located predominantly on the head and face, is a congenital benign organoid nevus.

【Etiology and Pathogenesis】

The etiology is still unclear, but a tumor suppressor gene (PTCH) deletion has been associated with these skin lesions in some cases.

【Clinical Manifestations】

Nearly all sebaceous nevi present at birth or in early childhood. They occur most commonly on the scalp, forehead and post-auricular area. The lesion is usually a solitary, oval or band-like, yellowish to skin-colored waxy plaque, that is otherwise asymptomatic.

The skin lesion changes clinically and histologically as the patient ages. In childhood, the skin lesion is velvety, pink to tan, hairless and remains the same size without symptoms. In adolescence, the plaque becomes thicker and more verrucous on the surface (Fig. 26-10).

In adults, about 20% of patients may develop benign or malignant tumors, which typically show new nodules or masses growing on the non-progressing sebaceous nevus.

第九节　皮脂腺痣

皮脂腺痣(sebaceous nevus)是一种主要发生于头面部的先天性的良性器官样痣。

【病因及发病机制】

病因不明。已发现部分病例的皮损内有肿瘤抑制基因 PTCH 的缺失。

【临床表现】

几乎所有的皮脂腺痣均发生于新生儿期或者幼儿期,好发部位为头皮、前额及耳后,常为单发的椭圆形或带状蜡样光泽的斑块,黄色或肤色,无症状。

随着年龄增长,皮损形态及组织结构均发生改变。在儿童期,斑块几乎不长大,表面柔软、无毛发,粉色至黄褐色,无自觉不适,至青春期,皮损逐渐增厚呈疣状(图 26-10)。

成年后,约 20%的患者在本病的基础上发生良性或恶性的皮肤肿瘤,表现为在先前稳定的皮脂腺痣皮损上又出现新的结节或肿块。

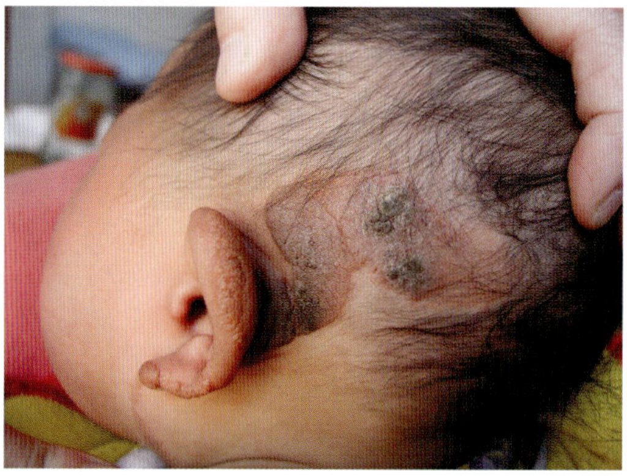

Fig. 26-10　Sebaceous nevus(图 26-10　皮脂腺痣)

【Histopathology】

The epidermis shows verrucous or papillomatous hyperplasia, in which the hair follicles and sebaceous glands are abundant, ranging in their development from immature to mature states in the dermis. Ectopic apocrine glands are commonly observed in the deep dermis beneath sebaceous glands in some adult cases.

【Diagnosis and Differential Diagnosis】

Clinical diagnosis is usually straightforward. The lesion

【组织病理】

表皮呈疣状增生或乳头状瘤样增生,真皮内见不同发育阶段的毛囊、大量不同成熟程度的增生的皮脂腺,部分成人病例在真皮深部皮脂腺下方可见异位的顶泌汗腺。

【诊断与鉴别诊断】

发生于头面部的单发的黄色斑块,

presents at birth and is always located on the scalp or the face as a single yellowish plaque without symptoms. Sebaceous nevus should be distinguished from juvenile xanthogranuloma, linear epidermal nevus (verrucous nevus), and aplasia cutis or syringocystadenoma papilliferum, etc.

无自觉症状，出生即有，临床上易诊断。皮脂腺痣通常需要与幼年性黄色肉芽肿、线状表皮痣(疣状痣)、皮肤再生不良和乳头状汗管囊腺瘤等相鉴别。

【Treatment】

Since malignant transformation may occur in some cases, the tumor should be removed early by excision.

【治疗】

一般建议早期手术切除皮损以防癌变。

Lin WANG (王琳)

Section Ten　Syringoma

第十节　汗　管　瘤

Syringoma is a benign skin adnexal tumor with ductal (syringeal) differentiation. It usually occurs on the periorbital area, especially on the eyelids of young females.

汗管瘤(syringoma)是向汗腺导管分化的良性皮肤附属器肿瘤，好发于青年女性眼眶周围，特别是眼睑。

【Etiology and Pathogenesis】

The etiology is still unclear. As some patients have a positive family history, it may have an autosomal dominant inheritance.

【病因及发病机制】

病因不明。部分患者有家族史，为常染色体显性遗传。

【Clinical Manifestations】

Syringoma appears mostly in young females. The skin lesions can occur on any part of the body, but the periorbital area, especially the eyelids, is the most common affected site. The forehead, cheek, neck, chest, abdomen and genital skin could also be involved. The papules tend to be in a group but do not coalesce with the size ranging from a sesame seed to a grain of rice, which are skin-colored, firm and hemispheric or flat (Fig. 26-11). Most patients are asymptomatic but may itch when the papules are on the external female genitalia.

【临床表现】

本病好发于青年女性，皮损可发生于身体的任何部位，但最多见于眼眶周围，特别是双侧眼睑，额部、面颊、颈胸部、腹部和外生殖器也较常见。皮损成群多发，为芝麻至米粒大小、肤色、坚实的半球形或扁平丘疹，密集而不融合(图26-11)。常无自觉症状，但发生于女性外阴可出现明显瘙痒。

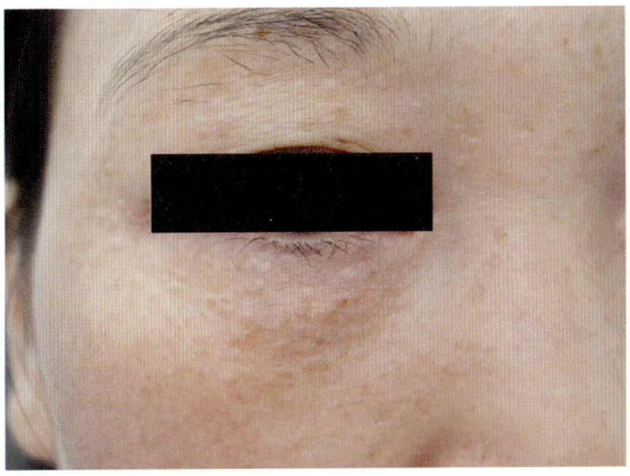

Fig. 26-11　Syringoma(图 26-11　汗管瘤)

【Histopathology】

The tumors are circumscribed and located in the superficial

【组织病理】

肿瘤位于真皮浅层，境界清楚，由胞

dermis. The epithelial tumor is composed of cells with pale or pinkish cytoplasm forming tubules and nests, which could be adenoid, cystic, comma or tadpole-shaped. Some of the tubules are filled with eosinophilic materials.

质淡染或粉红的上皮细胞组成管状或巢状结构,可呈腺样、囊样、逗号样或蝌蚪样,其腔内可有嗜酸性物质。

【Diagnosis and Differential Diagnosis】

The diagnosis of syringoma is straightforward if the tumors are on the eyelids, but it is not easy to make the diagnosis when they are located on the forehead, cheeks, trunk and external genitalia, and the condition should then be differentiated from verruca plana, multiple trichoepithelioma, milia, Fox-Fordyce disease, etc.

【诊断与鉴别诊断】

发生于眼睑的皮损颇具特征,易于诊断。但发生于额部、面颊、躯干、外阴的汗管瘤需要与扁平疣、多发型毛发上皮瘤、粟丘疹、大汗腺痒疹等疾病鉴别。

【Treatment】

No treatment is needed in general. The tumors may be treated with careful application of trichloroacetic acid, carbon dioxide laser, cryotherapy, electrocautery or fractional laser.

【治疗】

一般无需治疗。必要时可行三氯醋酸、二氧化碳激光、液氮冷冻、电灼、点阵激光等治疗。

Lin WANG (王琳)

Section Eleven　Dermatofibroma

第十一节　皮肤纤维瘤

Dermatofibroma is synonymous with fibrous histiocytomas, sclerosing hemangiomas, histiocytomas and nodular subepidermal fibrosis.

皮肤纤维瘤(dermatofibroma),又名纤维组织细胞瘤、硬化性血管瘤、组织细胞瘤、结节性表皮下纤维化等。

【Etiology and Pathogenesis】

The etiology is unknown. In some cases, onset has been linked to mild skin injuries such as insect bites.

【病因及发病机制】

病因不明,部分病例与皮肤微小损伤(如昆虫叮咬等)有关。

【Clinical Manifestations】

Dermatofibromas are encountered mostly in adults and tend to occur more commonly in females. The most commonly affected sites are the extremities and trunk. The tumor is usually a round or oval solid papule or nodule about 1 cm in diameter, typically reddish brown to yellowish-brown or dark brown in color and without subjective symptoms (Fig. 26-12). The lesion tends to adhere to the overlying skin, but not to the underlying subcutaneous fat, and is therefore mobile. The lesion usually grows slowly and persists for life and may present as a single tumor in most cases. Multiple dermatofibromas or even hundreds of lesions may be found occasionally.

【临床表现】

本病好发于成年人,女性较多见,好发部位为四肢和躯干。皮损为圆形或卵圆形坚实丘疹、结节,直径约 1 cm,棕红、黄褐、黑褐色(图 26-12),其上方与表皮粘连、下方与皮下脂肪组织不相连,可推动,一般无自觉症状。皮损生长缓慢,无自发消退倾向,常为单个,偶可多个,甚至达数百个。

【Histopathology】

The tumor is usually found without a clear boundary within the dermis. The major components of the proliferation are made up of fibrocytes, fibroblasts and variable collagen fibers; however other

【组织病理】

肿瘤位于真皮内,边界不清,由纤维细胞、纤维母细胞和多少不等的胶原纤维组成。部分病例肿瘤内含脂质和含铁

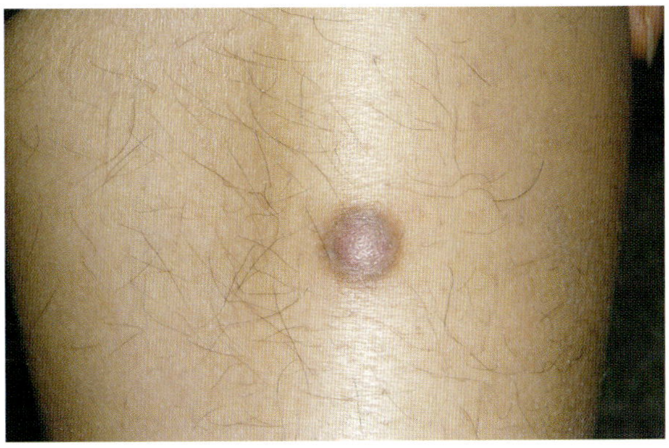

Fig. 26-12　Dermatofibroma(图 26-12　皮肤纤维瘤)

components such as lipids and hemosiderin can sometimes be observed. Hyperplasia of the overlying epidermis and hyperpigmentation of the basal cell layer are commonly seen as well, providing important clues for the diagnosis of dermatofibroma.

血黄素。肿瘤上方的表皮明显增生、基底层色素增加，此点对于诊断有重要意义。

【Diagnosis and Differential Diagnosis】

The clinical appearances of the lesion are distinctive and a diagnosis of dermatofibroma is not difficult, especially when histopathological evidence is taken into account. The disease should be distinguished clinically from nevocytic nevus, seborrheic keratosis, pigmented basal cell carcinoma and malignant melanoma, while histopathologically, keloid, tuberous xanthoma, fibrosarcoma and dermatofibrosarcoma protuberans may be confused with dermatofibroma.

【诊断与鉴别诊断】

根据皮肤纤维瘤的临床和病理特点容易诊断。临床上需要与痣细胞痣、脂溢性角化病、色素性基底细胞癌、恶性黑素瘤等相鉴别，组织病理上需要与瘢痕疙瘩、结节性黄瘤、纤维肉瘤、隆突性皮肤纤维肉瘤等相鉴别。

【Treatment】

The tumors usually do not require treatment. Surgical excision may be performed when necessary.

【治疗】

一般无需治疗，必要时行手术切除。

Lin WANG (王琳)

Section Twelve　Keloid

第十二节　瘢痕疙瘩

Keloid is an excessive response by the connective tissue to skin destruction or even to a very mild injury. It is a benign cutaneous tumor.

瘢痕疙瘩(keloid)为皮肤损伤(即便是轻微损伤)后，结缔组织过度增生而引起的良性皮肤肿瘤。

【Etiology and Pathogenesis】

Genetic predisposition has been noted in some cases. Other causative factors may be hormonal or immunological changes, even though it has not yet been shown how these factors affect the cellular signals that control the growth and proliferation of connective tissue.

【病因及发病机制】

瘢痕疙瘩的患者具有遗传易感性，此外，激素、免疫学因素等也参与发病，虽然这些因素是如何影响和控制结缔组织生长和增生的信号还不清楚。

【Clinical Manifestations】

The condition is more prevalent in young people under age 30, and is equally common in both sexes. The keloid usually arises as a result of mild injury, such as folliculitis, scratching, ear-piercing, tattooing or burning. Keloid can appear anywhere on the body, but most commonly on the chest, shoulders and back, less often on the neck, ear lobes and extremities, and only rarely on the face, palms or soles.

The skin lesions may be solitary or multiple. In the early stage, the lesion is a red firm small papule or nodule, rubbery in consistency with telangiectasia on the surface. After several months or years, the lesion will extend beyond the area of the original injury and then appears as claw-like extensions of the original lesion, and the surface gradually becomes smooth (Fig. 26-13). The patient may feel an itchy, twinge or tenderness during this period. Once the lesion reaches a stationary phase, it will look dull red and the symptoms will disappear.

【临床表现】

瘢痕疙瘩主要发生于30岁以下的人，男女发病率相似。轻微的皮肤损伤，如毛囊炎、皮肤抓破、穿耳、文身或灼伤后均可发病。可发生于皮肤任何部位，好发于胸前区、肩背部，亦常见于颈部、耳垂和四肢，很少发生于面部及掌跖部位。

皮损可单发或多发。初起皮损为小而坚实的红色丘疹、结节，呈橡皮样硬度，表面可有毛细血管扩张，持续数月至数年后，皮损超出原有的损伤范围，呈蟹足状向外伸展，皮损表面逐渐光滑(图26-13)，皮损有刺痒、刺痛、触痛。静止期皮损呈暗红色，自觉症状消失。

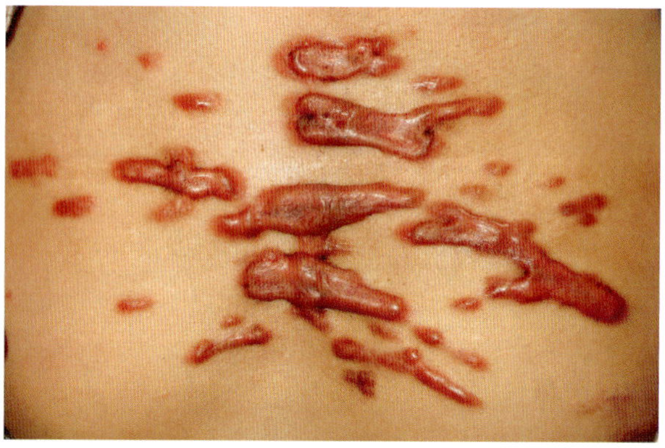

Fig. 26-13　Keloid(图 26-13　瘢痕疙瘩)

【Histopathology】

The tumor is located in the dermis and has an obscure boundary characterized by broad bundles of hyperplastic collagenous fibers which are thicker than normal, enlarged, homogeneous and brightly eosinophilic, in which some fibroblasts and a large number of mucopolysaccharides can be found. The superficial collagen bundles lie parallel to the epidermis, but the deeper ones are interlaced in all directions.

【组织病理】

肿瘤位于真皮内，边界不清，主要为增生、粗大、均质化、强嗜酸性的胶原纤维束构成，浅层胶原束与表皮平行排列，其下方胶原束则互相交织、排列紊乱，肿瘤内可有多少不等的增生的成纤维细胞、丰富的黏多糖。

【Diagnosis and Differential Diagnosis】

The diagnosis is based on the characteristic clinical features: the lesion follows a skin injury and appears commonly on the chest and back; as a smooth, bright red or dull red hard nodule or plaque with itching or pain.

Clinically, keloid should be distinguished from hypertrophic scars. The hypertrophic scar is often located at the flexor aspects of

【诊断与鉴别诊断】

根据临床特点，如皮损继发于皮肤损伤、好发于胸背部、呈红色或暗红色的质硬的表面光滑的结节或斑块，可伴有痒痛感，易于诊断。

临床上应该与增生性瘢痕鉴别，后者好发于关节屈侧和腹部，一般在原损

the joints and the abdomen. It arises as a red plaque on a previous injury, does not extend beyond the original wound, lacks the characteristic claw-like extensions and tends to flatten spontaneously several years later. Histopathologically, it should be distinguished from dermatofibroma, dermatofibrosarcoma protuberans and morphea-like basal cell carcinoma.

伤处长出红色斑块，不超过原有的损伤范围，无蟹足状生长，经数年后明显变平。组织病理学上应该与皮肤纤维瘤、隆突性皮肤纤维肉瘤、硬斑病样基底细胞癌等相鉴别。

【Treatment】

Treatment of keloid is a challenge since aggravation and recurrence are both quite common. The most effective treatment is intralesional injections of glucocorticoids, which should be repeated at intervals of 2-4 weeks. The lesion may flatten and the itching may cease, but there is usually a recurrence as soon as the injections stop. Surgical excision may be a good alternative when combined with intralesional glucocorticoid injections or radiation to reduce the risk of recurrence after the operation. Glucocorticoid creams or retinoic acid creams applied topically may also help relieve the symptoms.

【治疗】

该病治疗困难，因为常于治疗后加重和复发。糖皮质激素皮损内注射可获得较好的疗效，可每 2～4 周注射一次，皮损可逐渐变平，瘙痒症状减轻，但停药后有可能复发。亦可手术切除配合糖皮质激素皮损内注射或放射治疗，可减少复发。外用糖皮质激素霜、维 A 酸霜亦可缓解症状。

Lin WANG（王琳）

Section Thirteen　Congenital Vascular Malformations and Hemangiomas

Congenital vascular malformations and hemangiomas are a group of benign vascular dermatoses which are caused by angiopoiesis malformation or vascular dilation in the fetus. They frequently appear in infants or in early childhood. Congenital vascular malformations mainly include nevus flammeus and cavernous hemangioma, and most congenital hemangiomas are capillary hemangioma.

【Clinical Manifestations】

(1) Nevus flammeus: also known as port-wine nevus or nevus telangiectaticus, is a common congenital capillary malformation of the skin. It presents at birth or shortly after birth. The lesions are usually located on the scalp, face and neck, although they may appear anywhere on the skin and occasionally are spread over as much as half the body. The lesions are usually unilateral and may be single or multiple dark-red or bright-red patches with irregular borders (Fig. 26-14), and they will blanch under pressure. The lesion may spread gradually as the child grows, then cease its growth once the child reaches adulthood, but only rarely will it

第十三节　先天性血管畸形和血管瘤

先天性血管畸形（congenital vascular malformations）和血管瘤（hemangiomas）是在胎儿期血管形成组织畸形或原有血管扩张所致的一组良性的血管皮肤病，多发生于婴儿或儿童。先天性血管畸形主要包括鲜红斑痣和海绵状血管瘤，先天性血管瘤主要为毛细血管瘤。

【临床表现】

（1）鲜红斑痣（nevus flammeus）

鲜红斑痣又称为葡萄酒样痣（port-wine nevus）、毛细血管扩张痣，为常见的皮肤先天性毛细血管畸形，出生时即有或出生后不久发生，好发于头皮、面部和颈部，也可发生于身体其他部位，通常单侧发病，偶可非常广泛，累及半侧身体。皮损表现为一个或数个暗红色或鲜红色斑片，不高出皮面，边界不整齐（图 26-14），压之易褪色。可随人体发育而逐渐扩

spontaneously resolve. Vascular nodules or plaques may form as outgrowths on the primary lesions in some cases.

(2) Capillary hemangioma: it is also known as strawberry hemangioma, hemangioma simplex or infantile hemangioma, usually presents at birth or 3-4 weeks after birth. The lesions appear as single or multiple tumors that are commonly located on the head and neck, although they can be found anywhere on the body. The typical lesions are soft nodules or lobular plaques with smooth surfaces and sharp borders. They are bright red or dull red, and easily compressed (Fig. 26-15).

展,成年后停止生长,但极少消退。部分病例可在原有红斑上形成结节、斑块。

(2) 毛细血管瘤(capillary hemangioma) 毛细血管瘤又称为草莓状血管瘤(strawberry hemangioma)、单纯性血管瘤、婴儿血管瘤,出生时或出生后 3~4 周内发生,好发于头颈部,也可发生在身体的任何部位,单发或多发,表现为鲜红、暗红色结节或分叶状肿瘤,边缘清楚、表面光滑、质软、压之容易缩小(图 26-15)。

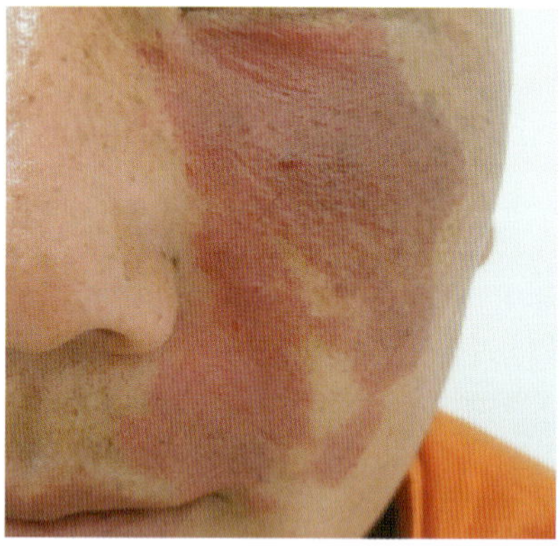

Fig. 26-14 Nevus flammeus
(图 26-14 鲜红斑痣)

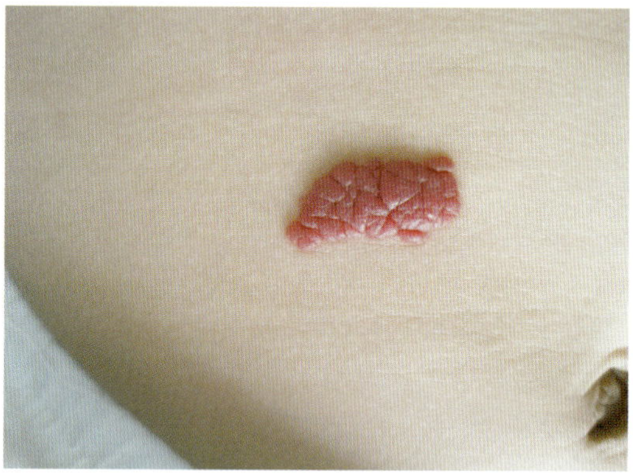

Fig. 26-15 Capillary hemangioma
(图 26-15 毛细血管瘤)

Capillary hemangioma grows fast in the first year of life, and slows down gradually thereafter. Approximately 70% of patients with this type of hemangioma can undergo spontaneous remission by age seven, but in some cases cavernous hemangioma may be concurrently found below the capillary hemangioma.

(3) Cavernous hemangioma: it is also known as venous malformation. The age of onset and the predilection sites are similar to those for strawberry hemangioma, but cavernous hemangioma will present as single or multiple subcutaneous masses. The tumors are often light-violet or blue, or even skin-colored if the tumor is deep-seated. The leisions may be elevated nodules or lobular masses with vague borders. These are soft and flexible, and can be shrunk when pressed, as with a sponge (Fig. 26-16).

Cavernous hemangioma tends to grow continuously until adult life, and may compress the internal organs when deep-seated structures are involved. However, in most cases such patients are asymptomatic, these hemangiomas might only be discovered during surgery or autopsy. A few cases involving internal hemorrhage have been reported. Ulcerations followed by infections also occur occasionally. This type of hemangioma has no tendency towards spontaneous regression.

毛细血管瘤在一岁以内生长较快,以后生长速度逐渐变慢,约 70%患儿的血管瘤在 7 岁以前自然消退。部分病例在其下方合并海绵状血管瘤。

(3) 海绵状血管瘤(cavernous hemangioma) 又称为静脉畸形,其发病年龄、好发部位等与草莓状血管瘤相似,表现为单个或数个淡紫色或蓝色皮下肿块,若发生部位较深,则肿瘤表面为正常皮肤颜色。可高出皮面,呈结节状、分叶状,边界不甚清楚,柔软而有弹性,压之可缩小,似海绵(图 26-16)。

海绵状血管瘤直至成年仍存在不断增大的倾向,影响或压迫其下面的重要器官。侵犯内脏者,一般无自觉症状,偶在尸检或外科手术中发现,间或有内出血的报告。海绵状血管瘤也可发生破溃继发感染,无自然消退倾向。

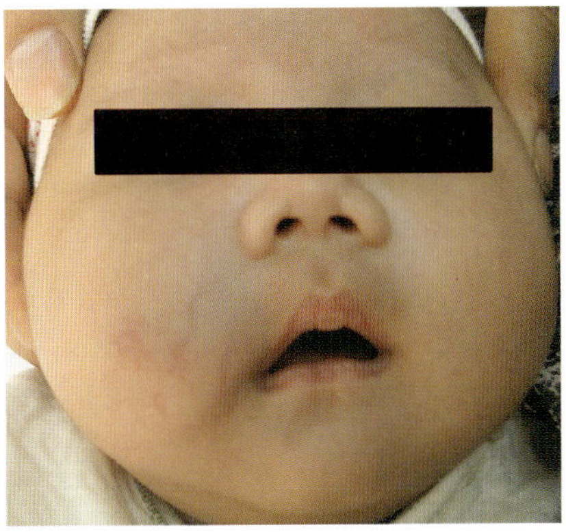

Fig. 26-16　Cavernous hemangioma(图 26-16　海绵状血管瘤)

A severe sub-type of cavernous hemangioma, the so called Kasabach-Merritt syndrome, is accompanied by thrombocytopenia and purpura. It frequently appears in infants.

Whenever two or three of the types of vascular malformation or hemangioma described above is found in one tumor mass, it is termed a mixed hemangioma.

【Histopathology】

(1) Nevus flammeus: there are dilated capillaries with variable sizes of lumina and full of erythrocytes in the superficial dermis.

(2) Capillary hemangioma: the tumor has a typical lobular architecture in the dermis, and the histopathological features vary with the lesion's evolution. In the growth phase, there is considerable proliferation of capillary endothelial cells, with only a few capillary lumina, and the endothelial cells are usually large, with mitoses common among them. However, these endothelial cells become more flat and the capillary lumina become wider as the condition proceeds into the maturation phase. Finally, in the involution phase, it will manifest as progressive fibrosis with disappearance of the capillaries.

(3) Cavernous hemangioma: the tumor mass is located in the dermis and subcutaneous layers. It usually has an obscure boundary and no capsule around it. The major components of the tumor are dilated vessels, which have variable sized lumens and variable vessel wall thicknesses. The endoepithelial cells are flat and the infiltration of some lymphocytes can be seen among the tumors.

【Diagnosis and Differential Diagnosis】

Given the clinical manifestations and age of onset, it is not difficult to diagnose congenital vascular malformations and hemangiomas. But clinicians should pay attention to possible coexisting hemangiomas located in deeper tissue and internal

海绵状血管瘤的一种严重类型，即伴有血小板减少和紫癜者，称为 Kasabach-Merritt 综合征(Kasabach-Merritt syndrome)，大多见于婴儿。

上述两种或三种类型的血管畸形和血管瘤可同时存在，称为混合性血管瘤。

【组织病理】

(1) 鲜红斑痣　真皮浅部可见管腔大小不一、扩张的毛细血管，管腔内充满红细胞。

(2) 毛细血管瘤　肿瘤在真皮内呈分叶状生长，其组织病理学特点随肿瘤的发展阶段不同而有差别。生长期可见毛细血管内皮细胞增生明显，胞体较大，核分裂象易见，血管腔小而不清楚。成熟期表现为毛细血管内皮细胞变平、管腔增大。退变期逐渐发生纤维化、毛细血管消失。

(3) 海绵状血管瘤　肿瘤位于真皮和皮下脂肪组织内，边界不清，无包膜，由大小不等的扩张的血管组成，血管壁厚薄不一，血管腔的内皮细胞扁平，间质内有较多的淋巴细胞浸润。

【诊断与鉴别诊断】

根据其发病年龄和典型的临床表现，先天性血管畸形和血管瘤诊断一般不难，应注意有无合并其他深部组织或内脏血管瘤，必要时进行组织活检以明

organs. Biopsy can be performed to confirm the pathology when necessary.

Histopathologically, congenital hemangiomas should be differentiated from other soft connective tissue tumors that present with abundant blood vessels, such as angiokeratoma, angioleiomyoma, hemangiofibroma and angiolipoma, etc.

【Treatment】

The therapeutic strategies should be based on the clinical types, symptoms and locations of the hemangiomas.

(1) Nevus flammeus: pulsed dye laser treatments have been used with satisfactory results, and usually without scarring, but the treatments may need to be repeated several times.

(2) Capillary hemangioma: pulsed dye laser treatments have been used with satisfactory results in this type of hemangioma as well. Superficial X-rays or patches containing phosphorus-32 or strontium-90 or other β emitters can also be helpful. Intralesional glucocorticoids or oral prednisone may also be used, but surgical excision should be considered when necessary. Recently oral propranolol (inderal) has been demonstrated to be effective for capillary hemangioma, especially for the severe patients or cases with special location involvement.

(3) Cavernous hemangioma: superficial X-rays, phosforus-32 or strontium-90 or other β emitter patches can be used for superficial lesions. Intralesional injection of sclerosing agents has achieved a good success rate, but excision is recommended when the tumor is large.

确诊断。

先天性血管瘤需要与组织病理学上富于血管的软组织肿瘤相鉴别，如血管角皮瘤、血管平滑肌瘤、血管纤维瘤、血管脂肪瘤等。

【治疗】

治疗方案应根据血管瘤类型、临床症状、病变部位等确定。

(1) 鲜红斑痣　脉冲染料激光治疗效果较好，一般不留瘢痕，但需多次反复治疗。

(2) 毛细血管瘤　脉冲染料激光治疗效果较好，浅层 X 线、同位素磷 32 或锶 90 贴敷、β 射线贴敷等治疗也有帮助，糖皮质激素皮损内注射或泼尼松口服也可使用，必要时可手术切除。近年发现，口服普萘洛尔(心得安)用于治疗毛细血管瘤取得了良好效果，特别适合重度、皮损部位特殊的患者。

(3) 海绵状血管瘤　浅表皮损者可采用浅层 X 线、同位素磷 32 或锶 90 贴敷、β 射线贴敷等治疗，局部注射硬化剂也有较好的效果，较大的海绵状血管瘤可手术切除。

Lin WANG (王琳)

Section Fourteen　Lipoma

Lipoma, composed of mature fat cells, is one of the most common benign tumors of the skin. It may occur in any age, but is most commonly found on middle-aged females (age 40-50). Family histories of multiple lipomas are often seen.

【Clinical Manifestations】

Lipomas appear most commonly on the trunk, although they can be found anywhere on the body. The tumors may be single or multiple and of variable sizes. The nodules may be small but can be as big as a child's head. Usually, the tumor is round or lobulated with a wide base, and is soft and movable, with normal skin on its surface (Fig. 26-17). Patients typically have no subjective symptoms, but movement restriction or pain may occur when the

第十四节　脂　肪　瘤

脂肪瘤(lipoma)是由成熟脂肪细胞构成的最常见的皮肤良性肿瘤之一，可发生于任何年龄，多见于 40～50 岁，女性多见，多发性损害病例可有家族史。

【临床表现】

脂肪瘤可发生于身体任何部位，但主要见于躯干。肿瘤可单发或多发，大小不一，可为小的结节或至小儿头大小，通常基底较宽，圆形或分叶状，质地较软，活动性好，表面皮肤正常(图 26-17)，多无自觉症状，偶尔当肿瘤较大压迫周围组织结构时可引起活动受限或疼痛。

tumor grows big enough to press on the surrounding tissues. The development of lipomas is not related to food or nutritional status of the patients.

发病与饮食及全身营养状况无关。

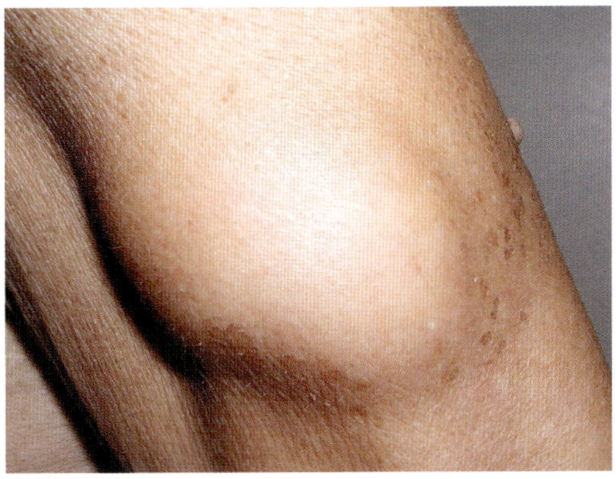

Fig. 26-17 Lipoma(图 26-17 脂肪瘤)

Lipoma usually grows slowly and fully stops after attaining a certain size. Transformations into malignancy are extremely rare in lipomas, but calcification, necrosis and liquefaction may develop. Lipoma has been described as one of the symptoms of Gardner's syndrome, in which other pathological changes such as multiple osteoma, epidermal cysts, colon polyps, fibrosarcomas will also present.

脂肪瘤通常逐渐长大,但长到一定程度时即保持大小不变,极少发生恶变。极少数病例可发生钙化、坏死、液化。脂肪瘤亦可为 Gardner 综合征的症状之一,此时可合并其他病变,如多发性骨瘤、表皮囊肿、结肠息肉、纤维肉瘤等。

【Histopathology】

Lipoma is located in subcutaneous adipose tissue. It is an encapsulated, lobulated tumor containing normal fat cells that are bound together in clusters by strands of connective tissue. Based on the stromal components of lipomas, this disease can be subdivided histopathologically into fibrolipoma, angiolipoma and myolipoma, all of which are categorized as hamartomas.

【组织病理】

脂肪瘤位于皮下脂肪组织内,包膜清楚,常由结缔组织分隔成大小不等的小叶。肿瘤细胞为成熟的脂肪细胞。组织病理学上脂肪瘤根据其间质成分的不同可分为纤维脂肪瘤、血管脂肪瘤以及肌脂肪瘤等亚型,这些均属错构瘤。

【Diagnosis and Differential Diagnosis】

Lipoma should be suspected if the tumor is soft, lobulated, mobile and growing slowly on the trunk or upper limbs. The pathology can be confirmed by biopsy if necessary. Lipoma should be distinguished from epidermal cysts, hibernomas and cysticercosis cutis, but biopsy and histopathological examination will be useful for differentiation.

【诊断与鉴别诊断】

发生于躯干、上肢的皮下肿块,生长缓慢,质地较软,呈分叶状,可推动,应怀疑本病。活检可明确诊断。脂肪瘤应该与表皮囊肿、冬眠瘤、皮肤猪囊虫病等相鉴别,活检和组织病理检查容易区别这些疾病。

【Treatment】

Treatment of lipoma is not necessary in most cases unless the patient requests it, or the tumor presents with other symptoms. In such cases, simple excision can be used to remove the tumor.

【治疗】

脂肪瘤一般不需治疗。若患者要求治疗或肿瘤有症状时可采用手术切除。

Lin WANG (王琳)

Section Fifteen Nevocytic Nevi

Nevocytic nevi, also known as pigmented nevi or melanocytic nevi, are the most common benign tumors in humans. Nevocytes originate from the neural crest of the embryonic ectoderm and become nevus during migration to the epidermis.

【Clinical Manifestations】

The majority of nevi begin to appear in childhood, adolescence, or sometimes at birth, and increase in number as the patient grows older. There appears to be no gender bias in their formation. Nevocytic nevi can be found anywhere on the body surface (both on skin and on mucous membranes) and the number of nevi varies from only a few to dozens or even hundreds. The skin lesions vary in size and are morphologically quite diverse, appearing as macules, maculopapules, papules, or as papillary, nodular, polypoid, or even with peduncle or hairs on them. The color of nevi may be skin-colored, brown, dark brown, bluish-black or black depending on the amount of melanin in the nevi (Fig. 26-18). Nevocytic nevi are classified into junctional nevi, intradermal nevi and compound nevi according to the position of the nevocytes in the skin.

第十五节　痣细胞痣

痣细胞痣(nevocytic nevi)，又名色素痣、黑素细胞痣，是人类最常见的良性皮肤肿瘤。痣细胞起源于胚胎期外胚叶的神经嵴，在向表皮移行过程中发展而来。

【临床表现】

大多数痣发生于儿童期和青春期，也可出生时即有，无性别差异，随年龄增长而增多。身体任何部位的皮肤、黏膜均可发生，数目不定，可为数个、数十个甚至数百个。临床表现多样，大小不等，如斑疹、斑丘疹、丘疹、乳头状、结节状、息肉样或有蒂，可有毛发贯穿。根据痣细胞内色素含量不同，颜色可呈肤色、棕褐色、深褐色、蓝黑色、黑色等(图 26-18)。根据痣细胞在皮内的位置不同，其可分为交界痣、皮内痣和复合痣。

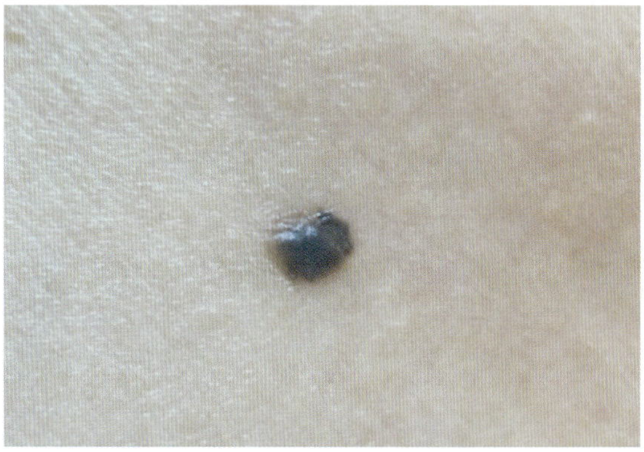

Fig. 26-18　Nevocytic nevi(图 26-18　痣细胞痣)

Junctional nevus, commonly found in children, is a light to dark brown macule or maculopapule, several millimeters in diameter or larger. Usually it has a regular border, a smooth surface with no hair, and can be located anywhere including the palms and soles and the genitalia. Intradermal nevus, commonly observed in adults, can be found at any place on the skin, but there is a predilection for the head and neck. The lesions are dome-shaped papules or nodules with a smooth or papillary appearance, sometimes with a pedicel or hair. They can be skin-colored, brown or black. Compound nevus is usually present in older children and adults. This resembles junctional nevus except that it's slightly elevated.

交界痣多见于儿童，为直径几毫米或更大的深浅不等的褐色斑疹、斑丘疹，通常表面光滑无毛，边缘规则，可见于身体任何部位(包括掌跖或外阴部)。皮内痣常见于成人，可发生于身体任何部位，但头颈部最常见，皮损为圆顶形丘疹、结节，呈皮色、棕色或黑褐色，表面光滑或呈乳头状，偶有蒂或含毛发。复合痣多见于较大儿童和成人，外观似交界痣，但常突出皮面。

Nevocytic nevi grow slowly without symptoms, and the malignant transformation is quite rare. But the junctional nevi, located at areas that are prone to irritation (such as the palms, soles, genitalia, armpits, groin or beltline), have a greater risk of transforming into malignancy. Signs that suggest malignant changes in a nevocytic nevus include the following: ① asymmetry of the lesion; ② border irregularity; ③ color variegation within the same lesion, ④diameter>6 mm, or diameter enlarging; ⑤evolution (any change in the appearance, symptoms such as pain, pruritus, bleeding, crusting, etc).

痣细胞痣发展缓慢，多无自觉症状，发生恶变的可能性小，但发生在掌跖、生殖器、腋窝、腹股沟、腰周等易摩擦部位的交界痣较易恶变。提示痣细胞痣恶变的表现包括：①损害不对称；②边缘不规则；③色泽不均匀；④直径大于 6 mm 或直径不断增大；⑤进展(外表的改变，或出现下列症状，如疼痛、瘙痒、出血、结痂等)。

【Histopathology】

Nevocyte nests are found in the dermis and epidermis as well. The nevocytes are polygonal, round or oval. The nevocytes adjacent to the epidermis are particularly larger than those in the deeper dermis and contain more melanin.

The nevocytic nests of a junctional nevus are well-circumscribed, located in the lower epidermis and bulge downward into the dermis resembling "tears", with a large amount of melanin. The nevocyte nests for intradermal nevus are located in the dermis, where the nevocytes in the superior part are larger, nested and contain only a moderate amount of melanin, whereas the nevocytes in the deeper dermis are smaller, spindle-shaped and contain even less melanin. For compound nevus, the nevocytic nests appear in the dermis and epidermis, and have histopathological features of both junctional nevus and intradermal nevus simultaneously.

【组织病理】

表皮和/或真皮内有成巢的痣细胞，痣细胞常呈多角形、圆形或卵圆形。近表皮的痣细胞较大、色素较多，深部的痣细胞逐渐变小、色素减少。

交界痣的痣细胞巢界限清楚，痣细胞位于表皮下部或向下突入真皮，表皮处的痣细胞呈"泪滴"状进入真皮，细胞内含大量色素。皮内痣痣细胞巢位于真皮内，真皮上部的痣细胞较大、呈巢状、含中等量色素，而真皮中下部痣细胞较小、以梭形细胞为主，色素很少。复合痣痣细胞巢位于表皮内和真皮内，同时具有交界痣和皮内痣的组织病理学特点。

【Diagnosis and Differential Diagnosis】

The diagnosis of nevocytic nevi is easy to establish according to the clinical features and histopathological examination. Nevocytic nevi should be differentiated clinically from lentigo, seborrheic keratosis, blue nevus, actinic keratosis, pigmented basal cell carcinoma and malignant melanoma. Histopathological examination can confirm the diagnosis.

【诊断与鉴别诊断】

根据临床特征和组织病理学检查结果，容易诊断。临床上需要与雀斑样痣、脂溢性角化病、蓝痣、日光角化病、色素性基底细胞癌、恶性黑素瘤等相鉴别，组织病理学检查可明确诊断。

【Treatment】

No treatment is required for nevocytic nevi in most cases, but nevi located in chronically irritated areas of the skin should be removed as early as possible. Another indication for excision with a safety margin is when the nevi show warning signs of malignant transformation described above.

【治疗】

一般不需要治疗。发生在易摩擦部位的痣宜早期手术切除，若痣出现上述恶变征象，应立即扩大切除。

Lin WANG (王琳)

Section Sixteen　Malignant Melanoma

Malignant melanoma (MM), also named melanoma, which originates from melanocytes, is a highly aggressive malignant tumor. It is the third most common cutaneous malignancy. It arises most frequently in the skin, but can also be found in the mucous membrane that borders the skin, choroid of the eye globe, meninges, etc.

【Etiology and Pathogenesis】

The etiology of MM is unknown. Known significant risk factors include race, genetic predisposition, exposure to sunlight, trauma or irritation, viruses and immunological disturbance.

【Clinical Manifestations】

MM frequently affects persons older than 30 years, but may occasionally be seen in children. There is no sex predilection. The early manifestation of MM is a black macule appearing on normal skin, or some change in an existing nevocytic nevus (e. g., sharp increase in size, ulceration, bleeding, and pain). The MM lesion may gradually progress to plaques, nodules and ulceration.

MM are classified into two categories: MM in situ, and invasive MM. MM in situ is also known as intraepidermal MM, and is characterized by atypical melanocytes confined to the epidermis. Invasive MM can be subdivided into four types according to their onset, clinical course, histopathological changes and prognosis as follows: acral lentiginous melanoma, lentigo maligna melanoma, nodular malignant melanoma and superficial spreading melanoma.

(1) Malignant melanoma *in situ*:

MM *in situ* has two major subtypes-lentigo maligna and superficial spreading malignant melanoma *in situ*.

① Lentigo maligna: it typically occurs in the elderly on sun-exposed skin, most commonly on the face (Fig. 26-19). The lesion begins with an irregular macule and extends gradually to form a patch several centimeters in diameter. The color of the lesion is generally uneven and could be light brown or brown, although some dark-brown to black spots or even hypopigmentation may also be seen on the lesion. The hypopigmentation may result from regression of the tumor. The spread and darkening of the lesion is usually very slow and may take 5-20 years to become an invasive melanoma or lentigo maligna melanoma.

② Superficial spreading malignant melanoma *in situ*: often

第十六节　恶性黑素瘤

恶性黑素瘤(malignant melanoma, MM),又称为黑素瘤(melanoma),是起源于黑素细胞的恶性程度较高的肿瘤,占皮肤恶性肿瘤发病率的第三位。多发生于皮肤,亦可见于邻近皮肤的黏膜、眼球脉络膜和软脑膜等处。

【病因及发病机制】

病因不明,可能与种族、遗传易感性、日光照射、创伤刺激、病毒、免疫紊乱等因素有关。

【临床表现】

本病好发于 30 岁以上的人,偶见于儿童,无明显性别差异。恶性黑素瘤早期表现是在正常皮肤上出现黑色斑疹,或原有的痣细胞痣发生变化,如迅速增大、破溃、出血、疼痛等。随着病情的发展,损害表现为斑块、结节、溃疡等。

恶性黑素瘤分为原位恶性黑素瘤和侵袭性恶性黑素瘤两大类。原位恶性黑素瘤又名表皮内恶性黑素瘤,其特征为非典型的黑素细胞局限于表皮内。侵袭性恶性黑素瘤根据其发病方式、病程、组织病理学表现及预后等的不同,一般分为肢端雀斑样黑素瘤、恶性雀斑样黑素瘤、结节性恶性黑素瘤、浅表扩散性恶性黑素瘤四型。

(1) 原位恶性黑素瘤

原位恶性黑素瘤主要有两种类型,即恶性雀斑样痣和浅表扩散性原位恶性黑素瘤。

①恶性雀斑样痣(lentigo maligna):好发于老年人的日光暴露部位,最常见于面部(图 26-19)。皮损初为边缘不规则的斑疹,逐渐向周围扩大,形成直径为数厘米的淡褐色、褐色斑片,色素分布不均匀,其上可见深褐色至黑色小斑点或色素减退,色素减退系肿瘤自行消退所致。此型原位恶性黑素瘤扩大、颜色加深的过程十分缓慢,经过 5～20 年发生侵袭性生长,成为恶性雀斑样黑素瘤。

②浅表扩散性原位恶性黑素瘤

occurs on the unexposed skin of middle-aged patients, most commonly on the back and legs. The cutaneous lesion may present as a pigmented macule or barely raised papule whose border is sharp and irregular. Pigment variegation within the perimeter demonstrates a mixture of colors, ranging from a dark brown to black, to dark blue-gray, to a pink or gray-white color. Most lesions are less than 2. 5 cm in diameter(Fig. 26-20). The tumor tends to grow fast and evolves into invasive superficial spreading malignant melanoma within 1-5 years.

(superficial spreading malignant melanoma *in situ*)：好发于中年人的非日光暴露部位，以背部及小腿多见，皮损为界限清楚而不规则的色素性斑疹或微隆起的丘疹，颜色斑驳，可由深褐色、黑色、深蓝灰色、粉红色、灰白色等多种颜色构成，直径很少超过 2. 5 cm(图 26-20)。肿瘤生长较快，经过 1～5 年即发展成侵袭性浅表扩散性恶性黑素瘤。

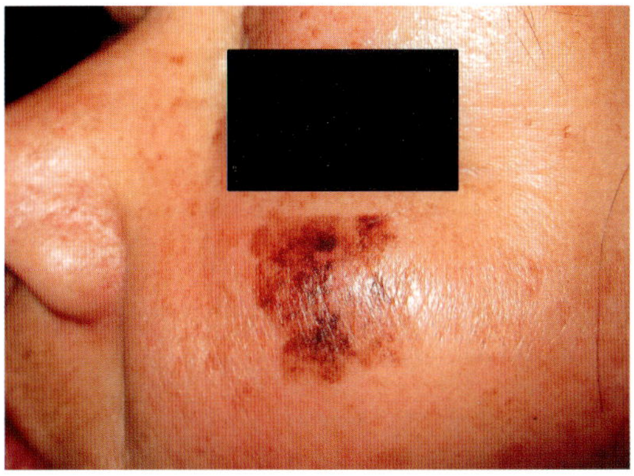

Fig. 26-19　Lentigo maligna
(图 26-19　恶性雀斑样痣)

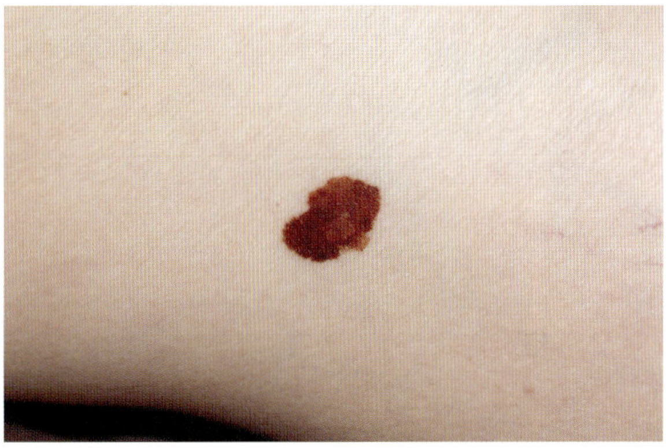

Fig. 26-20　Superficial spreading malignant melanoma *in situ*
(图 26-20　浅表扩散性原位恶性黑素瘤)

(2) Invasive malignant melanoma:

①Acral lentiginous melanoma (ALM): is the most common type of skin MM in Asians. The most frequent site is the sole of the foot, followed by the palm and nail unit (Fig. 26-21). In its early phase, the lesion presents as a brown or black macule or patch with an irregular saw-teeth-like edge and color variegation. When the tumor is in the vertical growth phase, the lesion presents as a dark-blue or black papule or nodule, or sometimes as verrucous hyperplasia. ALM progresses rapidly and tends to ulcerate, bleed and metastasize. The prognosis is poor once metastasis occurs. However, early non-metastatic lesions can be cured.

(2) 侵袭性恶性黑素瘤

①肢端雀斑样黑素瘤(acral lentiginous melanoma)：本病为亚洲人皮肤恶性黑素瘤中最常见的类型，足底是最常见的发病部位，其次为手掌和甲单位(图 26-21)。皮损在早期通常表现为褐色或黑色的斑疹、斑片，色素沉着不均匀，边缘明显不规则、呈锯齿状。当肿瘤发展至垂直生长期后，表现为深蓝色或黑色丘疹、结节，有时呈疣状增生。此型进展快，极易发生溃疡、出血和转移，一旦转移则预后差，但未发生转移者可以治愈。

②Lentigo maligna melanoma (LMM): is a rare type. It typically occurs on the chronically sun exposed cutaneous surfaces of the elderly, most commonly on the face, and occasionally on the neck, back, forearms or legs. The lesion is an irregular patch that can be as large as several centimeters in diameter. The lesion has color variegation which may be brown, dark-brown or black. The lesion gradually enlarges peripherally with single or multiple black-blue papules or nodules forming inside (Fig. 26-22). LMM evolves very slowly and can metastasize in the late stage, most frequently to the local regional lymph nodes. The prognosis is better than other MM types.

②恶性雀斑样黑素瘤(lentigo maligna melanoma)：一种较少见的恶性黑素瘤，好发于老年人的慢性日光损伤部位，最常见于面部，也可见于颈部、背部、前臂、小腿等。皮损为数厘米大的不规则的斑片，棕色、深褐色或黑色，色素沉着不均匀，逐渐向周围扩大，皮损内形成一个或多个蓝黑色丘疹或结节(图 26-22)。此型生长缓慢，晚期可发生转移，多倾向于向局部区域性淋巴结转移，较其他型预后好。

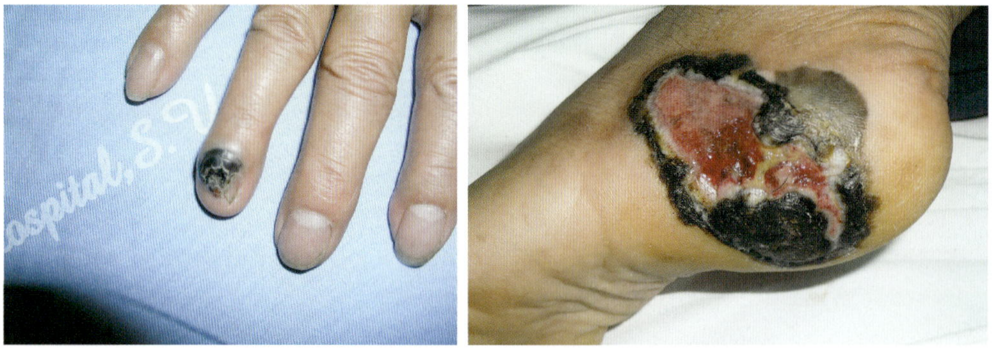

(a)　　(b)

Fig. 26-21　Acral lentiginous melanoma(图 26-21　肢端雀斑样黑素瘤)

③Nodular malignant melanoma: often occurs on the head, neck, trunk and lower legs. The lesion starts as an elevated, variably pigmented papule or nodules. The lesion is symmetrical and well demarcated, and sometimes can be surrounded by a narrow ring of erythema. The color can be black, bluish-black, or dark brown. It can rapidly grow to form a plaque and can ulcerate. It can present as a polypoid, mushroom-like or cauliflower-like nodule (Fig. 26-23). This type of MM usually metastasizes early and the prognosis is poor.

③结节性恶性黑素瘤(nodular malignant melanoma):本病好发于头颈部、躯干、小腿下部,皮损初起为隆起的色素性丘疹、结节,对称,界限清楚,有时周围绕以红晕,呈黑色、蓝黑色或暗褐色,生长迅速,可形成斑块及溃疡,或增生呈息肉样、蕈样或菜花样结节(图 26-23)。此型常早期发生转移,预后差。

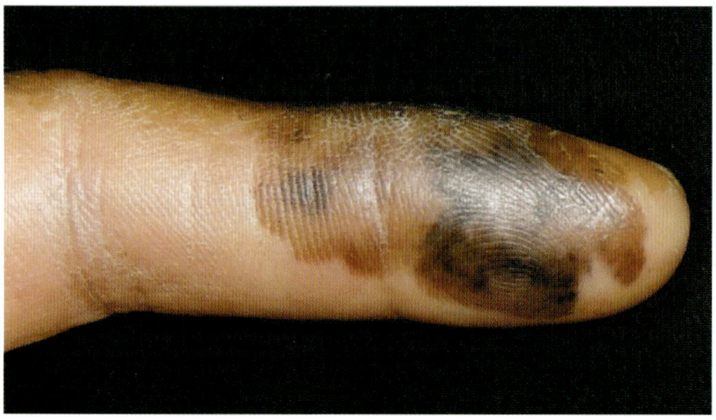

Fig. 26-22　Lentigo maligna melanoma
(图 26-22　恶性雀斑样黑素瘤)

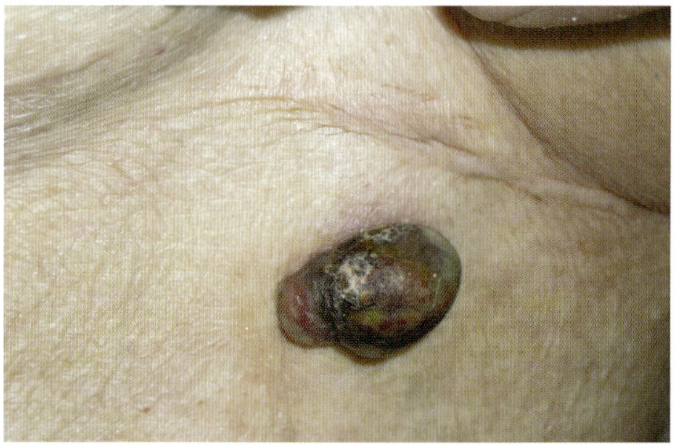

Fig. 26-23　Nodular malignant melanoma
(图 26-23　结节性恶性黑素瘤)

④Superficial spreading melanoma(SSM): is the most common type of MM worldwide except Asian. This type of MM usually arises from superficial spreading MM *in situ*. It is often found on the trunk and lower legs. The lesion is a macule or patch with an irregular shape, and is variable in size, ranging from a few millimeters to several centimeters in diameter. The color varies from tan to brown or even black and shows variegation. The tumor develops gradually and invasive nodules may develop from underneath. Bleeding, erosion and ulceration may occur (Fig. 26-24). The SSM grows slowly, metastasizes late and has a better prognosis than nodular malignant melanoma.

④浅表扩散性黑素瘤(superficial spreading melanoma):全球(虽然在亚洲并非如此)最常见的恶性黑素瘤,常由浅表扩散性原位恶性黑素瘤发展而来,好发于躯干和小腿。皮损开始为斑疹或斑片,形态不规则,大小不等,直径从几毫米到几厘米。其颜色多变,从浅棕色至深棕色甚至黑色不等。肿瘤逐渐发展,其表面形成侵袭性生长的结节,易出血、糜烂、溃疡(图 26-24)。该类型肿瘤生长较慢,转移也较迟,较结节性恶性黑素瘤预后好。

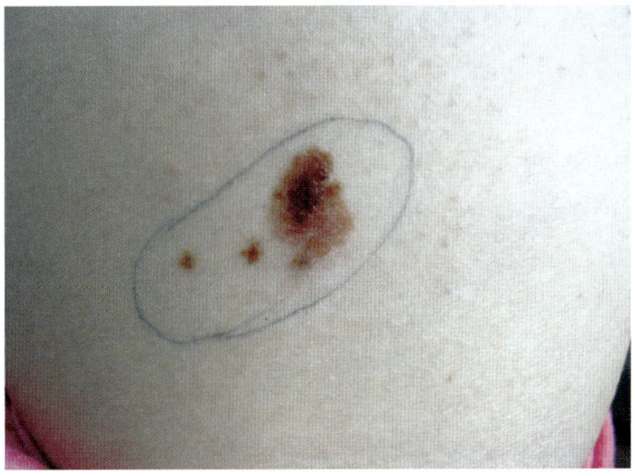

Fig. 26-24　Superficial spreading melanoma(图 26-24　浅表扩散性黑素瘤)

In addition,MM can also be found in the mucosal areas such as fossa orbitalis, nasal cavity, oral cavity, genital organs, urethra, anus,etc. A typical lesion is usually a heterogeneously pigmented macule or patch, or a nodule, and is often associated with hemorrhaging,pain and obstructive symptoms.

此外,恶性黑素瘤还发生在眼眶、鼻腔、口腔、生殖器、尿道和肛门等黏膜部位,典型皮损表现为色素不均匀的斑疹、斑片或结节,常伴有出血、疼痛、阻塞等表现。

【Histopathology】

The atypical melanocytes of MM *in situ* are confined to the epidermis. The tumor cells can be found not only in the upper part of the epidermis but also extend into the epithelia of hair follicles or sweat ducts. These atypical melanocytes exhibit a variation in morphology such as epithelioid or spindle-shaped,and the infiltrate is either dispersed or clustered. They are characterized by abundant cytoplasm and sometimes contain varying amounts of melanin. There is usually a distinct inflammatory response consisting of patchy aggregations of lymphocytes and melanophages within the papillary dermis.

MM usually occurs in the epidermal-dermal junction,and the tumor cells can extend through the basal cell membrane and invade downward into the dermis and also upward into the epidermis at the same time. The atypical melanocytes infiltrate as nests or diffusely into the dermis and adipose layer,and extend in both the horizontal and vertical directions. Although these atypical melanocytes usually vary in shape and size,the majority of the tumor cells are spindle-shaped and epithelioid. They have atypical hyperchromatic nuclei, large nucleoli and abundant cytoplasm. Mitoses are easily found. Varying amounts of melanin in the cells may also be present. Immunohistochemically, the atypical melanocytes express S100 protein,HMB-45 and Mart-1.

【组织病理】

原位恶性黑素瘤的非典型黑素细胞局限于表皮内,瘤细胞不仅见于表皮上部,而且可沿毛囊、汗腺导管向下扩展。瘤细胞散在或成簇状分布,形态多样,包括上皮样细胞和梭形细胞,瘤细胞的胞质丰富、含有多少不等的黑素。真皮乳头内有明显的片状聚集的淋巴细胞和噬色素细胞浸润。

恶性黑素瘤大多发生在表皮真皮交界处,该处瘤细胞增生,可突破基膜向下侵入真皮,瘤细胞也可向上方侵犯表皮。肿瘤呈巢状或弥漫性浸润,沿水平和垂直方向扩展,深达真皮和皮下脂肪层。瘤细胞大小和形态呈多样性,以梭形细胞和上皮样细胞为主,瘤细胞胞质丰富,核大深染、核仁明显、核分裂象易见,胞质内含有多少不等的黑素。免疫组化标记肿瘤细胞表达 S100 蛋白、HMB-45 和 Mart-1。

【Diagnosis and Differential Diagnosis】

The diagnosis of MM can be established easily according to the clinical features and histopathological changes, but it is almost always necessary to do an immunohistochemical staining,since the

【诊断与鉴别诊断】

根据皮损特点和组织病理学改变,恶性黑素瘤的诊断不难。由于误诊会导致严重后果,常需要做免疫组织化学标

consequences of a misdiagnosis are of serious concern.

A wide variety of skin diseases should be differentiated from MM. MM should be clinically differentiated from nevocytic nevi, blue nevus, lentigo, actinic keratosis, seborrheic keratosis, dermatofibroma, pyogenic granuloma, juvenile melanoma, pigmented basal cell carcinoma, and nail bed hemorrhage. Histopathologically, MM should be differentiated from juvenile melanoma, spindle cell squamous cell carcinoma, fibrosarcoma, Kaposi's sarcoma, and epithelioid sarcoma.

记以帮助确诊。

本病应和许多疾病进行鉴别。临床上应与痣细胞痣、蓝痣、雀斑样痣、日光性角化病、脂溢性角化病、皮肤纤维瘤、化脓性肉芽肿、幼年性黑素瘤、色素型基底细胞癌、甲床下出血等相鉴别;组织病理学上主要应与幼年性黑素瘤、梭形细胞鳞癌、纤维肉瘤、Kaposi 肉瘤、上皮样肉瘤等相鉴别。

【Treatment】

The early diagnosis and early selection of a therapeutic strategy are extremely important for the prognosis of MM. The primary therapeutic approach is surgical excision, and the excisional range depends on the type, depth and location of the tumor. In the more advanced stages, chemotherapy and radiotherapy should be considered. Immunotherapy may also be effective, including interferon, interleukin-2, tumor necrosis factor and Bacillus Calmette-Guérin vaccine.

【治疗】

早期诊断及合理治疗对于恶性黑素瘤的预后至关重要。早期完整手术切除是皮肤恶性黑素瘤的首选治疗,切除的范围应根据肿瘤的类型、深度和部位等综合确定。晚期恶性黑素瘤可行化疗、放疗。免疫疗法的方法很多,如干扰素、白细胞介素-2、肿瘤坏死因子、卡介苗等,有一定疗效。

【Prognosis】

MM is highly aggressive and highly prone to metastasis. While early melanomas can be cured with surgical excisions, metastatic melanoma has an extremely poor prognosis since no curative therapy exists at present. For metastatic melanoma, the frequent sites of metastasis are local regional lymph nodes, followed by the liver, lungs, central nervous system, bone and skin. The likelihood of metastasis of a melanoma is primarily determined by several factors, among which the most important is the Breslow thickness of the tumor, followed by the presence or absence of histopathological ulceration and the number of mitotic figures. For advanced melanoma, the number of lymph nodes involved and the elevated serum lactate dehydrogenase (LDH) are also important prognostic factors.

【预后】

恶性黑素瘤具有高度侵袭性,易发生转移,早期黑素瘤采用手术切除可以治愈,但转移性黑素瘤目前还没有治愈的方法,因而预后很差,转移性黑素瘤的常见转移部位包括区域淋巴结、肝脏、肺部、中枢神经系统、骨和皮肤。其转移与许多因素有关,但最重要的是 Breslow 肿瘤的厚度、病理上是否有溃疡及核分裂的数量。对进展性黑素瘤,累及的淋巴结的数量和血清乳酸脱氢酶(LDH)的水平也是重要的预后因素。

Lin WANG (王琳)

Section Seventeen　Granuloma Fungoides

Granuloma fungoides, also known as mycosis fungoides (MF), is a low grade primary cutaneous T-cell lymphoma.

第十七节　蕈样肉芽肿

蕈样肉芽肿(granuloma fungoides),又称为蕈样霉菌病(mycosis fungoides, MF),是一种原发于皮肤的低度恶性的 T 细胞淋巴瘤。

【Etiology and Pathogenesis】

The cause of MF is unknown, but it is believed that hereditary,

【病因及发病机制】

病因尚不清楚。遗传、感染和环境

infectious and environmental factors may contribute to its occurrence.

因素可能与本病的发生、发展有关。

【Clinical Manifestations】

MF commonly affects elderly people, but the condition can occur at any age, including adolescents and children. It is more common in males than in females with a ratio of about 2 : 1. Usually MF exhibits an indolent clinical course, often requiring years or even decades to develop into a tumor. MF can be divided into three phases clinically: the patch stage(erythematous stage), the plaque stage and the tumor stage.

(1) Patch stage(erythematous stage): this is the early stage of MF. The lower abdomen, buttocks, upper thighs and the breasts are preferentially affected. The skin lesions usually present as erythematous patches with a few scales (Fig. 26-25). The lesions may clinically resemble a variety of dermatoses, including psoriasis, eczema, lichen simplex chronicus (neurodermatitis), ichthyosis, poikiloderma, parapsoriasis, and pityriasis rosea. Occasionally, several different types of skin lesions may be seen on a single patient. Pruritus is usually mild or may not be present, although it can be severe in rare cases. This stage usually lasts for years or even decades before progressing to the plaque stage.

【临床表现】

本病通常发生于老年人，但可发生于任何年龄，包括青年人，甚至儿童。男性多于女性，男女之比约为 2 : 1。临床过程迁延，经过数年，甚至数十年才进展为肿瘤。临床上可分为 3 期：斑片期（红斑期）、斑块期和肿瘤期。

（1）斑片期（红斑期） 红斑期为 MF 的早期，皮损好发于下腹部、臀部、大腿和女性的乳房，常为红色斑片，伴少量鳞屑（图 26-25）。皮损可类似许多皮肤病，如银屑病、湿疹、慢性单纯性苔藓（神经性皮炎）、鱼鳞病、皮肤异色症、副银屑病、玫瑰糠疹等，有时一人身上同时有多种不同类型的皮损。患者常有轻度瘙痒或无瘙痒，但有的瘙痒剧烈。在进展为斑块期之前，此期通常可持续存在数年至数十年。

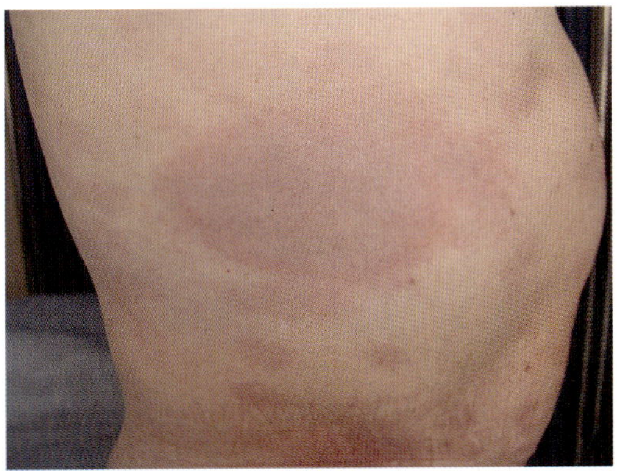

Fig. 26-25 Granuloma fungoides-patch stage(图 26-25 蕈样肉芽肿-斑片期)

(2) Plaque stage: this stage frequently follows the patch stage, but some patients do not go through an obvious patch stage and present at the full-blown plaque stage at the very beginning. The lesions are dull red infiltrated plaques with irregular shapes, elevated margins and sharp edges (Fig. 26-26). Occasionally, old lesions can spontaneously resolve completely, but most lesions will continue to grow to the tumor stage.

(3) Tumor stage: this stage will be marked by an exophytic hypertrophic growth, which can be dark brown or purple or red in color, appearing at the margins of the existing infiltrated plaques or as *de novo* lesions on apparently healthy skin. Ulcerations often

（2）斑块期 斑块期常由斑片期转化而来，也有部分患者斑片期不明显，而似乎一开始即为斑块期。皮损常表现为暗红色浸润性斑块、形态不规则、边缘高起、边界清楚（图 26-26）。陈旧皮损有时可自行消退而不留痕迹。但大多数皮损继续发展、增生而进入肿瘤期。

（3）肿瘤期 这一期以皮损外生性增生为特点，皮损呈深棕色或紫色或红色，可发生于原有的浸润性斑块的边缘或直接发生于正常皮肤上。此期肿瘤常

occur on the tumors at this stage (Fig. 26-27).

发生溃疡(图 26-27)。

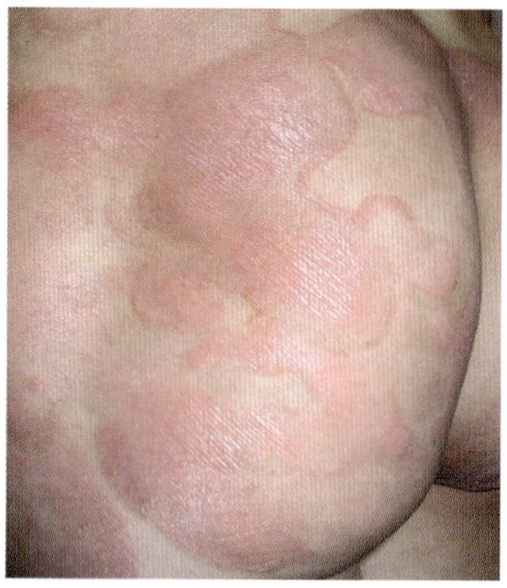

Fig. 26-26 Granuloma fungoides-plaque stage
(图 26-26 蕈样肉芽肿-斑块期)

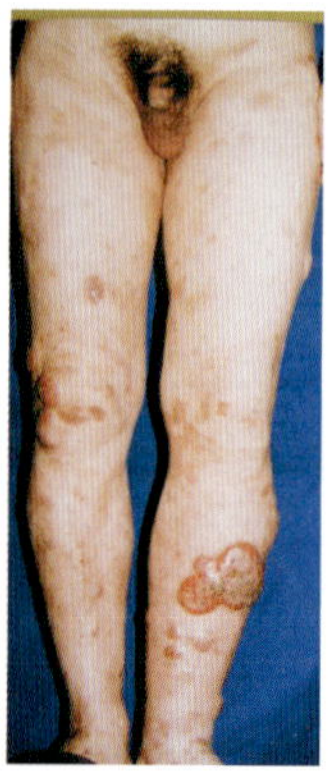

Fig. 26-27 Granuloma fungoides-tumor stage
(图 26-27 蕈样肉芽肿-肿瘤期)

Multiple organs may be involved in the advanced stages of MF, such as the lymph nodes, lungs, liver, spleen, bone marrow and kidneys. Patients often die from the disease within a few years.

晚期 MF 还可累及淋巴结和肺、肝、脾、骨髓、肾脏等多个器官系统。患者常在数年内死亡。

【Histopathology】

【组织病理】

(1) Patch stage (erythematous stage): the histopathological diagnosis of early MF is difficult because there are no specific histopathological changes. Nevertheless, the following features may provide important clues for diagnosis: lymphocytes with perinuclear haloes scattered among the keratinocytes, lymphocytes colonized in a linear configuration at the basal layer of the epidermis, the lymphocytes are atypical with larger indented hyperchromatic nuclei in the high power field, the infiltrated lymphocytes in the epidermis are larger than those in the dermis, and finally collagen fiber bundles in the papillary layer of the dermis are hyperplastic and their orientation is parallel to the epidermis above.

(1) 斑片期(红斑期) 早期缺乏特异性组织病理学改变,诊断困难。以下特点可为诊断提供重要的参考依据:淋巴细胞散在分布于角质形成细胞间,核周有空晕;淋巴细胞在表皮基膜带呈线状分布;淋巴细胞核有异型性,表现为在高倍镜下核稍大、不规则、染色质深;在表皮内浸润的肿瘤性淋巴细胞较同时浸润在真皮内者为大;真皮乳头层的胶原纤维束增生,其排列方向与表皮表面平行。

(2) Plaque stage: this stage retains the histopathological features of the patch stage, although the lymphocytes (especially in the epidermis) may appear more atypical. The atypical lymphocytes tend to gather in clusters within the epidermis-a pattern known as Pautrier microabscesses. At this stage there is dense infiltration with lymphocytes in the papillary layer of the dermis.

(2) 斑块期 此期保留了斑片期的组织病理学特点,但淋巴细胞特别是表皮内的淋巴细胞有明显的异型性,可见表皮内成簇的异型淋巴细胞的聚集,即 Pautrier 微脓肿形成,真皮乳头层有密集的淋巴细胞浸润。

(3) Tumor stage: epidermotropism is not obvious and may even disappear in this stage. The atypical lymphocytes infiltration spreads throughout the dermis in a nodular or diffuse pattern and even into the subcutaneous tissue.

(3) 肿瘤期 亲表皮现象(向表皮性)可以不明显或不存在,整个真皮甚至皮下组织有成团或弥漫性浸润的异型淋巴细胞。

Under immunohistochemical staining, the neoplastic cells of MF exhibit mature peripheral T-cell markers such as $CD3^+$, $CD4^+$, $CD5^+$, and $CD8^-$ T-cell phenotypes. Monoclonal T-cell receptor (TCR) α/β and TCR γ gene rearrangement can be detected by polymerase chain reaction or Southern blot in most cases.

MF 的肿瘤细胞用免疫组化染色标记显示为成熟外周 T 细胞,大多数病例的免疫表型为 CD3、CD4、CD5 阳性,CD8 阴性。多数病例用聚合酶链反应(PCR)或 Southern 杂交能检测出有克隆性 TCR α/β 和 TCR γ 的 T 细胞受体基因重排。

【Diagnosis and Differential Diagnosis】

It is difficult to establish a diagnosis of MF in the patch stage (erythematous stage) because both skin lesions and histopathological changes are nonspecific. The physician should suspect MF when the chronic pruritus resists conventional treatments for all common skin disorders. Multiple biopsies and multi-position biopsies may also be necessary for an early diagnosis. In contrast to the early stage of MF, the diagnosis of MF in the plaque or tumor stage will be easier, based on their clinical manifestations and histopathological features. Detection of $CD4^+$ tumor cells by immunohistochemical staining and monoclonal TCR gene rearrangement assays should provide support in confirming the diagnosis.

In the patch stage, MF often clinically simulates a variety of dermatoses, including psoriasis, parapsoriasis, eczema, lichen simplex chronicus (neurodermatitis) and ichthyosis. Because of this potential for confusion, histopathology is the most important method for differentiation.

【诊断与鉴别诊断】

斑片期(红斑期)的皮损及组织病理改变均无特异性,往往难以做出诊断,临床上对拟诊为其他慢性瘙痒性皮肤病但常规治疗无效者,应考虑 MF 的可能,必要时应多次及多部位取材,以利于早期诊断。斑块期及肿瘤期根据临床表现结合组织病理学特征可做出诊断。瘤细胞免疫组化标记为 CD4 阳性以及 T 细胞受体基因克隆性重排检测对确诊有重要帮助。

本病在斑片期时,临床上可以模拟许多皮肤病,包括银屑病、副银屑病、湿疹、慢性单纯性苔藓(神经性皮炎)和鱼鳞病,因而组织病理学检查是最重要的鉴别手段。

【Treatment】

The aims of MF treatment are to control the symptoms and to slow the progression of the tumor. In the early stage, immunotherapy and topical therapy should be applied. The former is a systemic treatment using interferon, Bacillus Calmette-Guérin vaccine, and transfer factor; the latter therapy includes glucocorticoids, retinoids, dilute solutions of nitrogen mustard, electron beam irradiation on the entire body and photochemotherapy (PUVA). In the tumor stage, chemotherapies such as cyclophosphamide, chlorambucil and methotrexate are often required. The therapeutic effects of chemotherapies can be further improved by applying them in combination with topical therapies.

【治疗】

治疗目的是减轻患者的症状,延缓疾病进程。早期皮损以增强患者免疫力和局部治疗为主,前者可用干扰素、卡介苗或转移因子等,局部治疗可选用糖皮质激素、维 A 酸或氮芥外用,全身电子束照射、光化学疗法(PUVA)等有一定疗效。肿瘤期患者应采用化疗(如环磷酰胺、苯丁酸氮芥、甲氨蝶呤等),与局部治疗联用可获更好疗效。

【Prognosis】

The most important prognostic indicator for MF is the clinical stage of the disease when first treated. The patient may have an aggressive clinical course when skin lesions are generalized, with lymph node and visceral involvement, or when large cell transformation occur in cases of MF. Patients usually die of systemic involvements or infections.

【预后】

临床分期是 MF 最重要的预后指标。患者皮损累及的范围大、淋巴结和内脏受累、大细胞转化均为预后不良的因素。患者通常死于多系统累及和继发感染。

Lin WANG (王琳)

Chapter Twenty-seven Sexually Transmitted Diseases

第二十七章 性传播疾病

Section One Syphilis

第一节 梅 毒

Syphilis is a chronic and systemic contagious sexually-transmitted disease caused by *Treponema pallidum*.

梅毒（syphilis）是由苍白密螺旋体（又名梅毒螺旋体）引起的一种慢性全身性感染的性传播疾病。

【Etiology】

The pathogen of syphilis, *Treponema pallidum*, is a delicate spiral facultative anaerobe. The living organism is motile and can be recognized under dark field microscopy by its characteristic movements: rotation, flexion, serpentine motion (undulation) and sidewinding. The organism is easily killed *in vitro* by heat, drying, soaps and antiseptics in a short period; however, it may survive for several hours on moist household appliances or towels. Even though the optimum temperature for *Treponema pallidum* growth is 37 ℃, it can resist cold and survive at 0 ℃ for 48 hours, and furthermore, it has been noted that specimens excised from syphilitic lesions retain their infectivity when kept at −78 ℃ for several years.

【病因】

梅毒的病原体为苍白密螺旋体（梅毒螺旋体），是一种细小的螺旋状兼性厌氧微生物。活的螺旋体在暗视野显微镜下可以观察到特征性的三种运动方式：旋转、伸缩、蛇行。梅毒螺旋体在人体外很容易死亡，煮沸、干燥、肥皂水及一般消毒剂均可短期内将其杀死。在潮湿的器具或毛巾上可存活数小时。梅毒螺旋体的最适温度是 37 ℃，但耐寒力强，0 ℃可存活 48 h，梅毒病损的切除标本在−78 ℃低温冰箱内保存数年仍具有传染性。

【Route of Infection】

Humans are the only known hosts for *Treponema pallidum*. The common routes of transmission of syphilis are summarized as follows.

(1) Sexual contact: this accounts for more than 95% of cases. Untreated patients have the highest infectivity for 1-2 years after infection.

(2) *In utero*: this generally occurs after the fourth month of pregnancy, resulting in miscarriage, premature labor and fetal death, or the bringing to term of a congenital syphilitic infant. *In utero* transmission occurs primarily in mothers who are themselves in the early stage of syphilis and only rare when the mother is in the later stage.

(3) Maternal birth canal: the fetus acquires the infection when passing through the birth canal of mother with syphilis. Chancre (described in primary syphilis) usually develops on the wounds of head and shoulders, which makes this mode of transmission distinguishable from congenital (*in utero*) syphilis.

(4) Transfusion: this occasionally occurs in people who receive blood transfusions containing *Treponema pallidum*.

(5) Non-sexual contact: though quite rare in reality (but often incorrectly attributed), infection may be spread either directly by

【传染途径】

人是梅毒螺旋体的唯一宿主。其传播途径常见有以下几种。

（1）性接触传染　占 95%以上。未经治疗的患者，感染后 1～2 年内具有强传染性。

（2）胎盘传染　多发生在妊娠 4 个月以后，导致流产、早产和死胎或分娩胎传梅毒儿。胎盘传染主要发生在早期梅毒孕妇，晚期较少。

（3）产道传染　梅毒孕妇在分娩时，新生儿通过产道时发生感染，常在头部、肩部擦伤处发生硬下疳（见一期梅毒中的描述），是区别于胎传梅毒的标志。

（4）输血感染　个别患者可因输入有传染性的梅毒患者的血液而被感染。

（5）非性接触传染　少数患者可因与梅毒患者皮肤黏膜发生直接接触而被

close contact with syphilitic patients (e. g., kissing, nursing and even hand-shaking), or else indirectly by contact with contaminated towels, bedding, razors or other medical appliances.

感染,包括接吻、哺乳、握手等;也可因接触带有梅毒螺旋体的毛巾、被褥、剃刀、医疗器械而间接被感染,但经这些途径传染的病例极少。

【Stages of Syphilis】

Syphilis can be classified into acquired (postnatal) syphilis and congenital (placenta transmitted) syphilis based on the mode of transmission, or can be divided into early syphilis and late syphilis according to the clinical course of the disease. Early syphilis is defined as the first two years after infection and late syphilis is infection for more than two years.

【梅毒的分期】

梅毒根据传染途径的不同可分为获得性(后天)梅毒和胎传(先天)梅毒,又可根据病程长短分为早期梅毒和晚期梅毒。前者病程在 2 年以内,后者在 2 年以后发病。

【Clinical Manifestations】

1. Acquired syphilis (postnatal syphilis)

1) Primary syphilis

Chancre is the main symptom of primary syphilis and the incubation period is 2-4 weeks. Primary syphilis is acquired via direct sexual contact with the infectious lesions of a person with syphilis. This chancre is a painless skin inflammation occurring at the points of contact with the infected lesion(s). The lesion first presents as a miliary sized, red, elevated papule. The typical chancre is a 1-2 cm round or oval, well-demarcated, superficial ulcer with elevated margin and a smooth and clean surface exuding serous fluids, which harbors large amounts of highly contagious *Treponema pallidum*. Apparent infiltration in this painless chancre may cause the lesion to be more palpable and give a cartilage-like hardness. Atypical chancre can occasionally present as multiple, deep, painful, or purulent exudant. The genital chancre is commonly located on the labia majora, labia minora, vagina or cervix in women; and on the penis, coronary sulcus, or glans and prepuce in men (Fig. 27-1). Extragenital chancre may occur on the anus, lips, tongue, breasts and fingers. The lesion usually heals spontaneously in 3-8 weeks without treatment.

Inguinal or regional lymphadenopathy may occur 1-2 weeks after the chancre appearance, and usually involves several lymph nodes (unilateral or bilateral) that become swollen, firm, isolated, mobile and painless without ulceration or suppuration. The overlying skin of the enlarged lymph nodes shows no redness, swelling or warmness.

2) Secondary syphilis

When primary syphilis is left untreated, or the course of treatment is interrupted or terminated prematurely, the person is likely to develop secondary syphilis, in which treponemas enter the

【临床表现】

一、获得性梅毒(后天梅毒)

(一)一期梅毒

一期梅毒的主要症状为硬下疳(chancre),潜伏期一般为 2～4 周,常通过直接性接触具有传染性的梅毒患者产生,是发生在梅毒螺旋体侵入部位的无痛性炎症反应。初起为粟粒大小、高出皮面的红色丘疹,典型硬下疳表现为 1～2 cm 的圆形或椭圆形浅在性溃疡,界限清楚、边缘隆起、基底平坦、表面光滑,有少量浆液分泌物,内含大量梅毒螺旋体,具有很强的传染性;触诊浸润明显,呈软骨样硬度,无明显疼痛。硬下疳也可不典型,表现为多个溃疡、深溃疡、溃疡表面有脓性渗出液、自觉疼痛等。通常好发于外生殖器,女性好发于大小阴唇、阴道、子宫颈,男性多见于阴茎、冠状沟、龟头包皮(图 27-1)。生殖器外的发病部位有肛门、唇、舌、乳房、手指等处。通常 3～8 周硬下疳可不治自愈。

硬下疳出现后 1～2 周,腹股沟或患处附近淋巴结可肿大,多累及数个,可为单侧或双侧,无痛,相互孤立不粘连,质硬,不发生化脓或破溃,其表面皮肤无红热或肿胀。

(二)二期梅毒

一期梅毒未经治疗或治疗不彻底,螺旋体由淋巴系统进入血液循环形成螺旋体菌血症,引起皮肤、黏膜、骨骼、内

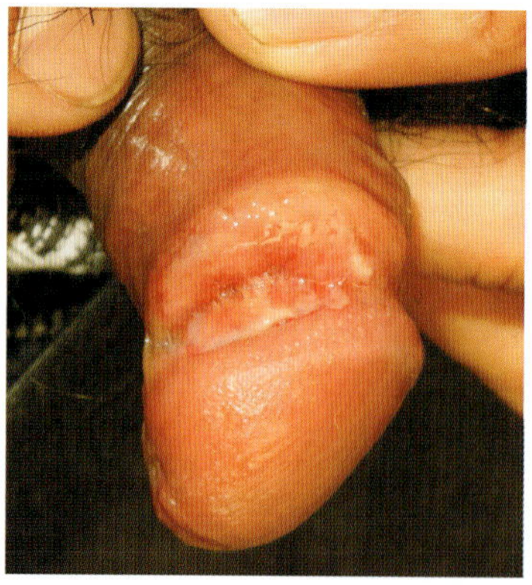

Fig. 27-1　Chancre(图 27-1　硬下疳)

bloodstream via the lymphatic system and cause bacteremia, affecting the skin, mucosa, skeleton, internal organs, cardiovascular and nervous systems. It usually occurs 4-6 weeks after the primary chancre resolves, but may occasionally occur concurrently with the chancre.

脏、心血管系统及神经系统损害,称为二期梅毒,常发生于硬下疳消退后 4～6 周,偶尔可与硬下疳同时出现。

Many types of cutaneous and mucosal lesions can be seen in secondary syphilis. Their common characteristics are summarized as follows: ① the rashes are more diffused and often symmetrical (except in cases of condylomata lata), bronze-colored, most commonly appearing on the palms and soles; ②all skin and mucosal lesions and the secretions are highly infectious and harbor a large population of treponemal organisms; ③ most patients are asymptomatic, except for pruritus in cases of condylomata lata; however, the objective symptoms are prominent; ④the lesions are less destructive, but highly infectious, and can resolve in a few weeks even if untreated; ⑤syphilis seropositive.

二期梅毒有多种皮肤黏膜损害,其共同特征为:①皮损泛发对称(除扁平湿疣外),多呈铜红色,好发于掌跖;②皮损和分泌物中有大量的梅毒螺旋体,传染性强;③皮疹一般无任何自觉症状(唯扁平湿疣可有痒感),而客观症状明显;④皮疹破坏性弱但传染性强,不经治疗持续数周可自行消退;⑤梅毒血清反应阳性。

(1) Skin rashes: the skin rashes for secondary syphilis vary in appearance, including macula, maculopapule, papule, papulosquamous rash, follicular rash and pustular eruptions, among which macular and papular syphilids are the most common. These rashes are usually diffused and symmetrical and can present alone or along with other types of rash. The lesions of recurrent secondary syphilis are fewer in number and circumscribed and they often present with weird shapes such as rings or crescents.

(1) 皮疹　呈多形性,包括斑疹、斑丘疹、丘疹、丘疹鳞屑疹、毛囊疹及脓疱疹等,常泛发对称。最常见的是斑疹和丘疹,常为一种或多种类型同时存在。二期复发梅毒,皮损局限,数目较少,皮损形态奇异,常呈环状或弓形。

①Macular syphilids (roseola syphilitica): these are the earliest lesions of secondary syphilis. They are round or oval, 1-2 cm sized, rose or brownish-red colored, non-confluent macules occurring mostly on the trunk and proximal extremities. The dark copper-colored infiltrative macules covered with collarette scales on the surface especially on the palms and soles are characteristic for this form of syphilids (Fig. 27-2 to Fig. 27-4).

①斑疹性梅毒疹(梅毒玫瑰疹):最早出现的二期梅毒疹,圆形或椭圆形,直径为 1～2 cm,玫瑰色或褐红色,互不融合,好发于躯干及四肢近端,尤其是掌跖部位的暗铜红色深在的浸润斑表面有衣领样鳞屑具有特征性(图 27-2 至图 27-4)。

②Papular syphilids: this type of syphilids arises a little later

②丘疹性梅毒疹:较斑疹性梅毒疹

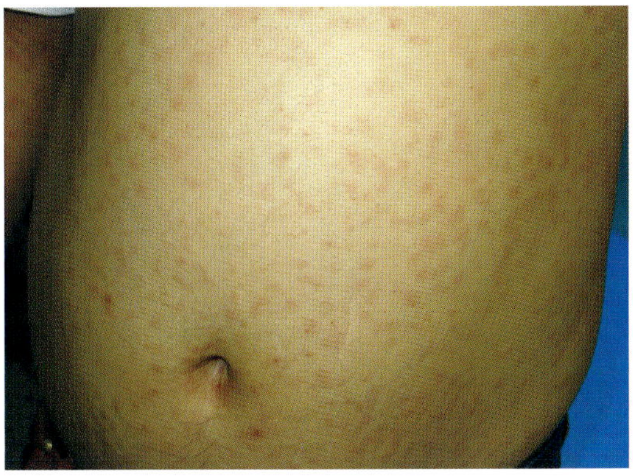

Fig. 27-2　Macular syphilids-on the trunk
(图 27-2　斑疹性梅毒疹-躯干部)

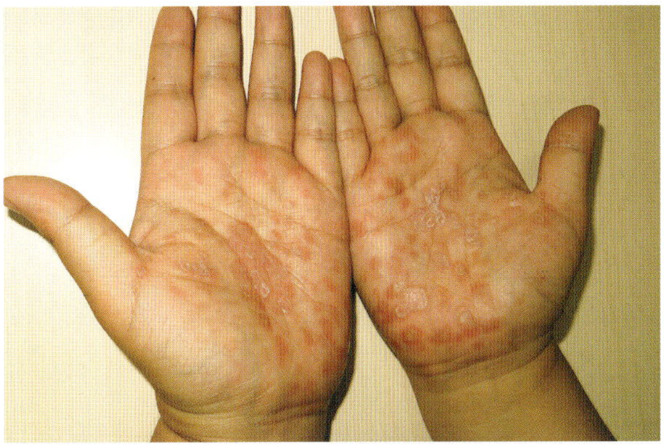

Fig. 27-3　Macular syphilids-on the palms
(图 27-3　斑疹性梅毒疹-手掌)

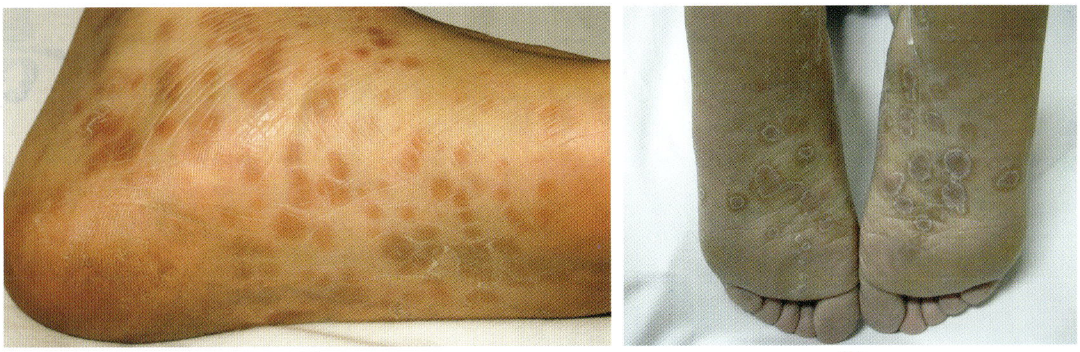

(a)　(b)

Fig. 27-4　Macular syphilids-on the soles(图 27-4　斑疹性梅毒疹-足底)

than the macular syphilids. They are typically 2-5 mm or larger in size, flesh or yellowish-red colored, slightly raised and firm papules. The surface of the papules is smooth or covered with adherent scales. Papules are frequently distributed on the face, the trunk and the flexures of the extremities (Fig. 27-5).

Condylomata lata: a special type of papular syphilids that generally occurs in the intertriginous moist areas, particularly the anogenital areas, armpit and groin (Fig. 27-6). The typical lesions are moist flat-topped papules that may enlarge or coalesce into grayish flat or lobular verrucous lesions. The bases are wide and sessile with copper-red infiltration around the rashes.

③Pustular syphilids: this is a rare type of secondary syphilids that only occurs in those persons in very poor health.

(2) Mucosal lesions: they are commonly present as pharyngitis or mucous patches on the tongue, throat or genitals. Mucous patches are the most characteristic mucosal lesions, which are round or oval grayish patches with a clear border and a moist surface. A narrow erythema band may be found around the periphery and a superficial ulcer can be seen after the grayish necrotic membrane is peeled.

出现稍晚，直径为 2～5 mm 或略大，为肉红色或黄红色、略高出皮面坚实的丘疹，表面光滑或被覆有粘连性鳞屑，皮疹好发于颜面、躯干、四肢屈侧(图 27-5)。

扁平湿疣(condylomata lata)：是丘疹性梅毒疹的特殊类型，好发于肛周、生殖器、腋窝、腹股沟等皱褶、多汗部位(图 27-6)。初起为表面湿润的扁平丘疹，随后扩大或融合成灰白色扁平或分叶状的疣状损害。其基底宽而无蒂，周围有铜红色浸润。

③脓疱性梅毒疹：罕见，多见于身体衰弱者。

(2) 黏膜损害　多见于舌、咽、喉或生殖器黏膜，表现为咽炎及黏膜斑。黏膜斑为特征性黏膜损害，呈圆形或椭圆形、灰白色的斑片，边缘清楚，表面潮湿，周边有狭小的红斑带，剥去灰白色坏死膜，可见浅表性溃疡。

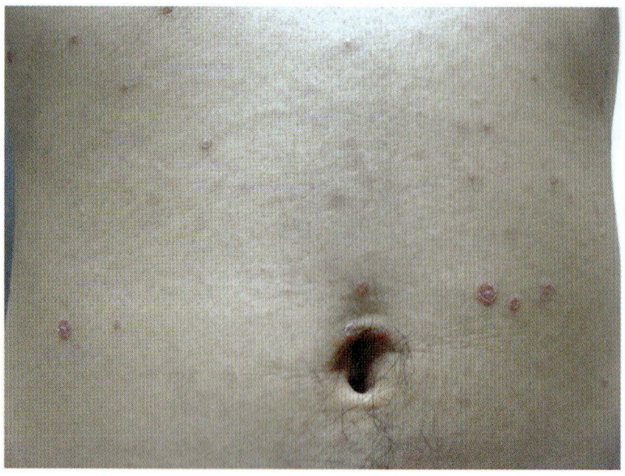

Fig. 27-5 Papular syphilids(图 27-5 丘疹性梅毒疹)

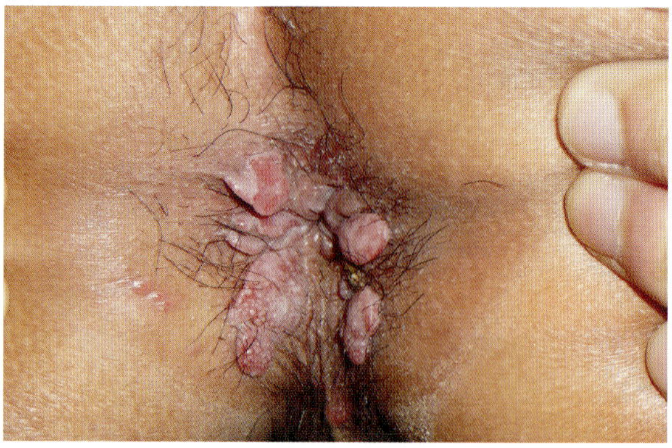

Fig. 27-6 Condylomata lata(图 27-6 扁平湿疣)

(3) Syphilitic alopecia: this is a relatively late development of the disease and it can present as syphilitic alopecia areata or diffuse alopecia. Syphilitic alopecia areata mimics alopecia areata with many 0.5 cm alopecic spots which are referred to moth-eaten or honeycomb alopecia (Fig. 27-7). In diffuse alopecia, the alopecia area is larger and the hair is thin and of variable length. The hair loss is not restricted to the scalp, and can extend to the eyebrows, eyelashes, beard and pubic hair. The hair loss is not permanent, and the hair will regrow in the affected area with or without treatment.

(3) 梅毒性脱发　通常发生较晚，表现为梅毒性斑秃或弥漫性秃发。梅毒性斑秃表现类似斑秃，为多个0.5 cm左右的秃发斑，呈虫蚀状或蜂窝状(图 27-7)；弥漫性面积较大，头发稀疏，长短不齐。梅毒性脱发不仅累及头发，还可累及眉毛、睫毛、胡须和阴毛。这种脱发为非永久性，及时治疗(有的甚至未经治疗)也可再生。

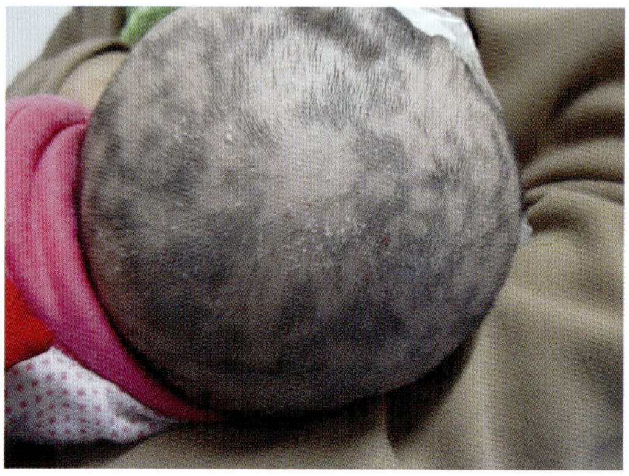

Fig. 27-7 Syphilitic alopecia(图 27-7 梅毒性脱发)

(4) Nail involvement: nail involvement includes changes on the nail plate (syphilitic onychia) or periungual tissue (syphilitic paronychia). Nail plate manifestations include the following: onychodystrophy, nail pitting, onycholysis and onychogryphosis. In syphilitic paronychia, painful violaceous inflammatory indurations appear around nail folds, but rarely transform into abscesses.

(4) 梅毒甲损害　包括甲板损害(甲床炎)和甲周组织损害(甲沟炎)。甲板损害表现为甲变形、甲凹陷、甲剥离、嵌甲；甲沟炎表现为甲襞周围痛性紫色炎性硬结，但很少出现脓肿。

3) Tertiary or late syphilis

About 40% of untreated or incompletely treated patients with early syphilis will develop tertiary syphilis after a latent period of 2-4 years. Besides the cutaneous, mucosal and bone lesions, other systems (especially the cardiovascular and central nervous systems) may be involved, which may be life threatening.

(三) 三期梅毒(晚期梅毒)

早期梅毒未经治疗或治疗不充分，经过一定潜伏期，一般为2～4年，约有40%梅毒患者发生三期梅毒，除在皮肤、黏膜、骨出现梅毒损害外，还会侵犯其他系统，特别是心血管系统及中枢神经系统等重要器官，可危及生命。

There are many documented forms of tertiary syphilis, but all have the following characteristics in common: ①the lesions appear asymmetrically, are few in number and tend to be more localized, but their destruction is more pronounced, and when healed, they leave atrophic scars; ② the subjective symptoms are mild, but the objective symptoms are severe; ③treponemas are usually not found in the lesions, indicating less or no infectivity at this stage; ④positive rate for *Treponema pallidum* detection in serologic tests is low.

三期梅毒损害类型很多，其共同点是：①损害分布不对称，局限，数目少但破坏性大，愈后留有萎缩性瘢痕；②自觉症状很轻但客观症状严重；③损害内梅毒螺旋体少，传染性弱或无传染性；④梅毒血清阳性率低。

(1) Cutaneous and mucosal lesions of tertiary syphilis: the late cutaneous lesions include nodular syphilids, gumma and syphilitic joint-articular nodules. Tertiary mucosal lesions are likely to appear as saddle nose, perforation of the palate and nasal septum caused by gummatous lesions on the tongue, palate and nasal septum mucosa. Among these manifestations at the late stage, nodular syphilids and gummata are the two major types.

(1) 三期梅毒皮肤黏膜损害　晚期皮肤损害有结节性梅毒疹、树胶样肿及近关节结节。晚期黏膜损害多表现为口舌、上腭及鼻中隔黏膜树胶肿，导致上腭及鼻中隔穿孔和马鞍鼻。其中以结节性梅毒疹和树胶肿最常见。

①Nodular syphilids: the lesions frequently occur on the head and face, the back and the extensors of the limbs. The nodules are 0.2-1.0 cm in size, copper-colored, firm and tend to form clusters. The surface of the nodules is smooth or covered with thin scales. The healing process will leave superficial atrophic scars and hyperpigmentation with new lesions occurring at the periphery.

①结节性梅毒疹：好发于头面部、背部及四肢伸侧，直径为 0.2～1.0 cm，簇集、坚硬的铜红色小结节，表面光滑或附有薄鳞屑。愈后留下浅表萎缩性瘢痕和色素沉着，边缘可出现新损害。

② Gummata: also known as syphilitic gummata, are the hallmark and the most destructive lesions of tertiary syphilis. The lesion is often solitary and occurs most commonly on the legs although any part of the body can be involved. Usually, the lesions begin with deep subcutaneous nodules, which gradually enlarge and affect the skin above them to form dark red infiltrated plaques. The central parts of the lesions gradually become softened and ulcerated which lead to the formation of deep punched-out ulcers with steep sides and a gummy exudate.

②树胶肿：又称为梅毒性树胶肿，是三期梅毒的特征性表现，也是破坏性最大的一种损害。可发生在全身各处，以小腿多见，常单发。初起为皮下深在结节，逐渐增大与皮肤粘连，形成表面呈暗红色的浸润斑块，中央逐渐软化、破溃呈穿凿性，侧壁陡峭，有黏稠树胶状脓汁流出。

③ Syphilitic joint-articular nodules: also known as syphilitic fibromas, which are rarely seen. They usually occur near the elbow, knee, hip, ischium and other joints, appearing as pea to walnut-sized, round or oval, painless subcutaneous fibrous nodules. They are firm, mobile and grow slowly and symmetrically with normal skin surface. In general, the subjective symptoms are not obvious.

③梅毒性近关节结节：又称梅毒性纤维瘤。此型少见，发生于肘、膝、髋及坐骨关节或其他关节附近的豌豆至胡桃大小、圆形或椭圆形、无痛性皮下纤维结节，生长缓慢，对称分布，质地坚硬，与周围组织无粘连，表面皮肤正常，无明显自觉症状。

④ Tertiary mucosal lesions: a gumma on the hard palate usually leads to perforation near the central part of the hard palate thus resulting in the perforation between oral cavity and nasal cavity, and producing one of the characteristic symptoms of tertiary syphilis. Gummata are also commonly formed at the nasal septum

④晚期黏膜损害：硬腭的结节性树胶肿往往使硬腭近中央部发生穿孔，造成口腔与鼻腔间穿孔，为三期梅毒的特征性表现。鼻中隔亦常形成树胶肿，出现鼻中隔穿孔，形成鞍鼻。

and may cause perforation of the nasal septum or saddle nose afterwards.

(2) Late bone syphilis: presents most commonly asperiostitis of the long bones, or rarely as gummatous osteoarthritis. Osteocope (or bone pain), most often worsened at night, is a suggestive symptom. This is a chronic condition and can develop into pathological fractures, bone perforation, joint deformity or stiffness in severe cases.

(2) 晚期骨梅毒　最常见的是长骨的骨膜炎，其次为树胶肿性骨关节炎。骨骼疼痛、夜间加重具有诊断意义。病程缓慢，可致病理性骨折、骨穿孔、关节畸形或强直等严重病变。

(3) Late cardiovascular syphilis: generally occurs after the infection which has run a course of 10-20 years. It can manifest as a wide spectrum of possible cardiovascular symptoms such as syphilitic aortitis simplex, syphilitic aortic incompetence, syphilitic coronary stenosis or choke, syphilitic aortic aneurysm and myocardial syphilitic gumma.

(3) 晚期心血管梅毒　多发生在感染后 10～20 年。临床上有单纯性梅毒性主动脉炎、梅毒性主动脉瓣关闭不全、梅毒性冠状动脉狭窄或阻塞、梅毒性主动脉瘤及心肌梅毒树胶肿五种类型。

(4) Late neurosyphilis: generally develops within 3-20 years of infection. It can manifest as any combination of meningovascular neurosyphilis, myelophthisis, dementia paralytica and optic atrophy.

(4)晚期神经梅毒　多在感染后 3～20 年发病，主要有脑膜血管型神经梅毒、脊髓痨、麻痹性痴呆、视神经萎缩等严重神经梅毒。

2. Congenital syphilis (placenta transmitted syphilis)

Congenital syphilis is acquired in uterus from the mother who usually has early stage syphilis at the time of birth. Infection through the placenta generally occurs after the fourth month of gestation. The outcomes of prenatal syphilis can be fetal death, miscarriage or a syphilitic infant. According to the time of onset, congenital syphilis can be divided into early congenital syphilis, late congenital syphilis and congenital latent syphilis. All resemble acquired syphilis except that the precursor chancre (lesion of primary syphilis) does not appear.

二、先天梅毒(胎传梅毒)

梅毒可由早期梅毒孕妇经胎盘传给胎儿，通常约在怀孕 4 个月后经胎盘传染，胎儿可发生死亡、流产或分娩出先天梅毒儿。根据胎儿发病时间的不同，先天梅毒可分为早期先天梅毒、晚期先天梅毒和先天潜伏梅毒，其经过与后天梅毒相似，特点是不发生硬下疳(一期损害)。

1) Early congenital syphilis

Early congenital syphilis occurs during the first 2 years of life. The newborn is usually premature, dystrophic, marasmic (due to severe malnutrition) and irritable. The face is wrinkled and drawn, resembling that of an old man. In severe cases, there is secondary anemia and fever of varying degrees.

(1) Cutaneous and mucosal lesions: usually appear after the third week of life, including macula, papule, bulla and pustule, which resemble those of acquired secondary syphilis. The macular rashes are commonly seen on the palms and soles, perioral areas and buttocks. The lesions on the perioral and perianal areas usually coalesce into infiltrated dark red patches with radial fissures on the surface, and characteristic radial scars after healing. Condylomata lata can be readily found in the vulva, perianal areas and other intertriginous folds of the body. Grayish mucous patches may be seen in the oral cavity.

(一) 早期先天梅毒

2 岁以内发病者为早期先天梅毒，婴儿通常早产，有营养障碍、消瘦、烦躁等症状，面部皮肤干皱脱水呈老人貌，严重者出现不同程度的贫血及发热。

(1) 皮肤黏膜损害　皮损多在出生后 3 周出现，与后天二期梅毒大致相似，有斑疹、丘疹、大疱及脓疱等类型。斑疹多见于掌跖、口周、臀部，在口周及肛周斑疹常融合成深红色浸润性斑，形成放射状皲裂，愈后遗留的放射状瘢痕具有特征性。间擦部位如外阴及肛周常发生扁平湿疣，口腔可见灰白色黏膜斑。

Syphilitic rhinitis commonly appears within the first 2 months after birth, and this is a specific symptom of congenital syphilis. The initial manifestation of nasal mucosa involvement is catarrhal, and in progressive cases ulcers will develop.

(2) Early congenital bone syphilis: includes osteochondritis, periostitis and syphilitic dactylitis.

(3) Early congenital visceral syphilis: may manifest as a general enlargement of the lymph nodes, splenohepatomegaly, nephrotic syndrome, anemia, etc.

(4) Early congenital neurosyphilis: the clinical manifestations of early congenital neurosyphilis may not become evident until 3-6 months of life, at which meningitis is mostly often encountered. About one third of all neurosyphilis cases show cerebral edema of varying degrees, and these resemble the symptoms of secondary acquired syphilis.

梅毒性鼻炎多在出生后 2 个月内发生，为先天梅毒特殊症状。初期为鼻黏膜卡他症状，病情加剧后鼻黏膜出现溃疡。

(2) 早期先天骨梅毒　包括：①骨软骨炎；②骨膜炎；③梅毒性指炎。

(3) 早期先天内脏梅毒　常有全身淋巴结肿大、肝脾肿大、肾病综合征、贫血等症状。

(4) 早期先天神经梅毒　在出生后 3～6 个月出现明显的临床症状，以脑膜炎多见，约 1/3 患者可有不同程度的脑水肿，症状与二期获得性梅毒相似。

2) Late congenital syphilis

Late congenital syphilis generally presents first after age two, and new symptoms continue to appear until age 13-14. The progress of the disease resembles late acquired syphilis-i. e. , most patients are asymptomatic-but others may present with keratitis, bone and nervous system impairments, and, even more rarely, cardiovascular syphilis.

(1) Cutaneous or mucous membrane syphilids: are not common in this type of syphilis, but gummata are often seen on the hard palate or nasal septum mucosa.

(2) Ocular syphilis: about 90% of ocular syphilis is interstitial keratitis. It begins with intense pericorneal inflammation and soon extends into the cornea to form a characteristic diffused, cloudy cornea that leads to permanent partial or complete opacity of the cornea and ablepsia if persistent.

(3) Bone syphilis: periostitis and gumma are the two common types of bone syphilis. Periostitis affects the tibia mostly and gummatous lesions are more likely found in the long bones and in the skull. Another less frequent lesion is arthritis (Clutton joints), which usually manifests itself as a bilateral effusive, painless swelling and slight stiffness of the knee joints.

(4) Neurosyphilis: asymptomatic neurosyphilis can be seen in 1/3-1/2 of all late stage congenital syphilis cases, and this generally occurs in adolescence. Cranial nerve lesions are usually involved, especially the auditory or optical nerves.

(5) The developmental defects (stigmata) of late congenital syphilis include: ①Hutchinson teeth appearing on the central upper incisors, characterized by peg-shaped, cylindrical malformation with its cutting edge narrower than the base. The dental arrangement is

(二) 晚期先天梅毒

晚期先天梅毒多在 2 岁以后发病，到 13～14 岁才有多种症状相继出现，损害大致与晚期后天梅毒相似，绝大部分为无症状感染，其中以角膜炎、骨和神经系统损害最为常见，心血管梅毒罕见。

(1) 皮肤黏膜梅毒　发病率低，以树胶肿多见，好发于硬腭、鼻中隔黏膜。

(2) 眼梅毒　约 90%为间质性角膜炎，初起有明显的角膜周围炎，继之出现特征性、弥漫性角膜混浊，反复发作导致永久性部分或全部角膜混浊，引起失明。

(3) 骨梅毒　骨膜炎和树胶肿常见，骨膜炎常累及胫骨，而长骨和颅骨多发生树胶肿。罕见的一种骨损害称为 Clutton 关节，其特点为双侧渗出性、无痛性膝关节肿胀，轻度强直。

(4) 神经梅毒　1/3～1/2 晚期先天梅毒患者发生无症状神经梅毒，常常延至青春期发病，以脑神经损害为主，尤以听神经、视神经损害多见。

(5) 发育缺陷体征（标志性损害）①哈钦森牙：见于上中切牙，表现为半月形门齿，上宽下窄，牙体短而厚呈柱状，齿列不齐，间距稀疏。②桑葚齿：第一臼

irregular with wide spaces between the teeth. ②Mulberry molar is usually seen on the first molar. This is a hyperplastic lesion, in which the flat occlusal surface of teeth is covered with a group of little knobs resembling a mulberry or raspberry. ③ Thickening of sternoclavicular joints, resulting from bone warts at the junction between sternum and clavicle. ④Interstitial keratitis begins with acute keratitis and the cornea soon becomes opaque, resulting in partial or complete ablepsia. ⑤Nerve deafness generally occurs in school-aged children, starting with vertigo and progressing to complete hearing loss. ⑥ The Hutchinson triad, which comprises Hutchinson teeth, nerve deafness and interstitial keratitis.

齿常见，是一种增生性损害，牙齿的咬合面上覆盖较多细小的球形小体，形如桑葚。③胸锁关节增厚征：胸骨与锁骨连接处发生骨疣所致。④间质性角膜炎：初起为急性角膜炎，继之角膜混浊，部分或完全失明。⑤神经性耳聋：多发于学龄儿童，先有眩晕，随之听力丧失。⑥哈钦森三联征：哈钦森齿、神经性耳聋和间质性角膜炎合称为哈钦森三联征(Hutchinson triad)。

3) Congenital latent syphilis

Congenital latent syphilis has no clinical signs except the positive serological tests for syphilis.

(三) 先天潜伏梅毒

先天潜伏梅毒无临床症状，梅毒血清反应阳性。

3. Latent syphilis

Patients with this form of syphilis have an infectious history of syphilis, but either show no clinical signs at all, or else preexisting clinical signs have disappeared, leaving only seropositivity. Latent syphilis includes congenital and acquired latent syphilis, both of which can be further divided into early latent syphilis (less than 2 years after initial infection) and late latent syphilis (more than 2 years after the initial infection). Early latent syphilis includes: a. those who have a clear history of high-risk sexual behavior within 2 years but without such behavior earlier than 2 years ago; b. those whose manifestations are in line with the clinical features of primary or secondary syphilis but have had no diagnosis or treatment in the past 2 years; c. those whose sexual partners have clear histories of early syphilis infection in the past 2 years. Late latent syphilis also includes those patients whose infection has lasted more than 2 years but the actual stage of the disease could not be determined.

三、潜伏梅毒

凡有梅毒感染史，无临床症状或临床症状已消失，除梅毒血清阳性外，无任何阳性体征称为潜伏梅毒。潜伏梅毒包括先天潜伏梅毒和后天潜伏梅毒，均可分为早期潜伏梅毒(感染 2 年以内)和晚期潜伏梅毒(感染 2 年以上)。早期潜伏梅毒包括：a. 在过去 2 年内有明确的高危性行为史，而 2 年前无高危性行为史。b. 在过去 2 年内，有符合一期或二期梅毒的临床表现，但未得到诊断和治疗者。c. 在过去 2 年内，性伴侣有明确的梅毒感染史。晚期潜伏梅毒也包括病程＞2 年，无法判断病程者。

【Histopathology】

The main pathologic features of syphilis include: ①endangeitis, presenting as endothelial cell swelling and hyperplasia; ②perivasculitis, showing as the infiltration of abundant lymphocytes and plasmocytes; ③besides the changes described above, granulomatous infiltration of epithelioid cells and macrophages in late syphilitic patients.

【组织病理】

梅毒的基本病变主要有：①血管内膜炎，血管内皮细胞肿胀、增生；②血管周围炎，有大量淋巴细胞、浆细胞浸润；③晚期梅毒除上述变化外，还有上皮样细胞和巨噬细胞肉芽肿性浸润。

【Diagnosis and Laboratory Findings】

The information required for a diagnosis of syphilis is typically collected from the detailed medical history, the clinical manifestations, and the laboratory findings including dark-field microscopy of the skin lesions, serological tests, and most often

【诊断和实验室检查】

梅毒的诊断须结合详细的病史、临床表现以及有关的实验室检查，如皮损的梅毒螺旋体暗视野检查、梅毒血清学试验(包括非梅毒螺旋体试验的初筛检

preliminary screening with a nontreponemal test and confirmation with a treponemal-specific test, and cerebrospinal fluid examination.

(1) *Treponema pallidum* dark field examination: is the most reliable technique for diagnosis of cutaneous and mucosal syphilis in the early stages.

(2) Serological testing: is also necessary for the diagnosis of syphilis, especially in cases of latent syphilis. The serum containing the antibody against *Treponema palladium* forms an aggregation with various nontreponemal antigens that can be detected by the so called nontreponemal antigen tests such as the rapid plasma reagin (RPR), unheated serum reagin (USR), and Venereal Disease Research Laboratory (VDRL) tests. Several specific treponemal antigens that can be monitored by these named treponemal antigen tests such as *Treponema pallidum* particle agglutination (TPPA) test, *Treponema pallidum* hemagglutination assay (TPHA), and fluorescent treponemal antibody absorption (FTA-ABS) test. Compared with nontreponemal antigen tests, the treponemal antigen tests are more sensitive and specific even in late stage or latent syphilis.

(3) Cerebrospinal fluid examination: it may be helpful in confirming neurosyphilis. The measurement consists of cell counting and protein ratio measurement, VDRL aggregation detection, PCR determination and colloidal gold testing.

(4) Molecular biologic techniques: they based on *Treponema palladium* DNA detection and have also been applied successfully to diagnose congenital syphilis and neurosyphilis.

【Treatment】

General principles of treatment: ①early detection and prompt and sustained regular treatment are required in order to achieve the best outcome; ② a sufficient dose of each drug, strictly following therapeutic guidelines, as irregular treatment puts patients at risk for recurrence and may promote the early appearance of late-stage syphilis; ③adequate follow-up after treatment; ④all sexual partners of patient should be examined and treated at the same time.

(1) Early syphilis (including primary, secondary and early latent syphilis):

①Penicillin remains the first choice for treatment of all stages of syphilis. Patients with primary, secondary and early latent syphilis can be treated effectively with an intramuscular injection of 2.4 MU of benzathine penicillin G split into two injections on each buttock once a week for 2 weeks; or 0.8 MU of penicillin G

查和梅毒螺旋体特异性试验的确证检查)及脑脊液检查。

(1) 梅毒螺旋体暗视野显微镜检查　早期梅毒皮肤黏膜损害最可靠的诊断方法。

(2) 梅毒血清学试验　诊断梅毒必需的检查方法，对潜伏梅毒血清学诊断尤为重要。患者的血清中含有针对梅毒螺旋体的抗体，能与各种非螺旋体抗原和特异性梅毒螺旋体抗原产生凝集反应，前者能通过所谓的非梅毒螺旋体抗原血清试验，如快速血浆反应素试验(RPR)、血清不加热的反应素试验(USR)、性病研究实验室(VDRL)试验加以检测，后者可通过梅毒螺旋体抗原血清试验如梅毒螺旋体颗粒凝集(TPPA)试验、梅毒螺旋体血凝试验(TPHA)和荧光梅毒螺旋体抗体吸收(FTA-ABS)试验加以检测，梅毒螺旋体抗原血清试验更敏感、特异，尤其适用于晚期和潜伏期梅毒。

(3) 脑脊液检查　用于诊断神经梅毒，包括细胞计数、蛋白定量、VDRL 试验、PCR 检测和胶体金试验。

(4)分子生物学技术检测　基于梅毒螺旋体 DNA 检测的分子生物学技术，已成功地用于先天梅毒和神经梅毒的诊断。

【治疗】

治疗的一般原则：①及早发现，及时正规治疗，愈早治疗效果愈好；②剂量足够，疗程规则。不规则治疗可增大复发的风险及促使晚期损害提前发生；③治疗后要经过足够时间的追踪观察；④对所有性伴侣同时进行检查和治疗。

(1) 早期梅毒(包括一期、二期及早期潜伏梅毒)

①青霉素依然是治疗各期梅毒的首选药物。一期、二期及早期潜伏梅毒可采用如下方案得到有效治疗：苄星青霉素 G(长效西林)240 万 U，分两侧臀部肌注，每周 1 次，共 2 次；或普鲁卡因青霉素

procaine intramuscular injection once a day for 15 days. Alternatively, intramuscular or intravenous injection of 0.5～1 g of ceftriaxone can be applied once a day for 10 days.

②In penicillin-allergic patients, tetracycline 0.5 g orally four times a day or doxycycline 0.1 g orally twice a day for 15 days is effective. Erythromycin is an acceptable alternative, at the same dosage as tetracycline.

(2) Late syphilis (including tertiary cutaneous, mucosal and bone syphilis, late latent syphilis and latent syphilis with uncertain status) and secondary relapsing syphilis:

①Patients with tertiary syphilis, late latent syphilis and secondary relapsing syphilis can be given an intramuscular injection of 2.4 MU of benzathine penicillin G split into two injections on each buttock once a week for 3 weeks; or of 0.8 MU of penicillin G procaine intramuscularly once a day for 20 days. If another course is considered, there should be a 2 week interval between the episodes.

②In penicillin-allergic patients, tetracycline 0.5 g orally four times a day(prohibited for patients with liver and/ or renal failure) or doxycycline 0.1 g orally twice a day for 30 days or erythromycin (at the same dosage as tetracycline) is recommended.

(3) Syphilitic patients with cardiovascular symptoms: should be treated in hospital. Treatment for syphilis should not start until the cardiovascular symptoms (including heart failure) have been controlled. To avoid Jarisch-Herxheimer reaction, prednisone 10 mg orally twice a day for 3 days is recommended before penicillin for these patients. Usually, penicillin G crystalline begins with a small dose and is gradually increased. The recommended regimens include penicillin G crystalline intramuscular 0.1 MU once for the first day, 0.1 MU twice for the second day, 0.2 MU twice for the third day. From the fourth day, the treatments are list as follow: penicillin G procaine intramuscular 0.8 MU once a day for 15 days, which is considered as one course. A minimum of two episodes of treatment are required, with a 2 week interval between the episodes; or an intramuscular injection of benzathine penicillin G 2.4 MU split into two injections on each buttock once a week for 3 weeks. Again, doxycycline or erythromycin is an appropriate choice for patients with an allergy to penicillin.

(4) Neurosyphilis or ocular syphilis patients: should be admitted to the hospital. Prednisone may be used as mentioned above to avoid Jarisch-Herxheimer reaction. Penicillin G crystalline should be administered, 18.0 MU to 24.0 MU a day which can be given as 3.0 MU to 4.0 MU intravenously every 4 hours for 10-14

G,80 万 U,1 次/天,肌内注射(简称肌注),连续 15 天。替代方案:头孢曲松 0.5～1 g,1 次/天,肌注或静脉给药,连续 10 天。

②对青霉素过敏者可使用盐酸四环素 0.5 g,4 次/天,连服 15 天;或多西环素 0.1 g,2 次/天,连服 15 天;或红霉素,用法同盐酸四环素。

(2) 晚期梅毒(包括三期皮肤、黏膜、骨骼梅毒,晚期潜伏梅毒或不能确定病期的潜伏梅毒)及二期复发梅毒

①苄星青霉素 G,240 万 U,分两侧臀部肌注,每周 1 次,连续 3 周;或普鲁卡因青霉素 G,80 万 U,1 次/天,肌注,连续 20 天为一个疗程。也可考虑给第 2 个疗程,疗程间停药 2 周。

②对青霉素过敏者可口服盐酸四环素 0.5 g/次,4 次/天,连服 30 天(肝、肾功能不全者禁用);或多西环素 0.1 g,2 次/天,连服 30 天;或红霉素,用法同盐酸四环素。

(3) 有心血管症状的梅毒患者　应住院治疗,心血管症状(包括心力衰竭),应予以控制后,再开始抗梅毒治疗。为避免吉海反应,青霉素注射前一日口服泼尼松,10 mg/次,2 次/天,连续 3 天。水剂青霉素 G 应从小剂量开始,逐渐增加剂量。首日 10 万 U,1 次/天,肌注;次日 10 万 U,2 次/天,肌注;第三日 20 万 U,2 次/天,肌注。自第四日起按下列方案治疗:普鲁卡因青霉素 G,80 万 U,肌注,1 次/天,连续 15 天为一个疗程,共 2 个疗程(或更多),疗程间停药 2 周;或苄星青霉素 G 240 万 U,分为双侧臀部肌注,每周 1 次,共 3 次。对青霉素过敏者,可选用多西环素或红霉素。

(4) 神经梅毒、眼梅毒患者　应住院治疗,为避免吉海反应,可按上述方法口服泼尼松。水剂青霉素 G,每日 1800 万～2400 万 U,静脉滴注,即每次 300 万～400 万 U,每 4 h 一次,连续 10～14 天,

days (if necessary, followed by benzathine penicillin G 2.4 MU intramuscularly once a week for 3 weeks) or penicillin G procaine 2.4 MU once a day, together with probenecid 0.5 g orally four times a day for 10-14 days, followed by benzathine penicillin G 2.4 MU intramuscularly once a week for 3 weeks if necessary. Doxycycline or erythromycin is recommended for penicillin-allergic patients.

(5) Pregnant women with syphilis: should be carefully treated with penicillin. The dosage for the individual patient depends on the stage of the syphilis. A major concern in pregnant patients is that the use of tetracycline or doxycycline should be prohibited, since these drugs can lead to complications in the pregnancy. Penicillin G procaine 0.8 MU intramuscularly once a day for 10 days is recommended for most patients, but the course may be extended longer if necessary. Erythromycin 0.5 g orally four times a day for 15 days for early syphilis, and for 30 days for secondary relapsing syphilis and late syphilis are recommended for patients with penicillin allergy. Usually, two entire courses are required for the mother, the first in her first trimester and the second in the third trimester. Additionally, the newborn should receive penicillin treatment after delivery.

(6) Congenital (placenta transmitted) syphilis:

①Early congenital syphilitic children should be evaluated by a CSF examination. The course of treatment depends very much on the CSF testing results in these cases. Penicillin G crystalline 0.1-0.15 MU/kg intravenously each day split into three injections in every 8 hours or penicillin G procaine 0.05 MU/kg intramuscularly once a day for 10-14 days should be prescribed when the CSF reveals an abnormal range. If CSF tests are normal, benzathine penicillin G 0.05 MU/kg is given once a day in two doses and injected intramuscularly into each buttock.

②Children with late congenital syphilis are recommended to administer penicillin G crystalline 0.15 MU/kg a day split into equal dosage every 4-6 hours intravenously or intramuscularly; or penicillin G procaine 0.05 MU/kg intramuscularly each day, both treatments to last for 10-14 days. A second course of treatment may be needed in some cases. If CSF tests are normal, benzathine penicillin G 0.05 MU/kg is given once a day split into two doses and injected intramuscularly into each buttock. Erythromycin is the best alternative choice for children allergic to penicillin. Tetracycline is forbidden for children younger than 8 years old.

(7) Syphilis patients with HIV infection: should be treated with benzathine penicillin G 2.4 MU intramuscularly once a week for three weeks or with benzathine penicillin G 2.4 MU

必要时，继以苄星青霉素 G 240 万 U，1 次/周，肌注，连续 3 次。或普鲁卡因青霉素 G 240 万 U，1 次/天，同时口服丙磺舒每次 0.5 g，4 次/天，共 10～14 天，必要时，继以苄星青霉素 G 240 万 U，1 次/周，肌注，连续 3 次。对青霉素过敏者，可选用多西环素或红霉素。

（5）妊娠梅毒患者　根据孕妇梅毒的分期不同，采用相应的青霉素方案进行治疗，应特别注意的是四环素、多西环素由于可导致妊娠并发症应禁服。普鲁卡因青霉素 G，80 万 U/天，肌注，连续 10 天，必要时可延长疗程。对青霉素过敏者，只选用红霉素治疗，每次 0.5 g 口服，4 次/天，早期梅毒连服 15 天，二期复发及晚期梅毒连服 30 天。妊娠初 3 个月与妊娠末 3 个月各进行一个疗程。但其所生婴儿应用青霉素补治。

（6）先天梅毒(胎传梅毒)

①早期先天梅毒推荐方案：对早期先天梅毒儿应进行脑脊液评估，治疗很大程度上取决于 CSF 检查结果。脑脊液异常者给予水剂青霉素 G，10 万～15 万 U/(kg·d)，静脉滴注每 8 h 一次，连续 10～14 天，或普鲁卡因青霉素 G，5 万 U/(kg·d)，肌注，1 次/天，连续 10～14 天。脑脊液正常者，苄星青霉素 G，5 万 U/(kg·d)，一次分两臀肌注。

②晚期先天梅毒推荐方案：水剂青霉素 G，15 万 U/(kg·d)，每 4～6 h 一次，静注或肌注，连续 10～14 天。或普鲁卡因青霉素 G，5 万 U/(kg·d)，肌注，连续 10～14 天为一个疗程。可考虑给予第二个疗程。脑脊液正常者，苄星青霉素 G，5 万 U/(kg·d)，一次分两侧臀肌注。对青霉素过敏者，红霉素是最佳选择。小于 8 岁儿童禁用四环素。

（7）合并 HIV 感染的梅毒患者　苄星青霉素 G 240 万 U 肌注，1 次/周，共 3 次；或苄星青霉素 G 240 万 U 肌注一次，

intramuscularly once, along with other effective antibiotics. It should be noted that: ① all HIV-infected patients should be screened by serological testing for syphilis; all syphilis patients should undergo HIV antibody screening; ② if routine syphilis serological testing is unable to diagnose, a lesion biopsy should be conducted for immunofluorescence staining or silver staining to find *Treponema pallidum*; ③ all syphilis patients with HIV infection should undergo CSF examination via lumbar puncture to exclude neurosyphilis; ④ whether the drug dose or treatment course for syphilis patients with HIV infection needs to increase remains uncertain at this point. A CSF examination is recommended for all the patients with primary, secondary or latent syphilis to exclude neurosyphilis. When CSF examination is not available or neurosyphilis cannot be ruled out, the neurosyphilis regimens should be applied to for those patients; ⑤ patients should be closely monitored and followed up.

同时加用其他有效的抗生素。应注意:①所有 HIV 感染者应做梅毒血清学筛查;所有梅毒患者应做 HIV 抗体筛查;②常规的梅毒血清学检查无法确定诊断时,可取皮损活检,做免疫荧光染色或银染色找梅毒螺旋体;③所有梅毒患者,凡合并 HIV 感染者,应考虑做腰椎穿刺检查脑脊液以排除神经梅毒;④梅毒患者合并 HIV 感染是否要加大剂量或疗程治疗梅毒仍不明确,对一期、二期及潜伏梅毒建议检查脑脊液以排除神经梅毒,若不能实现,则建议用神经梅毒治疗方案来进行治疗;⑤对患者进行密切监测及定期随访。

【Follow-up】

Syphilitic patients who have been treated sufficiently and regularly should nevertheless be followed up closely. Regular physical examination and nontreponemal antigen tests will indicate whether the syphilis is cured or relapses.

【随访】

梅毒患者经足量、规则治疗后还应定期体检及进行非梅毒螺旋体抗原血清试验检查,以了解是否治愈或复发。

Hong-xiang CHEN(陈宏翔), Meng-wen HE (何蒙文)

Section Two Gonorrhea

第二节 淋 病

Gonorrhea is a sexually transmitted disease (STD) caused by the bacterium *Neisseria gonorrhoeae*, which often affects the urogenital mucous membranes of men and women, occasionally but not always including the anus, rectum and oral mucosae. This is one of the most common STDs and passes from one person to another predominately by sexual intercourse, though newborns may be infected from an infected mother through contact with the birth canal. The usual symptom of gonorrhea is a purulent urethral discharge and dysuria in males; but the urethritis and/or cervicitis in females may be too mild to be symptomatic.

淋病(gonorrhea)是一种由奈瑟淋球菌引起的性传播疾病(STD),主要累及男女患者的泌尿生殖器官黏膜(也可感染肛门、直肠或口腔黏膜),是最常见的 STDs 之一,性传播是主要的传播方式,新生儿可通过患淋病母亲的产道而被感染。在男性,常出现化脓性尿道分泌物、排尿困难等症状。在女性,初起为轻微的尿道炎或宫颈炎,易被忽视。

【Etiology】

Neisseria gonorrhoeae is the responsible pathogen of gonorrhea. This is a gram-negative, orbicular-ovate or kidney-shaped diplococcus, usually seen in pairs and 0.6-0.8 μm in diameter. *Neisseria gonorrhoeae* does not survive for long outside the body and can be easily killed by many disinfectants, or by boiling or drying; however, it is quite resistant within the human

【病因】

病原菌为奈瑟淋球菌,是一种革兰阴性双球菌,呈卵圆形或肾形,成对排列,直径为 0.6～0.8 μm。奈瑟淋球菌离开人体后不易生长,消毒剂、煮沸、干燥均能致其死亡,但在人体器官中则相当稳定。急性期常位于多形核白细胞的胞

body. In acute cases, *Neisseria gonorrhoeae* is usually found intracellularly, in polymorphonuclear leukocytes; and in chronic cases it may be found outside polymorphonuclear cells.

质内，慢性期位于胞外。

【Clinical Manifestations】

The incubation period may range from 1-14 days, but averages 3-5 days. 1% - 5% of men and 80% of women infected with gonorrhea never show symptoms. Typical symptoms in infected males include purulent discharge from the urethra, along with painful and frequent urination. If women do have symptoms, they can be non-specific and misdiagnosed as a bladder or vaginal infection; common symptoms include abundant vaginal discharge, dysuria and lower abdominal pain.

【临床表现】

潜伏期一般为 1～14 天，平均为 3～5 天。临床上 1%～5%男性和 80%的女性感染后无明显的临床症状。在男性，症状主要表现为尿道流脓、尿痛、尿频。女性可为非特异性症状，易误诊为膀胱感染或阴道感染，女性淋病的症状为阴道分泌物增多、尿痛、下腹痛。

1) Gonorrhea in men

In men the urinary tract is primarily affected, and the sexual organs are involved later.

(1) Gonorrheal urethritis: usually an acute purulent inflammation occurs after 2-3 days incubation period, which gives rise to a prickling or burning sensation during urination. The urethral orifice may be obstructed by aggregated exudates. Approximately twenty-four hours later, a viscid, creamy yellow or greenish-yellow discharge of pus from the urethra may be observed (Fig. 27-8). The subjective symptoms may be worse by then, especially during erections and micturition.

(一) 男性淋病

男性淋病最初累及尿道器官，然后累及性器官。

(1) 淋病性尿道炎 经过 2～3 天的潜伏期后，急性化脓性炎症加剧了排尿时的针刺感和烧灼感，渗出物聚集堵塞尿道外口。约 24 h 后，尿道排出黏性、奶黄或黄绿色脓液(图 27-8)，主观症状加重，勃起和排尿时有明显疼痛。

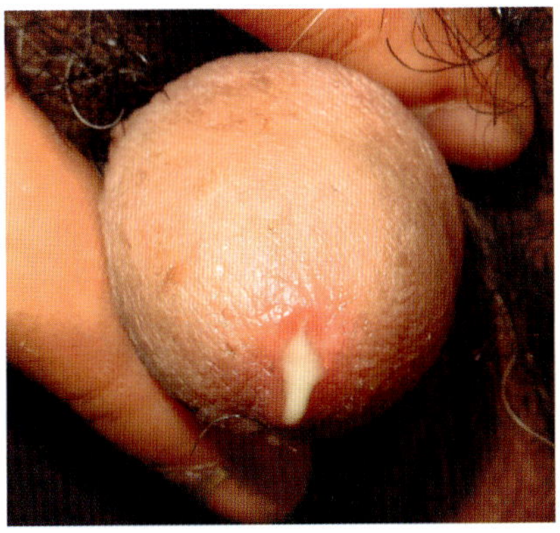

Fig. 27-8 Gonorrheal urethritis(图 27-8 淋病性尿道炎)

(2) Gonorrheal prostatitis: this is a complication of gonorrhea. It often occurs with urinary symptoms only and a pain localized to the urogenital area. The latter can progressively evolve into discomfort and bloating pain in the lower abdomen above pubic area and pelvic bone, rectal tenesmus and a constant urge to defecating. Unilateral or bilateral swellings of the prostate gland can be observed and may sometimes spread to the periprostatic tissue, which results in a more painful sensation during erection, ejaculation, or urination. Other severe complications are acute urinary retention, prostatic abscesses, etc.

(2) 淋病性前列腺炎 淋病的并发症，经常是仅有尿道症状和局部疼痛加重，进一步出现会阴部和耻骨上区坠胀不适感和直肠胀满、排便感。可发现单侧或双侧前列腺肿大，有时累及前列腺周围组织，勃起、射精或排尿时疼痛更明显。重者可并发急性尿潴留、前列腺脓肿等。

(3) Gonorrheal epididymitis: usually unilateral, this is an acute inflammation of the testicles that develops rapidly within hours, and then the swelling and pain increase in 1-2 days. The pain often radiates into the lower abdomen and groin area on the same side the testicle involved.

(4) Gonorrheal seminal vesiculitis or spermatocystitis: this is an inflammation of the seminal vesicles. The symptoms may not be distinguishable from those produced by the onset of acute prostatitis; however, semen mixed with blood or gonococci appearing in ejaculation may provide evidence of gonorrheal seminal vesiculitis.

(5) Gonococcal proctitis: here the rectum may be involved as a result of contamination by the infected genital discharge. Clinical signs include anal itching and burning sensations, tenesmus and rectal pain.

2) Gonorrhea in women

The most commonly involved sites of gonorrhea in women are the urethral orifice and the cervix.

(1) Gonorrheal urethritis: the typical clinical manifestation appears within 3-5 days after infection and is characterized by dysuria. Variable degrees of edema and erythema of the urethral meatus, purulent and/or mucopurulent discharge are present.

(2) Gonorrheal bartholinitis: this may occur when vaginal discharge spreads into the Bartholin's gland and is usually unilaterally involved. It is manifested by edema and erythema around the ductal orifice of the gland. When occlusion occurs, pseudoabscess or Bartholin's abscess can develop, accompanied by purulent related symptoms.

(3) Gonorrheal salpingitis: this is an infection of the fallopian tubes, mostly bilateral. In the acute stage, pain in the lower abdomen is common. Menstrual disorders can occur.

(4) Gonorrheal cervicitis: this is an inflammatory process developed in the mucosal layer of the cervical canal. Examination reveals edema and erythema of the vagina and part of the cervix. There may be a red crown around the external cervical orifice and a mucopurulent cervical discharge.

(5) Gonorrheal endometritis: this is the first stage of ascending gonorrhea with infection of the basal and functional layers of the endometrium. It is manifested by pain in the lower abdomen, high body temperature, and sometimes nausea and vomiting. The abdominal pain often has a spasmodic characteristic. Discharge is sanguine-purulent or mucopurulent. Uterus is painful when palpated. Chronic endometritis is characterized by menstrual disorders.

(3) 淋病性附睾炎　附睾的急性炎症，在数小时内迅速发展，常单侧发生，附睾肿大、疼痛明显，1～2天内加剧，同侧下腹部和腹股沟有反射性抽痛。

(4) 淋病性精囊炎　精囊的炎症，其症状有时与急性前列腺炎所致者无法区别，但自腺体排出的血精和淋球菌是确立本病诊断的唯一依据。

(5) 淋菌性直肠炎　直肠因受感染的生殖器排出物污染而被累及，轻者可有肛门瘙痒和烧灼感，重者可有里急后重和直肠疼痛。

(二) 女性淋病

女性淋病最常见的部位是尿道口和宫颈。

(1) 淋病性尿道炎　临床症状在感染后3～5天出现，表现为排尿困难，并出现不同程度的尿道口红斑、水肿、脓性或黏液脓性分泌物。

(2) 淋病性前庭大腺炎　通常为单侧，阴道分泌物中的淋球菌感染前庭大腺，引起导管外口周围红肿，当出现导管闭塞，可发展成假性脓肿或前庭大腺脓肿，并出现化脓性感染的症状。

(3) 淋病性输卵管炎　多为双侧输卵管感染，急性发作者常出现下腹痛，可出现月经紊乱。

(4) 淋病性宫颈炎　炎症性过程在宫颈管黏膜层发展，妇科检查示阴道和部分宫颈红肿，围绕宫颈外口有红冠，并出现黏液脓性宫颈分泌物。

(5) 淋病性子宫内膜炎　淋球菌逆行感染首先感染子宫内膜基底层和功能层，出现下腹痛、体温升高，有时有恶心、呕吐，腹痛常为间歇性，分泌物为血脓性或黏液脓性，并有子宫触痛，慢性子宫内膜炎表现为月经紊乱。

(6) Gonorrheal pelviperitonitis: this is a specific inflammation of the pelvic peritoneum and is a sequel to salpingo-oophoritis. The onset is usually acute. Severe lower abdominal pain, peritoneal irritation symptoms, vomiting, meteorism, constipation and high body temperature can all occur. Gonococcal inflammation is characterized by the tendency of adhesion process, which leads to localization of the inflammation in the pelvis.

(6) 淋病性盆腔腹膜炎 输卵管卵巢炎引起的盆腔腹膜的特殊炎症，多为急性发病，下腹部疼痛剧烈，可出现腹膜周围刺激症状、呕吐、腹胀、便秘、体温升高。淋菌性炎症倾向于粘连，导致骨盆炎症局限化。

3) Gonorrhea in children

(三) 儿童淋病

Mechanism of infection: babies can be infected by gonorrhea during delivery when a child passes through an infected birth canal or by intrauterine means through the amniotic fluid, or by nursing by the infected mother. Elder children may be infected if they share a bathtub or bath towel with a person infected with gonorrhea.

感染机制：出生时通过产道感染、宫内通过羊水感染、因患病母亲照管而感染，较大儿童因与淋病患者共用浴盆、浴巾而感染。

Ophthalmoblennorrhea in the newborn: the condition begins within 1-5 days of birth via a direct contact with gonococci in the birth canal. The initial symptoms include running eyes, photophobia and a mucoid secretion with crusted eyelids, which then is followed by pronounced swelling of the lids and abundant purulent discharge that is characteristic of the suppurative stage of gonorrheal conjunctivitis.

新生儿脓性眼炎：婴儿自淋球菌感染的产道出生后 1～5 天开始发病，起病症状表现为流泪、畏光、眼睑结有黏稠的脓性痂。睑板化脓，肿胀加重。病情进入淋病性结膜炎化脓期，有大量脓液形成。

Gonorrhea in young girls may manifest as edema and erythema of mucosal membranes accompanied by mucopurulent discharge, frequent and painful urination, and itching of the urethral tract. If the infection becomes more widespread and moves into the uterus or fallopian tubes, it may result in pelvic inflammatory disease (PID), which will typically cause a high fever.

幼女淋病表现为黏膜红肿，有黏液脓性分泌物、尿频和尿痛、瘙痒，如感染进一步扩散到子宫或输卵管，则引起盆腔炎症性疾病(PID)，常导致高热。

4) Disseminated gonococcal infection (DGI)

(四) 播散性淋球菌感染

Disseminated gonococcal infection (DGI), a rare serious complication of gonorrhea, is estimated to occur in 1%-3% of patients with gonorrhea. Clinical manifestations include skin lesions, arthralgias, tenosynovitis, arthritis, hepatitis, myocarditis, endocarditis and meningitis. DGI usually presents as an arthritis-dermatitis syndrome, in which patients experience migrating polyarthralgias primarily affecting the knees, elbows, and distal joints. Approximately 75% of DGI patients also show characteristic skin lesions consisting of discrete papules and pustules with a hemorrhagic tendency. If untreated, the arthritis tends to progress, involving more joints, such as those of the knee, ankle, elbow and wrist.

本病少见，是淋病的严重并发症，占淋病患者的 1%～3%。临床表现包括皮肤损害、关节痛、腱鞘炎、关节炎、肝炎、心肌炎、心内膜炎、脑膜炎，常出现关节炎-皮炎综合征，有迁移性多关节痛，累及膝、肘和末端关节。大约 75% 的患者有特征性皮炎，包括散在分布的丘疹和血性脓疱，若不处理，关节炎可发展至多个关节，包括膝、踝、肘、腕关节。

【Laboratory Findings】

【实验室检查】

No matter what form gonorrhea may take, the diagnosis of gonorrhea is always confirmed by pathogen detection. The common diagnostic tests for gonorrhea are smear staining and culture.

不管是哪种类型的淋病，检出病原体则可以确诊，常用的方法包括直接涂片和细菌培养。

(1) Smear staining: purulent secretion collected from the urethra or cervix is smeared on a slide and gram stained. Examination under microscopy shows abundant polymorphonuclear leukocytes and intracellular gram-negative diplococci.

(2) Bacterial culture: the laboratory culture test involves placing samples of the discharge onto selective culture plates. The gonococcal colonies usually appear on the culture plates after an incubation period of 2-3 days as fine transparent dewdrops. The typical gram-negative diplococcus will be revealed under microscopy, and oxidase testing will be positive once they are seen. Sugar fermentation and fluorescent antibody examination can be performed for diagnostic confirmation when necessary. PCR for gonorrhea DNA may also be used for pathogen detection due to its high sensitivity.

(1) 直接涂片　取尿道或宫颈脓性分泌物涂片，进行革兰染色，镜下可见大量多形核白细胞，细胞内可见革兰阴性双球菌。

(2) 细菌培养　标本在选择性培养基上培养，经孵育 2～3 天后，淋球菌菌落在培养皿上呈现为精细透明状的露珠，镜检可见到典型的革兰阴性双球菌，氧化酶试验阳性，必要时可做糖发酵及荧光抗体检查加以确诊。亦可用聚合酶链反应检测淋球菌 DNA，其敏感性高。

【Diagnosis and Differential Diagnosis】

The typical clinical features found in the variety of forms of gonorrhea, together with laboratory findings and epidemiologic characteristics should provide a conclusive diagnosis. The most common conditions requiring differentiation from gonorrhea are non-gonococcal urethra genital infections that are normally caused by other bacteria, and vaginitis caused by *Candida albicans* or *Trichomonas vaginalis*.

【诊断与鉴别诊断】

应根据流行病学史、临床表现和实验室检查结果进行综合分析，慎重做出判断。本病需和其他细菌引起的非淋菌性泌尿生殖道感染，以及白色念珠菌或阴道毛滴虫引起的阴道炎相鉴别。

【Treatment】

Ceftriaxone in a single intramuscular injection of 0.25 g is the treatment of choice for uncomplicated gonococcal infection of the urethra, cervix, and rectum. Alternative parenteral single-dose regimens include ceftizoxime 1.0 g or cefotaxime 1.0 g intramuscularly. For persons who are allergic to penicillin or cephalosporin, a single intramuscular dose of spectinomycin 2.0 g (4.0g for cervicitis) or a single oral dose of azithromycin 2.0 g is an alternative regimen.

Ceftriaxone in a single intramuscular injection of 1.0 g is the treatment of choice for disseminated gonococcal infection. An alternative regimen is 2.0 g of spectinomycin administered intramuscularly twice daily for more than 10 days.

【治疗】

无并发症的淋菌性尿道炎、宫颈炎、直肠炎，可给予头孢曲松钠 0.25 g，一次肌注；或头孢唑肟 1.0 g，一次肌注；或头孢噻肟钠 1.0 g，一次肌注。对青霉素或头孢类过敏者，大观霉素 2.0 g(宫颈炎 4.0g)，一次肌注；或阿奇霉素 2.0 g，一次口服。

播散性淋病，可给予头孢曲松钠 1.0 g 肌注，或大观霉素 2.0 g，肌注，2 次/天，连续 10 天以上。

【Prognosis】

The prognosis for patients with gonorrhea is excellent if the diagnosis is made and treatment started promptly. The recovery is usually complete unless complications occur. Gonococcal pelvic inflammatory disease (PID) may cause infertility, scarred fallopian tubes (leading to a higher risk of ectopic pregnancy in women) and chronic (long-lasting) abdominal pain.

【预后】

如果淋病能得到及时诊断和治疗，预后良好，如无并发症通常能痊愈。淋菌性盆腔炎能导致不孕、输卵管瘢痕(输卵管妊娠的高危因素)和慢性(持久性)腹痛。

Hong-xiang CHEN(陈宏翔), Song ZHANG (张颂)

Section Three Chlamydial Urogenital Infection

Chlamydial urogenital infections are the most common sexually transmitted disease in the United States and Europe. Its prevalence is the highest in persons aged less than 25 years. The incidence rate in China and elsewhere has also been increasing in recent years. Many studies have shown that individuals infected with *Neisseria gonorrhoeae* are often co-infected with *Chlamydia trachomatis*.

第三节 衣原体泌尿生殖道感染

在美国和欧洲国家，衣原体泌尿生殖道感染（chlamydial urogenital infection）是最常见的性传播性疾病，其发病率在年龄小于25岁的人群中是最高的。在中国和其他地区，近年来其发病率一直不断升高。而且，有研究显示，淋球菌感染者经常同时合并有沙眼衣原体感染。

【Etiology】

This disease is caused by *Chlamydia trachomatis* (*C. trachomatis*) and its serovars, of which the D-K serotypes are specifically associated with sexually transmitted diseases(STDs).

【病因】

本病由沙眼衣原体所致，其中与STDs相关的主要是D-K型沙眼衣原体。

【Clinical Manifestations】

The incubation period from time of exposure to onset of symptoms is usually 1-3 weeks, but it can be as long as 6 weeks. Chlamydial infection is always under-diagnosed because the majority of infected individuals are asymptomatic.

Among male patients, *C. trachomatis* mainly induces urethritis. Symptoms, if present, include purulent or mucopurulent discharge, dysuria, urethral pruritus or irritation, and underwear stains. Complications among men infected with *C. trachomatis* include epididymitis, prostatitis, and Reiter's syndrome.

C. trachomatis can cause infections other than urethritis in female patients, such as vaginitis or purulent cervicitis, etc. Symptoms in women may include vaginal discharge, dysuria, abdominal pain or abnormal vaginal bleeding. Perianal, rectal and oral involvements are not uncommon, and may result in local pruritus, discharge or pain during defecation. Most (about 90%) of oral infections are asymptomatic, but some people may experience sore throat. *C. trachomatis* infection in females may develop a variety of complications, among which the most severe ones include chronic pelvic inflammatory disease (PID), ectopic pregnancy, and tubal infertility.

Infection of neonates by *C. trachomatis* results from perinatal exposure to the mother's infected cervix. The infection in neonates is most frequently recognized by conjunctivitis that develops within 5-12 days after birth. *C. trachomatis* can also cause subacute, afebrile pneumonia in neonates aged 1-3 months.

【临床表现】

通常潜伏期为1～3周，也可长达6周。衣原体感染常常难以发现，因为大多数感染者是无症状的。

在男性患者中，沙眼衣原体感染主要引起尿道炎，如有症状，常表现为脓性或黏液脓性尿道分泌物、排尿时有疼痛或烧灼感、尿道瘙痒或刺激、内裤污迹等。并发症包括附睾炎、前列腺炎、Reiter综合征等。

在女性患者中，沙眼衣原体感染不仅可引起尿道炎，还可引起其他部位的感染，如阴道炎、化脓性宫颈炎等。其症状常表现为白带增多、排尿时有疼痛或烧灼感、腹痛、阴道异常出血等。肛周、直肠、口咽部的感染也并非罕见。肛周、直肠的感染可出现局部瘙痒、分泌物形成和排便疼痛。大多数(约90%)的口咽部感染者是没有症状的，但也可出现喉痛。女性沙眼衣原体感染者可出现多种并发症，其中，最严重的包括慢性盆腔炎、异位妊娠、输卵管性不孕等。

新生儿沙眼衣原体感染源于在围产期与被感染的母体宫颈相接触。感染沙眼衣原体的新生儿最常见的症状是在出生后5～12天出现结膜炎。沙眼衣原体还能在其出生后1～3个月引起无发热症状的亚急性肺炎。

【Laboratory Findings】

For asymptomatic, chronic or persistent chlamydial infection, diagnosis may be difficult. Recently, cell culture, direct detection of the pathogen antigens via direct immunofluorescence or EIA (enzyme immunoassay) and DNA-based techniques such as nucleic acid hybridization or NAATs (nucleic acid amplification test) have become available for the detection of *C. trachomatis*. The introduction of these methods has certainly increased the likelihood of detecting chlamydial infection, among which NAATs offers the best sensitivity as well as the necessary specificity for diagnosis, and should therefore be applied whenever possible in clinical practice.

Specimens of urine, urethral or cervical swabs from female patients; urine or urethral swab specimens from male patients; or rectal swabs from patients who have perianal or rectal infections resulting from receptive anal intercourse, are all acceptable for the assays described above.

【实验室检查】

无症状的、慢性或持续性衣原体感染的诊断比较困难。然而，近年来沙眼衣原体细胞培养、直接检查病原体抗原的方法（如直接免疫荧光或酶联免疫分析（EIA）），以及DNA技术（如核酸杂交、核酸扩增试验（NAATs））等均可用来检测沙眼衣原体，这些方法的应用提高了对沙眼衣原体感染的检出率。其中，NAATs是最具有敏感性和特异性的检测，应尽可能应用于临床标本的检测。

沙眼衣原体女性泌尿生殖道感染者可通过检测尿液、尿道或宫颈拭子等标本进行诊断；男性感染者可通过检测尿液、尿道拭子等标本进行诊断；肛交致肛周、直肠感染者可通过检测直肠拭子标本进行诊断。

【Diagnosis】

Chlamydial urogenital infection should be diagnosed on the basis of symptoms, signs and laboratory findings. All patients who have been confirmed or suspected to have urethritis (cervicitis) should be tested for *C. trachomatis*. Also, patients who have been diagnosed with genitourinary chlamydial infections should be tested for other STDs.

【诊断】

诊断主要根据其症状、体征及实验室检查。所有确诊或疑诊为尿道炎（宫颈炎）的患者均应行沙眼衣原体检测。另外，确诊为沙眼衣原体泌尿生殖道感染者还应进行其他常见性传播性疾病的相关检测。

【Differential Diagnosis】

It is necessary to differentiate chlamydial urogenital infection from gonorrhea. The Gram stain test, culture and NAATs are all helpful for differentiation.

【鉴别诊断】

本病应与淋病相鉴别。革兰染色、病原体培养、NAATs等均有助于鉴别。

【Treatment】

Treatment should be initiated as soon as possible once the diagnosis is established. Additionally, treatment of sex partners will help to prevent reinfection of the patient as well as prevent transmission of the infection to other sexual partners.

Chlamydial infections in adults: azithromycin 1 g orally in a single dose is the recommended primary regimen, or else doxycycline 100 mg orally twice a day for 7 days. Alternative regimens include erythromycin 500 mg orally four times a day for 7 days, minocycline 100 mg orally two times a day for 10 days, ofloxacin 300 mg orally twice a day for 7 days, or levofloxacin 500 mg orally once daily for 7 days.

【治疗】

一经诊断，应尽早治疗。而且，性伴侣也应治疗，这有助于防止再感染患者和感染性伴侣。

成人衣原体感染治疗方案如下。

推荐方案：阿奇霉素1 g，口服，1次/天，或多西环素100 mg，口服，2次/天，连服7天。

备选方案：红霉素500 mg，口服，4次/天，连服7天；米诺环素100 mg，口服，2次/天，连服10天；氧氟沙星300 mg，口服，2次/天，连服7天；左氧氟沙星500 mg，口服，1次/天，连服7天。

Chlamydial infections in pregnant women: here the recommended primary regimen is azithromycin 1 g orally in a single dose, or amoxicillin 500 mg orally three times a day for 7 days. Alternative regimens include erythromycin 500 mg orally four times a day for 7 days, erythromycin 250 mg orally four times a day for 14 days, erythromycin ethylsuccinate 800 mg orally four times a day for 7 days, or erythromycin ethylsuccinate 400 mg orally four times a day for 14 days.

孕妇衣原体感染治疗方案如下。

推荐方案：阿奇霉素 1 g，口服，1 次/天，或阿莫西林 500 mg，口服，3 次/天，连服 7 天。

备选方案：红霉素 500 mg，口服，4 次/天，连服 7 天；红霉素 250 mg，口服，4 次/天，连服 14 天；琥乙红霉素 800 mg，口服，4 次/天，连服 7 天；琥乙红霉素 400 mg，口服，4 次/天，连服 14 天。

Ophthalmia neonatorum or infantile pneumonia caused by *C. trachomatis*: the recommended regimen is erythromycin or erythromycin ethylsuccinate 50 mg/(kg · d) orally, dividing into 4 doses daily for 14 days.

沙眼衣原体感染所致新生儿眼炎或婴儿肺炎治疗方案如下。

推荐方案：红霉素或琥乙红霉素 50 mg/(kg · d)，分 4 次口服，连服 14 天。

【Prognosis】

A patient with chlamydial urethritis (cervicitis) has a good prognosis and infection can be completely resolved in most cases for patients undergoing regular treatment. However, patients may have persistent symptoms when the infection is mixed with other pathogens, or when a non-infective etiology exists.

【预后】

衣原体性尿道炎（宫颈炎）预后较好，经正规治疗后，大多数患者炎症可消退。但合并其他病原体感染或有非感染性致病因素存在的患者，症状可持续存在。

Hong-xiang CHEN（陈宏翔），Song ZHANG（张颂）

Section Four　Condyloma Acuminatum

Condyloma acuminatum (CA), also known as genital warts, is an anogenital warty growth caused by some types of the human papilloma virus (HPV). Recently condyloma acuminatum has become one of the most common sexually transmitted diseases (STDs) in China.

第四节　尖锐湿疣

尖锐湿疣（condyloma acuminatum，CA），又称为生殖器疣，是由人乳头瘤病毒（human papilloma virus，HPV）感染所致的肛门生殖器疣状赘生物，为我国近年来最常见的性传播疾病（sexually transmitted diseases，STDs）之一。

【Etiology and Epidemiology】

The term HPV does not describe a single specific virus, but a group of double-stranded DNA viruses. Approximately 40 different types of HPV have been associated with human anogenital warts. Most cases are caused by strains 6, 11, 30, 42, 43, 44, 45, 51, 52 and 54, in which HPV-6 and HPV-11 in particular are responsible for about 90% of genital warts. On the other hand, HPV-16 and HPV-18 have been linked to approximately 70% of the cases of cervical cancer.

Sexual transmission is the main route of the disease. If risk factors such as multiple sexual parters, unsafe sexual behavior, infection history of the sex partner exist, the transmission rate among the sex partners is about 60%. However, a minority of

【病因及流行病学】

HPV 不是一种单一特异性病毒，而是一组双链 DNA 病毒，可感染生殖器部位的 HPV 亚型大约有 40 种。大部分生殖器疣由 HPV-6、11、30、42、43、44、45、51、52 和 54 型感染导致。约 90%生殖器疣的病原体为 HPV-6 和 HPV-11，而约 70%子宫颈癌由 HPV-16 和 HPV-18 感染所致。

性传播为该病最主要的传播途径，如有多名性伴侣、不安全性行为、性伴侣感染史等，在性伴侣间传播率约为 60%。少数人也可通过非性传播途径感染，如

patients may also be infected by non sexual means, such as by close indirect contact with an infected patient, particularly in the case of newborns, having an HPV-infected mother. Over 50% of people encounter this virus at least once in their lives, but repeated HPV infections with certain HPV strains may put patients at greater risk for the development of precancerous lesions and cancer.

与尖锐湿疣患者有密切的间接接触史、新生儿的母亲为HPV感染者等。超过50%的人群在其一生中至少感染过一次HPV,但持续的高危型HPV感染是发展为癌前病变及癌的高危因素。

【Clinical Manifestations】

Condyloma acuminatum is often asymptomatic, but some patients may report itching, foreign body sensation, and a feeling of constriction or burning. In females, the warts may occur on the outside or inside of the vagina, or on the cervix, or around the anus, including the labia majora, the labia minora, the vaginal orifice, the vagina itself, the clitoris, the meatus, the cervix, or the perianal areas. In males, they usually appear on the frenulum, corona, glans, meatus, or may be seen on the shaft of the penis and scrotum, or sometimes around the anus (Fig. 27-9, Fig. 27-10). Rarely, genital warts will develop in the mouth or throat, and may often be linked to specific sexual behaviour.

【临床表现】

尖锐湿疣通常无自觉症状,少数患者可自觉痒感、异物感、压迫感或灼痛感。女性皮损可发生于阴道内外、宫颈和肛周,多见于大小阴唇、阴道口、阴道、阴蒂、尿道口、子宫颈和肛周。男性则多见于系带、冠状沟、龟头、尿道口,亦可见于阴茎部、阴囊或肛周(图27-9,图27-10)。偶可见发生于口腔或喉部,常由特殊的性行为引起。

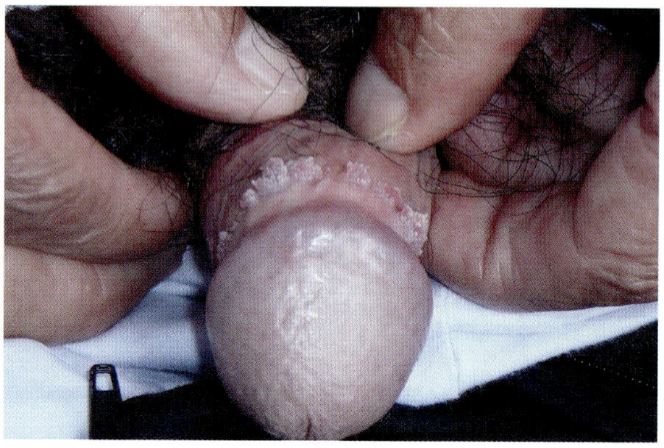

Fig. 27-9　Condyloma acuminatum-on the corona
(图27-9　冠状沟尖锐湿疣)

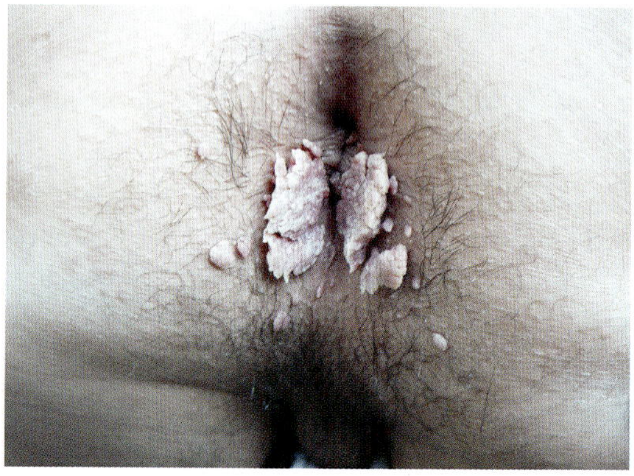

Fig. 27-10　Condyloma acuminatum-on the perianal region
(图27-10　肛周尖锐湿疣)

Condyloma acuminatum often occurs in clusters, and these clusters may either be very tiny in the genital area, or may grow into a large mass. Typically, the warts start with small slightly red papules, which are whitish when macerated. The lesions are usually multiple, especially on moist mucosal surfaces. Large cauliflower-like structures may form and may finally cover the entirety of the external genitalia.

尖锐湿疣通常表现为生殖器区域成簇分布的小赘生物,可融合成块。皮损初起为淡红色小丘疹,可因浸渍发白,常多发,在潮湿的皮肤黏膜表面尤为明显。大的菜花样赘生物最后可完全覆盖整个外生殖器。

【Histopathology】

Biopsy of the lesion area shows evidence of hyperkeratosis, acanthosis, papillomatosis and parakeratosis. Koilocytes are usually observed in the superficial epithelial cells. A chronic inflammatory infiltrate is often observed within the dermis.

【组织病理】

皮损部位活检示角化过度、棘层肥厚、乳头瘤状增生以及表皮角化不全,浅表上皮细胞内常可见空泡细胞,真皮层内通常有慢性炎性浸润。

【Diagnosis】

When the typical clinical features and histologic findings described above occur in individuals who have sexual contact or indirect contact with an infected person, along with a positive acetowhitening test, then condyloma acuminatum can be diagnosed.

【诊断】

如果患者曾与有感染史者发生性接触或间接接触，有典型皮损和组织病理学表现，醋酸白试验阳性，则可诊断为尖锐湿疣。

【Differential Diagnosis】

It is necessary to differentiate condyloma acuminatum from bowenoid papulosis of the genitalia, pseudocondyloma, pearly penile papules, and extramammary Paget's disease. Among them, bowenoid papulosis involves multiple benign proliferative lesions in the genital area which is also caused by HPV infection. This condition typically exhibits papules in sizes from a few millimeters to several centimeters across, and the colors vary significantly, from red to brown or various shades of brown (pigmented lesions). The surface of the lesions can be flat or verrucous. Bowenoid papulosis is often asymptomatic. The lesions may regress spontaneously in a few months. The histopathology of bowenoid papulosis is similar to those presented in Bowen's disease, which is characterized by circumscribed epidermal clusters of pleomorphic cells. Dyskeratotic cells can be easily found as well. Regardless clumped nuclei and abnormal mitoses in these pleomorphic cells, bowenoid papulosis usually shows a lesser degree of cytologic atypia than Bowen's disease.

【鉴别诊断】

本病需和生殖器鲍温样丘疹病、假性湿疣、珍珠状阴茎丘疹、乳房外 Paget 病等相鉴别。其中，鲍温样丘疹病也是一种由 HPV 感染引起的生殖器部位多发良性增生性病变，通常表现为数毫米到数厘米大小，红色、褐色或肤色色素沉着性丘疹，表面扁平或呈疣状，一般无自觉症状，数月后可自然消退。其与鲍温病具有类似的组织病理特征，即病灶性增生的表皮内成群分布具有异常细胞核和异常有丝分裂的异形细胞及角化不良细胞，但异型性常低于鲍温病。

【Treatment】

Curative treatment for condyloma acuminatum is still not available. Depending on the size and location of the warts, several medications can provide symptomatic relief for this infection, such as imiquimod, a tincture of 0.5% podophyllotoxin, an ointment of 5% 5-fluorouracil, trichloroacetic acid, etc. Small warts can be removed by cryosurgery, electrocautery, laser or photodynamic therapy. Surgery is occasionally used to remove large warts that can't be effectively treated with other treatments.

【治疗】

尖锐湿疣无根治疗法，可根据皮损大小和部位选择外用药物，如咪喹莫特、0.5%鬼臼毒素酊、5% 5-氟尿嘧啶软膏、三氯醋酸等。赘生物较小时可采用冷冻、电灼、激光或光动力疗法。手术治疗用于其他方法不能去除的巨大尖锐湿疣。

【Prognosis】

Condyloma acuminatum generally has a good prognosis. However, while the condition is manageable, most treatments are not able to completely eradicate the HPV, and the warts may reappear.

【预后】

大部分患者预后良好，但由于上述治疗方法不能完全清除 HPV 病毒，因此治疗后尖锐湿疣可复发。

Hong-xiang CHEN(陈宏翔), Ming-jing LI (李明静)

Section Five Genital Herpes

Genital herpes is a sexually transmitted disease (STD) caused by herpes simplex virus (HSV). The infection tends to recur and there is no permanent cure at present.

第五节 生殖器疱疹

生殖器疱疹(genital herpes, GH)是由单纯疱疹病毒感染引起的一种复发性、目前尚不能完全根治的性传播疾病。

【Etiology and Pathogenesis】

Genital herpes is caused by the infection of herpes simplex virus type Ⅰ (HSV-1) or type Ⅱ (HSV-2), which together approximately account for 85% of the primary infection and up to 98% of the recurrent lesions. Genital herpes is normally transmitted by skin to skin contact, especially during sexual activity. Herpes simplex virus enters the body through skin abrasions or susceptible mucosa. The replication of the virus will cause a balloon-like degeneration and focal necrosis in the affected cells and subsequently lymphocytic infiltration at affected area until re-epithelialization occur once viral replication is inhibited. HSV-2 (and rarely HSV-1) may invade the ganglia of sensory or autonomic nerve roots near the site of the first episode of HSV infection to cause a so called latent infection. Whenever the host's defense mechanisms decline for some reason, the virus is then reactivated and released from the nerve cells and migrates to the epidermal cells, leading to a new outbreak of herpes simplex infection.

【病因及发病机制】

由Ⅰ型单纯疱疹病毒(HSV-1)或Ⅱ型单纯疱疹病毒(HSV-2)(约占原发感染的 85%和复发损害的 98%)引起。生殖器疱疹主要通过皮肤的直接接触特别是性接触而传染。HSV 通过皮肤裂隙或易感黏膜进入体内，从而引起细胞的气球样变和局灶性坏死，随后出现淋巴细胞浸润。当病毒复制受抑时，损害出现上皮再生，但在初次感染的同时，HSV-2 (HSV-1 罕见)已进入感觉神经根或自主神经根的神经节产生潜伏性感染。当宿主的防御机制下降时病毒能被激活，从神经细胞中释放出来并到达表皮细胞，导致单纯疱疹复发。

【Clinical Manifestations】

This condition can be classified into primary and recurrent infections. The average incubation period for the primary infection is 6 days. Fever, headache, fatigue and myalgia may be evident. The classical local symptom is a mild burning or tingling sensation at first, then papules and blisters, single or clustered, appear on an erythematous base (Fig. 27-11), followed by the formation of punctate crusts or coalescent grouped erosions, or even ulcerations. Usually, the lesions last for 4-15 days and then become crusted. Scarring is rare once the infection goes into remission. Inguinal lymphadenopathy may be seen.

【临床表现】

可分为初发感染与复发感染。初发感染潜伏期平均为 6 天。全身症状有发热、头痛、乏力和肌痛。局部先有轻微烧灼感或轻微感觉异常，后在红斑上出现丘疹、水疱，单个或成簇(图 27-11)，继而形成点状结痂或融合的群集的糜烂，甚至溃疡；皮损持续 4～15 天，然后结痂，愈后一般不发生瘢痕，可伴腹股沟淋巴结肿大。

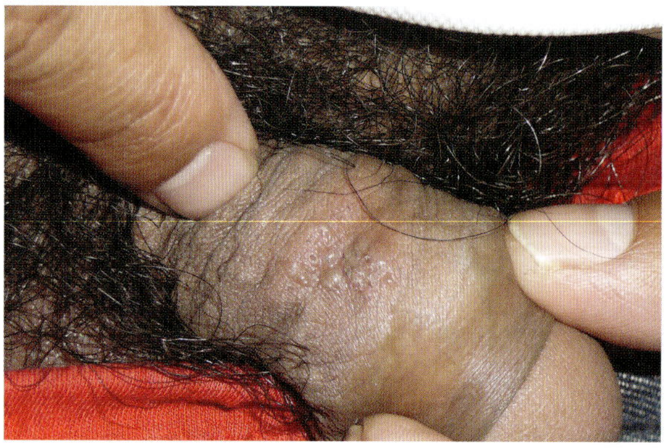

Fig. 27-11　Genital herpes(图 27-11　生殖器疱疹)

Lesions in males are mainly distributed on the foreskin of the penis, coronary sulcus, glans, penile shaft, and urethral meatus. In females, lesions can be found on the labia, clitoris, vagina or cervix. Symptoms such as itching, burning or tingling sensation may be

男性皮损主要分布在阴茎包皮、冠状沟、龟头及阴茎体、尿道口，女性皮损可分布在阴唇、阴蒂、阴道、宫颈。损害有瘙痒、灼热或刺痛等症状，在病程的前

present in the lesional areas, which gradually worsen within the first 6-7 days of the course and reach a peak between the 7th-11th days, then gradually subsiding afterwards. Viruses may be released through the entire course of the outbreak and will persist for 12 days on average from skin lesions and the cervix.

6～7天逐渐加重，在第7～11天达到高峰，然后逐渐消退。病程中有病毒排出，皮损和宫颈排放病毒时间平均为12天。

Recurrent herpes simplex infection is commonly induced by immune impairments in the host caused by skin trauma, menstruation, sun exposure, cold, malignancies, etc. Symptoms of pain and itching are usually milder in recurrent infections than in the primary infection. Before the outbreak, there can be radiating pain in the buttocks, thigh and hip, or partial numbness and a slight tingling sensation. Recurrence usually appears at the same sites as previous episodes. Blisters are often limited to one side of the body, and may be few in number in mild cases, or up to 15-20 lesions in severe cases. The course of recurrent infection is about 6-12 days with a virus release period of four days on average.

当患者存在导致免疫功能下降的因素(如皮肤创伤、月经、日晒、寒冷、恶性肿瘤等)时则出现复发感染，复发症状痛、痒比初发感染轻。发作前可有臀部、大腿和髋部的放射性疼痛，或局部有轻微的麻木和刺痒，每次复发往往发生在同一部位。水疱，常局限在一侧，轻者数个，重者15～20个，时间通常为6～12天。复发感染平均排毒时间为4天。

【Laboratory Findings】

【实验室检查】

The most reliable test for herpes is isolation of the HSV virus from cell cultures scraped from the base of the vesicles. The specificity is high for this assay, and it can distinguish between HSV-1 and HSV-2 and test the susceptibility of antiviral agents. However, some drawbacks limit its use, such as the time required (7-10 days), the labor required, and ultimately, the low sensitivity of the test. Giemsa or Wright-stained cytologic (Tzanck or Papanicolaou) smears of scrapings are also applied in clinics, but their low specificity and sensitivity are big concerns and not recommended for diagnostic confirmation.

在病灶部位底部取材，从细胞培养中分离病毒是诊断的金标准，其具有高度特异性，可区分HSV-1和HSV-2，以及检测抗病毒药物的敏感性。但也存在培养时间较长(7～10天)、人工消耗较大以及敏感性较差等缺点。而细胞学检查(Tzanck和巴氏涂片)的特异性及敏感性均较低，不建议用于诊断。

A rapid diagnosis may be made by direct immunofluorescence assay for antigen detection or polymerase chain reaction (PCR) for viral DNA. Serum specific antibody assays, particularly the most widely used HSV-2 antibody detection with reported sensitivities 80%-98% and specificities>96%, are useful for confirmation of the diagnosis in some circumstances. Serum antibodies against HSV may be transient negative during the acute phase and turn positive during the convalescent stage in primary HSV-1 or HSV-2 infection.

快速诊断方法包括直接免疫荧光法抗原检测及聚合酶链反应(polymerase chain reaction, PCR)检查病毒DNA。患者血清可进行抗体检测，应用最广泛的是HSV-2抗体检测，其敏感性为80%～98%，特异性>96%，在原发性HSV-1、HSV-2型感染中，可在急性期出现短暂的假阴性，而在恢复期血清转为阳性。

【Diagnosis】

【诊断】

The diagnosis is primarily based on the characteristic lesions of the genital blisters, erosions or crusts, symptoms of viral infection, sexual intercourse with infected partners, and laboratory findings.

主要根据生殖器特征性水疱、糜烂或结痂、病毒感染症状及不洁性交史，结合实验室检查可诊断。

【Differential Diagnosis】

【鉴别诊断】

The main differential diagnosis for HSV genital infection includes chancre and chancroid. Chancre is usually a single

本病主要与硬下疳、软下疳相鉴别。硬下疳为单个、质硬的无痛性溃疡，暗视

indurated painless ulcer. Dark field microscope examination of *Treponema pallidum* will usually be positive for chancre (although chancre is not always an indication of syphilis). Chancroid, on the other hand, which is caused by *Haemophilus Ducreyi*, is soft, with multiple painful ulcers.

野显微镜查梅毒螺旋体阳性(虽然硬下疳并非一定是梅毒);软下疳为质软的多发性溃疡,伴剧痛,由杜克雷嗜血杆菌引起。

【Treatment】

Acyclovir or famciclovir and other antiviral drugs can be given orally. It is important also to keep the affected areas clean and dry and prevent secondary infection. Topical 0.1% idoxuridine solution or 5% acyclovir ointment can also be of benefit.

【治疗】

采用口服阿昔洛韦或泛昔洛韦等抗病毒药物,保持局部干燥、清洁,防止继发感染,可试用0.1%碘苷或5%阿昔洛韦软膏。

【Prognosis】

The course of the initial infection is 16-20 days and of the recurrent infection is 6-10 days. Frequent relapses may occur in some patients. It has been suggested that HSV-2 infection is closely related to the occurrence of cervical cancer and to neonatal infections (via intrauterine, during or after delivery).

【预后】

初次感染病程为16～20天,复发感染病程为6～10天,部分患者可出现频繁复发。而HSV-2感染与子宫颈癌发生有密切关系,且HSV可使新生儿经子宫内、分娩和出生后感染,需引起注意。

Hong-xiang CHEN(陈宏翔), Ming-jing LI (李明静)

Section Six Acquired Immunodeficiency Syndrome (AIDS)

第六节 获得性免疫缺陷综合征(艾滋病)

Acquired immunodeficiency syndrome (AIDS) is a disease of the human immune system caused by the human immunodeficiency virus (HIV). HIV primarily infects T lymphocytes (T helper cells) and may compromise the human immune system partially or completely. As a result, the affected individuals will be susceptible to a variety of opportunistic infections and malignant tumors. AIDS is now a global pandemic disease. As of 2010, it has been estimated that 31.4 million-35.3 million people live with the disease worldwide, and that 1.6 million-2.1 million people have been died of AIDS.

获得性免疫缺陷综合征(艾滋病)(acquired immunodeficiency syndrome, AIDS)是由人类免疫缺陷病毒(human immunodeficiency virus, HIV)引起的免疫系统疾病,HIV主要侵犯T细胞,特别是辅助T细胞,使机体免疫功能部分或完全丧失,继而发生条件致病菌感染、恶性肿瘤等。目前,艾滋病在世界范围内流行。到2010年,全世界有3140万～3530万艾滋病患者,死亡患者达160万～210万。

【Etiology】

HIV is an RNA retrovirus, 110-120 nm in diameter. HIV-1 is composed of two copies of single-stranded RNA and reverse transcriptase and is enclosed by a conical capsid. The virus envelope spike is around the capsid, including the glycoproteins gp120 and gp41 that are the key to the virus-cell interaction.

【病因】

HIV属于RNA逆转录病毒,直径为100～120 nm。HIV-1由两条单链RNA、逆转录酶及包裹其外的病毒衣壳构成,在病毒最外层为包膜,包膜上有刺突,由病毒糖蛋白gp120和gp41组成,是与宿主细胞结合的部位。

【Pathogenesis】

The human immunodeficiency viruses, HIV-1 and HIV-2, both contain reverse transcriptase that allow the viral genome to be

【发病机制】

人类免疫缺陷病毒HIV-1和HIV-2,均含有逆转录酶,可以使病毒DNA复

incorporated into the chromosomes of the host cell. The main targets of HIV are the specific subsets of the T lymphocytes (helper/inducer cells) that express glycoprotein CD4 molecules on their surface. After the virus enters a T helper cell by binding to these molecules, the virus replicates within the T helper cells and eventually kills the cells. The depletion of $CD4^+$ T-cells will lead to the loss of cell-mediated immunity which is the hallmark of AIDS and the normal untreated outcome of the HIV infection. In turn this produces an increased incidence of a variety of opportunistic infections and secondary malignancies.

制整合进入宿主细胞染色体中，其主要靶细胞是表面有 $CD4^+$ 表位的辅助 T 细胞亚群，它们可以与病毒外膜结合。病毒在辅助 T 细胞中复制，导致宿主细胞死亡，$CD4^+$ T 细胞耗竭导致细胞免疫的丧失（HIV 感染的显著特征和未经治疗后的结果），随后各种条件性感染和继发性恶性肿瘤的发生率增加。

【Modes of Transmission】

AIDS patients and HIV-infected persons (specifically defined as those who harbor the virus but do not experience any symptoms of immunodeficiency) are the main reservoir of HIV and the main source of HIV infection. The three main transmission routes of HIV are sexual contact, including both homosexual and heterosexual contact, exposure to blood and blood products, and transfer from mother to fetus or newborn during the perinatal period.

【传染源及途径】

直接传染源是艾滋病患者及 HIV 感染者（携带有 HIV 病毒但没有免疫缺陷的症状者）。三条主要的传染途径是：性接触传播（同性与异性之间的性接触）；血液及血液制品传播；母婴传播（感染 HIV 的母亲在围生期传染给胎儿或新生儿）。

【Clinical Staging and Manifestations】

(1) Acute infection stage: the first stage of infection (usually 1-2 weeks post-exposure) is characterized by rapid viral replication that immediately leads to a marked decrease in circulating $CD4^+$ T-cells. During this period most individuals (80%-90%) develop symptoms as those of influenza-or mononucleosis-like illness.

(2) Clinically asymptomatic infection stage: a strong immune response reduces the number of viral particles in the peripheral blood, which then marks the start of the asymptomatic HIV infection stage or the clinical latency stage. Clinical latency can vary from two weeks to twenty years. As its name suggests, this phase of the infection is free of major symptoms, although there may be a persistent lymphadenopathy. The patients remain infectious at this stage even though the level of HIV in the peripheral blood drops to a very low level.

(3) Clinically Symptomatic Stage & AIDS: as the immune system undergoes progressively more serious damage from the virus over time, symptoms begin to develop. Initial manifestations often are fever, weakness and unexplained weight loss, lymphadenopathy, and recurring respiratory tract infections. When $CD4^+$ T-cell numbers decline below the critical level of 200 cells/μL, cell-mediated immunity deteriorates further and fails, leading eventually to the AIDS stage, which manifests as a variety of opportunistic infections or cancers, such as oral candidiasis, lung

【临床分期及表现】

(1) 急性感染期　感染的最初阶段（接触 HIV 后 1～2 周），HIV 大量复制，$CD4^+$ T 细胞急剧下降。有 80%～90% 的感染者在这一期表现为流感样或单核细胞增多症样症状。

(2) 临床无症状感染期　免疫防御系统减少血液中的病毒颗粒，出现临床无症状期或临床潜伏期。该期从两周到二十年不等，临床上没有任何表现，部分可出现持续性淋巴结肿大。此期感染者虽然外周血中的 HIV 水平很低，但仍有传染性。

(3) 临床症状感染期和艾滋病　随着时间的推移和患者免疫系统的破坏，临床症状逐渐表现出来，患者有发热、乏力和不明原因的体重下降、淋巴结肿大、反复呼吸道感染，当 $CD4^+$ T 细胞数量下降到 200 个/μL 以下，细胞介导的免疫反应丧失，即表现为 AIDS 期，患者常合并各种机会感染或肿瘤，如口腔念珠菌感染、肺结核、肺卡氏囊虫病、卡波西肉

tuberculosis, *Pneumocystis jiroveci* pneumonia or Kaposi's sarcoma.

瘤等。

(4) Cutaneous manifestations of HIV infection: skin lesions are seen in 90% of HIV-infected individuals. The common types of skin lesions are as follows.

①Oral hairy leukoplakia (OHL): it is seen in 20% of AIDS patients. This oral lesion is not severe itself, but is usually a specific sign of early HIV disease.

②Seborrheic dermatitis: it appears in 20%-80% of patients, often starting at an early stage of HIV infection.

③Psoriasis: the incidence of psoriasis is 5% in HIV infected patients. Psoriasis may be the first sign of the onset of HIV infection and is also a poor prognostic indicator of AIDS.

④Kaposi's sarcoma: the risk for Kaposi's sarcoma in HIV-infected patients is 20000 times more than that of the general population.

⑤Miscelaneous skin infections: these may include herpes simplex, herpes zoster, condyloma acuminatum, oral and cutaneous candidiasis, tinea, pityriasis versicolor, and facial and perianal warts, etc.

(4) HIV感染的皮肤病表现 90%的HIV感染者有皮肤的病变，比较重要的有以下几种。

①口腔毛状黏膜白斑：20%艾滋病患者伴发，其本身并不严重，但是HIV感染特异性相当高的早期体征。

②脂溢性皮炎：发生率为20%～80%，为HIV感染最初表现。

③银屑病：发生率为5%，可作为HIV感染的首发体征，也是预后差的标志。

④卡波西肉瘤：在HIV感染者中卡波西肉瘤的发生风险是正常人群的20000倍。

⑤各种皮肤感染：包括单纯疱疹、带状疱疹、尖锐湿疣、口腔和皮肤念珠菌感染、癣、花斑糠疹、面部及肛周疣等。

【Laboratory Findings】

Detection of HIV is important not only for confirmation of the diagnosis, but also to allow monitoring of the infection, which includes viral load measurement, HIV antigen detection and HIV isolation by cultures. In addition to HIV detection, there are many laboratory tests that should be carried out in order to keep track of the immunodeficiency, including peripheral complete blood count (CBC), $CD4^+$ T lymphocytes count and chemistry panels (kidney function and liver function tests). Finally, microbial identification of the specific opportunistic infections is especially necessary in the later stages of HIV infection.

【实验室检查】

HIV检测的重要性不仅在于确诊，而且有利于监测感染，HIV检测包括检测病毒负载水平、检测HIV抗原、分离培养HIV病毒等。除HIV检测外，还应进行一系列实验室检查监测免疫缺陷状态，免疫缺陷的实验室检查包括外周血细胞计数、$CD4^+$ T细胞计数、生化检查(如肝肾功能检查)。应进行条件致病微生物检查，特别是HIV感染的晚期。

【Diagnosis】

Diagnosis depends on contact history, clinical symptoms and laboratory examination. The last includes detection of HIV, $CD4^+$ T lymphocytes counts and microbial detection of any opportunistic infections.

【诊断】

诊断依靠病史、临床症状及实验室检查。其中后者包括HIV检测、$CD4^+$ T细胞计数及相关机会感染微生物检测。

【Treatment】

There is currently no vaccine or cure for HIV or AIDS. Current medications for HIV infection are used to control the reproduction of the virus and to slow or halt the virus' assault on the patient's immune system. The recommended regimen is known as highly active antiretroviral therapy (HAART), which combines three or more anti-HIV medications in a daily treatment, sometimes

【治疗】

目前无疫苗和特效疗法，目前治疗HIV感染的药物主要是控制病毒复制、减缓或阻止病毒对患者的免疫系统的攻击。常用方法是采用高效抗逆转录病毒治疗(HAART)，也就是每天联合3种或以上的药物，即所谓的“鸡尾酒”疗法，包

referred to as a "cocktail", consisting of nucleoside analogue reverse transcriptase inhibitors (NARTIs or NRTIs), protease inhibitors (PIs) and non-nucleoside reverse transcriptase inhibitors (NNRTIs).

括核苷类逆转录酶抑制剂(NARTIs 或 NRTIs)、蛋白酶抑制剂(PIs)、非核苷类逆转录酶抑制剂(NNRTIs)。

【Prevention】

Since there is no cure or vaccine today for HIV, it is fortunate indeed that the virus itself is not particularly virulent, and that relatively simple preventive measures can be employed to prevent its spread. Three things must be done in order to slow or reverse the spread of HIV: the first is to promote widespread awareness and education about HIV and its modes of transmission, the second is to establish HIV counseling and monitoring programs, and the third is to provide antiretroviral treatment to those patients actually infected.

【预防】

对于 HIV 感染，目前尚无疫苗和特效疗法，所幸的是该病毒本身并非特别具有致命性，而且一些相对简单的方法可以防止其扩散。有 3 个方面可以减慢或改变 HIV 的扩散：首先要重视宣教，认识艾滋病，了解传播途径；其次是要开展艾滋病病毒咨询和监测工作；再次是提供抗逆转录病毒治疗。

Hong-xiang CHEN(陈宏翔), Ming-jing LI (李明静), Ya-ting TU (涂亚庭)

English-Chinese Index
英汉对照索引

References
参考文献

[1] 樊尚荣，张慧萍. 2010年美国疾病控制中心生殖器疱疹治疗指南[J]. 中国全科医学，2011，14(5A)：1402-1403.

[2] 黄长征. 皮肤性病学[M]. 3版. 北京：科学出版社，2016.

[3] 黄长征. 英汉皮肤性病学(English-Chinese Dermatovenereology)[M]. 武汉：华中科技大学出版社，2010.

[4] 李伯埙，王俊民，肖生祥. 皮肤病临床与组织病理学[M]. 北京：世界图书出版公司，2015.

[5] 马晓蕾，周城，蔡林，等. 生物制剂治疗银屑病的研究进展[J]. 临床皮肤科杂志，2012，41(9)：577-579.

[6] 孙建方，高天文. 皮肤组织病理学[M]. 北京：人民卫生出版社，2013.

[7] 王芳，李毓，莫莹，等. 药疹临床类型和致敏药谱最近七年与过去十年的对比变化[J]. 实用医学杂志，2011，27(21)：3932-3933.

[8] 吴志华. 临床皮肤性病学[M]. 北京：人民军医出版社，2011.

[9] R. B. 奥多姆，W. D. 詹姆斯，T. G. 伯杰. 安德鲁斯临床皮肤病学[M]. 徐世正，译. 11版. 北京：科学出版社，2015.

[10] 杨慧兰. 病毒性皮肤病学[M]. 北京：人民军医出版社，2008.

[11] 赵辨. 中国临床皮肤病学[M]. 南京：江苏科学技术出版社，2009.

[12] 张建中，高兴华. 皮肤性病学[M]. 北京：人民卫生出版社，2015.

[13] 张学军. 皮肤性病学[M]. 8版. 北京：人民卫生出版社，2013.

[14] 张学军. 皮肤性病学高级教程[M]. 北京：人民军医出版社，2010.

[15] 中国疾病预防控制中心，性病控制中心，中华医学会皮肤性病学分会性病学组. 梅毒、淋病、生殖器疱疹、生殖道沙眼衣原体感染诊疗指南(2014)[J]. 中华皮肤科杂志，2014，47(5)：365-372.

[16] 中国中西医结合学会皮肤性病专业委员会性病学组. 生殖器疱疹中西医结合诊疗指南[J]. 中国中西医结合皮肤性病学杂志，2009，8(6)：382-383.

[17] 中华医学会感染病学分会艾滋病学组. 艾滋病诊疗指南[J]. 中华传染病杂志，2011，29(10)：629-640.

[18] 中华医学会皮肤性病学分会性病学组，中国医师协会皮肤科分会性病亚专业委员会. 尖锐湿疣临床诊疗与防治指南(一)[J]. 中国艾滋病性病，2015，21(2)：172-174.

[19] 中华医学会皮肤性病学分会性病学组，中国医师协会皮肤科分会性病亚专业委员会. 尖锐湿疣临床诊疗与防治指南(二)[J]. 中国艾滋病性病，2015，21(3)：260-262.

[20] 中华医学会皮肤性病学分会. 中国荨麻疹诊疗指南(2014版)[J]. 中华皮肤科杂志，2014，47(7)：514-516.

[21] 麦基，卡隆赫，格兰特尔. 皮肤病理学：与临床的联系[M]. 朱学骏，孙建方，译. 3版. 北京：北京大学医学出版社，2007.

[22] 博洛格尼，乔伊佐，拉皮尼. 皮肤病学[M]. 朱学骏，王宝玺，孙建方，等译. 2版. 北京：北京大学医学出版社，2011.

[23] Alam M, Ratner D. Cutaneous squamous-cell carcinoma[J]. N Engl J Med, 2001, 344(13): 975-983.

[24] Ale IS, Maibach HI. Irritant contact dermatitis[J]. Rev Environ Health, 2014, 29(3): 195-206.

[25] Aslam I, Sandoval LF, Feldman SR. What's new in the topical treatment of allergic skin diseases[J]. Curr Opin Allergy Clin Immunol, 2014, 14(5): 436-450.

[26] Badgwell C, Rosen T. Cutaneous sarcoidosis therapy updated [J]. J Am Acad Dermatol, 2007, 56(1): 69-83.

[27] Ball NJ, Kho GT, Martinka M. The histologic spectrum of cutaneous sarcoidosis: a study of twenty-eight cases [J]. J Cutan Pathol, 2004, 31(2): 160-168.

[28] Bandow GD, Koo JY. Narrow-band ultraviolet B radiation: a review of the current literature [J]. Int J Dermatol, 2004, 43(8): 555-561.

[29] Bernard P. Management of common bacterial infections of the skin [J]. Curr Opin Infect Dis, 2008, 21(2): 122-128.

[30] Beutler BD, Cohen PR, Lee RA. Prurigo pigmentosa: literature review [J]. Am J Clin Dermatol, 2015, 16(6): 533-543.

[31] Bienvenu B. Treatment of subcutaneous calcinosis in systemic disorders [J]. Rev Med Interne, 2014, 35(7): 444-452.

[32] Bolognia JL, Jorizzo JL, Schaffer JV. Dermatology [M]. 3rd ed. Oxford: Elsevier Health Sciences, 2012.

[33] Boursiquot JN, Gérard L, Malphettes M, et al. Granulomatous disease in CVID: retrospective analysis of clinical characteristics and treatment efficacy in a cohort of 59 patients [J]. J Clin Immunol, 2013, 33(1): 84-95.

[34] Brzeziska-WcisoL, Bergler-CzopB, Wciso-DziadeckaD, et al. New aspects of the treatment of alopecia areata[J]. Postepy Dermatol Alergol, 2014, 31(4): 262-265.

[35] Burns T, Breathnach S, Cox N, et al. Rook's textbook of dermatology[M]. 8th ed. Oxford: Wiley-Blackwell, 2010.

[36] Calonje E, Brenn T, Lazar A, et al. Pathology of the skin-with clinical correlations[M]. 4rd ed. Oxford: Elsevier Limited, 2012.

[37] Cavallini M, Cirillo P, Fundarò SP, et al. Safety of botulinum toxin A in aesthetic treatments: asystematic review of clinical studies [J]. Dermatol Surg, 2014, 40(5): 525-536.

[38] Centers for Disease Control. Sexually transmitted diseases treatment guidelines. Morbidity and mortality weekly report (MMWR): recommendations and reports, 64(No. RR-3)[R]. Atlanta: CDC, 2015.

[39] Cerroni L. Skin lymphoma-the illustrated guide [M]. 4th ed. New York: John Wiley & Sons, Ltd. , 2014.

[40] Cholewiński M, Derda M, Hada śE. Parasiticdiseasesin humans transmitted by vectors [J]. Ann Parasitol, 2015, 61(3): 137-157.

[41] Chuong CM1, Nickoloff BJ, Elias PM, et al. What is the 'true' function of skin? [J]. Exp Dermatol, 2002, 11(2): 159-187.

[42] Cohen AD, Andrews ID, Medvedovsky E, et al. Similarities between neuropathic pruritus sites and lichen simplex chronicus sites [J]. IMAJ, 2014, 16(2): 88-90.

[43] Dadabhoy I, Butts JF. Parasiticskin infections for primary care physicians [J]. Prim Care, 2015, 42 (4): 661-675.

[44] Das S, Reynolds RV. Recent advances in acne pathogenesis: implications for therapy[J]. Am J Clin Dermatol, 2014, 15(6): 479-488.

[45] Del Rosso JQ. Management of cutaneous rosacea: emphasis on new medical therapies[J]. Expert Opin Pharmacother, 2014, 15 (14): 2029-2038.

[46] Eads TJ, Hood AF, Chuang T-Y, et al. The diagnostic yield of histologic examination of seborrheic keratoses [J]. Arch Dermatol, 1997, 133(11): 1417-1420.

[47] Elder DE. Lever's histopathology of the skin [M]. 11th ed. Philadelphia: Wolters Kluwer, 2015.

[48] Elias PM. Skin barrier function [J]. Curr Allergy Asthma Rep, 2008, 8(4): 299-305.

[49] Elston DM, Stratman EJ, Miller SJ. Skin biopsy: biopsy issues in specific diseases [J]. J Am AcadDermatol, 2016, 74(1): 1-16.

[50] Feily A, Mehraban S. Treatment modalities of necrobiosis lipoidica: a concise systematic review [J]. Dermatol Reports, 2015, 7 (2): 5749.

[51] Feldman SR. Principles of topical treatment: advancement in gel vehicle technology [J]. J Drugs Dermatol, 2014, 13(4): 423-7.

[52] Fernandez-Faith E, McDonnell J. Cutaneous sarcoidosis: differential diagnosis [J]. Clin Dermatol, 2007, 25(3): 276-287.

[53] Ferrer M, Bartra J, Giménez-Arnau A, et al. Management of urticaria: not too complicated, not too simple [J]. Clin Exp Allergy, 2015, 45(4): 731-743.

[54] Fine J D, Bruckner-Tuderman L, Eady R A J, et al. Inherited epidermolysis bullosa: updated recommendations on diagnosis and classification[J]. J Am Acad Dermatol, 2014, 70(6): 1103-1126.

[55] Fleury J, Guillet G. Treatment of bromidrosis[J]. Ann Dermatol Venereol, 2012, 139(5): 404-408.

[56] Goldsmith LA, Katz SI, Gilchrest B, et al. Fitzpatrick's dermatology in general medicine[M]. 8th ed. New York: McGraw-Hill Education, 2012.

[57] Gupta AK, Richardson M, Paquet M. Systematic review of oral treatments for seborrheic dermatitis[J]. J Eur Acad Dermatol Venereol, 2014, 28(1): 16-26.

[58] Griffiths H, Barker J, Bleiker T, et al. Rook's textbook of dermatology [M]. 9th ed. Oxford: Blackwell Science Ltd. , 2016.

[59] Gronhagen CM, Tey HL. Primary localized cutaneous amyloidosis: a clinical diagnosis [J]. Skinmed, 2014, 12(4): 257-258.

[60] Hartman-Adams H, Banvard C, Juckett G. Impetigo: diagnosis and treatment [J]. Am Fam Physician, 2014, 90(4): 229-235.

[61] Hiroshi Shimizu. Textbook of dermatology [M]. Hokkaido: Nakayama Shoten Publishers, 2007.

[62] Iaccarino L, Ghirardello A, Bettio S, et al. The clinical features, diagnosis and classification of dermatomyositis [J]. J Autoimmun, 2014, 48(49): 122-127.

[63] Inghammar M, Rasmussen M, Linder A. Recurrent erysipelas—risk factors and clinical presentation [J]. BMC Infect Dis, 2014, 18(14): 270.

[64] James WD, Berger TG, Elston DM, et al. Andrews' diseases of the skin: clinical dermatology[M]. 12th ed. Oxford: Elsevier Health Sciences, 2015.

[65] Jean L Bolognia, Joseph L Jorizzo and Ronald P Rapini. Dermatology [M]. 2 nd ed. Oxford: Elsevier Limited, 2008.

[66] Jewell JR, Myers SA. Topical therapy primer for nondermatologists [J]. Med Clin North Am, 2015, 99(6): 1167-1182.

[67] Juan CK, Chen HJ, Shen JL, Kao CH. Lichen Simplex chronicus associated with erectile dysfunction: a population-based retrospective cohort study [J]. PloS One, 2015, 10(6): 1-11.

[68] Krilis M, Miyakis S. Cytophagic histiocytic panniculitis with haemophagocytosis in a patient with familial multiple lipomatosis and review of the literature [J]. Mod Rheumatol, 2012, 22(1): 158-162.

[69] Kullberg BJ, Arendrup MC. Invasive candidiasis [J]. N Engl J Med, 2015, 373(15): 1445-1456.

[70] Kumaresan M, Rai R, Raj A. Dermatitis artefacta [J]. Indian Dermatol Online J, 2012, 3(2): 141-143.
[71] Kuo CF, Yu KH, See LC, et al. Risk of myocardial infarction among patients with gout: a nationwide population-based study [J]. Rheumatology, 2013, 52(1): 111-117.
[72] Lacey CJ, Woodhall SC, Wikstrom A, et al. 2012 European guideline for the management of anogenital warts [J]. J Eur Acad Dermatol Venereol, 2013, 27(3): 263-270.
[73] Lachapelle JM. Allergic contact dermatitis: clinical aspects [J]. Rev Environ Health, 2014, 29(3): 185-194.
[74] Lee JH, Son SW, Cho SH. A comprehensive review of the treatment of atopic eczema [J]. Allergy Asthma Immunol Res, 2016, 8(3): 181-190.
[75] Lu S, Lu C, Zhang J, et al. Chromoblastomycosis in Mainland China: a systematic review on clinical characteristics [J]. Mycopathologia, 2013, 175(5-6): 489-495.
[76] Lyons JJ, Milner JD, Stone KD. Atopic dermatitis in children: clinical features, pathophysiology, and treatment [J]. Immunol Allergy Clin North Am, 2015, 35(1): 161-183.
[77] Marks Jr JG, Miller JJ. Lookingbill and Marks' principles of dermatology[M]. 4th ed. Amsterdam: Elsevier, 2006.
[78] Misery L, Brenaut E, Le Garrec R, et al. Neuropathic pruritus[J]. Nat Rev Neurol, 2014, 10(7): 408-416.
[79] Morrison LK, Rapini R, Willison CB, et al. Infection and panniculitis [J]. Dermatol Ther, 2010, 23(4): 328-340.
[80] Mosca M, Tani C, Vagnani S, et al. The diagnosis and classification of undifferentiated connective tissue diseases [J]. J Autoimmun, 2014, 48(49): 50-52.
[81] Neena Khanna. Illustrated synopsis of dermatology & sexually transmitted disease [M]. 3rd ed. Amsterdam: Elsevier, 2009.
[82] Northrup H, Krueger DA, International Tuberous Sclerosis Complex Consensus Group. Tuberous sclerosis complex diagnostic criteria update: recommendations of the 2012 international tuberous sclerosis complex consensus conference[J]. Pediatr Neurol, 2013, 49(4): 243-254.
[83] Oliveira EV, Pozetti AC, Pozetti EM, et al. Primary systemic amyloidosis associated with multiple myeloma [J]. An Bras Dermatol, 2012, 87(1): 119-122.
[84] Omi T, Numano K. The role of the CO_2 laser and fractional CO_2 laser in dermatology [J]. Laser Ther, 2014, 23(1): 49-60.
[85] Ortega-Hernandez OD, Shoenfeld Y. Mixed connective tissue disease: an overview of clinical manifestations, diagnosis and treatment [J]. Best Pract Res Clin Rheumatol, 2012, 26(1): 61-72.
[86] Patel R, Alderson S, Geretti A, et al. European guideline for the management of genital herpes(2010)[J]. Int J STD AIDS, 2011, 22(1): 1-10.
[87] Patil MM, Kamalanathan S, Sahoo J, et al. Pretibial myxedema [J]. QJM, 2015, 108(12): 985.
[88] Pedrosa AF, Lisboa C, Gonçalves Rodrigues A. Malassezia infections: a medical conundrum[J]. J Am Acad Dermatol, 2014, 71(1): 170-176.
[89] Phiske MM. An approach to acanthosis nigricans [J]. Indian Dermatol Online J. 2014, 5(3): 239-249.
[90] Ramdass P, Mullick S, Farber HF. Viral skin diseases [J]. Prim Care. 2015, 42 (4): 517-567.
[91] Ridky TW. Nonmelanoma skin cncer [J]. J Am Acad Dermatol, 2007, 57(3): 484-501.
[92] Rodriguez-Carreon AA, Rodriguez-Lobato E, Rodriguez-Gutierrez G, et al. Actinic prurigo [J]. Skinmed, 2015, 13(4): 287-295.
[93] Romero R, Nygaard I. CDC updates guidelines for treating sexually transmitted diseases [J]. AmJ Obstet Gynecol, 2015, 213(2): 117-118.
[94] Rogers M, McCrossin I, Commens C. Epidermal nevi and the epidermal nevus syndrome: a review of 131 cases [J]. J Am Acad Dermatol, 1989, 20(3): 476-488.
[95] Rossi R, Mori M, Lotti T. Actinic keratosis [J]. Int J Dermatol, 2007, 46(9): 895-904.
[96] Rousso DE, Kim SW. A review of medical and surgical treatment options for androgenetic alopecia [J]. JAMA Facial Plast Surg, 2014, 16(6): 444-450.
[97] Sanguinetti M, Posteraro B, Lass-Flörl C. Antifungal drug resistance among *Candida* species: mechanisms and clinical impact [J]. Mycoses, 2015, 58 Suppl 2: 2-13.
[98] Stashak AB, Brewer JD. Management of hyperhidrosis [J]. Clin Cosmet Investig Dermatol, 2014, 7: 285-299.
[99] Tchernev G. Cutaneous sarcoidosis: the "great imitator": etiopathogenesis, morphology, differential diagnosis, and clinical management [J]. Am J Clin Dermatol, 2006, 7(6): 375-382.
[100] Tempark T, Shwayder TA. Perioral dermatitis: a review of the condition with special attention to treatment options [J]. Am J Clin Dermatol, 2014, 15(2): 101-113.

[101] van den Hoogen F, Khanna D, Fransen J, et al. 2013 classification criteria for systemic sclerosis: an American College of Rheumatology/European League against Rheumatism Collaborative initiative [J]. Ann Rheum Dis, 2013, 72(11): 1747-1755.

[102] Warrington R, Watson W, Kim HL, et al. An introduction to immunology and immunopathology[J]. Allergy Asthma Clin Immunol, 2011, 7 Suppl 1: S1.

[103] Weedon D. Skin Pathology[M]. 3rd ed. Oxford: Elsevier Limited, 2010.

[104] Workowski KA, Bolan GA, Centers for Disease Control and Prevention. Sexually transmitted diseases treatment guidelines (2015)[J]. MMWR Recomm Rep, 2015, 64(03): 1-137.

[105] Workowski KA, Berman S, Centers for Disease Control and Prevention. Sexually transmitted diseases treatment guidelines (2010)[J]. MMWR Recomm Rep, 2010, 59(12): 1-110.

[106] Xin H, Matt D, Qin JZ, et al. The sebaceous nevus: a nevus with deletions of the PTCH gene [J]. Cancer Res, 1999, 59(8): 1834-1836.

[107] Yanardağ H, Pamuk ON, Karayel T. Cutaneous involvement in sarcoidosis: analysis of the features in 170 patients [J]. Respir Med, 2003, 97(8): 978-982.

[108] Zak A, Zeman M, Slaby A, et al. Xanthomas: clinical and pathophysiological relations [J]. Biomed Pap Med Fac Univ Palacky Olomouc Czech Repub, 2014, 158(2): 181-188.

[109] Zouboulis CC. The skin as an endocrine organ[J]. Dermatoendocrinol, 2009, 1(5): 250-252.

[110] Zuberbier T, Asero R, Bindslev-Jensen C, et al. EAACI/GA(2)LEN/EDF/WAO guideline: definition, classification and diagnosis of urticaria [J]. Allergy, 2009, 64(10): 1417-1426.

[111] Zuberbier T, Aberer W, Asero R, et al. The EAACI/GA(2)LEN/EDF/WAO guideline for the definition, classification, diagnosis, and management of urticaria: the 2013 revision and update [J]. Allergy, 2014, 69(7): 868-887.